■ Neurobiology of Personality Disorders

T0177574

Neurobiology of Personality Disorders

EDITED BY

Christian Schmahl, MD
Professor of Experimental Psychopathology
Medical Director
Department of Psychosomatic Medicine
and Psychotherapy
Central Institute of Mental Health
Mannheim, Germany

K. Luan Phan, MD
UI CDR Endowed Professor
Professor of Psychiatry
University of Illinois at Chicago
Chicago, Illinois

Robert O. Friedel, MD
Distinguished Clinical Professor of Psychiatry
Virginia Commonwealth University
Professor Emeritus
University of Alabama at Birmingham
Birmingham, Alabama

WITH

Larry J. Siever, MD
Professor of Psychiatry
James J. Peters Veterans Affairs Medical Center
Icahn School of Medicine at Mount Sinai
New York, New York

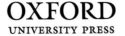

OXFORD
UNIVERSITY PRESS

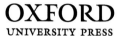

OXFORD
UNIVERSITY PRESS

Oxford University Press is a department of the University of Oxford. It furthers
the University's objective of excellence in research, scholarship, and education
by publishing worldwide. Oxford is a registered trade mark of Oxford University
Press in the UK and certain other countries.

Published in the United States of America by Oxford University Press
198 Madison Avenue, New York, NY 10016, United States of America.

© Oxford University Press 2018

CIP data is on file at the Library of Congress
ISBN 978–0–19–936231–8

9 8 7 6 5 4 3 2 1

Printed by Sheridan Books, Inc., United States of America

■ CONTENTS

SECTION III ■ Neurobiology of Categorical Diagnoses of Personality Disorder

SECTION IV ■ Implications for Diagnostic Systems and Treatment

■ PREFACE

The aim of this book is to outline the principles of neural science that mediate personality and to describe what is currently known about how these biological processes are impaired in individuals with personality disorders (PDs). We started with this book a few years ago, we were convinced that a new book is needed in this area for two reasons. First, there is a high prevalence of PDs in the general population with current estimates ranging from 9% to 15%. These disorders cause a substantial amount of human suffering and harm, not only to the individuals and families directly affected but also to the population at large. Antisocial personality disorder (AsPD) and borderline personality disorder (BPD) illustrate this point clearly. Second, these disorders are known to have a heritability rate that is generally in excess of 50%, strongly suggesting that the behavioral disturbances caused by PDs have a significant biomedical etiology. However, with the exception of BPD, little is known about the biological nature of personality and PDs and the effective treatment of the latter. The principles of the biological nature of medical disorders have served well as the foundation in other disciplines in medicine and psychiatry but have received relatively little attention in the areas of personality, temperament, and PDs.

This book is structured in four sections:

I. Foundations of Neurobiology of Personality (Chapters 1–6)
II. Critical Domains/Dimensions of Brain Function/Circuits for Personality and Its Disorders (Chapters 7–11)
III. Neurobiology of Categorical Diagnoses of Personality Disorder (Chapters 12–15)
IV. Implications for Diagnostic Systems and Treatment (Chapters 16–18)

Chapter 1, "Neurocircuitry of Affective, Cognitive, Regulatory Systems" by Annmarie McNamara and Luan Phan, provides a review and synthesis of the neurocircuitry involved in affect, cognition, and their interactions as it relates to regulatory functions. The chapter first gives an overview regarding structure and function of key brain regions, that is, prefrontal and cingulate regions, insula, and subcortical regions, as well as other temporal-parietal-occipital regions. Following this overview, the chapter proceeds with summarizing key neuroscientific findings as organized by cognitive processes and their relevance for emotion. The overall aim of the chapter is to provide a better understanding of cognitive-emotional interactions at the neurocircuit level.

Chapter 2, "The Fundamentals of Brain Neurotransmission" by Robert Friedel and Stephen Stahl, provides an introduction, review, and synthesis of the neurochemical and neurotransmitter systems that underlie brain function. In addition, it describes which and how psychoactive agents used in PDs target these systems by describing their mechanism(s) of action. It provides the reader a primer to better understand the pathophysiology and treatment of PDs discussed in the book.

Chapter 3, "Genetics of Personality Disorders" by Ted Reichborn-Kjennerud and Kenneth Kendler, reviews the evidence for genetic contributions to the etiology of PDs defined in the fifth edition of the *Diagnostic and Statistical Manual of Mental Disorders* (*DSM-5*). The following topics are discussed: the evidence for genetic influences on DSM PDs from family and twin studies using quantitative genetic methods; multivariate quantitative models exploring the influence of shared genetic factors on the comorbidity between PDs and the comorbidity between PDs and other clinical disorders; studies on the extent to which common genetic factors influence PDs and normal personality traits, and PDs and pathological personality trait domains; stability of genetic influences on PDs; molecular genetics of PDs and gene environment interplay (i.e., both gene–environment correlation and gene × environment interaction); and future directions in the exploration of genetic influences on PDs.

Chapter 4, "Cognitive Neuroscience Approaches to Personality Disorders" by Andrew Poppe and Angus MacDonald, describes a cognitive neuroscience approach to understanding the psychological and neural processes that underlie personality and behavior. It reviews the different neuroimaging tools and approaches that can be used to investigate brain structure and function. The chapter provides the reader an appreciation of how understanding brain structure and function in vivo can serve as a bridge between molecular/genetic and symptom-based data to enrich the pathophysiology of PDs.

Chapter 5, "Minding the Emotional Thermostat: Integrating Social Cognitive and Affective Neuroscience Evidence to Form a Model of the Cognitive Control of Emotion" by Bryan Denny and Kevin Ochsner, takes a social-cognitive-affective neuroscience approach to describe the processes and systems that give rise to emotion and the volitional control of emotion. It introduces and syntheses the brain structures involved in emotion processing and regulation, with a particular focus on the role of cognitive strategies such as reappraisal. It provides a critical framework for understanding the underlying behavioral and neural basis for the affect dysregulation observed across PDs.

Chapter 6, "The Neurobiology of Attachment and Mentalizing: A Neurodevelopmental Perspective" by Patrick Luyten and Peter Fonagy, addresses the neurobiology of attachment and mentalizing from a developmental psychopathology perspective. Neurobiologically, the attachment system is underpinned by the brain's reward system comprised mainly of the nucleus accumbens, hippocampus, and amygdala and mesocortical pathways. The neuromodulators dopamine, oxytocin, and vasopressin play a key role in the processes of attachment, and it appears that the cannabinoid and opioid systems are also involved. Abnormalities in the normal function of these systems have been found to dysregulate normal attachment behaviors.

Chapter 7, "Emotion Regulation" by Katja Bertsch, Harold Koenigsberg, Inga Niedtfeld, and Christian Schmahl, describes the processes and systems implicated in the regulation of emotions. It reviews several implicit and explicit forms including attention, habituation, and reappraisal. It describes multiple behavioral sequelae to emotion dysregulation such as avoidance and self-harm behaviors. The chapter synthesizes the evidence of altered emotion processing and regulation across multiple PDs, and introduces emotion regulation as a target for psychotherapy for PDs.

Chapter 8, "The Clinical Neuroscience of Impulsive Aggression" by Royce Lee, Jennifer Fanning, and Emil Coccaro, first delineates the social information processing model of impulsive aggression and its neurobiological underpinnings, with a special focus on ventral prefrontal-amygdala, frontostriatal, and frontoparietal circuits. In these circuits, structural as well as functional alterations have been associated with aggression. A large body of basic and clinical research has examined the role of neurotransmitters (glutamate, GABA) and neuromodulators (monoamines and neuropeptides) in mediating impulsive aggression.

Chapter 9, "Social Cognition in Personality Disorders" by Stefanie Lis, Nicole Derish, and Mercedes Perez-Rodriguez, focuses on alterations in social cognition, which are increasingly recognized as core illness features in the PDs. Despite the significant disability caused by social cognitive dysfunction, treatments for this symptom dimension are lacking. This chapter describes the evidence demonstrating abnormalities in social cognition and attachment in schizotypal personality disorder (SPD), BPD, APD, and avoidant personality disorder (AvPD), as well as the neurobiology of social cognition.

Chapter 10, "Attachment in Personality Disorders" by Mercedes Perez-Rodriguez, Nicole E. Derish, Nerea Palomares, Sukhbir Kaur, Armando Cuesta-Diaz, and Stefanie Lis, focuses on attachment theory which suggests that early relationships with significant others play a critical role in later interpersonal relationships. Attachment styles have a significant impact on social functioning. This chapter describes definitions and measures of attachment and briefly reviews the neurobiology of attachment. Then it describes the evidence demonstrating abnormalities in attachment in PDs. Finally, the psychotherapeutic implications of different attachment styles are reviewed, and attachment-focused treatments for PDs are described.

Chapter 11, "Suicide and Non-Suicidal Self Injury: Prevalence in Patients with Personality Disorders" by Paul Soloff and Christian Schmahl, reviews current data on the prevalence of suicidal behavior and nonsuicidal self-injury (NSSI) in patients with PDs, the characteristics of attempters versus completers, and the epidemiology of NSSI in BPD. In addition, it presents explanatory models for suicide and NSSI. Also, there are comprehensive discussions of the neurobiological mechanisms involved in both suicidality and NSSI focusing on the structural and functional neuroimaging of emotion dysregulation, impulsivity, executive cognitive deficits, affective interference and cognitive function, and the endogenous opioid system.

Chapter 12, "The Neurobiology and Genetics of Schizotypal Personality Disorder" by Daniel Rosell and Larry Siever, focuses on the neurobiology of SPD or attenuated schizophrenia-spectrum traits present among the general population. The chapter first characterizes the SPD construct, then turns to the genetics and development of SPD, followed by a review of studies employing nonimaging, laboratory measures. Then anatomical, functional, and neurochemical imaging findings are discussed.

Chapter 13, "The Neurobiological Basis of Borderline Personality Disorder" by Robert Friedel, Christian Schmahl, and Marijn Distel, provides an overview of the biological underpinnings of BPD. The material in this chapter is presented in five sections: one describing the structure of genetic and environmental risk factors for BPD and four describing our current knowledge about the anatomy and pathophysiology of symptoms in each of the four domains of the disorder (i.e., affective dysregulation, impulsive aggression, disturbances of perception and cognition, and interpersonal impairments). The chapter concludes with a discussion of the clinical, research, and educational implications of this information.

Chapter 14, "Neurobiology of Antisocial Personality Disorder" by Michael Baliousis, Najat Khalifa, and Birgit Völlm, describes the high heritability of APD. Prevalence in quantitative genetic studies in children with strong callous-unemotional traits suggest that psychopathic tendencies are under extremely strong genetic influence. The results of genome-wide association and candidate gene studies are reported in detail. Neurobiological studies evaluating brain structure, electrophysiological aberrations, and generalized neuropsychological studies of individuals with APD compared to controls are also reviewed.

Chapter 15, "The Neurobiological Basis of Avoidant Personality Disorder" by Theresa Wilberg and Kenneth Silk, reviews quantitative genetic studies that estimate a high prevalence of the disorder and molecular genetic studies that suggest aberrations in neurotransmitter functioning. Neuroimaging studies have evaluated regions of activity levels and functional connectivity in subjects with AvPD compared to individuals in the general population. They suggest a significant decrease in the behavioral activation system that is sensitive to rewarding stimuli and an increase in the behavioral inhibition system that is associated with risk assessment, avoidance, and negative emotions. These studies are consistent with the aberrations observed in the molecular genetic and neurochemical activity of the neurotransmitter systems related to these functions.

Chapter 16, "Established and Novel Pharmacological Approaches to the Treatment of Personality Disorders" by Charles Schulz and Robert Friedel, first reviews the current knowledge on medication for patients with PDs and then considers a number of novel pharmacological approaches that may yield additional beneficial results in the treatment of these disorders. A special emphasis of the chapter is laid on the role of clozapine in the treatment of PDs as well as new findings in the areas of pharmacogenetics and epigenetics.

Chapter 17, "Neurobiological Underpinnings of Psychosocial Treatments in Personality Disorders" by Marianne Goodman, Jennifer Chen, and Erin Hazlett, first reviews general concepts of psychotherapy that are most relevant to personality dysfunction. The authors then discuss current neuroscientific mechanisms and theories that are related to the psychotherapeutic mechanisms utilized in the treatment PDs. Emphasis is placed on the neurobiological basis of learning, memory consolidation, neural plasticity, epigenetic processes, neuroendocrinological mechanisms, and the contributions of current functional neuroimaging techniques.

Chapter 18, "Conclusions and Future Directions" by Christian Schmahl, K. Luan Phan, and Robert O. Friedel summarizes the most important findings and gives an outlook on what we think is important for future research in PDs and their neurobiological underpinnings.

Unfortunately, during the course of preparing the book, Larry became very seriously ill and could not continue to work with Bob and me on this endeavor, which had relied heavily on him in his capacity as lead editor. We were therefore very grateful that Luan Phan, a distinguished expert in the neurobiology of psychiatric disorders, stepped in and helped us to get this volume off the ground. With some temporal delay we are now very glad that this book gives a timely overview of what is known about the neurobiological foundations of the mechanisms behind and the treatment of PDs.

We dedicate this book to Larry Siever, who is truly a pioneer in this field and inspired us tremendously in or own research, which is always aimed at improving the lives of those suffering from PDs. We also thank all authors of individual chapters, and we are very grateful that we were able to attract, with Larry's assistance, such a broad array of distinguished experts in the field. It is a sad duty and fills us with deep regret that Ken Silk and Chuck Schulz, two highly valued colleagues and friends, who contributed significantly to this volume as chapter authors, passed away and could not enjoy, as we do, this book's publication.

■ CONTRIBUTORS

Michael Baliousis
Division of Psychiatry and
    Applied Psychology
School of Medicine
University of Nottingham
Nottingham, UK

Katja Bertsch
Department of General Psychiatry
Medical Faculty Heidelberg
Heidelberg, Germany

Jennifer Chen
Mental Illness Research, Education, and
    Clinical Center
James J. Peters Veterans Affairs
    Medical Center
Bronx, NY

Emil F. Coccaro
Clinical Neuroscience Research Unit
Department of Psychiatry & Behavioral
    Neuroscience
University of Chicago
Pritzker School of Medicine
Chicago, IL

Armando Cuesta-Diaz
Department of Psychiatry
Icahn School of Medicine at Mount Sinai
New York, NY

Bryan T. Denny
Department of Psychiatry
Icahn School of Medicine at Mount Sinai
New York, NY

Nicole E. Derish
Department of Psychiatry
Icahn School of Medicine at Mount Sinai
New York, NY

Marijn Distel
Department of Psychiatry
EMGO Institute for Health and Care
    Research and Neuroscience Campus
    Amsterdam
VU University Medical Centre
Amsterdam, The Netherlands

Jennifer R. Fanning
Clinical Neuroscience Research Unit
Department of Psychiatry & Behavioral
    Neuroscience
University of Chicago
Pritzker School of Medicine
Chicago, IL

Peter Fonagy
Research Department of Clinical,
    Educational and Health Psychology
University College London
London, UK

Marianne Goodman
Icahn School of Medicine
    at Mount Sinai
New York, NY
Mental Illness Research, Education,
    and Clinical Center
James J. Peters Veterans Affairs
    Medical Center
Bronx, NY

Erin A. Hazlett
Icahn School of Medicine at Mount Sinai
New York, NY
Mental Illness Research, Education,
    and Clinical Center
James J. Peters Veterans Affairs
    Medical Center
Bronx, NY

Sukhbir Kaur
Department of Psychiatry
Icahn School of Medicine at Mount Sinai
New York, NY

Kenneth S. Kendler
Virginia Institute for Psychiatric and
    Behavioral Genetics
Department of Psychiatry
Department of Human and
    Molecular Genetics
Virginia Commonwealth University
Richmond, VA

Najat Khalifa
Division of Psychiatry and Applied
    Psychology
School of Medicine
University of Nottingham
Nottingham, UK

Harold Koenigsberg
Professor of Psychiatry
Icahn School of Medicine at Mount Sinai
New York, NY

Royce Lee
Clinical Neuroscience Research Unit
Department of Psychiatry
    & Behavioral Neuroscience
University of Chicago
Pritzker School of Medicine
Chicago, IL

Stefanie Lis
Institute of Psychiatric and
    Psychosomatic Psychotherapy
Central Institute of Mental Health
Medical Faculty Mannheim
Heidelberg University
Heidelberg, Germany

Patrick Luyten
Faculty of Psychology and Educational
    Sciences
University of Leuven
Leuven, Belgium

Angus W. MacDonald III
Department of Psychology
University of Minnesota
Saint Paul, MN

Annmarie MacNamara
Department of Psychiatry
University of Illinois at Chicago
Chicago, IL

Inga Niedtfeld
Department of Psychosomatic Medicine
    and Psychotherapy
Central Institute of Mental Health
Medical Faculty Mannnheim
Heidelberg University
Heidelberg, Germany

Kevin N. Ochsner
Department of Psychology
Columbia University
New York, NY

Nerea Palomares
Department of Psychiatry
Icahn School of Medicine at Mount Sinai
New York, NY
Institute of Health Research of the
    Hospital Clinico San Carlos
Madrid, Spain

M. Mercedes Perez-Rodriguez
Department of Psychiatry
Icahn School of Medicine
    at Mount Sinai
Mental Health Patient Care Center
Mental Illness Research Education and
    Clinical Center
James J. Peters Veterans Affairs
    Medical Center
New York, NY
Autonoma University of Madrid
Fundacion Jimenez Diaz Hospital
Madrid, Spain

Andrew Poppe
Department of Psychology
University of Minnesota
Saint Paul, MN

Ted Reichborn-Kjennerud
Department of Mental Disorders
Norwegian Institute of Public Health
Institute of Clinical Medicine
University of Olso
Olso, Norway

Daniel R. Rosell
Department of Psychiatry
Icahn Medical School of Medicine at
    Mount Sinai
New York, NY

S. Charles Schulz (dec.)
Professor of Psychiatry
University of Minnesota
Minneapolis, MN

Larry J. Siever
Professor of Psychiatry
James J. Peters Veterans Affairs Medical
    Center
Icahn School of Medicine
    at Mount Sinai
New York, NY

Kenneth Silk (dec.)
Professor of Psychiatry
University of Michigan
Ann Arbor, MI

Paul Soloff
Department of Psychiatry
University of Pittsburgh School of
    Medicine
Pittsburgh, PA

Stephen M. Stahl
Neuroscience Education Institute
Carlsbad, CA

Birgit Völlm
Division of Psychiatry and Applied
    Psychology
School of Medicine
University of Nottingham
Nottingham, UK

Theresa Wilberg
Oslo University Hospital
Division of Mental Health and Addiction
Department of Research and
    Development
Oslo, Norway

Foundations of Neurobiology of Personality

1 Neurocircuitry of Affective, Cognitive, and Regulatory Systems

■ ANNMARIE MACNAMARA
AND K. LUAN PHAN

■ INTRODUCTION: APPROACH TO NEUROCIRCUITRY OF EMOTION AND COGNITION

In this chapter, we provide a review and synthesis of the neurocircuitry involved in affect, cognition, and their interactions as it relates to regulatory functions. We deliberately consider cognition and emotion together, under one umbrella (Lane, Nadel, Allen, & Kaszniak, 2002). That is, instead of first discussing the neural circuitry implicated in cognition and then discussing the neural circuitry implicated in emotion (or vice versa), we take a more integrated, functional perspective. This integrative approach recognizes that emotion and cognition—psychological processes and neural systems—are intertwined such that they interact and overlap in terms of response systems and neural substrates (Dolcos, Iordan, & Dolcos, 2011; Pessoa, 2010, 2013; Ray & Zald, 2012).

Here we define emotion as a multilayered, coordinated response to a stimulus that an organism *appraises* as having relevance to its goals (Frijda, 1987; Gross & Thompson, 2007). Appraisals give a situation meaning and therefore are intertwined with emotion in the vast majority of (if not all) cases (Lazarus, 2000). For instance, a single situation can elicit any number of different emotions (or may fail to elicit emotion), depending on the meaning ascribed to the situation. In addition, there are other reasons to conceptualize emotion within a cognitive framework, including the role of other cognitive processes such as attention in emotion elicitation, the utility of cognitive neuroscience techniques for studying emotion, and the goal of parsimony (e.g., there is no evidence to date that the brain systems implicated in cognition and emotion differ on a fundamental level; Lane et al., 2002). Therefore, in what follows, we begin by outlining a framework derived from the cognitive neuroscience literature (Baars & Gage, 2013) that we believe is amenable to conceptualizing both cognitive and affective processes and their interactions at the neural level.

■ AN INTEGRATIVE FRAMEWORK

Figure 1.1 depicts a framework for understanding the cognitive and affective processes that take place between the time sensory input is received and the time a behavioral

A Cognitive-Affective Framework

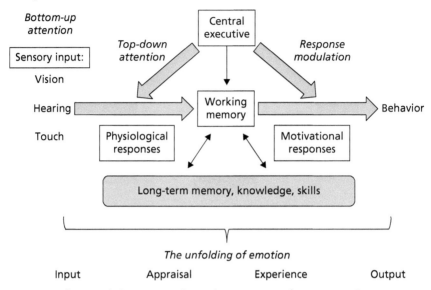

Figure 1.1 A framework for conceptualizing the integration of cognition and emotion.

response is enacted. An example may be helpful in conceptualizing this framework. Consider the dual role (as mother and driver) of a woman driving in busy traffic with her young children in the backseat. All of a sudden, the children begin shouting and fighting with each other. The mother's attention is automatically drawn to her children's shouts; her heart rate increases. Her working memory (WM) is filled with the sounds and words of her children (replacing its prior contents). The mother feels the urge to turn around to try to break up the fighting, but, as the driver, she knows that she must keep her hands on the steering wheel and her eyes on the road. In order to effectively navigate in traffic, the woman directs her attention to the car in front of her, to avoid rear-ending it. She then speaks calmly to her children and keeps her hands on the wheel.

This example illustrates the way in which sensory input is attended, given meaning and modulated by a series of cognitive and/or affective processes before guiding behavioral action/inaction (Figure 1.1). These processes unfold over time, may be automatic or voluntary, and draw upon prior experiences and knowledge to contextualize and shape response. In the next section we present the "lay of the land" in terms of the key neural regions involved in cognitive and affective response, before moving on to a summary of findings organized by process.

▪ BRAIN STRUCTURE-FUNCTION TOPOLOGY: A GENERAL GEOGRAPHY

Historically, neuroscientists tended to pursue a "locationist" approach in which they sought to map psychological functions to particular brain regions. However, in recent years it has become increasingly clear that such an approach is likely insufficient in understanding the vast number of complex and integrative functions performed by the brain. For example, studies of the same task or psychological process have often yielded sparse overlap between the neural regions involved (McGonigle et al., 2002; Poeppel, 1996). On the other hand, meta-analytic work has suggested that the same neural regions may be engaged by a number of seemingly different cognitive paradigms (e.g., Cabeza & Nyberg, 2000). Thus, more recent neuroscientific approaches have moved away from a locationist approach and have instead stressed the importance of brain regions working in concert as "circuits" and "networks" to influence psychological process—an issue to which we return briefly at the end of this chapter. Put differently, the psychological function of a brain region may be defined, at least in part, by the circuit of brain regions with which it fires (McIntosh, 2004). With this as a caveat, the following section is organized by broad neural regions because we felt it important to have a basic understanding of these regions before beginning to contemplate how these regions work together at the neural circuit level to implement cognitive and affective processing.

Prefrontal Regions

The prefrontal cortex (PFC) is located anterior to the brain's motor areas and is involved in most higher level cognitive tasks (Cabeza & Nyberg, 2000). The PFC is extremely well connected to the association and limbic cortices (Siddiqui, Chatterjee, Kumar, Siddiqui, & Goyal, 2008). These connections are essential for feed-forward and feedback circuits. All prefrontal connections are reciprocal, except for the basal ganglia and pontine nuclei, to which the PFC sends some unreciprocated signals (Fuster, 2008). The lateral PFC (lPFC) is connected to the lateral thalamus, the dorsal caudate nucleus, and the neocortex (Fuster, 2008). The orbital and medial regions of the PFC are primarily connected to the medial thalamus, hypothalamus, the amygdala, and limbic and medial temporal cortex, including the hippocampus. Traditionally, the PFC was thought of as subdivided into units or modules that each served a particular function. However, functional neuroimaging and electrocortical studies have failed to confirm a prefrontal map of cognitive or affective function. In other words, no "double dissociations" of area and function have been observed in the PFC (Fuster, Stuss, & Knight, 2013, p. 20).

The lPFC is involved in language, attention, memory, response conflict, novelty processing, temporal ordering, explicit memory, reality monitoring, and metamemory, among other functions. The dorsolateral prefrontal cortex (dlPFC; see Figure 1.2) is implicated in a diverse set of processes, including active maintenance of WM information, modifying behavior in line with task demands or goals, and representing past events, current goals, and predictions about the future as well as emotion regulation. The dlPFC is part of the *dorsal* frontoparietal network believed to be involved in top-down, goal-directed response selection (Corbetta, Patel, & Shulman, 2008; Corbetta & Shulman, 2002). The ventrolateral PFC (vlPFC; see Figure 1.2) has been associated with semantic processing, categorization of objects, representation of feature-based information for abstract categories, response selection, and inhibition of response. The vlPFC is part of the *ventral* frontoparietal network believed to be involved in directing attention to salient environmental stimuli (Corbetta et al., 2008; Corbetta & Shulman, 2002).

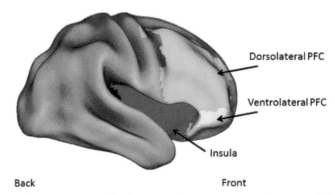

Figure 1.2 Key brain regions involved in cognitive-affective processing (lateral view).

The medial PFC (mPFC) is commonly activated during emotional tasks (Phan, Wager, Taylor, & Liberzon, 2004) and has been associated with the cognitive aspects of emotion processing. Specifically, the mPFC may integrate affective estimations of the stimulus generated by the amygdala and ventral striatum with valuations from other regions of the brain, including medial temporal regions (e.g., the hippocampus) which represent historic information (such as previous encounters with the stimulus) and the lPFC, which relays information about current goals. By contextualizing the affective valuation of a stimulus in terms of prior experience and current behavioral goals, the mPFC contributes to adaptive behavior.

For instance, the dorsomedial PFC (dmPFC; see Figure 1.3) has been associated with self-awareness and perspective taking (Miller & Cummings, 2007). Evidence suggests that patients with damage to the dmPFC show significant changes in the way they subjectively experience emotion (Hornak et al., 2003). Moreover, greater changes in emotion have been related to poorer social adjustment (Hornak et al., 2003), underscoring the relationship between subjective awareness of emotion and effective social behavior. Perspective-taking functions of the dmPFC include theory of mind (e.g., predicting the contents of other's minds based on comparison with

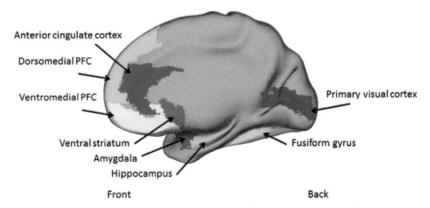

Figure 1.3 Key brain regions involved in cognitive-affective processing (medial view).

one's own mind), mentalizing and empathy (Miller & Cummings, 2007). The dmPFC may achieve these and other perspective-taking functions by momentarily subduing a person's own perspective, thereby enabling him or her to infer another's point of view (Decety & Jackson, 2004).

Lesions studies suggest that the ventromedial PFC (vmPFC; see Figure 1.3) is associated with personal and social decision-making (Bechara, Tranel, & Damasio, 2000). The vmPFC has also been associated with the retrieval of information from long-term memory, as well as metacognitive processes (Schnyer, Nicholls, & Verfaellie, 2005). The vmPFC is implicated in fear extinction and its successful recall (Kalisch et al., 2006; Milad, Wright, et al., 2007). More broadly, the vmPFC may provide "somatic markers" that enable individuals to learn from environmental experience (Damasio, Everitt, & Bishop, 1996). In other words, the vmPFC may permit association of current contingencies with prior affective events (e.g., facilitating modulation of response to stimuli that may have been previously associated with negative outcomes).

The orbitofrontal cortex (OFC), at times also referred to as the vmPFC, has been shown to play a key role in social and emotional behavior. The ventral PFC, emerging from the OFC, projects to the limbic system and is especially well connected to the amygdala and anterior cingulate. Therefore, the OFC is well positioned to integrate internal and external sensory information in order to guide behavior (Lindquist, Wager, Kober, Bliss-Moreau, & Barrett, 2012). In line with this notion, the OFC has been linked to the expectation of reward as well as the anticipation and processing of outcomes, as well as reversal learning (Fellows & Farah, 2003; Hornak et al., 2004; Kringelbach & Rolls, 2004; Schoenbaum, Takahashi, Liu, & McDannald, 2011) and emotional perspective taking (Hynes, Baird, & Grafton, 2006). Damage to the OFC has been shown to result in inappropriate social behavior (e.g., Beer, John, Scabini, & Knight, 2006; Eslinger & Damasio, 1985).

Cingulate Regions

The cingulate cortex is comprised of the posterior and anterior cingulate. The functions of the posterior cingulate are not well understood; however, its most widely known role is as part of the default mode network (DMN; Leech & Sharp, 2014), which comes on-line when an individual is engaged in internal tasks such as daydreaming, retrieving memories, or envisioning other's perspectives. The posterior cingulate cortex has also been associated with emotional salience (Maddock, Garrett, & Buonocore, 2003) and the retrieval of autobiographical memory (Maddock, Garrett, & Buonocore, 2001). The anterior cingulate cortex (ACC; see Figure 1.3) can be thought of as "a nexus of information processing and regulation in the brain" (Margulies et al., 2007, p. 579): it is centrally located and involved in a wide variety of motor, cognitive, and affective tasks. It is believed to be involved in monitoring and evaluating the outcomes of actions (Botvinick, Cohen, & Carter, 2004)—including error detection (Gehring & Fencsik, 2001; Lorist, Boksem, & Ridderinkhof, 2005)—and is more likely to be activated during effortful tasks (Paus, Koski, Caramanos, & Westbury, 1998). The ACC has long been thought to play a critical role in emotion processing, though knowledge of its precise role in this context remains uncertain. It has traditionally been divided into caudal-dorsal and rostral-ventral regions, which show anatomical differences and differing patterns of connectivity with the rest of the brain (Margulies et al., 2007). Initial accounts suggested that the dorsal region of the ACC (dACC) was associated with cognitive control and cognitive processing, whereas the more ventral region (vACC) was associated with emotion processing (Bush, Luu, & Posner, 2000); however, this cognitive/affective division has since been called into question (e.g., Etkin, Egner, & Kalisch, 2011). For example, many emotional processes have been found to recruit caudal-dorsal and mPFC regions (Etkin & Wager, 2007; Mechias, Etkin, & Kalisch, 2010).

Insular Region

The insular cortex (see Figure 1.2) has been associated with visceral states, interoceptive awareness, and the experience of negative emotion in general (Phan, Wager, et al., 2004). For instance, insula activation has been found during: processing of fearful faces and facial expressions of disgust (Calder, Lawrence, & Young, 2001; Phillips et al., 1997), fear conditioning (Sehlmeyer et al., 2009), script-induced sad mood (Liotti et al., 2000; Reiman et al., 1997), and aversive interoceptive experiences (Critchley, Wiens, Rotshtein, Öhman, & Dolan, 2004; Paulus & Stein, 2006). Evidence from animal and human studies suggests that the insula may be particularly important for "internally generated" emotions (Lane et al., 1997). For instance, it has been shown to play a role in anticipatory anxiety (Paulus & Stein, 2006) and guilt (Shin et al., 2000). Via its connections to the amygdala, the insula is positioned to communicate somatic sensations elicited by emotional stimuli (Augustine, 1996; Craig, 2002) and may therefore have played an important role evolutionarily, for signaling internally sensed danger or changes in homeostasis (Lane et al., 1997). The insula may also contribute to cognitive functions, including inhibition, error processing, conflict, feedback, and switching (Chang, Yarkoni, Khaw, & Sanfey, 2013).

Subcortical Regions

Regions of the brain that lie beneath the cortex are referred to as subcortical. Evidence suggests that these regions are not simply "slaves" to top-down modulation by cortical structures (as once thought), but rather substantially influence cortical processing (e.g., Johnson, 2005). Key amongst the subcortical structures is the amygdala (see Figure 1.3), a phylogenetically old "alarm" system implicated in the detection and perception of stimuli relevant to an organism's goals. Because some studies have shown that the amygdala is especially sensitive to threat-related information (e.g., Calder et al., 2001; Phan, Wager, Taylor, & Liberzon, 2002), the amygdala has been characterized as a neural structure whose function is to protect the organism from danger (Amaral, 2002). Nevertheless, damage to the amygdala does not necessarily change the subjective experience of fear (Phelps & Anderson, 1997), and the amygdala appears to play a prominent role in positively valenced processes such as reward (Baxter & Murray, 2002; Everitt et al., 1999; Holland & Gallagher, 2004) and positive expectation (Paton, Belova, Morrison, & Salzman, 2006). Moreover, according to a recent meta-analysis of nearly 400 studies, comparable levels of amygdala activation were observed for all types of emotional stimuli (including fear, disgust, sadness, anger, mixed negative, happiness, humor, sex, positive mixed) compared to nonemotional stimuli; however, fear-inducing and disgusting stimuli were found to be more likely to activate the amygdala relative to happy stimuli (Costafreda, Brammer, David, & Fu, 2008; see also Fitzgerald, Angstadt, Jelsone, Nathan, & Phan,

2006; Sergerie, Chochol, & Armony, 2008). Therefore, while the amygdala may show some degree of specialization for threat-related stimuli, it also appears to play a more general role in salience detection, via the processing of both positively and negatively valenced arousing stimuli.

The basal ganglia consists of a network of deep brain nuclei associated with a number of diverse functions, including control of voluntary movement, procedural learning, habitual behaviors, and certain cognitive and affective functions (Chakravarthy, Joseph, & Bapi, 2010; Utter & Basso, 2008). Within the basal ganglia are the striatum (caudate nucleus and putamen), the substantia nigra, and the nucleus accumbens, among other structures. The ventral striatum (see Figure 1.3) consists of the nucleus accumbens and the olfactory tubercle (Ubeda-Bañon et al., 2007); some texts also include ventromedial parts of the caudate and the putamen (Martin, 2012). In both animals and humans, the ventral striatum has been shown to be involved in learning which stimuli predict reward, and it has been shown to activate in response to both abstract stimuli (e.g., previously neutral cues paired with reward) and intrinsically pleasant stimuli (e.g., smiling faces; Knutson & Cooper, 2005; O'Doherty, 2004; Schultz, 2007). Although the ventral striatum was originally studied in the context of drug-related (Koob, 1999) and rewarding (Knutson, Fong, Adams, Varner, & Hommer, 2001) stimuli, it has also been shown to activate in response to the emotional intensity and self-relatedness of stimuli, irrespective of valence (e.g., Phan, Taylor, et al., 2004).

The hippocampus (see Figure 1.3) communicates with the neocortex (a part of the cerebral cortex) via the entorhinal cortex (Amaral & Lavenex, 2007). The hippocampus has been implicated in the consolidation of declarative information (e.g., facts, events, semantic knowledge) from short-term to long-term memory (Duvernoy, Cattin, & Risold, 2013; Eichenbaum, 2004) and in spatial memory (Burgess, Maguire, & O'Keefe, 2002). It has also been shown to play a key role in emotional memory, including in extinction learning and retention (Bouton, Westbrook, Corcoran, & Maren, 2006; Ji & Maren, 2007; Milad, Wright, et al., 2007). Animal research has indicated that the hippocampus is involved in spatial navigation, prompting the "cognitive map" theory (O'Keefe & Nadel, 1978). However, more recent research has suggested that the hippocampus' function might best be described as essential to the integration of objects and contexts (Lech & Suchan, 2013)—of which spatial memory may be just one example (Eichenbaum, 2000; Kumaran & Maguire, 2005).

Temporal-Parietal-Occipital Regions

The temporal lobe contains the fusiform gyrus (see Figure 1.3), which is involved in face perception (Kanwisher, McDermott, & Chun, 1997; Sergent, Ohta, & MacDonald, 1992). Temporal regions are also associated with high-level sensory processing and language recognition (e.g., Chao, Haxby, & Martin, 1999; Spitsyna, Warren, Scott, Turkheimer, & Wise, 2006). The primary auditory cortex, which shows a tonotopic organization, is in the temporal lobe (Gazzaniga, Ivry, & Mangun, 2013).

The parietal lobe integrates sensory information of different modalities, including spatial sense, touch, and vision. Parietal regions have also been implicated in episodic retrieval (Wagner, Shannon, Kahn, & Buckner, 2005; Yazar, Bergström, & Simons, 2012) as well as in spatial perception/selective attention (Behrmann, 2004; Petersen & Posner, 2012). A frontoparietal network has been found to play a role in the initiation and adjustment of top-down control (Dosenbach, Fair, Cohen, Schlaggar, & Petersen, 2008).

The primary visual cortex (V1; see Figure 1.3), sometimes referred to as the striate cortex because it appears striped to the naked eye, is located in the occipital cortex. After visual information is received in the retina and transmitted to the optic nerve, it is relayed to the lateral geniculate nucleus of the thalamus and then on to V1. (Note: all sensory processing is routed through the thalamus to the cortex, with the exception of some olfactory inputs.) Surrounding the striate region is a large area dedicated to visual processing that is known as the extrastriate cortex, to denote that it is anterior to the striate cortex (Gazzaniga, 2010).

■ BRAIN STRUCTURE-FUNCTION SPECIALIZED TOPOLOGY: EMOTION IN THE CONTEXT OF COGNITION

The previous section provided an overview of some of the key neural regions implicated in the cognitive and affective processes discussed in the following sections. In what follows, we summarize key neuroscientific findings as organized by cognitive processes and their relevance for emotion. It is our hope that by approaching the literature from two perspectives—that is, region and process—the reader will be left with a more complete and flexible view of the critical neurocircuitry involved in cognitive *and* affective processing. Our choice of processes reflects the key stages involved in responding to a stimulus, from the time of sensory input to behavioral response/output, and was guided by our cognitive affective framework, outlined in Figure 1.1. We note that these stages are not discrete, that each process affects another, and that these processes may occur in a simultaneous or ongoing/overlapping fashion.

Perception

Perception refers to the organization, identification, and interpretation of incoming sensory information in the service of orienting to or representing the environment. Depending on the stimulus modality, different sensory cortices are activated; here we focus primarily on the perception of visual stimuli (which begins in the occipital cortex), because of their widespread use in experiments investigating cognitive and affective processing.

Some research has sought to identify neural networks involved in the processing of particular categories of stimuli—for example, faces. Face perception may be one of the most developed forms of human visual processing, with good reason: the accurate perception of faces allows a person to distinguish friend from foe and to glean information necessary for effective social interaction (e.g., identity, emotion, gaze, attractiveness). Current models of face perception propose an initial encoding stage, after which different neural pathways are involved in determining the identity of a face versus analyzing facial expression (Haxby, Hoffman, & Gobbini, 2000, 2002).

Of relevance to emotion, a subcortical route for threat detection has been proposed, whereby fearful or threatening facial features trigger activation in the amygdala via the superior colliculus and pulvinar thalamus, yielding rapid but coarse identification of threat (LeDoux, 1996; Morris, Öhman, & Dolan, 1999; Öhman, 2002). However, despite evidence of amygdala involvement in the rapid identification of threatening faces, several studies have found that emotional faces of positive valence also lead to greater activation in the amygdala and Fusiform Face Area (FFA) compared to neutral faces (Breiter et al., 1996; Morris et al., 1998; Vuilleumier, Armony, Driver, & Dolan, 2001, 2003; Vuilleumier, Richardson, Armony, Driver, & Dolan, 2004). Therefore, both the FFA and the amygdala seem to be implicated in the prioritized perception of positively and negatively valenced emotional faces (but see Adolphs, Tranel, Damasio, & Damasio, 1994, 1995, for studies of amygdala damage).

Salient visual stimuli such as faces have often been used in neuroscientific work because of widespread interest in socioemotional processing and because of their availability in standardized databases (e.g., the Penn 3D facial emotion stimuli, Gur et al., 2002; the Nim Stim Face Stimulus Set, MacArthur Research Network on Early Experience and Brain Development, 2002). In addition, emotional and neutral photographic *scenes*, such as those available in the International Affective Picture System (IAPS; Lang, Bradley, & Cuthbert, 2008) have also been commonly used in functional magnetic resonance imaging (fMRI) studies of affective processing (see Sabatinelli et al., 2011, for a meta-analysis comparing perception of emotional faces versus scenes). Compared to neutral IAPS, emotional IAPS (both pleasant and unpleasant) have been found to elicit increased activity in the occipital and inferotemporal cortex, superior parietal visual areas, amygdala, insula, ACC, superior frontal gyrus, and mPFC (Bradley et al., 2003; Britton, Taylor, Sudheimer, & Liberzon, 2006; Britton, Phan, et al., 2006; Hariri, Tessitore, Mattay, Fera, & Weinberger, 2002; Sabatinelli, Bradley, Fitzsimmons, & Lang, 2005; Sabatinelli, Bradley, Lang, Costa, & Versace, 2007).

An important question is whether the neural substrates of emotional perception differ from those involved in nonemotional perception. In support of the notion that these processes may overlap considerably, evidence now suggests that emotional stimuli seem to affect processing in the primary visual cortex (Damaraju, Huang, Barrett, & Pessoa, 2009) and that emotion modulates core aspects of visual perception, from contrast sensitivity (Phelps, Ling, & Carrasco, 2006) to visual awareness (Anderson, Siegel, Bliss-Moreau, & Barrett, 2011). Moreover, several recent meta-analyses of emotion processing have found that emotional stimuli consistently activate visual regions (Kober et al., 2008), even when these stimuli are not visual (Lindquist et al., 2012). While one possibility is that emotional stimuli are simply more visually complex than nonemotional stimuli, evidence suggests that pictorial complexity is unlikely to explain emotion-related effects in the amygdala or visual cortex (e.g., Taylor, Liberzon, & Koeppe, 2000). A more likely explanation may be that neuroanatomical connections between the visual cortex and regions of the brain involved in emotion processing (e.g., the amygdala, OFC; Amaral & Price, 1984; Barrett & Bar, 2009; Pessoa & Adolphs, 2010) allow limbic regions to boost activation in the ventral stream while viewing emotional stimuli (Duncan & Barrett, 2007)—a process that, historically, may have facilitated survival via early detection of motivationally relevant (e.g., life-threatening) stimuli in the environment (e.g., Öhman & Mineka, 2001).

Learning and Memory

Declarative memory (i.e., memories that can be consciously recalled) is thought to involve a pathway from the neocortex (i.e., the association cortex, in particular) to the parahippocampus and then to the hippocampus. The main outputs of the parahippocampus and hippocampus are back to the neocortex; therefore, this pathway is bidirectional. Procedural memory (i.e., skills, habits, associative learning), on the other hand, operates via a pathway extending from the neocortex to the striatum and cerebellum—two routes that mediate different types of motor memory. This pathway involves projections back to the cortex as well as to the brainstem motor nuclei (Eichenbaum, 2012). Emotional memory is thought to involve a path from the cortex to the amygdala, which projects to the hypothalamus and several hormonal and autonomic outputs. The medial temporal lobe also plays a key role in the formation of emotional memories (e.g., Murty, Ritchey, Adcock, & LaBar, 2010). In what follows, we have chosen to focus on the neurocircuitry of one particular form of memory—fear learning (and extinction), selected because it (a) bridges both cognitive and emotional domains and (b) may have translational relevance to the study of psychopathology and its treatment (e.g., Lissek et al., 2005; Milad & Quirk, 2012).

The amygdala plays a primary role in the acquisition of fear responses via classical conditioning (e.g., Moscarello & LeDoux, 2013). Evidence for the central role of the amygdala in fear conditioning comes from studies of rats, in which amygdala lesions have been found to impair fear conditioning and the expression of conditioned fear responses. Stimulation of the amygdala immediately after training can also impair the acquisition of conditioned fear responses (e.g., Gold, Hankins, Edwards, Chester, & McGaugh, 1975), and injection of certain pharmacological agents into the amygdala have also been found to increase or decrease fear conditioning (e.g., McGaugh & Cahill, 1997; McGaugh, 2000).

What other areas of the brain are involved in fear learning besides the amygdala? In a recent review, Sehlmeyer and colleagues (2009) reported that the insula and ACC were also activated across a range of fear conditioning tasks. In addition, hippocampal activation was observed, but this was stronger during trace conditioning, in which there is a delay between the conditioned stimulus (CS) offset and the unconditioned stimulus (US) onset (as compared to delay conditioning, in which CS presentation overlaps with or coterminates with US presentation).

The insular cortex may be involved in fear conditioning via its role in receiving and relaying sensory (e.g., visual) information to the amygdala (Turner & Zimmer, 1984). For instance, lesions to the caudal insular cortex have been found to interfere with the retention of fear-potentiated startle elicited by a visual CS (Rosen et al., 1992), and temporary inactivation of the insular cortex has been found to impair retention of inhibitory avoidance learning (Bermudez-Rattoni, Introini-Collison, & McGaugh, 1991).

The dACC may be involved in the expression of fear more generally rather than fear learning per se. For example, in a recent study performed in humans, cortical thickness in the dACC correlated positively with conditioned fear responses to the CS (as measured by skin conductance responses). In a separate group of participants, the authors also found that dACC activity was positively correlated with differential SCR (CS+ relative to the CS–) during fear conditioning (Milad, Quirk, et al., 2007). Nevertheless, more work is needed to confirm this hypothesis and fully understand the role of the dACC in fear learning (Milad & Quirk, 2012).

Evidence suggests that the hippocampus is involved in storing *contextual* fear memory. For example, experiments using rats have indicated that hippocampal lesions performed one-day post-training abolish conditioned fear to diffuse contextual cues but not to discrete cue tones (Anagnostaras, Maren, & Fanselow, 1999; Maren, Aharonov, & Fanselow, 1997). However, when hippocampal lesions are made 28 days after training, a substantive amount of contextual conditioning is retained (Kim & Fanselow, 1992). In addition, hippocampal lesions administered prior to training have been found to block contextual fear conditioning but not fear conditioning to cue tone (Phillips & LeDoux, 1992). Finally, when a single CS signals different outcomes depending on the context in which it is presented, the hippocampus may play a key role in using contextual clues to regulate the recall of CS memories (Maren, 2001).

Fear extinction—which has been conceptualized as a form of *implicit* emotion regulation (Ochsner, Silvers, & Buhle, 2012)—was once thought of as the "forgetting" of CS-US pairing but is now believed to involve the active formation of new memories that inhibit a prior CS association (Bouton, 2002; Myers & Davis, 2002). A number of brain regions have been implicated in extinction, key amongst them the amygdala, the hippocampus, and the PFC (Sotres-Bayon, Bush, & LeDoux, 2004). In line with the idea that extinction is not the erasure of a fear memory, evidence suggests that although the responses of many amygdala cells return to preconditioning levels during extinction, certain populations of cells in the amygdala do not seem to lose their elevated levels of activation (Repa et al., 2001). Moreover, the protein N-methyl-D-aspartate (NMDA) and NMDA-dependent plasticity have been shown to be important in learning and memory, and neural activity in the amygdala that leads to this plasticity may play a key role in extinction (Davis, 2011; see also Falls, Miserendino, & Davis, 1992).

The hippocampus' involvement in extinction likely stems from its role in the formation of contextual memories. For instance, when CS-US pairings have been made in a variety of contexts and then extinction training is performed in only one of these contexts, fear responding is typically extinguished only in that context (Bouton & Bolles, 1979; Bouton & Ricker, 1994). However, when the Gamma-aminobutyric acid receptor agonist muscimol is infused into the hippocampus prior to extinction training, animals later exhibit freezing (a fear response) in all contexts, including the one in which the CS was extinguished (Corcoran, Desmond, Frey, & Maren, 2005).

In 2000, Quirk, Russo, Barron, and Lebron set out to better understand the role of the vmPFC in extinction. They administered lesions of the infralimbic cortex (the rat homologue of the vmPFC) and found no impairments in extinction learning; however, the following day, rats with vmPFC lesions failed to retrieve their extinction memory at the start of the experiment. As a result of this work, it became clear that understanding the neurobiology of extinction would require accurately distinguishing between the various stages of extinction (Quirk & Mueller, 2008). Since this time, experiments in humans have replicated these results, showing that the vmPFC increases in activation during extinction *recall*—that is, the retention of fear extinction memory after a delay (Phelps, Delgado, Nearing, & LeDoux, 2004; see also Kalisch et al., 2006)—and correlates positively with the magnitude of extinction recall (Milad, Wright, et al., 2007). In addition to the vmPFC, the hippocampus also activates during extinction recall (Milad, Wright, et al., 2007) and, as noted, plays a key role in contextual gating of extinction (Bouton et al., 2006; Ji & Maren, 2007).

Central Executive

The notion of a central executive originated more than 160 years ago, when scientists made initial attempts to understand the function of the prefrontal cortices (Harlow, 1848; Luria, 1966). The central executive is charged with supervisory control over all voluntary actions (Luria, 1966)—functions that are often referred to as "executive functioning". One problem with this concept, however, is that ever since its initial definition (Pribram, 1973), the notion of executive functioning has been conflated with the functions of the PFC and vice versa (Barkley, 2012). However, executive functioning is not entirely a function of the PFC. For example, the PFC has extensive connections to many other regions of the brain, including the basal ganglia, the limbic system, and the cerebellum (Fuster, 2008), and the PFC engages in other processes that are not typically thought of as executive functions (e.g., simple/automatic sensory processes, speech, olfactory identification; Barkley, 2012).

Since its early definition as "what the PFC does," executive functioning has been conceptualized in a number of different models (see Barkley, 2012). Despite disagreement between these various psychological theories of the central executive, there has been a reasonable degree of convergence as to the large-scale neural networks that may underlie supervisory control in the brain (e.g., Chen et al., 2013; Sridharan, Levitin, & Menon, 2008). That is, research has identified a fronto-parietal central executive network, whose key nodes include the dlPFC and the posterior parietal cortex (Dosenbach et al., 2007, 2008; Seeley et al., 2007), as well as a cingulo-opercular/salience network, whose key nodes include the vlPFC, anterior insula (together referred to as the fronto-insular cortex; Dosenbach et al., 2007; Seeley et al., 2007; Sridharan et al., 2008) and ACC. Together, these networks are believed to be involved in supporting a large number of higher order cognitive functions, including attention, WM, and decision-making. In what follows, we outline work that examined the neurocircuitry underlying three such processes: attention, WM, and action monitoring.

On a daily basis, people find themselves in environments containing an overwhelming number of stimuli. This "information overload" necessitates a system that can prioritize—that is, bias—the processing of some stimuli above others. Two attentional systems are generally thought to bias sensory signals. A *dorsal* frontoparietal network is believed to modulate the sensory processing of particular locations or features of stimuli that are relevant to task goals. A *ventral* frontoparietal network is believed to be involved in detecting unexpected or unattended stimuli and in shifting attention.

The dorsal attention network is believed to involve bilateral regions of the brain and includes the intraparietal sulcus (IPS) and the frontal eye fields (FEF), both of which include retinotopically organized subregions (Silver & Kastner, 2009). The IPS and FEF are active in tasks that require participants to overtly or covertly (i.e., without moving their head or eyes) direct attention to a particular location. The dorsal frontoparietal network is also active when target *features* are cued, for example when participants are alerted as to the color of an upcoming target stimulus (Ptak, 2012).

The ventral attention network includes the temporoparietal junction (TPJ) and the ventral frontal cortex—regions that tend to respond when motivationally salient stimuli occur unexpectedly (e.g., outside the focus of spatial attention). Some researchers have proposed that the ventral attention system may be right-lateralized because unexpected stimuli have been found to preferentially activate temporoparietal regions in the right hemisphere (Corbetta et al., 2008; Corbetta & Shulman, 2002). However, *bilateral* TPJ activation has been observed in tasks involving attentional reorienting and the processing of odd/infrequent stimuli (Downar, Crawley, Mikulis, & Davis, 2000; Geng & Mangun, 2011; Vossel, Weidner, Thiel, & Fink, 2008).

Evidence of separable dorsal and ventral attention systems has come from task-related activation as well as from functional activation observed while participants are at rest (Fox, Corbetta, Snyder, Vincent, & Raichle, 2006; He et al., 2007). Structural work has also supported the notion of different white matter tracts for ventral and dorsal attention networks (Umarova et al., 2010). Finally, effective connectivity work (Bressler, Tang, Sylvester, Shulman, & Corbetta, 2008) and transcranial magnetic stimulation work (Ruff et al., 2006, 2008) has provided evidence of the *directionality* of effects in dorsal and ventral attention systems (e.g., by showing that IPS and FEF influence visual activity in a top-down manner).

Emotional stimuli represent a particular kind of behaviorally relevant stimuli. Evolutionarily, it is likely that organisms that attended preferentially to emotional stimuli would have had a survival advantage; thus it is likely that attention has evolved in this direction (e.g., Öhman & Mineka, 2001). A critical question, however, is whether the brain mechanisms involved in emotional attention are distinct from or overlap (fully or partly) with those involved in nonemotional forms of attention.

In a recent review, Pourtois and colleagues (2013) suggested that emotion exerts attentional influences via distinct neural systems that differ from (i.e., do not overlap with) those involved in nonemotional attention. Despite having different neural origins, however, emotional and nonemotional attentional influences on gain control mechanisms might affect the same sensory pathways and might therefore interact in this common final pathway. Evidence in support of distinct emotional and nonemotional attention brain mechanisms comes from a variety of sources. For instance, work that has modulated endogenous, exogenous, and emotional attention simultaneously has reported additive results for each type of attention (Brosch, Pourtois, Sander, & Vuilleumier, 2011). Additionally, studies of patients with brain lesions have found differences between these forms of attention—for example, neglect (Fox, 2002; Grabowska et al., 2011; Vuilleumier & Schwartz, 2001) versus amygdala damage (Anderson & Phelps, 2001; Benuzzi et al., 2004; Rotshtein et al., 2010; Vuilleumier et al., 2004).

The amygdala is a candidate region for emotional attention (Pourtois et al., 2013), because of its strong bidirectional connections to the sensory cortices—particularly for early visual regions (Amaral, Behniea, & Kelly, 2003; Catani, Jones, Donato, & Ffytche, 2003; Gschwind, Pourtois, Schwartz, Ville, & Vuilleumier, 2012) but also for other stimulus modalities (Yukie, 2002). Moreover, as noted, lesion studies suggest that the amygdala is implicated in emotional attention. For instance, in one study in which individuals with amygdala lesions failed to show emotional modulation of face processing in the visual cortex (Vuilleumier et al., 2004), decrements were observed primarily on the same side as amygdala lesions, which fits with evidence from anatomical studies on direct-feedback connections from the amygdala (Amaral et al., 2003). Thus, the amygdala may exert gain control effects on perceptual processing in the visual cortex, much like spatial attention can bias visual processing via top-down attentional modulation exerted by fronto-parietal regions (Corbetta & Shulman, 2002; Pourtois et al., 2013).

For emotional attention to be effective, it must be able to alert the organism to the presence of an emotionally evocative stimulus in the absence of awareness. On one hand, a number of studies in brain-damaged and healthy participants have found that emotional stimuli can be processed at least to some extent without voluntary attention or even conscious awareness (e.g., Carretié, Hinojosa, Mercado, & Tapia, 2005; Morris et al., 1999; Tamietto & de Gelder, 2010; Vuilleumier et al., 2002; Whalen et al., 1998; Williams & Mattingley, 2004). Of note, this property is not unique to emotional stimuli; nonemotional stimuli can also be processed without awareness (e.g., Dehaene et al., 1998; Kouider & Dehaene, 2007). However, on the other hand, task demands can strongly modulate amygdala activity (e.g., Erk, Abler, & Walter, 2006; Ferri, Schmidt, Hajcak, & Canli, 2013; also see section on Emotion Regulation) and when a task is difficult enough, attention to emotional distracters may be completely abolished (e.g., Pessoa, McKenna, Gutierrez, & Ungerleider, 2002). Thus, while emotional stimuli *can* be processed without voluntary attention (e.g., Phaf & Kan, 2007), highly demanding tasks appear to be able to completely attenuate neural response to these stimuli in both the amygdala and sensory cortices (despite these stimuli being clearly visible in the stimulus presentation; Pessoa, 2005; Pourtois et al., 2013).

After capturing attention, a stimulus gains entry into WM (or short-term memory; Smith & Jonides, 1999). WM is typically distinguished from long-term memory in that it is thought of as storing an immediately accessible but limited amount of information for a shorter time and is likely facilitated by different neurobiological mechanisms. Importantly, WM interacts with long-term memory in several ways. First, WM is likely the "gateway" to long-term memory, in that any information that enters long-term memory must first be held in WM. Second, information from long-term memory can be held in WM; thus, WM likely plays a critical role in memory retrieval.

In recent years, a number of neuroimaging studies have attempted to elucidate the neurobiological correlates of WM. In a meta-analysis of 189 WM studies, Rottschy and colleagues (2012) reported a "core" set of neural regions that activated across a variety of WM tasks, contrasts and task phases (i.e., encoding, maintenance, recall). These regions included the inferior frontal gyrus (IFG), anterior insula, IPS, and (pre-)supplementary motor area (SMA). Significantly, these findings were similar to results observed in previous meta-analyses (Owen, McMillan, Laird, & Bullmore, 2005; Wager & Smith, 2003). However, because these brain regions have been implicated in a number of other tasks—e.g., motor tasks involving orientation (Marangon, Jacobs, & Frey, 2011) and movement planning (Bortoletto & Cunnington, 2010); tasks involving switching (Wager, Jonides, & Reading, 2004) and response inhibition (Nee, Wager, & Jonides, 2007)—it seems unlikely that these brain regions are specific to WM (or indeed, to any particular psychological function). Instead, they might represent even more fundamental aspects of cognition implicated in a number of higher order processes (Rottschy et al., 2012).

Only a few neuroimaging studies have investigated emotion's effects on WM. In one study, Waugh and colleagues (Waugh, Lemus, & Gotlib, 2014) examined the neural regions activated when participants deliberately maintained an affective state in memory. Participants performed two tasks, each of which involved viewing sequentially presented pairs of pleasant, neutral or unpleasant IAPS pictures. In one task, participants were required to maintain the emotion elicited by the first picture for comparison with that elicited by the second picture. In another task, participants simply rated their emotional response to the second picture. Results showed that maintaining an affective state in WM increased activity in the dmPFC, a region associated with explicit emotion generation (Mechias et al., 2010; Ochsner et al., 2004) as well as in the lPFC, a region implicated in WM maintenance (e.g., Smith & Jonides, 1998). Simply viewing and rating unpleasant pictures resulted in longer lasting activation in the rostral mPFC, a region associated with the generation of primary appraisals of emotional stimuli (Roy, Shohamy, & Wager, 2012; Wager et al., 2009). Therefore, active versus passive maintenance of affect may be differentially represented by dorsal and ventral regions of the mPFC, as well as by regions implicated in the WM maintenance of non-affective information.

Flexible, adaptive behavior requires action monitoring—that is, the constant, effortful monitoring of ongoing actions and outcomes related to these actions as well as adjustments in behavior and learning (see Ridderinkhof, Ullsperger, Crone, & Nieuwenhuis, 2004, for a meta-analysis). While action monitoring can include a number of functions—including response conflict and detection of unfavorable outcomes—here we focus on the neural correlates of error-monitoring.

Work using event-related potentials has identified the error-related negativity (ERN), a negative-going component that peaks approximately 50ms after error commission and is generated in the ACC (Brázdil, Roman, Daniel, & Rektor, 2005; Holroyd, Dien, & Coles, 1998; Miltner et al., 2003). Although the ERN was discovered more than 20 years ago (Falkenstein, Hohnsbein, Hoormann, & Blanke, 1991; Gehring, Coles, Meyer, & Donchin, 1995), there is still considerable controversy over its functional significance. One line of thinking suggests that the ERN signals conflict detection (Yeung, Botvinick, & Cohen, 2004)—for example, between the simultaneous activation of both an erroneous (but prepotent) response and a correct response. Another line of thinking suggests that the ERN is a reinforcement learning signal that indicates that outcomes are worse than expected (Holroyd & Coles, 2002). More recently, Hajcak and Foti (2008) proposed that the ERN might signify the affective response to errors (see also Proudfit, Inzlicht, & Mennin, 2013). First, the ACC is connected to both limbic and prefrontal brain regions and is therefore ideally situated to integrate affective and cognitive information. Second, evidence indicates that the ERN is larger in individuals who are more sensitive to negative information (see Moser, Moran, Schroder, Donnellan, & Yeung, 2013, for a meta-analysis in anxiety) and evidence of increased defensive activation (i.e., eyeblink startle; Lang, Davis, & Öhman, 2000) has been observed following errors as opposed to correct responses (Hajcak & Foti, 2008; Riesel, Weinberg, Moran, & Hajcak, 2013). Therefore, errors appear to elicit an affective, motivational response, which could be reflected in the ERN (but see Moser et al., 2013; Moser, Moran, Schroder, Donnellan, & Yeung, 2014, for an alternative interpretation focused on compensation).

There is evidence that modulation of activity in the ACC is linked to subsequent changes in performance. For instance, trial-level analysis has indicated that larger ERN amplitudes (Gehring, Goss, Coles, Meyer, & Donchin, 1993) and increased ACC activity (Garavan, Ross, Murphy, Roche, & Stein, 2002; Kerns et al., 2004) are related to greater post-error slowing (believed to signal a change in the speed/accuracy trade-off; Botvinick, Braver, Barch, Carter, & Cohen, 2001). In addition, error-*preceding* trials have been found to be characterized by an electrocortical *positivity* occurring in the time window of the ERN (Ridderinkhof, Nieuwenhuis, & Bashore, 2003). This error-preceding positivity is thought to indicate a temporary disengagement of the conflict-monitoring system, which could result in a control adjustment failure and, subsequently, an error (Ridderinkhof et al., 2004).

While the posterior medial frontal cortex has been consistently implicated in action monitoring and has even been linked to subsequent adjustments in performance, the neural mechanisms that implement these performance adjustments are less well-understood. In the studies described, lateral prefrontal cortex (lPFC) activity was increased on trials with the greatest behavioral adjustments post-error and on correct, high-conflict trials (which also tend to be followed by response slowing; Botvinick et al., 2001). In addition, greater mPFC activity on error trials predicted lPFC activity on subsequent trials (Kerns et al., 2004). Therefore, one possibility is that the mPFC functions as a monitor and the lPFC implements subsequent changes in behavior (Botvinick et al., 2001; Ridderinkhof et al., 2004).

Cognitive Appraisal-Reappraisal

Emotion regulation refers to goal-directed changes in the nature, duration, or magnitude of emotional responses, including initiating new emotions (Gross & Thompson, 2007). There are many ways of modulating emotional response, including situation selection, attentional deployment, and cognitive reappraisal (Gross & Thompson, 2007). However, cognitive reappraisal is by far the most commonly studied of these strategies. Cognitive reappraisal involves changing the meaning of emotional stimuli, such as when a person distances himself from the stimulus (e.g., by reminding himself that a gory film is "just a movie") or reinterprets the meaning of the stimulus (e.g., by telling himself that the protagonist in a gory film will likely survive). Cognitive reappraisal is a complex technique relying on a variety of higher order cognitive processes, including those involved in language and WM, and may overlap with other, incidental forms of emotion regulation, such as affect labelling (Burklund, Creswell, Irwin, & Lieberman, 2014; Lieberman et al., 2007; Taylor, Phan, Decker, & Liberzon, 2003). In many studies of reappraisal, appraisal and reappraisal may occur simultaneously, because participants are typically provided with instructions to reappraise an upcoming stimulus (e.g., an unpleasant picture) prior to its presentation.

According to Ochsner and colleagues (2012), cognitive reappraisal begins in the dlPFC and posterior PFC, as well as inferior parietal regions of the brain involved in selective attention and WM. These regions of the brain are thought to be involved in directing attention to stimulus attributes that are most relevant to the reappraisal and in holding reappraisal goals and reappraisal content online. Next, dorsal regions of the ACC are believed to be involved in monitoring the extent to which affect is changing in line with an intended regulation goal. The vlPFC then comes online to help select reappraisals from memory and inhibit initial appraisals of stimuli. Finally, the dmPFC may also be involved in reappraisal, particularly when appraisal of emotional states (self or others') is involved.

In terms of reappraisal's effects on neural measures of emotion processing, reductions in amygdala activity have been observed more consistently than in any other region (Buhle et al., 2013). However, it is worth noting that most studies of reappraisal have used negative stimuli, which may be more likely to activate the amygdala than positive stimuli (e.g., Calder et al., 2001; Phan, Wager, Taylor, & Liberzon, 2002). Additionally, visual stimuli tend to be the stimuli of choice in most emotion regulation studies, which—given extensive connections between the amygdala and the visual system—may contribute to the preponderance of amygdala findings. Finally, evidence of amygdala deactivation during reappraisal is likely due at least in part to targeting of this area as a region of interest in many studies (Buhle et al., 2013).

Just over a decade ago, the first fMRI studies of emotion regulation were performed. At that time, having no prior work to draw upon, researchers hypothesized that the modulation of affect via emotion regulation would involve the same cognitive control systems implicated in the control of nonemotional processes such as memory, attention, and other types of thoughts (Ochsner, Bunge, Gross, & Gabrieli, 2002). This initial hypothesis has, for the most part, turned out to be correct (Ochsner et al., 2012). However, despite relative clarity on the neural regions involved in cognitive reappraisal, there has been less consensus about the neural pathways underlying emotion regulation.

How do lateral frontal regions, which are not well connected to the amygdala anatomically—exert their effects on subcortical regions? There are at least two possible pathways. First, frontal regions that *are* well-connected to the amygdala—such as the vmPFC—might mediate the effects of more lateral frontal regions, such as the vlPFC, to modulate activity in the amygdala/striatum (Diekhof, Geier, Falkai, & Gruber, 2011; Etkin et al., 2011). Second, prefrontal regions might modulate activity in the amygdala/striatum via lateral temporal regions of the brain implicated in visual perception and semantic processing; the amygdala might then "see" and respond to the imagined/reappraised stimulus (Ochsner et al., 2012).

The first possibility has received some support. For example, work by Banks, Eddy, Angstadt, Nathan, and Phan (2007) found that activation of the dlPFC, dmPFC, ACC, and OFC covaried with amygdala activity during reappraisal and, moreover, that the strength of amygdala coupling with the OFC and dmPFC predicted the degree to which reappraisal was successful in reducing negative affect. Additionally, two studies (Johnstone, Reekum, Urry, Kalin, & Davidson, 2007; Urry et al., 2006) found that although reappraisal of negative pictures did not reduce amygdala activity, vmPFC activity was negatively correlated with amygdala activity during the task. Moreover, results showed that the vmPFC mediated activity between the left vlPFC or left dmPFC and the amygdala, such that activity in the vmPFC was positively related to activity in the left vlPFC or left dmPFC, and negatively related to activity in the amygdala. Therefore, regions of the prefrontal cortex such as the OFC and the vmPFC—a region implicated in extinction and reversal learning (Milad, Wright, et al., 2007; Schiller & Delgado, 2010; Schiller, Levy, Niv, LeDoux, & Phelps, 2008)—might mediate lateral prefrontal-subcortical connections during reappraisal.

On the other hand, recent meta-analytic work supports the second possibility. Buhle and colleagues (2013) conducted a meta-analysis of 48 studies of reappraisal including studies of both down- and upregulation, as well as both negative and positive stimuli. In line with prior work, results showed that reappraisal activates a number of neural regions implicated in cognitive control, including the posterior dmPFC, bilateral dlPFC, vlPFC, and posterior parietal cortex. In addition, downregulation of emotional response was found to reduce activation in the amygdala and ventral striatum. However, Buhle and colleagues found no evidence that the vmPFC plays a crucial role in reappraisal (also see Kalisch, 2009; but see Diekhof et al., 2011), contradicting the notion that the vmPFC might play an intermediary role between lateral prefrontal regions and the amygdala/striatum during reappraisal. Instead, because Buhle and colleagues observed reappraisal-related modulation of a large region in the left, posterior temporal cortex, Buhle and colleagues suggest a key role for the temporal lobe in reappraisal. The temporal lobe is involved in semantic (Olson, Plotzker, & Ezzyat, 2007) and perceptual (Allison, Puce, & McCarthy, 2000; Wheaton, Thompson, Syngeniotis, Abbott, & Puce, 2004) judgment; therefore, its activation during reappraisal could reflect semantic and perceptual changes to stimulus representation, which could lead to modulation of amygdala/striatum activity.

In sum, there is fairly clear evidence that emotion regulation involves increased activation of domain-general cognitive control regions and, in many studies, modulation of amygdala activity (but see Johnstone et al., 2007; Phan et al., 2005; Urry et al., 2006, for studies that have not found amygdala modulation). However, understanding the pathway(s) by which activation of lateral frontal regions leads to changes of activity in subcortical regions during emotion regulation will require further work.

■ TOWARD UNDERSTANDING AT THE NEUROCIRCUIT LEVEL

At the beginning of this chapter, we alluded to a paradigm shift that is now emerging within cognitive affective neuroscience: what began with function-region mapping is now headed toward understanding at the neural systems level, in which emphasis is increasingly being placed on the interaction of diverse neural regions distributed across the brain. This shift has been spearheaded in part by recent conceptual and methodological developments (Menon, 2011), including the revelation that the human brain is inherently organized into distinct functional networks (e.g., Bressler & Menon, 2010); the discovery of task-positive and task-negative networks in the brain (Fox et al., 2005; Greicius & Menon, 2004; Honey, Kötter, Breakspear, & Sporns, 2007); the identification of the DMN (Qin & Northoff, 2011; Raichle et al., 2001); the discovery of the salience network and frontoparietal interactions that underlie attention and cognitive control (Chen et al., 2013; Seeley et al., 2007; Sridharan et al., 2008); graph-theory techniques, which have become important in understanding whole-brain architecture (Minati, Varotto, D'Incerti, Panzica, & Chan, 2013; Sporns, 2011); and finally increased knowledge of how development affects information-processing biases in the brain (Fan et al., 2011; Hwang, Hallquist, & Luna, 2013; Vogel, Power, Petersen, & Schlaggar, 2010).

A neurocircuit approach encompasses the idea that neural networks are comprised of "nodes" (regions) and "edges" (connections; Sporns, 2011). Dysfunction (e.g., in the case of psychopathology) is believed to arise from abnormalities within these nodes and/or edges—either of which may propagate to the entire network or to subnetwork(s) within the broader network (Menon, 2011). Neural networks can be assessed by measuring structural (e.g., diffusion tensor imaging) and/or functional connectivity (e.g., fMRI). Next we give examples of studies that have taken a neurocircuit approach by measuring functional or effective connectivity during fMRI studies of cognitive and affective processing.

In one study, Kanske and Kotz (2011a, 2011b) set out to determine whether emotional stimuli can facilitate conflict resolution and how this takes place at the neurocircuit level. To do so, they used a conflict resolution task that involved the presentation of emotional stimuli. Results showed that the dACC activated in response to conflict and the amygdala activated in response to emotional stimuli; however, the vACC activated specifically when conflict and emotion coincided. Moreover, emotion reduced reaction times and increased functional connectivity between the vACC, the amygdala, and the dACC. Therefore, the results suggest that the vACC is central to emotional conflict resolution and that it might facilitate this process by boosting the dACC while downregulating amygdala activity (Kanske & Kotz, 2011b; see also Etkin, Egner, Peraza, Kandel, & Hirsch, 2006).

In another study, Ichikawa and colleagues (2011) used effective connectivity analysis (which permits interrogation of *directional* effects) to examine the neurocircuitry of emotion and action monitoring. Building on the idea that errors are perceived as aversive, Ichikawa and colleagues asked participants to either increase or decrease their affective response to errors made on a cognitive (continuous performance) task or to respond naturally to their errors. Results showed that greater negative affective response to errors was associated with reduced task performance but only when participants were asked to respond naturally to their errors (not when they were asked to regulate their affective response). In addition, the neuroimaging results revealed that a region extending from the dACC to the SMA (involved in response inhibition) was associated with error processing, while the rostral ACC (rACC)/mPFC was associated with error prevention (as defined by conjunction analysis). Trial-by-trial analysis revealed that emotion regulation modulated connectivity between the rostral and dorsal ACC. That is, during regulation of the affective response to errors, greater earlier rACC/mPFC activation during error prevention/regulation was found to reduce activity in the SMA, which in turn led to greater rACC/mPFC regulatory activity on the subsequent trial. Therefore, cingulate activity and connectivity predicted error commission, and—more broadly—emotion appeared to affect error commission, even on an ostensibly neutral/cognitive task.

In addition to task-based functional and effective connectivity, we note that non-task-based approaches provide essential and complementary methods for investigating neurocircuit level function and dysfunction. Such approaches (e.g., Anticevic et al., 2014; Cole, Anticevic, Repovs, & Barch, 2011) may be particularly important when, for instance, certain forms of psychopathology impose limits on the utility of task-based analysis (e.g., when ceiling or floor effects are observed) or when individual or temporal variation in task performance makes it difficult to adjust task difficulty to an appropriate level (Menon, 2011).

■ CONCLUSION

Over the past century, neuroscience research has generated continuously evolving views of how emotion and cognition are represented and instantiated in the brain. In the past two decades, however, this research has begun to suggest that the traditional view of emotion and cognition as inhabiting separate realms in the brain—which has facilitated substantial progress in understanding specific features of behavior to-date—may nevertheless be inaccurate (Pessoa, 2013). Evidence in support of a more integrated relationship between emotion and cognition in the brain has come from both structural and functional neuroscientific work. For instance, the amygdala has long been thought of as occupying a highly specialized niche as the "fear center" of the brain. However, one of the most defining features of the amygdala is its extensive array of connections to virtually all areas of the cortex (i.e., all but eight areas; Young, Scannell, Burns, & Blakemore, 1994; see also Barbas, 1995; Swanson, 2003). Moreover, its connectivity to other, more "provincial" regions of the brain that are central to additional, functionally specialized networks (Pessoa, 2008) demarcates the amygdala as a "connector" hub (Guimerà & Nunes Amaral, 2005), ideally situated for the integration of cognition and emotion (Pessoa, 2010). In other words, the widespread connectivity of the amygdala with diverse regions of the brain makes it unlikely that it is charged with such a narrow functional role (Amaral & Price, 1984). The amygdala—despite its reputation—may actually play a central and varied role in both cognitive and affective brain functions.

Understanding of the anatomy of the PFC has also progressed considerably over the past two decades. Some of this work has refined understanding of the close relationships between the PFC and bodily functions (e.g., Bechara, Damasio, & Damasio, 2000). For instance, it is now known that significant regions of the PFC are connected to brain stem nuclei that are charged with controlling autonomic and endocrine function essential to the maintenance of bodily homeostasis (Pessoa, 2010). Likewise, the PFC is known to be intricately connected to the cingulate, orbitofrontal, and insular cortices, as well as to the amygdala—regions that play key roles in emotion processing. Therefore, knowledge of *vertical* as well as *horizontal* (e.g., prefrontal-parietal) interactions in the frontal cortex may be important in furthering understanding of PFC function (Pessoa, 2010).

Functional studies have also highlighted the extent to which emotion and cognition are integrated in the brain. For instance, the anterior insula is commonly associated with emotion and interoception (e.g., Paulus & Stein, 2006) yet appears to be recruited in most cognitive tasks (Van Snellenberg & Wager, 2009; see also Chang et al., 2013). Likewise, the amygdala has been implicated in cognitive processes such as attention and decision-making, even in rodents (Floresco, Onge, Ghods-Sharifi, & Winstanley, 2008; Holland & Gallagher, 1999). A recent study in humans found that participants with greater amygdala activation showed faster reaction times on a WM task—despite the fact that stimuli used in this study were nonemotional (Schaefer et al., 2006). Finally, contrasting aversively conditioned cues (CS+) with neutral cues (CS−) activates multiple regions in the frontal cortex, including the IFG, ACC, middle frontal gyrus, and anterior insula (Pessoa, 2009), underlining the extent to which affective and nonaffective processes share common neural and attentional resources.

Going forward, it is likely that both basic and clinical research will be called upon to go beyond basic descriptions of emotion-cognition interactions (which have traditionally been described as being mutually antagonistic) in order to begin to characterize how these systems are *integrated* at a systems level in the brain (Pessoa, 2010, 2013). In so doing, a more accurate and complete description of how emotion and cognition jointly contribute to the control of mental processes and behavior may be achieved.

■ REFERENCES

Adolphs, R., Tranel, D., Damasio, H., & Damasio, A. (1994). Impaired recognition of emotion in facial expressions following bilateral damage to the human amygdala. *Nature*, 372(6507), 669–672. doi:10.1038/372669a0

Adolphs, R., Tranel, D., Damasio, H., & Damasio, A. R. (1995). Fear and the human amygdala. *J Neurosci*, 15(9), 5879–5891.

Allison, T., Puce, A., & McCarthy, G. (2000). Social perception from visual cues: role of the STS region. *Trends Cogn Sci*, 4(7), 267–278. doi:10.1016/S1364-6613(00)01501-1

Amaral, D. G. (2002). The primate amygdala and the neurobiology of social behavior: implications for understanding social anxiety. *Biol Psychiatry*, *51*(1), 11–17.

Amaral, D. G., Behniea, H., & Kelly, J. L. (2003). Topographic organization of projections from the amygdala to the visual cortex in the macaque monkey. *Neuroscience*, *118*, 1099–1120.

Amaral, D. G., & Lavenex, P. (2007). Hippocampal Neuroanatomy. In P. Anderson, R. Morris, D. Amaral, T. Bliss, & J. O'Keefe (Eds.), *The hippocampus book* (pp. 37–114). New York: Oxford University Press.

Amaral, D. G., & Price, J. L. (1984). Amygdalo-cortical projections in the monkey (Macaca fascicularis). *J Comp Neurol*, *230*, 465–496.

Anagnostaras, S. G., Maren, S., & Fanselow, M. S. (1999). Temporally graded retrograde amnesia of contextual fear after hippocampal damage in rats: within-subjects examination. *J Neurosci*, *19*(3), 1106–1114.

Anderson, A. K., & Phelps, E. A. (2001). Lesions of the human amygdala impair enhanced perception of emotionally salient events. *Nature*, *411*(6835), 305–309. doi:10.1038/35077083

Anderson, E., Siegel, E. H., Bliss-Moreau, E., & Barrett, L. F. (2011). The visual impact of gossip. *Science*, *332*(6036), 1446–1448. doi:10.1126/science.1201574

Anticevic, A., Hu, S., Zhang, S., Savic, A., Billingslea, E., Wasylink, S., . . . Pittenger, C. (2014). Global resting-state functional magnetic resonance imaging analysis identifies frontal cortex, striatal, and cerebellar dysconnectivity in obsessive-compulsive disorder. *Biol Psychiatry*, *75*(8), 595–605. doi:10.1016/j.biopsych.2013.10.021

Augustine, J. R. (1996). Circuitry and functional aspects of the insular lobe in primates including humans. *Brain Res Rev*, *22*(3), 229–244.

Baars, B. J., & Gage, N. M. (2013). *Fundamentals of cognitive neuroscience: a beginner's guide*. New York: Academic Press.

Banks, S. J., Eddy, K. T., Angstadt, M., Nathan, P. J., & Phan, K. L. (2007). Amygdala–frontal connectivity during emotion regulation. *Soc Cogn Affect Neurosci*, *2*(4), 303–312. doi:10.1093/scan/nsm029

Barbas, H. (1995). Anatomic basis of cognitive-emotional interactions in the primate prefrontal cortex. *Neurosci Biobehav Rev*, *19*(3), 499–510. doi:10.1016/0149-7634(94)00053-4

Barkley, R. A. (2012). Problems with the concept of executive functioning. In *Executive functions: what they are, how they work, and why they evolved* (pp. 1–36). New York: Guilford Press.

Barrett, L. F., & Bar, M. (2009). See it with feeling: affective predictions during object perception. *Philos Trans R Soc Lond B Biol Sci*, *364*(1521), 1325–1334. doi:10.1098/rstb.2008.0312

Baxter, M. G., & Murray, E. A. (2002). The amygdala and reward. *Nat Rev Neurosci*, *3*(7), 563–573. doi:10.1038/nrn875

Bechara, A., Damasio, H., & Damasio, A. R. (2000). Emotion, decision making and the orbitofrontal cortex. *Cereb Cortex*, *10*, 295.

Bechara, A., Tranel, D., & Damasio, H. (2000). Characterization of the decision-making deficit of patients with ventromedial prefrontal cortex lesions. *Brain*, *123*(11), 2189–2202. doi:10.1093/brain/123.11.2189

Beer, J. S., John, O. P., Scabini, D., & Knight, R. T. (2006). Orbitofrontal cortex and social behavior: integrating self-monitoring and emotion-cognition interactions. *J Cogn Neurosci*, *18*(6), 871–879. doi:10.1162/jocn.2006.18.6.871

Behrmann, M. (2004). Parietal cortex and attention. *Curr Opin Neurobiol*, *14*(2), 212–217. doi:10.1016/j.conb.2004.03.012

Benuzzi, F., Meletti, S., Zamboni, G., Calandra-Buonaura, G., Serafini, M., Lui, F., . . . Nichelli, P. (2004). Impaired fear processing in right mesial temporal sclerosis: a fMRI study. *Brain Res Bull, 63*(4), 269–281. doi:10.1016/j.brainresbull.2004.03.005

Bermudez-Rattoni, F., Introini-Collison, I. B., & McGaugh, J. L. (1991). Reversible inactivation of the insular cortex by tetrodotoxin produces retrograde and anterograde amnesia for inhibitory avoidance and spatial learning. *Proc Natl Acad Sci U S A, 88*(12), 5379–5382. doi:10.1073/pnas.88.12.5379

Bortoletto, M., & Cunnington, R. (2010). Motor timing and motor sequencing contribute differently to the preparation for voluntary movement. *NeuroImage, 49*(4), 3338–3348. doi:10.1016/j.neuroimage.2009.11.048

Botvinick, M. M., Braver, T. S., Barch, D. M., Carter, C. S., & Cohen, J. D. (2001). Conflict monitoring and cognitive control. *Psychol Rev, 108*(3), 624–652. doi:10.1037/0033-295X.108.3.624

Botvinick, M. M., Cohen, J. D., & Carter, C. S. (2004). Conflict monitoring and anterior cingulate cortex: an update. *Trends Cogn Sci, 8*(12), 539–546. doi:10.1016/j.tics.2004.10.003

Bouton, M. E. (2002). Context, ambiguity, and unlearning: sources of relapse after behavioral extinction. *Biol Psychiatry, 52*(10), 976–986.

Bouton, M. E., & Bolles, R. C. (1979). Contextual control of the extinction of conditioned fear. *Learn Motiv, 10*(4), 445–466. doi:10.1016/0023-9690(79)90057-2

Bouton, M. E., & Ricker, S. T. (1994). Renewal of extinguished responding in a second context. *Anim Learn Behav, 22*(3), 317–324. doi:10.3758/BF03209840

Bouton, M. E., Westbrook, R. F., Corcoran, K. A., & Maren, S. (2006). Contextual and temporal modulation of extinction: behavioral and biological mechanisms. *Biol Psychiatry, 60*(4), 352–360. doi:10.1016/j.biopsych.2005.12.015

Bradley, M. M., Sabatinelli, D., Lang, P. J., Fitzsimmons, J. R., King, W., & Desai, P. (2003). Activation of the visual cortex in motivated attention. *Behav Neurosci, 117*(2), 369–380. doi:http://dx.doi.org/10.1037/0735-7044.117.2.369

Brázdil, M., Roman, R., Daniel, P., & Rektor, I. (2005). Intracerebral error-related negativity in a simple go/nogo task. *J Psychophysiol, 19*(4), 244–255. doi:10.1027/0269-8803.19.4.244

Breiter, H. C., Etcoff, N. L., Whalen, P. J., Kennedy, W. A., Rauch, S. L., Buckner, R. L., . . . Rosen, B. R. (1996). Response and habituation of the human amygdala during visual processing of facial expression. *Neuron, 17*(5), 875–887. doi:10.1016/S0896-6273(00)80219-6

Bressler, S. L., & Menon, V. (2010). Large-scale brain networks in cognition: emerging methods and principles. *Trends Cogn Sci, 14*(6), 277–290. doi:10.1016/j.tics.2010.04.004

Bressler, S. L., Tang, W., Sylvester, C. M., Shulman, G. L., & Corbetta, M. (2008). Top-down control of human visual cortex by frontal and parietal cortex in anticipatory visual spatial attention. *J Neurosci, 28*(40), 10056–10061. doi:10.1523/JNEUROSCI.1776-08.2008

Britton, J. C., Phan, K. L., Taylor, S. F., Welsh, R. C., Berridge, K. C., & Liberzon, I. (2006). Neural correlates of social and nonsocial emotions: an fMRI study. *NeuroImage, 31*(1), 397–409. doi:10.1016/j.neuroimage.2005.11.027

Britton, J. C., Taylor, S. F., Sudheimer, K. D., & Liberzon, I. (2006). Facial expressions and complex IAPS pictures: common and differential networks. *NeuroImage, 31*(2), 906–919. doi:10.1016/j.neuroimage.2005.12.050

Brosch, T., Pourtois, G., Sander, D., & Vuilleumier, P. (2011). Additive effects of emotional, endogenous, and exogenous attention: behavioral and electrophysiological evidence. *Neuropsychologia, 49*(7), 1779–1787. doi:10.1016/j.neuropsychologia.2011.02.056

Buhle, J. T., Silvers, J. A., Wager, T. D., Lopez, R., Onyemekwu, C., Kober, H., . . . Ochsner, K. N. (2013). Cognitive reappraisal of emotion: a meta-analysis of human neuroimaging studies. *Cereb Cortex*, bht154. doi:10.1093/cercor/bht154

Burgess, N., Maguire, E. A., & O'Keefe, J. (2002). The human hippocampus and spatial and episodic memory. *Neuron, 35*(4), 625–641. doi:10.1016/S0896-6273(02)00830-9

Burklund, L. J., Creswell, J. D., Irwin, M. R., & Lieberman, M. D. (2014). The common and distinct neural bases of affect labeling and reappraisal in healthy adults. *Front Psychol, 5,* 221. doi:10.3389/fpsyg.2014.00221

Bush, Luu, & Posner. (2000). Cognitive and emotional influences in anterior cingulate cortex. *Trends Cogn Sci, 4*(6), 215–222.

Cabeza, R., & Nyberg, L. (2000). Imaging cognition II: an empirical review of 275 PET and fMRI studies. *J Cogn Neurosci, 12*(1), 1–47. doi:10.1162/08989290051137585

Calder, A. J., Lawrence, A. D., & Young, A. W. (2001). Neuropsychology of fear and loathing. *Nature Rev Neurosci, 2*(5), 352–363.

Carretié, L., Hinojosa, J. A., Mercado, F., & Tapia, M. (2005). Cortical response to subjectively unconscious danger. *NeuroImage, 24*(3), 615–623. doi:10.1016/j.neuroimage.2004.09.009

Catani, M., Jones, D. K., Donato, R., & Ffytche, D. H. (2003). Occipito-temporal connections in the human. *Brain, 126*(9), 2093–2107. doi:10.1093/brain/awg203

Chakravarthy, V., Joseph, D., & Bapi, R. (2010). What do the basal ganglia do? A modeling perspective. *Biol Cybern, 103*(3), 237–253. doi:10.1007/s00422-010-0401-y

Chang, L. J., Yarkoni, T., Khaw, M. W., & Sanfey, A. G. (2013). Decoding the role of the insula in human cognition: functional parcellation and large-scale reverse inference. *Cereb Cortex, 23*(3), 739–749. doi:10.1093/cercor/bhs065

Chao, L. L., Haxby, J. V., & Martin, A. (1999). Attribute-based neural substrates in temporal cortex for perceiving and knowing about objects. *Nature Neurosci, 2*(10), 913–919. doi:10.1038/13217

Chen, A. C., Oathes, D. J., Chang, C., Bradley, T., Zhou, Z.-W., Williams, L. M., . . . Etkin, A. (2013). Causal interactions between fronto-parietal central executive and default-mode networks in humans. *Proc Natl Acad Sci U S A, 110*(49), 19944–19949.

Cole, M. W., Anticevic, A., Repovs, G., & Barch, D. (2011). Variable global dysconnectivity and individual differences in schizophrenia. *Biol Psychiatry, 70*(1), 43–50. doi:10.1016/j.biopsych.2011.02.010

Corbetta, M., Patel, G., & Shulman, G. L. (2008). The reorienting system of the human brain: from environment to theory of mind. *Neuron, 58*(3), 306–324. doi:10.1016/j.neuron.2008.04.017

Corbetta, M., & Shulman, G. L. (2002). Control of goal-directed and stimulus-driven attention in the brain. *Nature Rev Neurosci, 3*(3), 201–215. doi:10.1038/nrn755

Corcoran, K. A., Desmond, T. J., Frey, K. A., & Maren, S. (2005). Hippocampal inactivation disrupts the acquisition and contextual encoding of fear extinction. *J Neurosci, 25*(39), 8978–8987. doi:10.1523/JNEUROSCI.2246-05.2005

Costafreda, S. G., Brammer, M. J., David, A. S., & Fu, C. H. Y. (2008). Predictors of amygdala activation during the processing of emotional stimuli: a meta-analysis of 385 PET and fMRI studies. *Brain Res Rev, 58*(1), 57–70. doi:10.1016/j.brainresrev.2007.10.012

Craig, A. D. (2002). How do you feel? Interoception: the sense of the physiological condition of the body. *Nature Rev Neurosci, 3*(8), 655–666.

Critchley, H. D., Wiens, S., Rotshtein, P., Öhman, A., & Dolan, R. J. (2004). Neural systems supporting interoceptive awareness. *Nature Neurosci, 7*(2), 189–195. doi:10.1038/nn1176

Damaraju, E., Huang, Y.-M., Barrett, L. F., & Pessoa, L. (2009). Affective learning enhances activity and functional connectivity in early visual cortex. *Neuropsychologia, 47*(12), 2480–2487. doi:10.1016/j.neuropsychologia.2009.04.023

Damasio, A. R., Everitt, B. J., & Bishop, D. (1996). The somatic marker hypothesis and the possible functions of the prefrontal cortex [and discussion]. *Philos Trans R Soc Lond B Biol Sci, 351*(1346), 1413–1420.

Davis, M. (2011). NMDA receptors and fear extinction: implications for cognitive behavioral therapy. *Dialogues Clin Neurosci, 13*(4), 463–474.

Decety, J., & Jackson, P. L. (2004). The functional architecture of human empathy. *Behav Cogn Neurosci Rev, 3*(2), 71–100. doi:10.1177/1534582304267187

Dehaene, S., Naccache, L., Le Clec'H, G., Koechlin, E., Mueller, M., Dehaene-Lambertz, G., van de Moortele, P. F., & Le Bihan, D. (1998). Imaging unconscious semantic priming. *Nature, 395*(6702), 597–600. PMID: 9783584.

Diekhof, E. K., Geier, K., Falkai, P., & Gruber, O. (2011). Fear is only as deep as the mind allows: a coordinate-based meta-analysis of neuroimaging studies on the regulation of negative affect. *NeuroImage, 58*(1), 275–285. doi:10.1016/j.neuroimage.2011.05.073

Dolcos, F., Iordan, A. D., & Dolcos, S. (2011). Neural correlates of emotion-cognition interactions: a review of evidence from brain imaging investigations. *J Cogn Psychol, 23*(6), 669–694. doi:10.1080/20445911.2011.594433

Dosenbach, N. U. F., Fair, D. A., Cohen, A. L., Schlaggar, B. L., & Petersen, S. E. (2008). A dual-networks architecture of top-down control. *Trends Cogn Sci, 12*(3), 99–105. doi:10.1016/j.tics.2008.01.001

Dosenbach, N. U. F., Fair, D. A., Miezin, F. M., Cohen, A. L., Wenger, K. K., Dosenbach, R. A. T., . . . Petersen, S. E. (2007). Distinct brain networks for adaptive and stable task control in humans. *Proc Natl Acad Sci U S A, 104*(26), 11073–11078. doi:10.1073/pnas.0704320104

Downar, J., Crawley, A. P., Mikulis, D. J., & Davis, K. D. (2000). A multimodal cortical network for the detection of changes in the sensory environment. *Nature Neurosci, 3*(3), 277–283. doi:10.1038/72991

Duncan, S., & Barrett, L. F. (2007). The role of the amygdala in visual awareness. *Trends Cogn Sci, 11*(5), 190–192. doi:10.1016/j.tics.2007.01.007

Duvernoy, H. M., Cattin, F., & Risold, P.-Y. (2013). *The human hippocampus: functional anatomy, vascularization and serial sections with MRI.* New York: Springer Science & Business.

Eichenbaum, H. (2000). Hippocampus: mapping or memory? *Curr Biol, 10*(21), R785–R787. doi:10.1016/S0960-9822(00)00763-6

Eichenbaum, H. (2004). Hippocampus: cognitive processes and neural representations that underlie declarative memory. *Neuron, 44*(1), 109–120. doi:10.1016/j.neuron.2004.08.028

Eichenbaum, H. (2012). Handbook of psychology, behavioral neuroscience. In I. B. Weiner, R. J. Nelson, & S. Mizumori (Eds.), *Memory systems* (pp. 551–573). New York: Wiley.

Erk, S., Abler, B., & Walter, H. (2006). Cognitive modulation of emotion anticipation. *Eur J Neurosci, 24*, 1227–1236.

Eslinger, P. J., & Damasio, A. R. (1985). Severe disturbance of higher cognition after bilateral frontal lobe ablation patient EVR. *Neurology, 35*(12), 1731–1741. doi:10.1212/WNL.35.12.1731

Etkin, A., Egner, T., & Kalisch, R. (2011). Emotional processing in anterior cingulate and medial prefrontal cortex. *Trends Cogn Sci, 15*(2), 85–93. doi:10.1016/j.tics.2010.11.004

Etkin, A., Egner, T., Peraza, D. M., Kandel, E. R., & Hirsch, J. (2006). Resolving emotional conflict: a role for the rostral anterior cingulate cortex in modulating activity in the amygdala. *Neuron, 51*(6), 871–882. doi:10.1016/j.neuron.2006.07.029

Etkin, A., & Wager, T. D. (2007). Functional neuroimaging of anxiety: a meta-analysis of emotional processing in PTSD, social anxiety disorder, and specific phobia. *Am J Psychiatry, 164*(10), 1476–1488. doi:10.1176/appi.ajp.2007.07030504

Everitt, B. J., Parkinson, J. A., Olmstead, M. C., Arroyo, M., Robledo, P., & Robbins, T. W. (1999). Associative processes in addiction and reward the role of amygdala-ventral

striatal subsystems. *Ann N Y Acad Sci, 877*(1), 412–438. doi:10.1111/j.1749-6632.1999.
tb09280.x

Falkenstein, M., Hohnsbein, J., Hoormann, J., & Blanke, L. (1991). Effects of crossmodal
divided attention on late ERP components. II. Error processing in choice reaction tasks. *Electroencephalogr Clin Neurophysiol, 78*(6), 447–455. doi:10.1016/
0013-4694(91)90062-9

Falls, W. A., Miserendino, M. J., & Davis, M. (1992). Extinction of fear-potentiated
startle: blockade by infusion of an NMDA antagonist into the amygdala. *J Neurosci,
12*(3), 854–863.

Fan, Y., Shi, F., Smith, J. K., Lin, W., Gilmore, J. H., & Shen, D. (2011). Brain anatomical networks in early human brain development. *NeuroImage, 54*(3), 1862–1871.
doi:10.1016/j.neuroimage.2010.07.025

Fellows, L. K., & Farah, M. J. (2003). Ventromedial frontal cortex mediates affective shifting
in humans: evidence from a reversal learning paradigm. *Brain, 126*(8), 1830–1837.
doi:10.1093/brain/awg180

Ferri, J., Schmidt, J., Hajcak, G., & Canli, T. (2013). Neural correlates of attentional deployment within unpleasant pictures. *NeuroImage, 70*, 268–277. doi:10.1016/
j.neuroimage.2012.12.030

Fitzgerald, D. A., Angstadt, M., Jelsone, L. M., Nathan, P. J., & Phan, K. L. (2006). Beyond
threat: amygdala reactivity across multiple expressions of facial affect. *NeuroImage,
30*(4), 1441–1448. doi:10.1016/j.neuroimage.2005.11.003

Floresco, S. B., Onge, J. R. S., Ghods-Sharifi, S., & Winstanley, C. A. (2008). Cortico-limbic-
striatal circuits subserving different forms of cost-benefit decision making. *Cogn Affect
Behav Neurosci, 8*(4), 375–389. doi:10.3758/CABN.8.4.375

Fox, E. (2002). Processing emotional facial expressions: the role of anxiety and awareness. *Cogn Affect Behav Neurosci, 2*(1), 52–63. doi:10.3758/CABN.2.1.52

Fox, M. D., Corbetta, M., Snyder, A. Z., Vincent, J. L., & Raichle, M. E. (2006). Spontaneous
neuronal activity distinguishes human dorsal and ventral attention systems. *Proc Natl
Acad Sci U S A, 103*(26), 10046–10051. doi:10.1073/pnas.0604187103

Fox, M. D., Snyder, A. Z., Vincent, J. L., Corbetta, M., Essen, D. C. V., & Raichle, M. E. (2005).
The human brain is intrinsically organized into dynamic, anticorrelated functional
networks. *Proc Natl Acad Sci U S A, 102*(27), 9673–9678. doi:10.1073/pnas.0504136102

Frijda, N. H. (1987). Emotion, cognitive structure, and action tendency. *Cogn Emot, 1*,
115–143.

Fuster, J. M. (2008). Anatomy of the prefrontal cortex. In *The prefrontal cortex* (4th ed., pp.
7–58). London: Elsevier.

Fuster, J. M., Stuss, D. T., & Knight, R. T. (2013). Cognitive functions of the prefrontal cortex.
In *Principles of frontal lobe function* (pp. 11–22). New York: Oxford University Press.

Garavan, H., Ross, T. J., Murphy, K., Roche, R. A. P., & Stein, E. A. (2002). Dissociable executive functions in the dynamic control of behavior: inhibition, error detection, and
correction. *NeuroImage, 17*, 1820–1829.

Gazzaniga, M. S. (2010). *The Cognitive Neurosciences*. Cambridge: MIT Press (4th ed., pp.
91–108).

Gazzaniga, M., Ivry, R. B., & Mangun, G. R. (2013). *Cognitive neuroscience: the biology of the
mind* (4th ed.). New York: W. W. Norton.

Gehring, W. J., Coles, M. G. H., Meyer, D. E., & Donchin, E. (1995). A brain potential manifestation of error-related processing. *Electroencephalogr Clin Neurophysiol Suppl, S44*,
261–272.

Gehring, W. J., & Fencsik, D. E. (2001). Functions of the medial frontal cortex in the processing of conflict and errors. *J Neurosci, 21*(23), 9430–9437.

Gehring, W. J., Goss, B., Coles, M. G. H., Meyer, D. E., & Donchin, E. (1993). A neural system for error detection and compensation. *Psychol Sci, 4*(6), 385–390. doi:10.1111/j.1467-9280.1993.tb00586.x

Geng, J. J., & Mangun, G. R. (2011). Right temporoparietal junction activation by a salient contextual cue facilitates target discrimination. *NeuroImage, 54*(1), 594–601. doi:10.1016/j.neuroimage.2010.08.025

Gold, P. E., Hankins, L., Edwards, R. M., Chester, J., & McGaugh, J. L. (1975). Memory interference and facilitation with posttrial amygdala stimulation: effect on memory varies with footshock level. *Brain Res, 86*(3), 509–513.

Grabowska, A., Marchewka, A., Seniów, J., Polanowska, K., Jednoróg, K., Królicki, L., . . . Członkowska, A. (2011). Emotionally negative stimuli can overcome attentional deficits in patients with visuo-spatial hemineglect. *Neuropsychologia, 49*(12), 3327–3337. doi:10.1016/j.neuropsychologia.2011.08.006

Greicius, M. D., & Menon, V. (2004). Default-mode activity during a passive sensory task: uncoupled from deactivation but impacting activation. *J Cogn Neurosci, 16*(9), 1484–1492. doi:10.1162/0898929042568532

Gross, J. J., & Thompson, R. A. (2007). Emotion regulation: conceptual foundations. In J. J. Gross (Ed.), *Handbook of emotion regulation* (pp. 3–26). New York: Guilford Press.

Gschwind, M., Pourtois, G., Schwartz, S., Ville, D. V. D., & Vuilleumier, P. (2012). White-matter connectivity between face-responsive regions in the human brain. *Cereb Cortex, 22*(7), 1564–1576. doi:10.1093/cercor/bhr226

Guimerà, R., & Nunes Amaral, L. A. (2005). Functional cartography of complex metabolic networks. *Nature, 433*(7028), 895–900. doi:10.1038/nature03288

Gur, R. C., Sara, R., Hagendoorn, M., Marom, O., Hughett, P., Macy, L., . . . Gur, R. E. (2002). A method for obtaining 3-dimensional facial expressions and its standardization for use in neurocognitive studies. *J Neurosci Methods, 115*, 137–143.

Hajcak, G., & Foti, D. (2008). Errors are aversive defensive motivation and the error-related negativity. *Psychol Sci, 19*(2), 103–108.

Hariri, A. R., Tessitore, A., Mattay, V. S., Fera, F., & Weinberger, D. R. (2002). The amygdala response to emotional stimuli: a comparison of faces and scenes. *NeuroImage, 17*(1), 317–323. doi:10.1006/nimg.2002.1179

Harlow, J. M. (1848). Passage of an iron rod through the head. *BMS, 39*(20), 389–393.

Haxby, J. V., Hoffman, E. A., & Gobbini, M. I. (2000). The distributed human neural system for face perception. *Trends Cogn Sci, 4*(6), 223–233. doi:10.1016/S1364-6613(00)01482-0

Haxby, J. V., Hoffman, E. A., & Gobbini, M. I. (2002). Human neural systems for face recognition and social communication. *Biol Psychiatry, 51*(1), 59–67. doi:10.1016/S0006-3223(01)01330-0

He, B. J., Snyder, A. Z., Vincent, J. L., Epstein, A., Shulman, G. L., & Corbetta, M. (2007). Breakdown of functional connectivity in frontoparietal networks underlies behavioral deficits in spatial neglect. *Neuron, 53*(6), 905–918. doi:10.1016/j.neuron.2007.02.013

Holland, P., & Gallagher, M. (1999). Amygdala circuitry in attentional and representational processes. *Trends Cogn Sci, 3*(2), 65–73.

Holland, P. C., & Gallagher, M. (2004). Amygdala–frontal interactions and reward expectancy. *Curr Opin Neurobiol, 14*(2), 148–155. doi:10.1016/j.conb.2004.03.007

Holroyd, C. B., & Coles, M. G. H. (2002). The neural basis of human error processing: reinforcement learning, dopamine, and the error-related negativity. *Psychol Rev, 109*(4), 679–709.

Holroyd, C. B., Dien, J., & Coles, M. G. (1998). Error-related scalp potentials elicited by hand and foot movements: evidence for an output-independent error-processing system in humans. *Neurosci Lett, 242*(2), 65–68.

Honey, C. J., Kötter, R., Breakspear, M., & Sporns, O. (2007). Network structure of cerebral cortex shapes functional connectivity on multiple time scales. *Proc Natl Acad Sci U S A, 104*(24), 10240–10245. doi:10.1073/pnas.0701519104

Hornak, J., Bramham, J., Rolls, E. T., Morris, R. G., O'Doherty, J., Bullock, P. R., & Polkey, C. E. (2003). Changes in emotion after circumscribed surgical lesions of the orbitofrontal and cingulate cortices. *Brain, 126*(Pt 7), 1691–1712. doi:10.1093/brain/awg168

Hornak, J., O'Doherty, J., Bramham, J., Rolls, E. T., Morris, R. G., Bullock, P. R., & Polkey, C. E. (2004). Reward-related reversal learning after surgical excisions in orbito-frontal or dorsolateral prefrontal cortex in humans. *J Cogn Neurosci, 16*(3), 463–478. doi:10.1162/089892904322926791

Hwang, K., Hallquist, M. N., & Luna, B. (2013). The development of hub architecture in the human functional brain network. *Cereb Cortex, 23*(10), 2380–2393. doi:10.1093/cercor/bhs227

Hynes, C. A., Baird, A. A., & Grafton, S. T. (2006). Differential role of the orbital frontal lobe in emotional versus cognitive perspective-taking. *Neuropsychologia, 44*(3), 374–383. doi:10.1016/j.neuropsychologia.2005.06.011

Ichikawa, N., Siegle, G. J., Jones, N. P., Kamishima, K., Thompson, W. K., Gross, J. J., & Ohira, H. (2011). Feeling bad about screwing up: emotion regulation and action monitoring in the anterior cingulate cortex. *Cogn Affect Behav Neurosci, 11*(3), 354–371. doi:10.3758/s13415-011-0028-z

Ji, J., & Maren, S. (2007). Hippocampal involvement in contextual modulation of fear extinction. *Hippocampus, 17*(9), 749–758. doi:10.1002/hipo.20331

Johnson, M. H. (2005). Subcortical face processing. *Nature Rev Neurosci, 6*(10), 766–774. doi:10.1038/nrn1766

Johnstone, T., Reekum, C. M. van, Urry, H. L., Kalin, N. H., & Davidson, R. J. (2007). Failure to regulate: counterproductive recruitment of top-down prefrontal-subcortical circuitry in major depression. *J Neurosci, 27*(33), 8877–8884. doi:10.1523/JNEUROSCI.2063-07.2007

Kalisch, R. (2009). The functional neuroanatomy of reappraisal: time matters. *Neurosci Biobehav Rev, 33*, 1215–1226.

Kalisch, R., Korenfeld, E., Stephan, K. E., Weiskopf, N., Seymour, B., & Dolan, R. J. (2006). Context-dependent human extinction memory is mediated by a ventromedial prefrontal and hippocampal network. *J Neurosci, 26*(37), 9503–9511. doi:10.1523/JNEUROSCI.2021-06.2006

Kanske, P., & Kotz, S. A. (2011a). Emotion speeds up conflict resolution: a new role for the ventral anterior cingulate cortex? *Cereb Cortex, 21*(4), 911–919. doi:10.1093/cercor/bhq157

Kanske, P., & Kotz, S. A. (2011b). Emotion triggers executive attention: anterior cingulate cortex and amygdala responses to emotional words in a conflict task. *Hum Brain Mapp, 32*(2), 198–208. doi:10.1002/hbm.21012

Kanwisher, N., McDermott, J., & Chun, M. M. (1997). The fusiform face area: a module in human extrastriate cortex specialized for face perception. *J Neurosci, 17*(11), 4302–4311.

Kerns, J. G., Cohen, J. D., MacDonald, A. W., Cho, R. Y., Stenger, V. A., & Carter, C. S. (2004). Anterior cingulate conflict monitoring and adjustments in control. *Science, 303*(5660), 1023–1026. doi:10.1126/science.1089910

Kim, J. J., & Fanselow, M. S. (1992). Modality-specific retrograde amnesia of fear. *Science, 256*(5057), 675–677. doi:10.1126/science.1585183

Knutson, B., & Cooper, J. C. (2005). Functional magnetic resonance imaging of reward prediction. *Curr Opin in Neurol, 18*(4), 411–417.

Knutson, B., Fong, G. W., Adams, C. M., Varner, J. L., & Hommer, D. (2001). Dissociation of reward anticipation and outcome with event-related fMRI. *NeuroReport, 12*(17), 3683–3687. doi:http://dx.doi.org/10.1097/00001756-200112040-00016

Kober, H., Barrett, L. F., Joseph, J., Bliss-Moreau, E., Lindquist, K., & Wager, T. D. (2008). Functional grouping and cortical-subcortical interactions in emotion: a meta-analysis of neuroimaging studies. *NeuroImage, 42*(2), 998–1031. doi:10.1016/j.neuroimage.2008.03.059

Kouider, S., & Dehaene, S. (2007). Levels of processing during non-conscious perception: a critical review of visual masking. *Philos Trans R Soc Lond B Biol Sci, 362*(1481), 857–875. Review. PMID: 17403642.

Koob, G. F. (1999). The role of the striatopallidal and extended amygdala systems in drug addiction. *Ann N Y Acad Sci, 877*(1), 445–460. doi:10.1111/j.1749-6632.1999.tb09282.x

Kringelbach, M. L., & Rolls, E. T. (2004). The functional neuroanatomy of the human orbitofrontal cortex: evidence from neuroimaging and neuropsychology. *Prog Neurobiol, 72*(5), 341–372. doi:10.1016/j.pneurobio.2004.03.006

Kumaran, D., & Maguire, E. A. (2005). The human hippocampus: cognitive maps or relational memory? *J Neurosci, 25*(31), 7254–7259. doi:10.1523/JNEUROSCI.1103-05.2005

Lane, R. D., Nadel, L., Allen, J. J. B., & Kaszniak, A. W. (2002). The study of emotion from the perspective of cognitive neuroscience. In R. D. Lane & L. Nadel (Eds.), *Cognitive neuroscience of emotion* (pp. 3–11). New York: Oxford University Press.

Lane, R. D., Reiman, E. M., Bradley, M. M., Lang, P. J., Ahern, G. L., Davidson, R. J., & Schwartz, G. E. (1997). Neuroanatomical correlates of pleasant and unpleasant emotion. *Neuropsychologia, 35,* 1437–1444.

Lang, P. J., Bradley, M. M., & Cuthbert, B. N. (2008). *International affective picture system (IAPS): affective ratings of pictures and instruction manual, Technical Report A-8.* University of Florida.

Lang, P. J., Davis, M., & Öhman, A. (2000). Fear and anxiety: animal models and human cognitive psychophysiology. *J Affect Disord, 61,* 137–159.

Lazarus, R. S. (2000). The cognition-emotion debate: a bit of history. In T. Dalgleish & M. Power (Eds.), *Handbook of cognition and emotion* (pp. 3–19). New York: Wiley.

Lech, R. K., & Suchan, B. (2013). The medial temporal lobe: memory and beyond. *Behav Brain Res, 254,* 45–49. doi:10.1016/j.bbr.2013.06.009

LeDoux, J. E. (1996). *The emotional brain: the mysterious underpinnings of emotional life.* New York: Simon & Schuster.

Leech, R., & Sharp, D. J. (2014). The role of the posterior cingulate cortex in cognition and disease. *Brain, 137*(1), 12–32. doi:10.1093/brain/awt162

Lieberman, M. D., Eisenberger, N. I., Crockett, M. J., Tom, S. M., Pfeifer, J. H., & Way, B. M. (2007). Putting feelings into words: affect labeling disrupts amygdala activity in response to affective stimuli. *Psychol Sci, 18*(5), 421–428. doi:10.1111/j.1467-9280.2007.01916.x

Lindquist, K. A., Wager, T. D., Kober, H., Bliss-Moreau, E., & Barrett, L. F. (2012). The brain basis of emotion: a meta-analytic review. *Behav Brain Sci, 35*(03), 121–143. doi:10.1017/S0140525X11000446

Liotti, M., Mayberg, H. S., Brannan, S. K., McGinnis, S., Jerabek, P., & Fox, P. T. (2000). Differential limbic–cortical correlates of sadness and anxiety in healthy subjects: implications for affective disorders. *Biol Psychiatry, 48*(1), 30–42. doi:10.1016/S0006-3223(00)00874-X

Lissek, S., Powers, A. S., McClure, E. B., Phelps, E. A., Woldehawariat, G., Grillon, C., & Pine, D. S. (2005). Classical fear conditioning in the anxiety disorders: a meta-analysis. *Behav Res Ther, 43*(11), 1391–1424. doi:10.1016/j.brat.2004.10.007

Lorist, M. M., Boksem, M. A. S., & Ridderinkhof, K. R. (2005). Impaired cognitive control and reduced cingulate activity during mental fatigue. *Cogn Brain Res, 24*(2), 199–205. doi:10.1016/j.cogbrainres.2005.01.018

Luria, A. R. (1966). *Higher cortical functions in man*. Oxford: Basic Books.

MacArthur Research Network on Early Experience and Brain Development. (2002). NimStim face stimulus set.

Maddock, R. J., Garrett, A. S., & Buonocore, M. H. (2001). Remembering familiar people: the posterior cingulate cortex and autobiographical memory retrieval. *Neuroscience, 104*(3), 667–676. doi:10.1016/S0306-4522(01)00108-7

Maddock, R. J., Garrett, A. S., & Buonocore, M. H. (2003). Posterior cingulate cortex activation by emotional words: fMRI evidence from a valence decision task. *Hum Brain Mapp, 18*(1), 30–41. doi:10.1002/hbm.10075

Marangon, M., Jacobs, S., & Frey, S. H. (2011). Evidence for context sensitivity of grasp representations in human parietal and premotor cortices. *J Neurophysiol, 105*(5), 2536–2546. doi:10.1152/jn.00796.2010

Maren, S. (2001). Neurobiology of Pavlovian fear conditioning. *Ann Rev Neurosci, 24*(1), 897–931. doi:10.1146/annurev.neuro.24.1.897

Maren, S., Aharonov, G., & Fanselow, M. S. (1997). Neurotoxic lesions of the dorsal hippocampus and Pavlovian fear conditioning in rats. *Behav Brain Res, 88*(2), 261–274. doi:10.1016/S0166-4328(97)00088-0

Margulies, D. S., Kelly, A. M. C., Uddin, L. Q., Biswal, B. B., Castellanos, F. X., & Milham, M. P. (2007). Mapping the functional connectivity of anterior cingulate cortex. *NeuroImage, 37*(2), 579–588. doi:10.1016/j.neuroimage.2007.05.019

Martin, J. (2012). *Neuroanatomy text and atlas* (4th ed.). New York: McGraw-Hill Medical.

McGaugh, J. L. (2000). Memory—a century of consolidation. *Science, 287*(5451), 248–251. doi:10.1126/science.287.5451.248

McGaugh, J. L., & Cahill, L. (1997). Interaction of neuromodulatory systems in modulating memory storage. *Behav Brain Res, 83*(1–2), 31–38. doi:10.1016/S0166-4328(97)86042-1

McGonigle, D. J., Howseman, A. M., Athwal, B. S., Friston, K. J., Frackowiak, R. S. J., & Holmes, A. P. (2002). Variability in fMRI: an examination of intersession differences. In *5th IEEE EMBS International Summer School on Biomedical Imaging, 2002* (p. 27). doi:10.1109/SSBI.2002.1233972

McIntosh, A. R. (2004). Contexts and catalysts. *Neuroinformatics, 2*(2), 175–181. doi:10.1385/NI:2:2:175

Mechias, M.-L., Etkin, A., & Kalisch, R. (2010). A meta-analysis of instructed fear studies: implications for conscious appraisal of threat. *NeuroImage, 49*(2), 1760–1768. doi:10.1016/j.neuroimage.2009.09.040

Menon, V. (2011). Large-scale brain networks and psychopathology: a unifying triple network model. *Trends Cogn Sci, 15*(10), 483–506. doi:10.1016/j.tics.2011.08.003

Milad, M. R., & Quirk, G. J. (2012). Fear extinction as a model for translational neuroscience: ten years of progress. *Ann Rev Psychol, 63*(1), 129–151. doi:10.1146/annurev.psych.121208.131631

Milad, M. R., Quirk, G. J., Pitman, R. K., Orr, S. P., Fischl, B., & Rauch, S. L. (2007). A role for the human dorsal anterior cingulate cortex in fear expression. *Biol Psychiatry, 62*(10), 1191–1194. doi:10.1016/j.biopsych.2007.04.032

Milad, M. R., Wright, C. I., Orr, S. P., Pitman, R. K., Quirk, G. J., & Rauch, S. L. (2007). Recall of fear extinction in humans activates the ventromedial prefrontal cortex and hippocampus in concert. *Biol Psychiatry, 62*(5), 446–454. doi:10.1016/j.biopsych.2006.10.011

Miller, B. L., & Cummings, J. L. (2007). *The human frontal lobes: functions and disorders.* New York: Guilford Press.

Miltner, W. H. R., Lemke, U., Weiss, T., Holroyd, C. B., Scheffers, M. K., & Coles, M. G. H. (2003). Implementation of error-processing in the human anterior cingulate cortex: a source analysis of the magnetic equivalent of the error-related negativity. *Biol Psychol, 64*(1–2), 157–166.

Minati, L., Varotto, G., D'Incerti, L., Panzica, F., & Chan, D. (2013). From brain topography to brain topology: relevance of graph theory to functional neuroscience. [Miscellaneous Article]. *Neuroreport, 24*(10), 536–543. doi:10.1097/WNR.0b013e3283621234

Morris, J. S., Friston, K. J., Büchel, C., Frith, C. D., Young, A. W., Calder, A. J., & Dolan, R. J. (1998). A neuromodulatory role for the human amygdala in processing emotional facial expressions. *Brain, 121*(1), 47–57. doi:10.1093/brain/121.1.47

Morris, J. S., Öhman, A., & Dolan, R. J. (1999). A subcortical pathway to the right amygdala mediating "unseen" fear. *Proc Natl Acad Sci U S A, 96*(4), 1680–1685. doi:10.1073/pnas.96.4.1680

Moscarello, J. M., & LeDoux, J. E. (2013). The contribution of the amygdala to aversive and appetitive pavlovian processes. *Emot Rev, 5*(3), 248–253. doi:10.1177/1754073913477508

Moser, J. S., Moran, T. P., Schroder, H. S., Donnellan, M. B., & Yeung, N. (2013). On the relationship between anxiety and error monitoring: a meta-analysis and conceptual framework. *Front Hum Neurosci, 7.* doi:10.3389/fnhum.2013.00466

Moser, J. S., Moran, T. P., Schroder, H. S., Donnellan, M. B., & Yeung, N. (2014). The case for compensatory processes in the relationship between anxiety and error monitoring: a reply to Proudfit, Inzlicht, and Mennin. *Front Hum Neurosci, 8.* doi:10.3389/fnhum.2014.00064

Murty, V. P., Ritchey, M., Adcock, R. A., & LaBar, K. S. (2010). fMRI studies of successful emotional memory encoding: a quantitative meta-analysis. *Neuropsychologia, 48*(12), 3459–3469. doi:10.1016/j.neuropsychologia.2010.07.030

Myers, K. M., & Davis, M. (2002). Behavioral and neural analysis of extinction. *Neuron, 36*(4), 567–584.

Nee, D. E., Wager, T. D., & Jonides, J. (2007). Interference resolution: insights from a meta-analysis of neuroimaging tasks. *Cogn Affect Behav Neurosci, 7*(1), 1–17.

O'Doherty, J. P. (2004). Reward representations and reward-related learning in the human brain: insights from neuroimaging. *Curr Opin Neurobiol, 14*(6), 769–776. doi:10.1016/j.conb.2004.10.016

O'Keefe, J., & Nadel, L. (1978). *The hippocampus as a cognitive map.* Oxford: Oxford University Press.

Ochsner, K. N., Bunge, S. A., Gross, J. J., & Gabrieli, J. D. E. (2002). Rethinking feelings: an fMRI study of the cognitive regulation of emotion. *J Cogn Neurosci, 14*(8), 1215–1229. doi:10.1162/089892902760807212

Ochsner, K. N., Ray, R. D., Cooper, J. C., Robertson, E. R., Chopra, S., Gabrieli, J. D. E., & Gross, J. J. (2004). For better or for worse: neural systems supporting the cognitive down- and up-regulation of negative emotion. *NeuroImage, 23*(2), 483–499. doi:10.1016/j.neuroimage.2004.06.030

Ochsner, K. N., Silvers, J. A., & Buhle, J. T. (2012). Functional imaging studies of emotion regulation: a synthetic review and evolving model of the cognitive control of emotion. *Ann N Y Acad Sci, 1251*(1), E1–E24. doi:10.1111/j.1749-6632.2012.06751.x

Öhman, A. (2002). Automaticity and the amygdala: nonconscious responses to emotional faces. *Curr Dir Psychol Sci, 11*(2), 62–66. doi:10.1111/1467-8721.00169

Öhman, A., & Mineka, S. (2001). Fears, phobias, and preparedness: toward an evolved module of fear and fear learning. *Psychol Rev, 108*(3), 483–522. doi:10.1037/0033-295X.108.3.483

Olson, I. R., Plotzker, A., & Ezzyat, Y. (2007). The Enigmatic temporal pole: a review of findings on social and emotional processing. *Brain, 130*(7), 1718–1731. doi:10.1093/brain/awm052

Owen, A. M., McMillan, K. M., Laird, A. R., & Bullmore, E. (2005). N-back working memory paradigm: a meta-analysis of normative functional neuroimaging studies. *Hum Brain Mapp, 25*(1), 46–59. doi:10.1002/hbm.20131

Paton, J. J., Belova, M. A., Morrison, S. E., & Salzman, C. D. (2006). The primate amygdala represents the positive and negative value of visual stimuli during learning. *Nature, 439*(7078), 865–870. doi:10.1038/nature04490

Paulus, M. P., & Stein, M. B. (2006). An insular view of anxiety. *Biol Psychiatry, 60*(4), 383–387. doi:10.1016/j.biopsych.2006.03.042

Paus, T., Koski, L., Caramanos, Z., & Westbury, C. (1998). Regional differences in the effects of task difficulty and motor output on blood flow response in the human anterior cingulate cortex: a review of 107 PET activation studies. *Neuroreport, 9*(9), R37–R47.

Pessoa, L. (2005). To what extent are emotional visual stimuli processed without attention and awareness? *Curr Opin Neurobiol, 15*(2), 188–196. doi:10.1016/j.conb.2005.03.002

Pessoa, L. (2008). On the relationship between emotion and cognition. *Nature Rev Neurosci, 9*(2), 148–158. doi:10.1038/nrn2317

Pessoa, L. (2009). How do emotion and motivation direct executive control? *Trends Cogn Sci, 13*(4), 160–166. doi:10.1016/j.tics.2009.01.006

Pessoa, L. (2010). Emergent processes in cognitive-emotional interactions. *Dialogues Clin Neurosci, 12*(4), 433–448.

Pessoa, L. (2013). *The cognitive-emotional brain: from interactions to integration.* Cambridge, MA: MIT Press.

Pessoa, L., & Adolphs, R. (2010). Emotion processing and the amygdala: from a "low road" to "many roads" of evaluating biological significance. *Nature Rev Neurosci, 11*, 773–783.

Pessoa, L., McKenna, M., Gutierrez, E., & Ungerleider, L. G. (2002). Neural processing of emotional faces requires attention. *Proc Natl Acad Sci U S A, 99*, 11458.

Petersen, S. E., & Posner, M. I. (2012). The Attention system of the human brain: 20 years after. *Ann Rev Neurosci, 35*, 73–89. doi:10.1146/annurev-neuro-062111-150525

Phaf, R. H., & Kan, K.-J. (2007). The automaticity of emotional Stroop: a meta-analysis. *J Behav Ther Exp Psychiatry, 38*(2), 184–199. doi:10.1016/j.jbtep.2006.10.008

Phan, K. L., Fitzgerald, D. A., Nathan, P. J., Moore, G. J., Uhde, T. W., & Tancer, M. E. (2005). Neural substrates for voluntary suppression of negative affect: a functional magnetic resonance imaging study. *Biol Psychiatry, 57*(3), 210–219. doi:10.1016/j.biopsych.2004.10.030

Phan, K. L., Taylor, S. F., Welsh, R. C., Ho, S.-H., Britton, J. C., & Liberzon, I. (2004). Neural correlates of individual ratings of emotional salience: a trial-related fMRI study. *NeuroImage, 21*(2), 768–780. doi:10.1016/j.neuroimage.2003.09.072

Phan, K. L., Wager, T. D., Taylor, S. F., & Liberzon, I. (2004). Functional neuroimaging studies of human emotions. *CNS Spectrums, 9*(4), 258–266.

Phan, K. L., Wager, T., Taylor, S. F., & Liberzon, I. (2002). Functional neuroanatomy of emotion: a meta-analysis of emotion activation studies in PET and fMRI. *Neuroimage, 16*, 331–348.

Phelps, E. A., & Anderson, A. K. (1997). Emotional memory: what does the amygdala do? *Curr Biol, 7*(5), R311–R314. doi:10.1016/S0960-9822(06)00146-1

Phelps, E. A., Delgado, M. R., Nearing, K. I., & LeDoux, J. E. (2004). Extinction learning in humans: role of the amygdala and vmPFC. *Neuron, 43*(6), 897–905. doi:10.1016/j.neuron.2004.08.042

Phelps, E. A., Ling, S., & Carrasco, M. (2006). Emotion facilitates perception and potentiates the perceptual benefits of attention. *Psychol Sci, 17*(4), 292–299. doi:10.1111/j.1467-9280.2006.01701.x

Phillips, M. L., Young, A. W., Senior, C., Brammer, M., Andrew, C., Calder, A. J., . . . David, A. S. (1997). A specific neural substrate for perceiving facial expressions of disgust. *Nature, 389*(6650), 495–498. doi:10.1038/39051

Phillips, R. G., & LeDoux, J. E. (1992). Differential contribution of amygdala and hippocampus to cued and contextual fear conditioning. *Behav Neurosci, 106*(2), 274–285.

Poeppel, D. (1996). A critical review of PET studies of phonological processing. *Brain Lang, 55*(3), 317–351. doi:10.1006/brln.1996.0108

Pourtois, G., Schettino, A., & Vuilleumier, P. (2013). Brain mechanisms for emotional influences on perception and attention: what is magic and what is not. *Biol Psychol, 92*(3), 492–512. doi:10.1016/j.biopsycho.2012.02.007

Pribram, K. H. (1973). The primate prefrontal cortex—executive of the brain. In K. H. Pribram & A. R. Luria (Eds.), *Psychophysiology of the frontal lobes* (pp. 293–314). New York: Academic Press.

Proudfit, G. H., Inzlicht, M., & Mennin, D. S. (2013). Anxiety and error monitoring: the importance of motivation and emotion. *Front Hum Neurosci, 7*. doi:10.3389/fnhum.2013.00636

Ptak, R. (2012). The frontoparietal attention network of the human brain action, saliency, and a priority map of the environment. *Neuroscientist, 18*(5), 502–515. doi:10.1177/1073858411409051

Qin, P., & Northoff, G. (2011). How is our self related to midline regions and the default-mode network? *NeuroImage, 57*(3), 1221–1233. doi:10.1016/j.neuroimage.2011.05.028

Quirk, G. J., & Mueller, D. (2008). Neural mechanisms of extinction learning and retrieval. *Neuropsychopharmacology, 33*(1), 56–72. doi:10.1038/sj.npp.1301555

Quirk, G. J., Russo, G. K., Barron, J. L., & Lebron, K. (2000). The role of ventromedial prefrontal cortex in the recovery of extinguished fear. *J Neurosci, 20*(16), 6225–6231.

Raichle, M. E., MacLeod, A. M., Snyder, A. Z., Powers, W. J., Gusnard, D. A., & Shulman, G. L. (2001). A default mode of brain function. *Proc Natl Acad Sci U S A, 98*(2), 676–682. doi:10.1073/pnas.98.2.676

Ray, R. D., & Zald, D. H. (2012). Anatomical insights into the interaction of emotion and cognition in the prefrontal cortex. *Neurosci Biobehav Rev, 36*(1), 479–501. doi:10.1016/j.neubiorev.2011.08.005

Reiman, E. M., Lane, R. D., Ahern, G. L., Schwartz, G. E., Davidson, R. J., Friston, K. J., . . . Chen, K. (1997). Neuroanatomical correlates of externally and internally generated human emotion. *Am J Psychiatry, 154*(7), 918–925.

Repa, J. C., Muller, J., Apergis, J., Desrochers, T. M., Zhou, Y., & LeDoux, J. E. (2001). Two different lateral amygdala cell populations contribute to the initiation and storage of memory. *Nature Neurosci, 4*(7), 724–731. doi:10.1038/89512

Ridderinkhof, K. R., Nieuwenhuis, S., & Bashore, T. R. (2003). Errors are foreshadowed in brain potentials associated with action monitoring in cingulate cortex in humans. *Neurosci Lett, 348*(1), 1–4. doi:10.1016/S0304-3940(03)00566-4

Ridderinkhof, K. R., Ullsperger, M., Crone, E. A., & Nieuwenhuis, S. (2004). The role of the medial frontal cortex in cognitive control. *Science, 306*(5695), 443–447. doi:10.1126/science.1100301

Riesel, A., Weinberg, A., Moran, T., & Hajcak, G. (2013). Time course of error-potentiated startle and its relationship to error-related brain activity. *J Psychophysiol, 27*(2), 51–59. doi:10.1027/0269-8803/a000093

Rosen, J. B., Hitchcock, J. M., Miserendino, M. J., Falls, W. A., Campeau, S., & Davis, M. (1992). Lesions of the perirhinal cortex but not of the frontal, medial prefrontal, visual, or insular cortex block fear-potentiated startle using a visual conditioned stimulus. *J Neurosci, 12*(12), 4624–4633.

Rotshtein, P., Richardson, M. P., Winston, J. S., Kiebel, S. J., Vuilleumier, P., Eimer, M., . . . Dolan, R. J. (2010). Amygdala damage affects event-related potentials for fearful faces at specific time windows. *Hum Brain Mapp, 31*(7), 1089–1105. doi:10.1002/hbm.20921

Rottschy, C., Langner, R., Dogan, I., Reetz, K., Laird, A. R., Schulz, J. B., . . . Eickhoff, S. B. (2012). Modelling neural correlates of working memory: a coordinate-based meta-analysis. *NeuroImage, 60*(1), 830–846. doi:10.1016/j.neuroimage.2011.11.050

Roy, M., Shohamy, D., & Wager, T. D. (2012). Ventromedial prefrontal-subcortical systems and the generation of affective meaning. *Trends Cogn Sci, 16*(3), 147–156. doi:10.1016/j.tics.2012.01.005

Ruff, C. C., Bestmann, S., Blankenburg, F., Bjoertomt, O., Josephs, O., Weiskopf, N., . . . Driver, J. (2008). Distinct causal influences of parietal versus frontal areas on human visual cortex: evidence from concurrent TMS–fMRI. *Cereb Cortex, 18*(4), 817–827. doi:10.1093/cercor/bhm128

Ruff, C. C., Blankenburg, F., Bjoertomt, O., Bestmann, S., Freeman, E., Haynes, J.-D., . . . Driver, J. (2006). Concurrent TMS-fMRI and psychophysics reveal frontal influences on human retinotopic visual cortex. *Curr Biol, 16*(15), 1479–1488. doi:10.1016/j.cub.2006.06.057

Sabatinelli, D., Bradley, M. M., Fitzsimmons, J. R., & Lang, P. J. (2005). Parallel amygdala and inferotemporal activation reflect emotional intensity and fear relevance. *NeuroImage, 24*(4), 1265–1270. doi:10.1016/j.neuroimage.2004.12.015

Sabatinelli, D., Bradley, M. M., Lang, P. J., Costa, V. D., & Versace, F. (2007). Pleasure rather than salience activates human nucleus accumbens and medial prefrontal cortex. *J Neurophysiol, 98*(3), 1374–1379. doi:10.1152/jn.00230.2007

Sabatinelli, D., Fortune, E. E., Li, Q., Siddiqui, A., Krafft, C., Oliver, W. T., . . . Jeffries, J. (2011). Emotional perception: meta-analyses of face and natural scene processing. *NeuroImage, 54*(3), 2524–2533. doi:10.1016/j.neuroimage.2010.10.011

Schaefer, A., Braver, T. S., Reynolds, J. R., Burgess, G. C., Yarkoni, T., & Gray, J. R. (2006). Individual differences in amygdala activity predict response speed during working memory. *J Neurosci, 26*(40), 10120–10128. doi:10.1523/JNEUROSCI.2567-06.2006

Schiller, D., & Delgado, M. R. (2010). Overlapping neural systems mediating extinction, reversal and regulation of fear. *Trends Cogn Sci, 14*(6), 268–276. doi:10.1016/j.tics.2010.04.002

Schiller, D., Levy, I., Niv, Y., LeDoux, J. E., & Phelps, E. A. (2008). From fear to safety and back: reversal of fear in the human brain. *J Neurosci, 28*(45), 11517–11525. doi:10.1523/JNEUROSCI.2265-08.2008

Schnyer, D. M., Nicholls, L., & Verfaellie, M. (2005). The role of VMPC in metamemorial judgments of content retrievability. *J Cogn Neurosci, 17*(5), 832–846. doi:10.1162/0898929053747694

Schoenbaum, G., Takahashi, Y., Liu, T.-L., & McDannald, M. A. (2011). Does the orbitofrontal cortex signal value? *Ann N Y Acad Sci, 1239*(1), 87–99. doi:10.1111/j.1749-6632.2011.06210.x

Schultz, W. (2007). Multiple dopamine functions at different time courses. *Ann Rev Neurosci, 30*(1), 259–288. doi:10.1146/annurev.neuro.28.061604.135722

Seeley, W. W., Menon, V., Schatzberg, A. F., Keller, J., Glover, G. H., Kenna, H., . . . Greicius, M. D. (2007). Dissociable intrinsic connectivity networks for salience processing and executive control. *J Neurosci, 27*(9), 2349–2356. doi:10.1523/JNEUROSCI.5587-06.2007

Sehlmeyer, C., Schöning, S., Zwitserlood, P., Pfleiderer, B., Kircher, T., Arolt, V., & Konrad, C. (2009). Human fear conditioning and extinction in neuroimaging: a systematic review. *PLoS ONE, 4*(6), e5865. doi:10.1371/journal.pone.0005865

Sergent, J., Ohta, S., & MacDonald, B. (1992). Functional neuroanatomy of face and object processing. a positron emission tomography study. *Brain, 115*(Pt 1), 15–36.

Sergerie, K., Chochol, C., & Armony, J. L. (2008). The role of the amygdala in emotional processing: a quantitative meta-analysis of functional neuroimaging studies. *Neurosci Biobehav Rev, 32*(4), 811–830. doi:10.1016/j.neubiorev.2007.12.002

Shin, L. M., Dougherty, D. D., Orr, S. P., Pitman, R. K., Lasko, M., Macklin, M. L., . . . Rauch, S. L. (2000). Activation of anterior paralimbic structures during guilt-related script-driven imagery. *Biol Psychiatry, 48*(1), 43–50. doi:10.1016/S0006-3223(00)00251-1

Siddiqui, S. V., Chatterjee, U., Kumar, D., Siddiqui, A., & Goyal, N. (2008). Neuropsychology of prefrontal cortex. *Indian J Psychiatry, 50*(3), 202–208. doi:10.4103/0019-5545.43634

Silver, M. A., & Kastner, S. (2009). Topographic maps in human frontal and parietal cortex. *Trends Cogn Sci, 13*(11), 488–495. doi:10.1016/j.tics.2009.08.005

Smith, E. E., & Jonides, J. (1998). Neuroimaging analyses of human working memory. *Proc Natl Acad Sci U S A, 95*(20), 12061–12068. doi:10.1073/pnas.95.20.12061

Smith, E. E., & Jonides, J. (1999). Storage and executive processes in the frontal lobes. *Science, 283*(5408), 1657–1661. doi:10.1126/science.283.5408.1657

Sotres-Bayon, F., Bush, D. E. A., & LeDoux, J. E. (2004). Emotional perseveration: an update on prefrontal-amygdala interactions in fear extinction. *Learn Mem, 11*(5), 525–535. doi:10.1101/lm.79504

Spitsyna, G., Warren, J. E., Scott, S. K., Turkheimer, F. E., & Wise, R. J. S. (2006). Converging language streams in the human temporal lobe. *J Neurosci, 26*(28), 7328–7336. doi:10.1523/JNEUROSCI.0559-06.2006

Sporns, O. (2011). The human connectome: a complex network. *Ann N Y Acad Sci, 1224,* 109–125. doi:10.1111/j.1749-6632.2010.05888.x

Sridharan, D., Levitin, D. J., & Menon, V. (2008). A critical role for the right fronto-insular cortex in switching between central-executive and default-mode networks. *Proc Natl Acad Sci U S A, 105*(34), 12569–12574. doi:10.1073/pnas.0800005105

Swanson, L. W. (2003). The amygdala and its place in the cerebral hemisphere. *Ann N Y Acad Sci, 985*(1), 174–184. doi:10.1111/j.1749-6632.2003.tb07081.x

Tamietto, M., & de Gelder, B. (2010). Neural bases of the non-conscious perception of emotional signals. *Nature Rev Neurosci, 11*(10), 697–709. doi:10.1038/nrn2889

Taylor, S. F., Liberzon, I., & Koeppe, R. A. (2000). The effect of graded aversive stimuli on limbic and visual activation. *Neuropsychologia, 38*(10), 1415–1425. doi:10.1016/S0028-3932(00)00032-4

Taylor, S. F., Phan, K. L., Decker, L. R., & Liberzon, I. (2003). Subjective rating of emotionally salient stimuli modulates neural activity. *NeuroImage, 18*(3), 650–659. doi:10.1016/S1053-8119(02)00051-4

Turner, B. H., & Zimmer, J. (1984). The architecture and some of the interconnections of the rat's amygdala and lateral periallocortex. *J Comp Neurol, 227*(4), 540–557. doi:10.1002/cne.902270406

Ubeda-Bañon, I., Novejarque, A., Mohedano-Moriano, A., Pro-Sistiaga, P., de la Rosa-Prieto, C., Insausti, R., . . . Martinez-Marcos, A. (2007). Projections from the posterolateral olfactory amygdala to the ventral striatum: neural basis for reinforcing properties of chemical stimuli. *BMC Neurosci, 8,* 103. doi:10.1186/1471-2202-8-103

Umarova, R. M., Saur, D., Schnell, S., Kaller, C. P., Vry, M.-S., Glauche, V., . . . Weiller, C. (2010). Structural connectivity for visuospatial attention: significance of ventral pathways. *Cereb Cortex, 20*(1), 121–129. doi:10.1093/cercor/bhp086

Urry, H. L., Reekum, C. M. van, Johnstone, T., Kalin, N. H., Thurow, M. E., . . . Davidson, R. J. (2006). Amygdala and ventromedial prefrontal cortex are inversely coupled during regulation of negative affect and predict the diurnal pattern of cortisol secretion among older adults. *J Neurosci, 26*(16), 4415–4425. doi:10.1523/JNEUROSCI.3215-05.2006

Utter, A. A., & Basso, M. A. (2008). The basal ganglia: an overview of circuits and function. *Neurosci Biobehav Rev, 32*(3), 333–342. doi:10.1016/j.neubiorev.2006.11.003

Van Snellenberg, J. X., & Wager, T. D. (2009). Cognitive and motivational functions of the human prefrontal cortex. In A. Christensen, E. Goldberg, & D. Bougakov (Eds.), *Luria's legacy in the 21st century* (pp. 30–61). New York: Oxford University Press.

Vogel, A. C., Power, J. D., Petersen, S. E., & Schlaggar, B. L. (2010). Development of the brain's functional network architecture. *Neuropsychol Rev, 20*(4), 362–375. doi:10.1007/s11065-010-9145-7

Vossel, S., Weidner, R., Thiel, C. M., & Fink, G. R. (2008). What is "odd" in Posner's location-cueing paradigm? neural responses to unexpected location and feature changes compared. *J Cogn Neurosci, 21*(1), 30–41. doi:10.1162/jocn.2009.21003

Vuilleumier, P., Armony, J. L., Clarke, K., Husain, M., Driver, J., & Dolan, R. J. (2002). Neural response to emotional faces with and without awareness: event-related fMRI in a parietal patient with visual extinction and spatial neglect. *Neuropsychologia, 40*(12), 2156–2166.

Vuilleumier, P., Armony, J. L., Driver, J., & Dolan, R. J. (2001). Effects of attention and emotion on face processing in the human brain: an event-related fMRI study. *Neuron, 30*(3), 829–841. doi:10.1016/S0896-6273(01)00328-2

Vuilleumier, P., Armony, J. L., Driver, J., & Dolan, R. J. (2003). Distinct spatial frequency sensitivities for processing faces and emotional expressions. *Nature Neurosci, 6*(6), 624–631. doi:10.1038/nn1057

Vuilleumier, P., Richardson, M. P., Armony, J. L., Driver, J., & Dolan, R. J. (2004). Distant influences of amygdala lesion on visual cortical activation during emotional face processing. *Nature Neurosci, 7*(11), 1271–1278. doi:10.1038/nn1341

Vuilleumier, P., & Schwartz, S. (2001). Emotional facial expressions capture attention. *Neurology, 56*(2), 153–158. doi:10.1212/WNL.56.2.153

Wager, T. D., Jonides, J., & Reading, S. (2004). Neuroimaging studies of shifting attention: a meta-analysis *NeuroImage, 22*(4), 1679–1693. doi:10.1016/j.neuroimage.2004.03.052

Wager, T. D., & Smith, E. E. (2003). Neuroimaging studies of working memory. *Cogn Affect Behav Neurosci, 3*(4), 255–274. doi:10.3758/CABN.3.4.255

Wager, T. D., Waugh, C. E., Lindquist, M., Noll, D. C., Fredrickson, B. L., & Taylor, S. F. (2009). Brain mediators of cardiovascular responses to social threat: Part I: Reciprocal dorsal and ventral sub-regions of the medial prefrontal cortex and heart-rate reactivity. *NeuroImage, 47*(3), 821–835. doi:10.1016/j.neuroimage.2009.05.043

Wagner, A. D., Shannon, B. J., Kahn, I., & Buckner, R. L. (2005). Parietal lobe contributions to episodic memory retrieval. *Trends Cogn Sci, 9*(9), 445–453. doi:10.1016/j.tics.2005.07.001

Waugh, C. E., Lemus, M. G., & Gotlib, I. H. (2014). The role of the medial frontal cortex in the maintenance of emotional states. *Soc Cogn Affect Neurosci*, nsu011. doi:10.1093/scan/nsu011

Whalen, P. J., Rauch, S. L., Etcoff, N. L., McInerney, S. C., Lee, M. B., & Jenike, M. A. (1998). Masked presentations of emotional facial expressions modulate amygdala activity without explicit knowledge. *J Neurosci, 18*(1), 411–418.

Wheaton, K. J., Thompson, J. C., Syngeniotis, A., Abbott, D. F., & Puce, A. (2004). Viewing the motion of human body parts activates different regions of premotor, temporal, and parietal cortex. *NeuroImage, 22*(1), 277–288. doi:10.1016/j.neuroimage.2003.12.043

Williams, M. A., & Mattingley, J. B. (2004). Unconscious perception of non-threatening facial emotion in parietal extinction. *Exp Brain Res, 154*(4), 403–406. doi:10.1007/s00221-003-1740-x

Yazar, Y., Bergström, Z. M., & Simons, J. S. (2012). What is the parietal lobe contribution to long-term memory? *Cortex, 48*(10), 1381–1382. doi:10.1016/j.cortex.2012.05.011

Yeung, N., Botvinick, M. M., & Cohen, J. D. (2004). The neural basis of error detection: conflict monitoring and the error-related negativity. *Psychol Rev, 111*(4), 931–959. doi:10.1037/0033-295X.111.4.939

Young, M. P., Scannell, J. W., Burns, G. A., & Blakemore, C. (1994). Analysis of connectivity: neural systems in the cerebral cortex. *Rev Neurosci, 5*(3), 227–250.

Yukie, M. (2002). Connections between the amygdala and auditory cortical areas in the macaque monkey. *Neurosci Res, 42*(3), 219–229. doi:10.1016/S0168-0102(01)00325-X

2 The Fundamentals of Brain Neurotransmission

■ ROBERT O. FRIEDEL
AND STEPHEN M. STAHL

■ INTRODUCTION

The purpose of this chapter is to provide information about the fundamental processes of brain neurotransmission. Focus will be placed on the neural networks. circuits, synaptic function, neurotransmitters, neuromodulators, and neuroreceptors that are especially related to personality disorders (PDs) and are discussed in subsequent chapters of this book. An increasing amount of data suggests that aberrant activity in pathways involved in PDs (Chapter 1) and the mechanisms of action of most psychotropic drugs are mediated by alterations in specific neurotransmitter receptor activity at key nodal points in these pathways. Therefore, it is essential to have a reasonable knowledge of the mechanisms of action of neurotransmitters and other substances that modulate neuronal activity throughout neural circuits and networks.

The material included in this chapter also provides a description of the mechanisms of action of medications that appear to reduce some of the symptoms of PDs. The material in this chapter is not intended to be comprehensive. (To obtain more comprehensive information on these topics in general, the reader is referred to Kandel, 2000; Stahl, 2013; Ledoux, 2002; Damasio, 1994; Krause-Utz et al., 2014). Rather, the intent here is to provide a broad overview that will serve as a framework for information presented in the following chapters. For purposes of clarity and coherency, some of the material overlaps with that presented on neural pathways in Chapter 1.

■ NEUROSCIENCE-BASED NOMENCLATURE

With the leadership of Joseph Zohar, the European College of Neuopsycho-pharmacology, American College of Neuropsychopharmacology, the Asian College of Neuropsychopharmacology, the International College of Neuropsychopharmacology, and the International Union of Basic and Clinical Pharmacology have approved and introduced a revised nomenclature for psychotropic drugs named the neuroscience-based nomenclature (NbN; Zohar et al., 2014, 2015). This system provides a significant shift from the current nomenclature of psychopharmacological medications because it emphasizes the pharmacological domains and modes of action of these medications rather than their indications (e.g., antipsychotics, antidepressants, anxiolytic, etc.). The NbN provides a framework with updated relevant and specific scientific, regulatory and clinical information, and as such facilitates and guides rationale and clear decisions for treatment selection. Such a change should clarify and improve the rationale for medication selection and increase medication compliance. The NbN is also intended to produce a nomenclature of psychopharmacology which coincides more closely with that employed in the other fields of medicine.

A major contention of the NbN is that although the current nomenclature of psychopharmacology may be more simple to apply, this simplicity comes at a significant cost. The cost is that it does not provide the clinician with the fundamental pharmacological information required to make well-informed choices when required during the evolving process of medication treatment. Also, the current system is confusing to patients who are prescribed "antipsychotics" when they are not psychotic, "antidepressants" when they are not depressed, and so on.

The specific expectations established for the NbN are that it should

1. Be based on contemporary scientific knowledge.
2. Help clinicians to make informed choices when working out the next "pharmacological step."
3. Provide a system that does not conflict with the use of medications.
4. Be future proof and to accommodate new types of compounds. (Zohar et al., 2015)

The NbN is relevant to and underscores the subject matter of this chapter. One of its authors (SMS) played a major role in conceptualizing and writing the NbN, and it has been applied whenever appropriate in the material presented. We believe that doing so will help the reader to understand simultaneously and more readily both sets of information.

■ FUNDAMENTAL PRINCIPLES OF NEURAL SCIENCE: A SELECTIVE OVERVIEW

Brain functions are determined primarily by the *location and activity levels* of neural circuits and networks. *Circuits* may be defined as a group of neurons that are linked by synaptic connections at subcortical nodes such as the thalamus, striatum, amygdala, and others and at cortical sites. By themselves, they may not produce a notable function, but they modulate the levels of activity at the synaptic nodes of the circuit. Multiple, integrated neural circuits that perform complex, specific functions, such as primary sensations such as vision and hearing, emotions, reasoning, motivation, and behaviors, are referred to as neural *networks* (Kandel, 2000, pp. 33–34). These networks are comprised of multiple neural circuits that are distributed to appropriate regions of the brain depending on the specific information they process related to their function. This concept is referred to as *distributed processing* and is central to understanding brain function (Kandel, 2000, p. 11). The most complex neural circuitry elucidated at this time is that describing the fear and anxiety systems (LeDoux & Pine, 2017). It serves as a model for using neuroscience to define the fundamental framework of the neural integration of emotions, motivations, thoughts, and behaviors.

The processes involved in the conscious recognition of activity in a neural network is a matter of considerable controversy. It appears to depend, in part, on the degree and breadth of the connections across cortical processing systems and on the pattern and synchronization of neural activity within the network (Crick & Koch, 2005; Panksepp, 2005).

Pertinent to our focus on PDs, there is now sound empirical evidence for the connectivity between negative affectivity, impulsivity, and disordered reasoning in individuals with these disorders. This connectivity is a function of the degree of integrated activity of the extended amygdala, the periaqueductal gray, and other subcortical emotion pathways and the ventromedial, dorsolateral, and anterior cingulate prefrontal cortical pathways (Whittle et al., 2006; Panksepp, 2005). Further clarification of the functions of these neural pathways, and others, is of particular importance in deepening our understanding of PDs because many of them have been found to be significantly and consistently altered in subjects with a number of these disorders compared to control subjects (Chapter 1; Mauchnik & Schmahl, 2010). Also, the functions of these brain regions, as described in the following chapters, are those characteristic of specific features of the core psychopathology of the disorders.

For example, the extended amygdala and other subcortical emotion systems appear to be primarily involved in the generation of nonconscious emotional processes and the physiological and behavioral responses associated with them. The projections of these subcortical systems to the ventromedial prefrontal cortex, and other brain areas, such as the insula, are thought to contribute in part to the conscious perceptions (feelings) of emotions (Damasio, 1994; Panksepp, 2005). The dorsolateral prefrontal cortex (DLPC) is known to be strongly related to working memory and executive functions. The anterior cingulate cortex (ACC), located on the medial aspect of the frontal lobe, interacts with the ventromedial and DLPF cortical areas in the perception and regulation (top-down control) of affect-, motivation-, and cognitive-driven behaviors. Though the evidence is preliminary, it has been suggested that a fourth system with connections to the anterior insula, a region of the cortex located deep in the fissure between the temporal and parietal lobes, is involved in the processes of attachment, interpersonal bonding, and trust that are typically disrupted in PDs (Seres et al., 2009).

Neuroimaging studies in subjects with borderline personality disorder (BPD) have consistently demonstrated alterations of structure and function in many of the brain regions discussed (Chapter 15; also see Krause-Utz et al. 2014). For example, subjects with BPD demonstrate decreased volume and increased activity in the amygdala and associated circuits compared to control populations. The DLPC and the ACC have also shown structural and functional alterations in subjects with BPD compared to controls. Therefore, it is now commonly accepted that *increased* activity of "bottom-up" subcortical emotion circuits and *decreased* "top-down" control by prefrontal circuits account for many of the affective, impulsive, and cognitive-perceptual symptoms that are characteristic of this PD. There is also increasing evidence that such brain disturbances predominate in the right hemisphere of subjects with BPD (Silbersweig et al., 2007; Meares et al., 2011).

Abnormalities have also been demonstrated in the underlying *biochemical processes* of the neural networks noted in subjects with PDs. For example, in subjects with BPD, data suggest that regional activity of serotonin (New et al., 2008), dopamine (Friedel, 2004), and mu-opioid binding potential (Prossin et al., 2010) are altered. Increased levels of the stimulatory transmitter glutamate are present in the ACC of subjects with BPD, which correlate positively with impulsivity ratings (Hoerst et al., 2010). Levels of the inhibitory transmitter GABA in the DLPC are inversely related to impulsivity in normal subjects (Boy et al., 2006). It is important to recognize that these alterations are correlative but not necessarily causative. For example, the increased levels of glutamate in the ACC noted may be secondary to an increased requirement for top-down control emanating from the ACC to subcortical brain areas that are hyperactive. If so, the correlation noted would still be found. Regardless of the precise meaning of these findings, they indicate that a disruption of chemical processes vital to normal function in critical neural networks may be responsible, in part, for the core symptoms of BPD and other PDs.

■ NEURONS, PROCESSING SITES, AND SYNAPTIC TRANSMISSION

Neurons and Information Processing Sites

It is estimated that the human brain contains 10^{11} (100 billion) neurons of many types. Almost all of these neurons have the same basic components, a cell body and fibers of two types—dendrites that receive information and a single axon that sends information mainly to the dendrites and less often to the cell bodies of the next neurons. The sites of these neuronal connections occur in subcortical nodes such as the basal ganglia, the hippocampal formation, the amygdala, and complex, multilayered cylindrical columns in the cortex (Amaral, 2000, pp. 329–332). These cortical columns are positioned perpendicularly to the surface of the cortex and vary in the cellular structure of their layers from one region of the brain to another depending on the function of that cortical region. Cortical columns may constitute the basic information processing units of the brain. Not surprisingly, the human cortex contains more of these units than any other species of animal. The multiple foldings of the cortex upon itself permits increased cortical area and the number of columns. Subcortical processing centers such as the basil ganglia, hypothalamus, and amygdala are also cites of concentrated, complex neural connections. Although they do not possess the clear, cytoarchitectural features of the cortex, their cellular structure is typically evident and informative of their various functions.

These cortical and subcortical neuronal connection sites serve as more than relay stations for impulses flowing to, from, and within the brain. They also serve as major processing centers where information from other sites are integrated, recoded, then sent on to other sites where they are further processed. The organization and degree of complexity of these sites progressively enhances the ability to fine-tune the information processed in the brain's networks. It is postulated that this system of information processing serves as the basis for the individuality of species and members of the same species (LeDoux, 2002, p. 36).

Synaptic Transmission

Once it is recognized that the location, level, and nature of activity in the architectonic pathways of the brain determine specific brain functions, the question then becomes what determines and regulates this activity within networks and subcortical and cortical sites to enable appropriate thinking, feeling, behavior, and storage of important memories? One answer to this question is proposed succinctly by the neuroscientist Joseph LeDoux (2002) in *Synaptic Self*: "I believe, in short, an answer to the question of how brains make us who we are can be found in synaptic processes that allow cooperative interactions to take place between the various brain systems that are involved in particular states and experiences, and for these interactions to be linked over time" (p. 32). In other words, it is mainly through temporal synaptic activity that the numerous types of neurons found in the brain are able to communicate with other neurons and ultimately carry out their sensory, motor, and cognitive functions and store memories for future use. These synaptic interactions are very similar in location and function from one individual to the next but vary qualitatively and quantitatively depending on differences in heritable factors and life experiences.

To understand the processes of interneuronal communication more precisely, it is necessary to know how synapses transmit information to their receptor neurons. At the distal sites of axons are *axon terminals* that serve as the first structure in the chemical connection with the dendrites or cell bodies of the next neuron at specific neuronal loci referred to as synapses. The cytoarchitecture of synapses is now well understood and provides insight into how communication between neurons occurs. Axon terminals contain *vesicles* that each carry numerous, specific neurotransmitters or neuromodulators that are released into the *synaptic cleft* upon stimulation by an action potential. On the postsynaptic side of the synaptic cleft is a *base plate* highly enriched in receptors that bind a specific neurotransmitter or neuromodulator. Multiple receptors have now been identified for each neurotransmitter and neuromodulator. For example, stimulatory neurotransmitter receptors receive information from glutamate projection neurons and are usually located on the dendrites of the neuron receiving their chemical signals. The inhibitory GABA receptors that receive information from local GABA interneurons are located closer to or on the cell body to block more effectively the stimulatory actions of the glutamate signals. Other synaptic sites are located on glutamate and GABA neurons that receive communications from neuromodulators that fine-tune the flow and processing of information. It is estimated that each brain neuron receives information from and connects to approximately 1,000 neurons.

Neurotransmitters

The most common neurons found in neural circuits and networks utilize one of two neurotransmitters: glutamate and GABA. Glutamate is the main stimulatory transmitter in the central nervous system (Table 2.1) and is primarily secreted by *association* neurons that project to other neurons over short to long distances. GABA is the main inhibitory transmitter in the brain (Table 2.1). Its cells are localized within a more spatially limited area of projection; many of them are referred to as interneurons because they bind with and inhibit the activity of other neurons in their immediate vicinity. Glutamate neurons and stimulatory neuromodulator neurons increase the likelihood that the next neurons will generate an action potential by decreasing the negative internal charge of their target neurons by regulating Na^+, K^+, and Ca^{++} ion channels, bringing the charge closer to the firing point that generates an all-or-nothing action potential in that neuron. GABA neurons inhibit the stimulatory actions of glutamate and other neuromodulator neurons by increasing their negative internal electrical charge by closing Na^+, K^+, and Ca^{++} ion channels or by opening Cl^- ion channels, thereby increasing the internal charge of the neuron and reducing the likelihood of stimulation of an action potential by glutamate or a stimulatory neuromodulator (Table 2.1). These actions may occur by a direct effect on the ion channels or an indirect effect by a second messenger (Siegelbaum et al., 2000).

TABLE 2.1. *Brain Neurotransmission Process*

I. Neurotransmitters	Receptor Type	Subtype	Activity	Mechanisms of Action	Functions
Glutamate					
	Ionotropic	kainite	Excitatory	Gates Na^+ & K^+ ion channels	Main stimulatory brain neurotransmitter
	Ionotropic	AMPA	Excitatory	Gates Na^+ & K^+ ion channels	"
	Ionotropic	NMDA	Excitatory	Gates Na^+, K^+ & Ca^{++} ion channels	"
	Metabotropic	PIP_2	Excitatory	Stimulates phospholipase C: increases IP_3 and DAG	
GABA					
Family					
$GABA_A$	Ionotropic		Inhibitory	Opens membrane Cl^- ion channels	Main inhibitory brain neurotransmitter
$GABA_B$	Metabotropic		Inhibitory	G protein-coupled: increases K^+ conductance and decreases Ca^{++} channel activity	"

II. Neuromodulators	Receptor Type	Subtype	Activity	Mechanisms of Action	Functions
Serotonin					
Family					
5–HT1A,B,D	Metabotropic	cAMP	Inhibitory	Inhibits adenyl cyclase: decreases levels of cAMP	Autoreceptors: decrease 5-HT release
5–HT2A,C	"	PIP_2	Excitatory	Activates phospholipase C: increases levels of IP_3 and DAG; inhibits D release; increases pyramidal cell glutamate release	Play role in obesity, mood and cognition; 5-HT2A inhibition reduces EPS and negative symptoms
5–HT3	Ionotropic		Excitatory	Gates Na^+ and K^+ channels	Regulates inhibitory interneurons in cortex; and vomiting via vagal nerve
5–HT4	Metabotropic	cAMP	Excitatory	Increases levels of cAMP	
5–HT5	"	cAMP	Inhibitory	Decreases levels of cAMP	
5–HT6	"	cAMP	Excitatory	Increases levels of cAMP	May regulate release of BDNF
5–HT7	"	cAMP	Excitatory	Increases levels of cAMP	May be linked to circadian rhythms, sleep and mood

Dopamine					
D1, D5	Metabotropic	cAMP	Excitatory	Activate adenyl cyclase; increase levels of cAMP	More prominent in cortex than D2; increase cortical activity; low affinity for antipsychotic agents
D2, D3, D4	"	cAMP	Inhibitory	Inhibit adenyl cyclase: decrease levels of cAMP	More common in subcortical nodes; high affinity for antipsychotic agents
Norepinephrine					
Family					
alpha$_1$	Metabotropic: Gq-coupled	PIP$_2$	Excitatory	Activates phospholipase C: increases levels of IP$_3$, DAG and Ca^{++}	Acts on postsynaptic membranes of post-autonomic ganglia projections: "fight or flight"
alpha$_2$	G/G$_o$-coupled	cAMP	Inhibitory	Inhibits adenyl cyclase: decreases levels of cAMP	Decrease presynaptic release of NE
beta$_{1,2,3}$	G$_s$-coupled	cAMP	Excitatory	Activate adenyl cyclase; increase levels of cAMP	Acts on postsynaptic membranes of post-autonomic ganglia projections: "fight or flight"
Acetylcholine					
Nicotinic: multifamily	Ionotropic		Excitatory	Activate postsynaptic cells: open Na$^+$, K$^+$ and Ca^{++} ion channels	Activate autonomic nervous system ganglia: prepare body to "rest, nourish and breed;" other multimodal brain functions
Muscarinic: five subtypes	Metabotrobic	PIP$_2$	Excitatory	Activates phospholipase C: increases levels of IP$_3$, DAG and Ca^{++}	Multimodal brain functions: e.g., memory formation (degeneration of ACh projections from nucleus basalis of Meynert in Alzheimer's)
Histamine					
H1	Metabotropic	PIP$_2$	Excitatory	Activates phospholipase C: increases levels of IP$_3$, and DAG, especially in hypothalamic and limbic regions	Promotes sympathetic activity: arousal; regulates endocrine function and body temperature; appetite inhibition; cognition
H2	Metabotropic	cAMP	Mainly excititory	Activates adenyl cyclase; increase levels of cAMP	Somatodendritic autoreceptor activity; controls firing rate
H3	Metabotrobic	cAMP	Inhibitory	Inhibits voltage-dependent calcium channels	Presynaptic autoreceptor activity: decrease ACh, 5-HT and NE release

Neuromodulators

Activity levels in glutamate and GABA neurons are also regulated by other less numerous but specifically distributed neural pathways that utilize *neuromodulators* (e.g., serotonin, dopamine, norepinephrine, acetylcholine, histamine, and neuropeptides; Table 2.1), as well as by circulating hormones. These substances modulate (fine-tune) the activity within circuits and networks by enhancing or diminishing the activity of glutamate and GABA neurons described. Neuromodulators are distinguished from neurotransmitters in a number of ways. While the vast majority of neurons in the brain are glutamatergic and GABAnergic neurons, there are relatively few neurons that secrete neuromodulators. For example, more than 50% of the brain's 10^{11} neurons secrete glutamate and somewhat fewer secrete GABA. However, it has been estimated that there are only 400 to 600 *thousand* dopaminergic neurons in the human brain (Bjorkland & Dunnett, 2007). Neuromodulators are less involved than neurotransmitters in the point-to-point transmission of information than they are in selectively tuning the processes of transmission. Finally, glutamate and GABA are fast-acting in contrast to neuromodulators that are slower acting, and the latter have longer-lasting effects.

The importance of synaptic function is underscored by the fact that most psychotropic drugs affect the activity levels of neurotransmitters and neuromodulators at their various synaptic sites of action.

Neuroreceptors

Neuroreceptors mediate neural activity by directly and rapidly affecting the stimulatory or inhibitory actions of glutamate and GABA on postsynaptic neurons or by enhancing or diminishing (modulating) the effects of these two neurotransmitters. Neurotransmitters and neuromodulators exert their actions by the chemical processes they trigger when they bind to their receptors. These are varied and complex and are discussed later. At this point, it is important to keep in mind that individual transmitters and modulators each have multiple receptors that have both different and similar biochemical mechanisms of action that cause downstream cascades of other biochemical actions. The mechanisms of action and purposes of these different receptors are not clear, but they appear to have evolved to increase the flexibility and adaptability of responses of the brain to its environment. Many of these receptors are discussed in connection with the neurotransmitters and modulators with which they bind.

At this point, a specific example of the importance of the interaction of neurotransmitter and neuromodulator activity on neuroreceptors may prove useful. Dopamine injected into the nucleus accumbens activates animals because it activates the neuronal pathway from the accumbens to the pallidum. This in turn facilitates cortically mediated motor movement. Novel, conditioned, and unconditioned stimuli are examples of events that stimulate dopamine release in the pallidum (LeDoux, 2002, pp. 247–248).

We next describe the mechanisms of action of the main types of neurotransmitter receptors.

Types of Brain Synapses

Two types of brain synapses have been determined: electrical and chemical. There are far fewer electrical synapses in the nervous system than chemical. Most of them transmit both hyperpolarizing and depolarizing currents. The main advantage of electrical synapses is their speed of action, which is required under certain circumstances.

For the most part, brain neurons communicate through chemical synapses. As stated, actions of neurotransmitters and neuromodulators on postsynaptic cells depend on the chemical responses of the receptors, not on the nature of the transmitters. In addition, as will be seen, multiple neurotransmitters utilize the same transmitter receptor cascades of biochemical activity that follow receptor activation. This is an example of evolutionary preservation that has retained certain processes because they have proven to be effective.

There are two main types of chemical receptors in the neuronal cell membrane: ionotropic and metabotropic. Ionotropic receptors directly gate ion channels, and metabotropic receptors gate ion channels indirectly through their metabolic effects on specific postsynaptic substances. The former produce more rapid signaling than the latter. Brain neurons have receptors of both types and must integrate the signals from many presynaptic neurons in order to fire properly. For example, it is estimated that 50 to 100 excitatory neurons are required to produce an action potential in a postsynaptic neuron.

▪ SPECIFIC NEUROTRANSMITTERS AND THEIR MECHANISMS OF ACTION

Glutamate

Glutamate neurons comprise more than 50% of the brain's 10^{11} neurons. Glutamate exerts its stimulatory effect on postsynaptic neurons by the chemical changes it causes in three different types of ionotropic receptors and one metabotropic receptor present in the postsynaptic membrane of these neurons (Table 2.1). The three ionotropic receptors are named for the glutamate agonists that bind to them: kainate and α-amino-3-hydroxy-5-methylisoxazole-4-propionic acid (AMPA) receptors regulate channels permeable to Na^+ and K^+. The N-methyl-D-aspartate (NMDA) receptor regulates channels permeable to Na^+, K^+, and Ca^{++}. The metabotropic glutamate receptor indirectly regulates ion channels by stimulating the metabolism of a secondary messenger, phosphatidylinositol 4,5-bisphosphate (PIP_2) to two chemically active metabolites, inositol-1,4,5 triphosphate (IP_3) and diacylglycerol (DAG). IP_3 mobilizes Ca^{++} from internal stores and DAG activates protein kinase C (PKC; Siegelbaum et al., 2000, pp. 236–238). All glutamate receptors are excitatory. Excessive action of glutamate (e.g., resulting from prolonged seizures) will kill neurons, an action referred to as glutamate excitotoxicity. There is emerging evidence that glutamate dysregulation is involved in BPD (see Chapter 15). Certain psychotropic drugs effective in treating BPD appear to exert their therapeutic effect by their action on glutamate receptors (Table 2.2).

GABA

GABA is the second most prevalent neurotransmitter in the brain. It exerts its inhibitory action by hyperpolarizing postsynaptic potentials by binding to $GABA_A$ and $GABA_B$ receptors (Table 2.1). $GABA_A$ receptors are ionotropic and open a Cl–ion channel. $GABA_B$ is metabotropic; it stimulates a second-messenger cascade that activates a K^+

TABLE 2.2. *Neurobiological Profiles of Medications Useful in Personality Disorders*

Medication	Current Nomenclature	NbN Nomenclature	PD: Symptom Targets	Receptor Effects	Mechanisms of Action	Therapeutic Actions	Side Effects
Antipsychotics							
Haloperidol; thiothixene	First-generation antipsychotics (FGAs)	Dopamine: D2 receptor antagonist	BPD: mood hyperreactivity and lability, harmful impulsivity; cognitive disturbances	**1°: D2 receptor antagonism** in mesolimbic, nigrostriatal, and tuberoinfundibular D pathways	Decreases D activity in the mesolimbic, nigrostriatal and tuberoinfundibular pathways	Reduces mood lability and hyperreactivity; decreases harmful, impulsive behavior and paranoid and split thinking	EPS, TD, **flattening of mood and dulling of cognitive activity, reward reduction,** hyperprolactinemia
Olanzapine—Evidence for efficacy in BPD of others in class: case study: ziprasidone IM experience: lurasidone little to none: iloperidone, iloperidone, perospirone, loxapine, sertindole, zotepine	Second-generation antipsychotics (SGAs)	Dopamine, serotonin: receptor antagonist (D2, 5-HT2)	"	**1°: D2, 5-HT2A receptor antagonism** in mesolimbic, nigrostriatal, and tuberoinfundibular pathways	Decreases D and increases 5-HT activity in the mesolimbic, mesocortical, nigrostriatal, and tubero-infundibular pathways, but functionally less in nigrostriatal pathway than FGAs; increases 5-HT activity	"	compared to FGAs: reduced EPS, TD, mood dulling, cognitive and reward reduction, and increased weight gain and metabolic syndrome
Aripiprazole	Atypical second-generation antipsychotic (ASGA)	Dopamine, serotonin: receptor partial agonist (D2, 5-HT1A)	BPD: same as FGA but appears to produce fewer extrapyramidal adverse reactions	**1°: D2, 5-HT1A receptor partial agonist and 5-HT2 antagonist** in mesolimbic, nigrostriatal, and tuberoinfundibular D and 5-HT2 pathways	"	Same as SGAs, but larger therapeutic effect sizes	"

Risperidone, clozapine others in class—little or no evidence of efficacy in personality disorders: asenapine, palliperidone	Second-generation antipsychotic (SGA)	Dopamine, serotonin, norepinephrine: receptor antagonist (D2, 5-HT2, NE α-2)	BPD and possibly AsPD: same as for SGAs; see Chapter 19 for more details, especially on clozapine	**1°: same as SGAs and NE autoreceptor antagonism 2°: clozapine: unknown**	Risperidone: same as SGAs and increases NE activity clozapine: unknown	"	risperidone: same as SGAs clozapine: potentially fatal neutropenia if not monitored
quetiapine	"	Multimodal: receptor antagonist (D2, 5-HT2) and reuptake inhibitor of NE (NET) (metabolite)	BPD: same as FGA but appears to produce fewer extrapyramidal adverse reactions	**1°: same as SGAs 2°: blocks NE reuptake**	Same as SGAs, plus increased NE activity	Same as SGAs, plus sedation at low doses but not at high doses	same as SGAs, but is abused, possibly because of stimulatory action of increased NE activity

Mood Stabilizers

Topiramate	Antiepileptic, mood stabilizer	Not defined	BPD: mood hyperreactivity and lability, harmful impulsivity	Affects voltage-gated sodium channels; high-voltage-activated calcium channels; GABA-A and ampa/kainate receptors; carbonic anhydrase isoenzymes	Inhibits glutamate activity	Reduces mood lability and hyperreactivity; decreases harmful, impulsive behavior	decreases weight gain caused by antipsychotics, dizziness, paraesthesia, somnolence, nausea, fatigue
Lamotrigene	"	Voltage-gated sodium ion channel blocker	"	Inhibits glutamate receptor activity		"	potential life-threatening skin reaction,

channel. Both actions hyperpolarize the postsynaptic neuron in a different manner but move it further from its trigger point of firing an action potential. A decrease in GABA activity has been demonstrated in subjects with BPD (Chapter 15). Some psychotropic drugs, especially mood stabilizers (Table 2.1), activate GABA receptors.

■   **SPECIFIC NEUROMODULATORS AND THEIR MECHANISMS OF ACTION**

Serotonin

As opposed to the ubiquitous distribution of glutamate and GABA neurons throughout the human brain, most neuromodulators arise in distinct loci in the brain stem and other sites and are distributed through specific pathways to their multiple receptor targets in cortical and subcortical structures. They are fewer in number than glutamate and GABA neurons by many orders of magnitude; each estimated at less than 1 million, a strikingly small number considering their importance in normal and disordered human brain function.

Serotonin (5-HT) neurons originate primarily in specific cell clusters in the brain stem termed the rostral and caudal raphé nuclei. The caudal cells project to the spinal cord where they appear to regulate pain pathways and innervate the gastrointestinal tract. The rostral neurons project widely to most cortical regions and subcortical structures in the brain. As noted, the effects of serotonin on brain function depend on the location and chemical actions of the 5–HT receptors to which it binds (Table 2.1). Fourteen distinct 5–HT receptors have now been described and grouped into seven families based on their specific mechanisms of action. The $5–HT_3$ family are ionotropic and gate Na^+ and K^+ channels that depolarize postsynaptic membranes and are thus excitatory. The other six families of 5–HT receptors are G-protein coupled metabotropic receptors that are either inhibitory (1, 5) or excitatory (4, 6, 7) by decreasing or increasing levels of cyclic adenosine monophosphate (cAMP), or excitatory (2) by stimulating phospholipase C thereby increasing levels of IP_3 and DAG. Effects of cAMP are mediated by specific pathways of protein kinase A (Taskén & Aandahl, 2004). The 5–HT receptors most often involved in the effects of psychiatric drugs (see following section) are 5-HT1A (inhibitory) and 5-HT2A (excitatory) receptors. As an aside, it is important to recognize that here the terms "excitatory" and "inhibitory" do not refer to their effects on brain function but on the postsynaptic neuron they innervate in the circuit, which may be either excitatory or inhibitory itself. The summation and integration of all of these receptor actions in neuronal circuits ultimately result in a network's action.

There is a significant amount of evidence derived from complementary research methods that demonstrate serotonergic dysfunction in BPD (Chapter 15).

Dopamine

Dopamine (D) neurons originate from two major cell clusters in the brain stem. Those from the substantia nigra, retrorubal, and ventral tegmental areas project primarily to the "limbic" structures such as the amygdala, lateral septum, and nucleus accumbens in the ventral striatum, basal forebrain, thalamus, and frontotemporal cortex. Cells from the hypothalamic cluster project in pathways to the autonomic regions in the lower brain stem and spinal cord. D neurons that project to the hypothalamus itself inhibit prolactin release. The D2 receptor antagonism of all first-generation antipsychotics (FGAs) and second-generation antipsychotics (SGAs) account for the elevation of prolactin levels observed as a result of treatment with most of the agents. Similar to acetylcholine and opposed to 5-HT and norepinephrine (NE), D neurons do not appear to project to the cerebellum.

At least five types of dopamine receptors have been described (Table 2.1). The D1 and D5 receptors are assigned to the D1-like family. These receptors are located mainly in the cerebral cortex and hippocampus and, like the metabotropic receptors of 5-HT, are coupled to G proteins that activate adenyl cyclase which converts adenosine triphosphate to cAMP, and both D1 and D5 receptors have a low affinity for antipsychotic drugs. The D2-like family of receptors, which includes D3 and D4 receptors, are found mainly on neurons in the caudate nucleus, putamen, nucleus accumbens, amygdala, and hippocampus. Compared to D1 and D5 receptors, there are relatively few D2, D3, and D4 receptors in the cerebral cortex. They *decrease* cAMP activity. The D2 receptor has the highest affinity for antipsychotic drugs of all dopamine receptors, and the level of affinity correlates inversely with the average daily dose required to achieve clinical efficacy.

As noted in Chapter 19, FGAs demonstrate a significant degree of D2 receptor affinity and antagonistic activity, whereas SGAs have a similar range of affinity for D2 receptors and a greater affinity for and antagonistic activity on 5-HT2A receptors. It is thought that one effect of the action of SGAs on 5-HT2A receptors is a decrease in extrapyramidal symptoms, which is a result of relative dopamine-induced activity of the nigrostriatal pathway. Dopamine dysregulation is involved in schizophrenia, attention deficit hyperactivity disorder (ADHD), drug addiction, most likely in the mesolimbic pathway, and Tourette's syndrome and Parkinson's disease in the nigostriatal pathway. SGAs, and to a lesser degree the FGAs, appear to be effective and important pharmacological agents in the treatment of some symptoms of BPD (Abraham & Calabrese, 2008; Feurino & Silk, 2010; Stoffers et al., 2010; Lieb et al., 2010) and schizoid personality disorder (Chapter 15).

Norepinephrine

NE neurons originate primarily in two clusters of cells located in the locus coeruleus and lateral tegmental area of the brain stem. Most arise in the nucleus coeruleus and project to the cortex, thalamus, hippocampus, and cerebellum. Those that arise in the lateral tegmentum innervate structures in the basal forebrain such as the hypothalamus and amygdala. There are few NE receptors in the striatum/nucleus accumbens. Three major NE receptors are present in the brain. Alpha 2 NE autoreceptors, located mainly on presynaptic terminals throughout the brain, inhibit the release of NE by inhibiting adenyl cyclase and thus cAMP levels (Table 2.1). Alpha 1 and beta 1, 2, and 3 NE receptors are all excitatory. Alpha 1 receptors increase IP_3 and CA^{++} levels by activating phospholipase C, and the three beta receptors increase cAMP levels by activating adenyl cyclase.

The main function of NE in the brain and body is to rapidly increase the state of alertness, arousal, and fight/flight activities. By its stimulatory effects on brain circuits and networks, NE enhances vigilance and other sensory activity, affective states, cognition, memory formation and retrieval, level of motor activity, and aggressive behavior and improves reaction time. Dysregulation of NE function is associated with some symptoms of BPD (Chapter 15), and with mood and anxiety disorders, posttraumatic stress disorder, and ADHD, all of which are more prevalent in individuals with BPD than in the general population.

Acetylcholine

Acetylcholine neurons in the brain arise from the brainstem neurotransmitter center and the basal forebrain. They are usually excitatory. The former project to the prefrontal cortex, basal forebrain, thalamus, hypothalamus, amygdala, and hippocampus. The basal forebrain site gives rise to the cells of the nucleus basalis of Meynert, the medial septal nucleus, and the diagonal band which appear to be associated with cognitive functions such as memory, reasoning, concentration, and decision-making. They are thought to be involved in Alzheimer's disease.

Acetylcholine has two types of receptors: nicotinic and muscarinic (Table 2.1). Nicotinic receptors are ionotropic; activating postsynaptic cells by gating (opening) Na^+, K^+, and Ca^{++} ion channels. Muscarinic receptors are metabotropic and also activating. They have five subtypes that are G protein-coupled and, like alpha 1 NE receptors, increase IP_3 and CA^{++} levels by activating phospholipase C.

Histamine

Compared to the two neurotransmitters and the four neuromodulators described, histamine neurons and their receptors in the brain may not appear to warrant the same level of attention in a selective overview focused on PDs. However, given their effects on core brain functions relevant to these disorders and their mechanisms of action that are similar to other neuromodulators, it seems justified to provide some basic information on histamine's effects on neurotransmission.

Histamine neurons arise solely from the tuberomammilary nucleus in the hypothalamus (Brown et al., 2001). They project to most regions of the brain but particularly to the ventral areas that include the hypothalamus, basal forebrain, and amygdala. As is the case with the other amine neuromodulators, histamine acts more slowly and has more lasting effects on postsynaptic polarization than do the neurotransmitters glutamate and GABA.

The postsynaptic H1 receptors (Table 2.1) are stimulatory and second messenger-linked to the activation of phospholipase C; therefore they increase levels of IP_3 and DAG. H2 receptors are also postsynaptic and stimulatory but are coupled to activation of adenyl cyclase and cANP. The H3 autoreceptors, unlike other amine modulators, mainly effect voltage-dependent Ca^{++} channels. Histamine also effects the NMDA glutamate receptor by its action at its polyamine binding site.

Histamine affects numerous brain functions that are mediated by its activity on brain circuits and pathways. For example, it is involved in sympathetic nervous system activation, secretion of stress-related hormones by the pituitary, the control of sleep-wake cycles, and appetite suppression. The weight gain observed with some psychoactive drugs is attributed to their H1 and H2 receptor antagonistic effects.

▪ MECHANISMS OF ACTION OF PSYCHOACTIVE AGENTS IN PDs

This material is intended to help the reader better understand the pathophysiology of PDs described later in this book. In addition, it will be useful in grasping the mechanisms by which certain psychoactive agents are thought to be effective in the pharmacological management of patients with some of the core symptoms of these disorders. This section describes the neurobiological profiles of the two major drug classes and the individual medications in these classes that have been found to be effective in the pharmacological treatment of individuals with certain PDs, especially BPD.

The first class of psychotropic drugs to be tested against a placebo in random controlled trials in subjects with PDs were the FGAs thiothixene (Brinkley et al., 1979) and haloperidol (Soloff et al., 1986). The mildly encouraging results of these studies rapidly resulted in further tests of SGAs and other classes of psychotropic agents (see Chapter 19). Early studies suggested that the SGAs appeared to help psychotic-like symptoms of BPD and a few other symptoms of the disorder and some symptoms of schizotypal personality disorder. Initially, a few selective serotonin reuptake inhibitors (SSRIs) were found helpful in the control of depressive and other emotional symptoms of BPD. These conclusions were incorporated into the guideline of the American Psychiatric Association (2001) on the treatment of BPD.

Subsequent studies have supported the efficacy of antipsychotic agents, mainly the SGAs, but not the SSRIs in the treatment of some core symptoms of BPD. However, antiepileptic drugs, now also referred to as mood stabilizers, have also been found to be efficacious in BPD even when the data from these studies are subjected to different statistical methods (Abraham & Calabrese, 2008; Feurino & Silk, 2010; Stoffers et al., 2010, Lieb et al., 2010). Therefore, we focus on the neurobiological basis of the psychopharmacological effects of these two classes of psychotherapeutic agents.

Antipsychotic Agents

The FGAs and SGAs have been demonstrated to bind avidly to and block the activity of D2 receptors. The therapeutic effects of these drugs on some symptoms of BPD (Table 2.2) are an important component of the evidence which supports the thesis that dopamine dysfunction occurs in pathways related to some D-dependent brain functions observed in the disorder (Friedel, 2004). The FGAs mainly block D2 receptors while the SGAs and other atypical antipsychotics are also 5-HT2A receptor antagonists. This is not surprising because 5-HT dysfunction has been shown repeatedly to be disturbed in subjects with BPD (see Chapter 15). These two mechanisms of action of the atypical antipsychotics suggest that these actions, and possibly others (Stahl, 2013, p. 130), present in SGAs are additive and may be synergistic. Although there are no reported head-to-head comparisons of a FGA with a SGA in subjects with BPD, it would appear that some data (e.g., the positive effects of clozapine in medication-resistant patients and clinical experience) seem to support patient-dependent differences in the efficacy of drugs in these classes (see Chapter 19).

The differences in receptor activity also provides a partial explanation of the differences in the side effects of FGAs and SGAs, as well as those between medications in each class. For example, with the exception of lurasidone, which one of the authors

(ROF) has found to be effective in a number of patients with BPD and which results in few side effects; most patients with BPD treated with SGAs experience significant weight gain, glucose intolerance, adverse metabolic effects on serum lipid levels, and elevation of prolactin levels. In subjects with schizophrenia treated with an SGA (especially aripiprazole), concomitant treatment with topiramate (see following section) results in a significant reduction in weight gain, fewer other critical side effects, and greater clinical improvement (Choi, 2015). These findings may be explained by the fact that, as a group, SGAs and their subclasses compared to FGAs appear to have a greater variety of other receptor actions in addition to their D2 and 5-HT2A antagonistic effects (Stahl, 2013, p. 130).

Mood Stabilizers

Two antiepileptics/mood stabilizers, topiramate, and lamotrigine (Table 2.2; Feurino & Silk, 2010; Stoffers et al., 2010; Lieb et al., 2010) appear to reduce symptoms in two dimensions of BPD. Topiramate was initially approved by the US Food and Drug Administration (FDA) as an antiepileptic in 1996 and Lamotrigine was approved for maintenance treatment of bipolar disorder in 2003. In BPD, these drugs have been found to reduce emotional lability and hyperreactivity, especially anger, a major criterion of the disorder, and aggressive-impulsivity (see Chapters 15 and 19). Consistent with their mechanisms of action (Table 2.2), they have not been found to ameliorate positive or negative cognitive symptoms in any mental disorder.

Topiramate

Topiramate, which has not yet been defined in the NbN nomenclature, appears to have multiple modes of action that include the voltage-gating of sodium channels, the high-voltage-activation of calcium channels, and effects on $GABA_A$ and AMPA/kainate receptors, all of which inhibit glutamate receptor activity (Table 2.2). Topiramate in conjunction with phentermine was also been approved by the FDA in 2012 for weight loss. Choi (2015) reviewed and evaluated by meta-analysis those studies that examined the combination of topiramate and atypical antipsychotics in patients with schizophrenia. The results suggest that the combination produces significantly less weight gain and other critical adverse side effects and is also more efficacious in clinical improvement. These findings were particularly robust when topiramate was combined with aripiprazole.

The most commonly occurring side effects of topiramate include dizziness, paraesthesia, somnolence, fatigue, and decreased mental alertness.

Lamotrigine

Lamotrigine is defined in the NbN as a voltage-gated sodium ion channel blocker; it inhibits glutamate receptor activity (Table 2.2). In acute bipolar depression its effects are primarily upon depressive cognitions and psychomotor slowing (Mitchell et al., 2013). As noted, in BPD there is evidence that lamotrigine, like topiramate, reduces emotional lability and hyperreactivity and aggressive-impulsivity (see Chapter 19). There is no substantial evidence that lamotrigine results in a synergistic effect when combined with an atypical antipsychotic agent in subjects with BPD.

Prescribing information for lamotrigine has a black box warning for potentially fatal skin reactions such as Stevens-Johnson syndrome with a prevalence estimated at 1 in 1,000. Common side effects include insomnia, myoclonic episodes, and congenital abnormalities such as cleft palate. The mechanisms of these effects are unknown.

■ **REFERENCES**

Abraham, P. F., & Calabrese, J. R. (2008 November). Evidenced-based pharmacologic treatment of borderline personality disorder: a shift from SSRIs to anticonvulsants and atypical antipsychotics?, *J Affect Disord 111*(1), 21–30. doi: 10.1016/j.jad.2008.01.024. Epub 2008 Mar 4. Review. PMID: 18304647.

Amaral, D. G. (2000). The anatomical organization of the central nervous system. In E. R. Kandel, J. H. Schwartz, & T. M. Jessell (Eds.), *Principles of neural science* (4th ed., pp. 317–336). New York: McGraw-Hill.

American Psychiatric Association. (2001). Practice guideline for the treatment of patients with borderline personality disorder. *Am J Psychiatry, 158*(Suppl.). https://www.ncbi.nlm.nih.gov/pubmed/11665545

Boy, F., Evans, C. J., Edden, R. A., Lawrence, A. D., Singh, K. D., Husain, M., & Sumner, P. (2006). Dorsolateral prefrontal gamma-aminobutyric acid in men predicts individual differences in rash impulsivity. *Biol Psychiatry, 70*, 866–872.

Björklund, A., & Dunnett, S. B. (2007). Dopamine neuron systems in the brain: an update. *Trends Neurosci, 30*(5), 194–202. Epub 2007 Apr 3. Review. PMID: 17408759.

Brinkley, J. R., Beitman, B. S., & Friedel, R. O. (1979). Low-dose neuroleptic regimens in the treatment of borderline patients. *Arch Gen Psychiatry, 36*, 319–326.

Brown, R. E., Stevens, D. R., & Haas, H. L. (2001). The physiology of brain histamine. *Prog Neurobiol, 63*, 637–672.

Choi, Y. J. (2015). Efficacy of adjunctive treatments added to olanzapine, or clozapine for weight control in patients with schizophrenia: a systematic review and meta-analysis. *Sci World J.* doi: 10.1155/2015/970730

Crick, F. C., & Koch C. (2005). What is the function of the claustrum. *Philos Trans R Soc Lond B Biol Sci, 360*(1458), 1271–1279. Review. PMID: 16147522.

Damasio, A. R. (1994). *Descartes' error: emotion, reason, and the human brain.* New York: Putnam Berkley Group.

Feurino, L. 3rd, & Silk, K. R. (2010). State of the art in the pharmacologic treatment of borderline personality disorder. *Curr Psychiatry Rep, 13*, 69–75.

Friedel, R. O. (2004). Dopamine dysfunction in borderline personality disorder: a hypothesis. *Neuropsychopharmacology, 29*(6), 1029–1039.

Hoerst, M., Weber-Fahr, W., Tunc-Sharka, N., Ruf, M., Bohus, M., Schmahl, C., & Ende, G. (2010). Correlation of glutamate levels in the anterior cingulate cortex with self-reported impulsivity in patients with borderline personality disorder. *Arch Gen Psychiatry, 67*, 946–954.

Kandel, E. R. (2000). The brain and behavior. In E. R. Kandel, J. H. Schwartz, & T. M. Jessell (Eds), *Principles of neural science* (4th ed., pp. 5–18). New York: McGraw-Hill.

Krause-Utz, A., Winter, D., Niedtfeld, I., & Schmahl, C. (2014). The latest neuroimaging findings in borderline personality disorder. *Curr Psychiatry Rep, 16*, 438.

LeDoux, J. (2002). *Synaptic self: how our brains become who we are.* New York: Viking Penguin.

LeDoux, J. E., & Pine, D. S. (2017). Using neuroscience to help understand fear and anxiety: a two-system framework. *Am J Psychiatry, 173*, 1083–1093.

Lieb, K., Völlm, B., Rücker, G., Timmer, A., & Stoffers, J. M. (2010). Pharmacotherapy for borderline personality disorder: cochrane systematic review of randomised trials. *Brit J Psychiatry, 196*, 4–12.

Mauchnik, J., & Schmahl, C. (2010). The latest neuroimaging findings in borderline personality disorder. *Curr Psychiatry Rep, 16*, 46–55.

Meares, R., Schore, A., & Melkonian, D. (2011). Is borderline disorder a particularly right hemispheric disorder? A study of P3a using single trial analysis. *Austral New Zeal J Psychiatry, 45*, 131–139.

Mitchell, P. B., Hadzi-Pavlovic, D., Evoniuk, G., Calabrese, J. R., & Bowden, C. L. (2013 Aug). A factor analytic study in bipolar depression, and response to lamotrigine. *CNS Spectr, 18*(4), 214–24. doi: 10.1017/S1092852913000291. Epub 2013 May 23. PMID: 23702258.

New, A. S., Goodman, M., Triebwasser, J., & Siever, L. J. (2008). Recent advances in the biological study of personality disorders. *Psychiatric Clin North Amer, 31*, 441–461.

Panksepp, J. (2005). Affective consciousness: core emotional feelings in animals and humans. *Cons Cog, 14*, 30–80.

Prossin, A. R., Love, T. M., Koeppe, R. A., Zubieta, J. K., & Silk, K. R. (2010). Dysregulation of regional endogenous opioid function in borderline personality disorder. *Am J Psychiatry, 167*, 925–933.

Seres, I., Unoka, Z., & Keri, S. (2009). The broken trust and cooperation in borderline personality disorder. *Neuroreport, 20*, 388–392.

Siegelbaum, S. A., Schwartz, J. H., & Kandel, E. R. (2000). Modulation of synaptic transmission: second messengers. In E. R. Kandel, J. H. Schwartz, & T. M. Jessell (Eds.), *Principles of Neural Science* (4th ed., pp. 229–252). New York: McGraw-Hill.

Silbersweig, D., Clarkin, J. F., Goldstein, M. (2007). Failure of frontolimbic inhibitory function in the context of negative emotion in borderline personality disorder. *Am J Psychiatry, 164*, 1832–1841.

Soloff, P. H., George, A., Nathan, R. S., Schulz, P. M., Ulrich, R. F., Perel, J. M. Progress in pharmacotherapy of borderline disorders. A double-blind study of amitriptyline, haloperidol, and placebo. *Arch Gen Psychiatry, 43*(7), 691–697.

Stahl, S. M. (2013). *Stahl's essential psychopharmacology: neuroscientific basis and practical applications* (4th ed.) New York: Cambridge University Press.

Stoffers, J., Völlm, B. A., Rücker, G., Timmer, A., & Lieb, K. (2010). Pharmacological interventions for borderline personality disorder. *Cochrane Database Syst Rev, 6*.

Taskén, K., & Aandahl, E. M. (2004). Localized effects of cAMP mediated by distinct routes of protein kinase A. *Physiol Rev, 84*, 137–167.

Whittle, S., Allen, N. B., Lubman, D. I., & Yucel, M. (2006). The neurobiological basis of temperament: towards a better understanding of psychopathology. *Neurosci Biobehav Rev, 30*, 511–525.

Zohar, J., Nutt, D., Kupfer, D., Moller, H. J., Yamawaki, S., Spedding, M., & Stahl, S. M. (2014). A proposal for an updated neuropsychopharmacological nomenclature. *Eur Neuropsychopharmacol, 24*, 1005–1014

Zohar, J., Stahl, S., Moller, H. J., Blier, P., Kupfer, D., Yamawaki, S., Uchida, H., Spedding, M., Goodwin, G. M., & Nutt, D. (2015). A review of the current nomenclature for psychotropic agents and an introduction to the neuroscience-based nomenclature. *Eur Neuropsychopharmacol, 25*, 2318–2325.

3 Genetics of Personality Disorders

■ TED REICHBORN-KJENNERUD
AND KENNETH S. KENDLER

In this chapter, we review the evidence for genetic contributions to the etiology of personality disorders (PDs) as defined by the *Diagnostic and Statistical Manual of Mental Disorders* (*DSM*; American Psychiatric Association, 2013). This diagnostic approach and some of the controversial issues associated with its development are briefly described in the first section. In the second section, we evaluate the evidence for genetic influence on *DSM* PDs from family and twin studies using quantitative genetic methods.

Studies that move beyond individual PDs, using multivariate quantitative models to explore the influence of shared genetic factors on the comorbidity between PDs and comorbidity between PDs and other clinical disorders are also reviewed, together with studies on the extent to which common genetic factors influence PDs and normal personality traits and PDs and pathological personality trait domains.

Stability of genetic influences on PDs over time are also examined.

In quantitative genetic studies of PDs, specific genetic variants are not addressed. This is the purpose of molecular genetic studies, which are reviewed in the third section. The fourth section deals with gene environment interplay, that is both gene-environment correlation and gene × environment interaction. In the final section, we discuss future directions in the exploration of genetic influences on PDs.

■ CLASSIFICATION OF PDs

A PD is defined, according to the American Psychiatric Association (2013), as an enduring pattern of inner experience and behavior that deviates markedly from the expectations of the individual's culture, is pervasive and inflexible, has an onset in adolescence or early adulthood, is stable over time, and leads to distress or impairment. The current official classification, in Section II (Diagnostic Criteria and Codes) of the fifth edition of the *DSM* (*DSM-5*), includes 10 categorical PD diagnoses grouped into three clusters based on descriptive similarities. Cluster A includes *paranoid, schizoid,* and *schizotypal* PDs. Individuals in this group often appears odd or eccentric. Cluster B includes *antisocial, borderline, histrionic,* and *narcissistic* and Cluster C, *avoidant, dependent,* and *obsessive–compulsive* PDs. Individuals with Cluster B PDs often appear dramatic, emotional, and erratic whereas individuals with disorders from Cluster C present with anxious and fearful traits.

Since PDs were introduced as diagnostic categories with the publication of the third edition of the *DSM* in 1980 (American Psychiatric Association, 1980), several controversial issues regarding their classification have remained unresolved (see Krueger, 2013; Widiger & Trull, 2007). Extensive co-occurrence between the *DSM* PDs has consistently been found in both clinical and community samples, challenging the validity of the classification. Co-occurrence is also extensive between PDs and other psychiatric disorders. Results from both clinical- and population-based studies indicate that stability over time and early age of onset, key features in the *DSM* definition, do not distinguish PDs from other mental disorders (Krueger, 2005). One of the most controversial and long-standing issues in the field of PD classification is whether PDs should be conceptualized dimensionally or as discrete categories (Krueger et al., 2007), and many authors have argued strongly in favor of a dimensional system of classification (e.g., Widiger & Simonsen, 2005).

The PD Workgroup for *DSM-5* proposed dramatic changes in PD classification and diagnosis (Krueger, 2013; Skodol, 2012), but it was not accepted by the American Psychiatric Association (Zachar et al., 2016). The fourth edition *DSM* (*DSM-IV*) categories, diagnoses, and criteria were therefore retained in their entirety in *DSM-5*, Section II (Diagnostic Criteria and Codes). An alternative model of classification, however, was included in Section III (Emerging Measures and Models). It defines PDs through impairments in functioning in the *self* and *interpersonal relationships* (Criterion A) and *pathological personality traits* (Criterion B). The latter is incorporated in a dimensional trait model of five broad higher-order domains—Negative Affectivity, Detachment, Antagonism, Disinhibition, and Psychoticism—as well as 25 lower-order trait facets (American Psychiatric Association, 2013). The dimensional trait model largely reflects maladaptive variants of normal personality trait dimensions, particularly the so-called Five Factor Model or "the Big Five" (Krueger et al., 2012; John, 1990).

◼ QUANTITATIVE GENETIC STUDIES

Family, adoption, and twin studies are used to quantify the relative contribution of genetic and environmental risk factors to the etiology of traits and disorders. Twin studies have been most widely used to examine the contribution of genetic variation to individual differences in risk for PDs. In the classical twin model, the total variance in a trait or disorder is accounted for by three latent variables: additive genetic, shared environment, and individual-specific environment. This implies that the genetic and environmental effects are not directly measured; that is, we do not know which specific genes or environmental factors influence the phenotype. Genetic effects are usually additive, so the independent effects of different alleles or loci act in an additive way to increase risk for the disorder or trait. While twin models can theoretically examine nonadditive effects (such as epistasis or dominance), the power to do this with realistic sample sizes is usually quite small (Neale et al., 1994). Heritability is defined as the proportion of variance in a trait or disorder in a population that can be attributed to genetic factors. Shared environment includes all environmental exposures that contribute to making the twins similar, and individual-specific or nonshared environment includes all environmental exposures that make them different, plus measurement error. Unreliability will therefore inflate estimates of nonshared environmental influences and deflate estimates of genetic influence. Methods that reduce measurement error will therefore yield higher estimates of the effects both of genetic and shared environmental factors.

Heritability of *DSM* PDs

Normal personality traits have consistently been found to be influenced by genetic factors with heritability estimates ranging from approximately 30% to 60%. A recent meta-analysis concluded that the heritability of personality, assessed across multiple measures and kinds of samples (twin, adoptee, and family) was .39 (.47 when using only twin studies; Vukasovic & Bratko, 2015).

Prior studies have suggested that familial/genetic factors contribute to the etiology of the three PDs making up the *DSM* Cluster A. Heritabilities are typically in the range of 35% to 60%. Only one population-based study of the *DSM-IV* Cluster A PDs, based on structured interviews, has been published. Heritability was estimated to be 21% for paranoid, 28% for schizotypal, and 26% for schizoid PD (Kendler et al., 2006). No shared environmental effects or sex differences were found. In a subsequent study, where unreliability of measurement was accounted for by using two measures differing in both time and mode of assessment, the estimated heritabilities were substantially higher (66% for paranoid, 55%–59% for schizoid, and 72% for schizotypal PD) in large part because of the relatively low reliability of these assessments (Kendler et al., 2007).

In Cluster B, the most widely studied PD using genetic epidemiological methods is antisocial PD. In a meta-analyses of 51 twin and adoption studies on antisocial behavior, based largely on records, self-report, and family report, Rhee and Waldman (2002) found that the variance could be most parsimoniously explained by additive genetic factors (32%), nonadditive genetic factors (9%), shared environmental factors (16%), and individual-specific environmental factors (43%). There were no significant differences in the magnitude of genetic and environmental influences for males and females. In a review of family studies on borderline PD, the disorder was found to aggregate in families (White et al., 2003), and a number of twin studies have demonstrated significant effect of genetic factors on this PD. However, heritability estimates vary considerably (ranging from 35% to 69%) probably due to methodological differences such as mode of measurement and sample ascertainment. Genetic effects are mostly additive, but one study found evidence for nonadditive influences on borderline PD (Distel et al., 2009). One study using self-report assessment of borderline personality traits found that heritability ranged from 31% at age 14 to 46% at age 24 (Bornovalova, Hicks, Iacono, & McGue, 2009), while another study calculated the heritability of borderline personality disorder (BPD) using a composite score from the Five Factor Model traits as 44% (Few et al., 2016). In a population-based twin study of all *DSM-IV* Cluster B PDs, heritability was estimated to be 38% for antisocial PD, 31% for histrionic PD, 24% for narcissistic PD, and 35% for borderline PD. No shared environmental influences or sex effects were found (Torgersen et al., 2008). Substantially higher heritability estimates were found using a different measurement at another point in time which made possible correction for measurement error: antisocial PD, 69%; BPD, 67%; narcissistic PD, 71%; histrionic PD, 63% (Torgersen et al., 2012). Higher heritability (51%–60%) has also been reported for borderline PD using different methods to control for unreliability of measurement (Distel et al., 2010; Kendler et al., 2011; Reichborn-Kjennerud et al., 2013).

All Cluster C PDs have also been found to be significantly influenced by genetic factors (Torgersen et al., 2000). In a population-based study of all *DSM-IV* Cluster C PDs, heritability estimates ranged from 27% for obsessive-compulsive PD to 35%

for avoidant PD. No shared environmental effects or sex differences were found (Reichborn-Kjennerud et al., 2007). In a subsequent study in the same data set where corrections for measurement error was performed, heritability was estimated to be 64% for avoidant and 66% for dependent PD (Gjerde et al., 2012), and in a longitudinal study over a 10-year period using structured interviews, the heritability corrected for measurement error was 67% for avoidant PD and 53% for obsessive-compulsive PD (Gjerde et al., 2015).

Taken together these studies indicate that all PDs are significantly influenced by genetic factors. Studies correcting for measurement error suggest that heritabilities probably exceed 50%.

Comorbidity between PDs

Multivariate analyses can examine the sources of comorbidity between PDs or between PDs and other psychiatric disorders, clarifying the degree to which they arise from genetic or familial sources (Krueger & Markon, 2006).

Cluster A PDs have been found to coaggregate in families of probands with schizophrenia (as described later), and substantial overlap in genetic liability has been indicated in twin studies (Kendler et al., 2006). Familial coaggregation has also been found for borderline PD and antisocial PD (White et al., 2003) and for borderline PD and all the other Cluster B PDs (Zanarini et al., 2009). A population-based twin study including all PDs within Cluster B indicated that borderline and antisocial PDs share genetic risk factors above and beyond those shared in common with the other Cluster B disorders (Torgersen et al., 2008). In a subsequent longitudinal study of antisocial and borderline PD in young adulthood, Reichborn-Kjennerud and coworkers (2015) found that genetic influences on both PDs remained completely stable over a 10 year period, The correlation between the genetic risk factors influencing antisocial and borderline PD was high (0.73). In another twin study of all Cluster C PDs, common genetic factors accounting for 83%, 48%, and 15% for, respectively, in avoidant, dependent, and obsessive–compulsive PD, suggesting that genetic effects for the latter PD appear to be relatively specific (Reichborn-Kjennerud et al., 2007a). Only one population-based multivariate twin study including all 10 *DSM-IV* PDs has been published (Kendler et al., 2008). The results indicated that the co-morbidity between the PDs can be explained by three genetic and three environmental factors. Figure 3.1 depicts the structure of the genetic factors. The first genetic factor (shown in red) had high loadings on PDs from all three clusters including paranoid, histrionic, borderline, narcissistic, dependent, and obsessive-compulsive PD. This factor probably reflects a broad vulnerability to PD pathology and/or negative emotionality and is related to genetic liability to the normal personality trait neuroticism. The second genetic factor (shown in green) was quite specific, with substantial loadings only on borderline and antisocial PD. This is consistent with the results from prior family and twin studies and suggests genetic liability to a broad phenotype for impulsive/aggressive behaviour. The third factor (shown in blue) identified had high loadings only on schizoid and avoidant PD. This might, in part, reflect genetic risk for schizophrenia spectrum pathology (see following sections). From the perspective of the Five Factor Model of normal personality, it reflects genetic liability for introversion. It is noteworthy that obsessive-compulsive PD had the highest disorder-specific genetic loading (shown in pink), which parallels prior findings that this PD shares little genetic and environmental

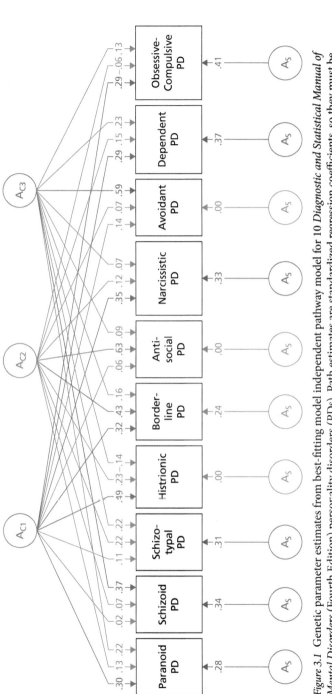

Figure 3.1 Genetic parameter estimates from best-fitting model independent pathway model for 10 *Diagnostic and Statistical Manual of Mental Disorders* (Fourth Edition) personality disorders (PDs). Path estimates are standardized regression coefficients, so they must be squared to obtain the proportion of variance accounted for in the dependent variable. A represents additive genetic effects. The subscripts C and S represent common factor and disorder-specific effects, respectively. The first, second, and third genetic common factors are indicated by the subscripts C1, C2, and C3. Paths with values of +0.28 or greater (which account for ≥8% of phenotypic variance) are colored with the first, second, and third common factors, indicated by red, green, and blue, respectively; the disorder-specific factors are shown in pink. Paths not exceeding the +0.28 or greater cutoff are depicted in black.

liability with the other Cluster C PDs. Taken together, these results indicate that genetic risk factors for *DSM-IV* PDs do not reflect the Cluster A, B, and C typology. However, this is reflected in the structure of the environmental risk factors, suggesting that the comorbidity of PDs within clusters is due to environmental experiences.

■ PDs AND COMMON MENTAL DISORDERS

A number of family and adoption studies have demonstrated increased risk for Cluster A PDs in relatives of schizophrenic and control probands. The results suggest that schizotypal PD has the closest familial relationship to schizophrenia, followed by paranoid and schizoid PD, and are consistent with the hypothesis that a common genetic risk factor for Cluster A PDs reflects—in the general population—the liability to schizophrenia (Kendler et al., 2006). The extended phenotype believed to reflect this genetic liability to schizophrenia is often described by the term "schizophrenia spectrum."

Family studies indicate that borderline PD and major depression share familial risk factors (Zanarini et al., 2009). Findings from a population-based twin study of major depression and dimensional representations of all 10 *DSM-IV* PDs indicate that all PDs were significantly associated with major depression in bivariate analyses. In a multivariate model including all 10 PDs, however, only paranoid PD from Cluster A, borderline PD from Cluster B, and avoidant PD from Cluster C and were independently and significantly associated with increased risk for major depression. All three PDs share genetic liability with major depression through a single common genetic factor. These results suggest that vulnerability to general PD pathology and major depression are likely to be closely related (Reichborn-Kjennerud et al., 2010).

Numerous family, adoption, and twin studies have demonstrated that antisocial PD, conduct disorder, and substance use disorders (often called externalizing disorders) share a common genetic liability. Results from a family twin study indicate that a highly heritable (80%) general vulnerability to all the externalizing disorders account for most of the familial resemblance. Disorder-specific vulnerabilities were detected for conduct disorder, alcohol dependence, and drug dependence but not for antisocial PD (Hicks et al., 2004). Similar results were found in a later twin/adoption study from the same group (Hicks et al., 2013).

Borderline PD is also closely related to the externalizing spectrum (Eaton et al., 2011) mostly through familial factors (Hudson et al., 2014). Shared genetic risk factors for substance use disorders and borderline PD have been found both in adolescence (Bornovalova et al., 2013) and in adulthood (Distel et al., 2012; Few et al., 2014). In a recent twin study, antisocial and borderline PD was found to be most closely related to alcohol use disorders (Long et al., 2017).

PDs in Cluster C often co-occur with anxiety disorders. There is an elevated risk for avoidant PD in relatives of individuals with social anxiety disorder (odds ratio of first-degree relative = 3.54; Isomura et al., 2015). In a cross-sectional study of females, avoidant PD and social phobia were found to be influenced by identical genetic factors, whereas the environmental factors influencing the two disorders appear to be uncorrelated. This suggests that an individual with high genetic liability will develop avoidant PD versus social phobia entirely as a result of environmental risk factors unique to each disorder (Reichborn-Kjennerud et al., 2007b). Analyses including also data from a follow-up assessment of the same sample 10 years later suggested that the relationship between social anxiety disorder and avoidant PD was best accounted for by a model with separate, although highly correlated ($r = .76$) and highly heritable ($r = .66$ and .71) latent factors for each disorders. The correlation between genetic risk factors influencing the two disorders was .84 (Torvik et al., 2016).

All studies mentioned have included a limited number of PDs and symptom disorders. To our knowledge, only one study has included all 10 PDs and a large number of common mental disorders using a genetically informative sample (Kendler et al., 2011). Four correlated underlying genetic factors reflecting shared genetic vulnerability were identified: internalizing and externalizing PDs and internalizing and externalizing axis I disorders. The internalizing PD factor had strong loadings on schizoid, schizotypal avoidant, and dependent PD in addition to dysthymia and social anxiety disorder. The externalizing PD factor influenced five PDs: histrionic, narcissistic, obsessive–compulsive, borderline, and paranoid. Antisocial PD was almost exclusively influenced by the other externalizing factor together with substance use disorders and conduct disorders. Although the four factors were correlated from .16 to .49 and some disorders had notable cross-loadings, a coherent underlying genetic structure that reflects two major dimensions emerged.

Stability Over Time

Longitudinal twin studies from adolescence to adulthood of antisocial behavior and antisocial PD traits (Lyons et al., 1995; Jacobson et al., 2002; Burt et al., 2007; Silberg et al., 2007) and borderline PD traits (Bornovalova et al., 2009), indicate that the contribution of genetic factors increases over time as new genetic effects are expressed, and the influence of shared environment decrease correspondingly, often approaching zero by early adulthood. Longitudinal studies of PDs in adulthood indicate that mean levels of most traits decrease substantially over time while rank order stability is generally moderate (Johnson et al., 2000; Nestadt et al., 2010; Hopwood et al., 2013; Morey & Hopwood, 2013). Very few studies have been performed on the stability of genetic and environmental influences on PDs in adulthood (Kendler et al., 2015; Reichborn-Kjennerud et al., 2015; Gjerde et al., 2015; Torvik et al., 2016). In a population-based sample, six PDs (two from each cluster) were studied over 10 years from early adulthood (mean age 28). The genetic correlations over time in the best fitting models were + 1.00 for paranoid, schizotypal, antisocial borderline, and avoidant PD, indicating no change in genetic influences over this period. Only for obsessive–compulsive PD was the genetic correlation estimated at less than unity although still quite high (0.72). Taken together these results suggest that the influence of genetic factors on PDs increase from adolescence to early adulthood and thereafter remain constant. The correlations between the environmental factors, on the other hand, were generally low, suggesting that most environmental risk factors were relatively transient in their effects on the symptoms of PD and appear to be the main source of change over time.

PDs and Normal Personality Traits

Several authors have argued that normal and abnormal personality can be considered within a single structural framework in which PDs represent extremes of normal personality traits. This implies that the etiological factors (genetic and environmental) underlying normal and pathological personality traits should be very similar if not identical. Two twin studies have investigated the relationship between borderline PD traits and normal personality. Distel et al. (2009) found that all genetic liability to borderline PD could be accounted for by genetic effects on normal personality traits as conceptualized in the Five Factor Model, and Kendler et al. (2011) found high genetic correlations between borderline personality traits and normal personality traits. We are aware of only one study including all 10 *DSM* PDs and the Big Five model of normal personality (Czajkowski et al., 2016). The results indicate that a moderate to substantial proportion of the genetic influence underlying *DSM* PDs are not shared with those underlying normal personality. This does not support the hypothesis that PDs can be best understood as extremes of normal personality.

PDs and Pathological Personality Traits

Pathological personality traits were introduced in *DSM-5* in 2013 as an alternative way to conceptualize PDs. Only a few quantitative studies using these measures have been published. South et al. (2016) found moderate genetic influences on pathological personality trait domains, ranging from 19% (antagonism in females) to 37% (detachment in males and females). The only clear evidence for sex differences was found for the antagonism scale, with greater genetic influences for men (26% vs. 19%). No evidence for shared environmental effects were detected.

In a study comparing genetic risk factors for the psychopathological trait domains and six *DSM* PDs measured concurrently (paranoid, schizotypal, antisocial, borderline, avoidant, obsessive–compulsive), the highest correlations between genetic risk factors for the PDs (measured as criteria counts) and one or more of the five domains exceeded 0.80 for paranoid, schizotypal, borderline, and avoidant. The highest genetic correlations with antisocial was 0.68 and with obsessive–compulsive 0.53 (Reichborn-Kjennerud et al., 2017). All genetic factors influencing the pathological personality trait domains in aggregate overlapped 100% for five of the six PDs measured (43% for obsessive–compulsive), indicating that these PDs appear to reflect—at the aggregate level—the same genetic factors as the pathological domains (Reichborn-Kjennerud et al., 2017).

In a twin study using short self-report measures of normative personality according to the Five Factor Model and pathological personality trait domains as defined by the alternative model of *DSM-5*, bivariate genetic and environmental correlations were calculated. As expected genetic correlations were high between neuroticism and negative affectivity (+0.83), conscientiousness and disinhibition (–0.83), extraversion and detachment (–0.76), and agreeableness and antagonism (–0.64). Openness had no substantial correlation with any of the pathological personality trait domains. Three of the domains (negative affectivity, detachment, and disinhibition) shared most of their genetic risk factors with genetic factors for normative personality traits in aggregate. Genetic factors underlying the other domains were shared to a lesser extent, suggesting that they might be located on separable continua rather than representing extremes of normative personality traits (Kendler et al., 2016).

■ MOLECULAR GENETIC STUDIES

The number of molecular genetic studies of PDs is limited compared to studies of other psychiatric disorders and normal personality traits and include mostly hypothesis-driven candidate gene association studies focusing on particular genes related to the neurotransmitter pathways, especially in the serotonergic and dopaminergic systems. No genome-wide association studies (GWAS) using categorical diagnoses and no studies using novel polygenic methods has been published. Although the number of genetic association studies are increasing exponentially, only a very small fraction of these positive results are replicated. Given the very small effect sizes expected for individual genetic variants on traits as complex as PDs, most of these candidate gene studies are likely very unpowered. We do, however, include these studies in our review for completeness although our judgement is that all of these results should be treated with considerable skepticism. Candidate gene studies on cluster A PDs build on results from quantitative genetic studies indicating that common genetic risk factors exist for schizophrenia, schizotypal PD and the other cluster A PDs. Consistent with the hypothesis that schizophrenia and related PDs are linked to dopaminergic dysfunction, Cluster A PDs have been found to be associated with a polymorphism in the gene coding for the dopamine-2 receptor (Rosmond et al., 2001). Significant associations have also been demonstrated between symptoms of schizotypy (schizotypal personality traits) and a number of other susceptibility genes for schizophrenia.

Significant associations with schizotypal personality traits have also been found in several studies with polymorphisms in the gene coding for catechol-O-methyltransferase (COMT), an enzyme involved in the degradation of catecholamines, and linked to the etiology of schizophrenia (Schurhoff et al., 2007).

Multiple lines of evidence suggest that dysfunction in the serotonin (5-HT) system is associated with impulsivity, aggression, affective liability, and suicide. Genes linked to the function of this neurotransmitter can, therefore, be considered possible candidate genes for borderline and antisocial PD. Kennedy and coworkers found that borderline PD was significantly associated with polymorphisms in the serotonin transporter gene (5-HTTLPR) and polymorphisms in the gene coding for the catabolic enzyme monoamine oxidase A (MAOA, involved in the regulation of biogenic amines like serotonin, norepinephrine, and dopamine), concluding that serotonin genes and their interaction may play a role in the susceptibility to borderline PD (Ni et al., 2009). Other groups have reported similar findings, including a significant relationship between the low-activity short 5-HTTLPR allele and both borderline and antisocial PD (Lyons-Ruth et al., 2007) and associations between polymorphisms in the MAOA gene and Cluster B PDs (Jacob et al., 2005). Tryptophan hydroxylase is the rate-limiting enzyme in the serotonin metabolic pathway. Two genes related to this enzyme (TPH1 and TPH2) have been associated with borderline PD (Wilson et al., 2009) and personality traits related to emotional instability as well as to Cluster B and C PDs (Gutknecht et al., 2007). Taken together, these findings provide some limited evidence that borderline and antisocial PDs, and possibly also the other Cluster B PDs are influenced by genes regulating the serotonergic system. However, two recent meta-analytic reviews of promising genes found no association between the polymorphisms TPH1, 5-HTTLPR, or Stin2 VNTR (all in the serotonin system) and borderline PD (Amad et al., 2014; Calati, Gressier, Balestri, & Serretti, 2013). One linkage study has been conducted for borderline PD features, indicating significant linkage on chromosome 9 (Distel et al., 2008). The finding has, however, not been replicated.

Variations in the COMT gene, previously implicated in the etiology of schizophrenia and Cluster A PDs, have also been found to contribute to genetic risk shared across a range of anxiety-related personality traits (Stein et al., 2005). Polymorphisms in the dopamine D3 receptor gene (DRD3) have been associated with symptoms of both avoidant and obsessive–compulsive PD. The association has been replicated for obsessive–compulsive symptoms, indicating that DRD3 may contribute to the development of obsessive–compulsive PD (Light et al., 2006).

To date, there have been very few molecular genetic studies of personality disorders that scan across the whole genome (i.e., GWAS). In the first GWAS of borderline PD, the authors found a promising association on chromosome 5 that corresponded to the SERINC5 gene; the SERINC5 protein is thought to play a role in myelination (Lubke et al., 2014). A GWAS study of adult antisocial behavior found that no associations with any polymorphisms reached statistical significance (Tielbeek et al., 2012); the closest associated gene, DYRK1A, is on chromosome 21 and is thought to play a role in mental retardation. Finally, a GWAS of antisocial PD found no significant associations, although the strongest associations were located at distinctive regions on chromosome 6 (Rautiainen et al., 2016).

■ GENE–ENVIRONMENT INTERPLAY

Since genes influence behavior, genetic factors can indirectly influence or control exposure to the environment. This is called *gene–environment correlation*. Genetic factors can also impact on an individual's sensitivity to the environment; that is, genetic factors may influence or alter an organism's responsiveness to environmental stressors. This is usually called *gene–environment interaction* (Rutter et al., 2006). Twin and adoption studies have provided much of the evidence for gene–environment correlations by demonstrating genetic influences for a number of measures of the environment. Overall, the evidence from twin and adoption studies suggests that gene–environment correlations are mediated by heritable personality traits and possibly PDs (Jaffee & Price, 2007; Rutter et al., 2006).

Gene–environment interaction between a number of different measures of adverse life events and genetic liability to antisocial behavior have been repeatedly demonstrated in a number of adoption and twin studies for several decades (Hicks et al., 2009; Rutter et al., 2006). Significant gene–environment interaction has also been demonstrated in quantitative studies of anxiety, mood, and schizophrenia spectrum disorders (Rutter et al., 2006) and well as normal personality (Krueger, South, Johnson, & Iacono, 2008; South, Krueger, Elkins, Iacono, & McGue, 2016). This work is only recently being extended to PDs (beyond antisocial behavior or antisocial PD per se). For instance, one study found lower heritability (24%) of borderline PD features among individuals with a history of exposure to sexual assault as compared to nonexposed individuals (47%; Distel, Middeldorp, Trull, Derom, Willemsen, & Boomsma, 2011).

Few studies of gene–environment correlation using measured genes and measured environments have been published. However, results confirm the existence of gene–environment correlation with measured genes in both the dopaminergic and serotonergic system and provide preliminary support for the finding that correlations are mediated by behavioral and personality characteristics (Jaffee & Price, 2007). Gene × environment interaction studies using identified susceptibility genes (i.e., measured G × E) rather than unmeasured latent genetic factors can provide more secure estimates (Rutter et al., 2006). Novel methods using aggregate genome-wide measures of genetic risk (Vinkhuyzen & Wray, 2015) have, however, not been applied to PDs.

Based on results from quantitative genetic studies showing gene–environment interaction for antisocial behavior, Caspi et al. (2002) studied the association between childhood maltreatment and a functional polymorphism in the promoter region of the MAOA gene on antisocial behavior, assessed through a range of categorical and dimensional measures using questionnaire and interview data plus official records. The results showed no main effect of the gene, a main effect for maltreatment, and a substantial and significant interaction between the gene and adversity. The maltreated children whose genotype conferred low levels of MAOA expression developed conduct disorder and antisocial personality more often than children with a high activity MAOA genotype (Caspi et al., 2002). Although several studies have replicated the original finding, some have not. In a recent meta-analysis, however, the original finding was confirmed. In addition, the findings were extended to include childhood (closer in time to the maltreatment), and the possibility of a spurious finding was ruled out by accounting for gene–environment correlation (Kim-Cohen et al., 2006). The interaction between MAOA and childhood maltreatment in the etiology of antisocial PD appears to be one of the few replicated findings in the molecular genetics of PDs.

Since the seminal Caspi et al. (2002) paper, several other measured G × E studies have been published. Many of these focus on borderline PD (for a review, see Amad et al., 2014), and while they investigate several different polymorphisms many focus on abuse as the environmental context. In a recent study, Hammen and colleagues (2015) found that the link between family functioning at age 15 and symptoms of borderline PD at age 20 was moderated by the oxytocin receptor gene. Carriers with the AA/AG genotypes had high levels of BPD symptoms only under negative family conditions but low levels of BPD symptoms under positive family conditions. Without replication, however, such results should be regarded as quite tentative.

■ FUTURE DIRECTIONS

Further studies in the genetics of PDs will certainly take several different directions. Using genetic-epidemiologic methods, future studies are likely to address a range of questions including (a) the developmental role of genes and environment in the etiology of PDs; (b) clarifying, using longitudinal studies, how the genetic and environmental factors predisposing to PDs relate to those of key clinical disorders such as major depression and alcohol use disorders interact; (c) evaluating more complex and complete etiologic models for PDs incorporating both genetic risks and a range of relevant environmental risks that will clarify the mediational pathways for genetic effects to PDs; and (d) clarification of the genetic and environmental structure of normative personality, abnormal personality traits, and PDs. Results from these latter studies may have an important impact on the ongoing debate about the best approach to the measurement and diagnosis of PDs that was a source of such controversy during *DSM-5*.

Two types of research questions are likely to arise using molecular genetic methods. The first is the search for individual risk variants using the methods of GWAS and potentially sequencing. Given the expected small effect sizes, current evidence suggests that, to have adequate power, such samples will require at least tens of thousands of subjects. Large-scale collaborative efforts—which would optimally agree on the best method of measurement—would likely be needed to accomplish this goal. The second is the use of polygenic risk scores (PRSs) that can be derived from such large-scale samples. Once generated from large samples, these PRSs can then be applied to other ethnically similar populations and provide a measure of genetic risk in any genotyped subjects in clinical or epidemiological samples. This will open up a range of research possibilities including further studies of gene–environment interaction and correlation and understanding how the PRS for PDs relate to those now well assessed for classical psychiatric disorders such as schizophrenia, autism, bipolar illness, and depression.

■ REFERENCES

Amad, A., Ramoz, N., Thomas, P., Jardri, R., & Gorwood, P. (2014). Genetics of borderline personality disorder: systematic review and proposal of an integrative model. *Neuroscience and Biobehav Rev, 40*, 6–19. doi:10.1016/j.neubiorev.2014.01.003

American Psychiatric Association. (1980). *Diagnostic and statistical manual of mental disorders*, 3rd ed. Washington, DC: American Psychiatric Association.

American Psychiatric Association. (2000). *Diagnostic and statistical manual of mental disorders*, 4th ed., text revision. Washington, DC: American Psychiatric Association.

American Psychiatric Association. (2013). *Diagnostic and statistical manual of mental disorders*, 5th ed. Arlington, VA: American Psychiatric Association.

Bornovalova, M. A., Hicks, B. M., Iacono, W. G., & McGue, M. (2009). Stability, change, and heritability of borderline personality disorder traits from adolescence to adulthood: a longitudinal twin study. *Dev Psychopathol, 21*, 1335–1353. doi:10.1017/S0954579409990186

Bornovalova, M. A., Hicks, B. M., Iacono, W. G., & McGue M. (2013). Longitudinal twin study of borderline personality disorder traits and substance use in adolescence: developmental change, reciprocal effects, and genetic and environmental influences. *Personal Disord, 4*, 23–32.

Burt, S. A., McGue, M., Carter, L. A., & Iacono, W. G. (2007). The different origins of stability and change in antisocial personality disorder symptoms. *Psychol Med, 37*, 27–38.

Calati, R., Gressier, F., Balestri, M., & Serretti, A. (2013). Genetic modulation of borderline personality disorder: systematic review and meta-analysis. *J Psychiatr Res, 47*, 1275–1287. doi:10.1016/j.jpsychires.2013.06.002

Caspi, A., McClay, J., Moffitt, T. E., Mill, J., Martin, J., Craig, I. W., . . . Poulton, R. (2002). Role of genotype in the cycle of violence in maltreated children. *Science, 297*, 851–854.

Distel, M. A., Hottenga, J. J., Trull, T. J., & Boomsma, D. I. (2008). Chromosome 9: linkage for borderline personality disorder features. *Psychiatr Gen, 18*, 302–307.

Distel, M. A., Middeldorp, C. M., Trull, T. J., Derom, C. A., Willemsen, G., & Boomsma, D. I. (2011). Life events and borderline personality features: the influence of gene-environment interaction and gene-environment correlation. *Psychol Med, 41*(4), 849–860. doi:10.1017/s0033291710001297

Distel, M. A., Rebollo-Mesa, I., Willemsen, G., Derom, C. A., Trull, T. J., Martin, N. G., & Boomsma, D. I. (2009). Familial resemblance of borderline personality disorder features: genetic or cultural transmission? *PLoS One, 4*, e5334.

Distel, M. A., Willemsen, G., Ligthart, L., Derom, C. A., Martin, N. G., Neale, M. C., Trull, T. J., & Boomsma, D. I. (2010). Genetic covariance structure of the four main features of borderline personality disorder. *J Personal Disord, 24*, 427–444.

Distel, M. A., Trull, T. J., de Moor, M. M., Vink, J. M., Geels, L. M., van Beek, J. H., . . . Boomsma, D. I. (2012). Borderline personality traits and substance use: genetic factors underlie the association with smoking and ever use of cannabis, but not with high alcohol consumption. *J Personal Disord, 26*, 867–879.

Eaton, N. R., Krueger, R. F., Keyes, K. M., Skodol, A. E., Markon, K. E., Grant, B. F., & Hasin, D. S. (2011). Borderline personality disorder co-morbidity: relationship to the internalizing-externalizing structure of common mental disorders. *Psychol Med, 41*, 1041–1050.

Few, L. R., Grant, J. D., Trull, T. J., Statham, D. J., Martin, N. G., Lynskey, M. T., & Agrawal, A. (2014). Genetic variation in personality traits explains genetic overlap between borderline personality features and substance use disorders. *Addiction, 109*, 2118–2127. doi:101111/add.12690

Few, L. R., Miller, J. D., Grant, J. D., Maples, J., Trull, T. J., Nelson, E. C., . . . Agrawal, A. (2016). Trait-based assessment of borderline personality disorder using the NEO Five-Factor Inventory: Phenotypic and genetic support. *Psychol Assess, 28*, 39–50.

Gjerde, L. C., Czajkowski, N., Røysamb, E., Orstavik, R. E., Knudsen, G. P., Ostby, K., . . . Reichborn-Kjennerud, T. (2012). The heritability of avoidant and dependent personality disorder assessed by personal interview and questionnaire. *Acta Psychiatr Scand, 126*, 448–457.

Gjerde, L. C., Czajkowski, N., Røysamb, E., Ystrom, E., Tambs, K., Aggen, S. H., . . . Knudsen, G. P. (2015). A longitudinal, population-based twin study of avoidant and obsessive–compulsive personality disorder traits from early to middle adulthood. *Psychol Med, 45*, 3539–3548.

Gutknecht, L., Jacob C, Strobel A, Kriegebaum, C., Müller, J., Zeng, Y., . . . Lesch, K. P. (2007). Tryptophan hydroxylase-2 gene variation influences personality traits and disorders related to emotional dysregulation. *Int J Neuropsychopharmacol, 10*, 309–320.

Hammen, C., Bower, J. E., & Cole, S. W. (2015). Oxytocin receptor gene variation and differential susceptibility to family environment in predicting youth borderline symptoms. *J Personal Disord, 29*, 177–192. doi:10.1521/pedi_2014_28_152

Hicks, B. M., Foster, K. T., Iacono, W. G., & McGue, M. (2013). Genetic and environmental influences on the familial transmission of externalizing disorders in adoptive and twin offspring. *JAMA Psychiatry, 70*, 1076–1083.

Hicks, B. M., Krueger, R. F., Iacono, W. G., Mcgue, M., & Patrick, C. J. (2004). Family transmission and heritability of externalizing disorders—a twin-family study. *Arch Gen Psychiatry, 61*, 922–928.

Hicks, B. M., South, S. C., Dirago, A. C., Iacono, W. G., & Mcgue, M. (2009). Environmental adversity and increasing genetic risk for externalizing disorders. *Arch Gen Psychiatry, 66*, 640–648.

Hopwood, C. J., Morey, L. C., Donnellan, M. B., Samuel, D. B., Grilo, C. M., McGlashan, T. H., . . . Skodol, A. E. (2013). Ten-year rank-order stability of personality traits and disorders in a clinical sample. *J Per, 81*, 335–344.

Hudson, J. I., Zanarini, M. C., Mitchell, K. S., Choi-Kain, L. W., & Gunderson, J. G. (2014). The contribution of familial internalizing and externalizing liability factors to borderline personality disorder. *Psychol Med, 44*, 1–11.

Isomura, K., Boman, M., Rück, C., Serlachius, E., Larsson, H., Lichtenstein, P., & Mataix-Cols, D. (2015). Population-based, multi-generational family clustering study of social anxiety disorder and avoidant personality disorder. *Psychol Med, 45*(8), 1581–1589. doi:10.1017/S0033291714002116

Jacob, C. P., Muller, J., Schmidt M, Hohenberger, K., Gutknecht, L., Reif, A., . . . Lesch, K. P. (2005). Cluster B personality disorders are associated with allelic variation of monoamine oxidase a activity. *Neuropsychopharmacology, 30*, 1711–1718.

Jacobson, K. C., Prescott, C. A., & Kendler, K. S. (2002). Sex differences in the genetic and environmental influences on the development of antisocial behavior. *Dev Psychopathol, 14*, 395–416.

Jaffee, S. R., & Price, T. S. (2007). Gene-environment correlations: a review of the evidence and implications for prevention of mental illness. *Mol Psychiatry, 12*, 432–442.

John, O. P. (1990). The "Big Five" factor taxonomy: dimensions of personality in the natural language and in questionnaires. In L. Pervin (Ed.), *Handbook of Personality Theory and Research* (pp. 66–100). New York: Guilford Press.

Johnson, J. G, Cohen, P., Kasen, S., Skodol, A. E., Hamagami, F., & Brook, J. S. (2000). Age-related change in personality disorder trait levels between early adolescence and adulthood: a community-based longitudinal investigation. *Acta Psychiatr Scand, 102*, 265–275.

Kendler, K. S., Czajkowski, N., Tambs K, Torgersen, S., Aggen, S. H., Neale, M. C., & Reichborn-Kjennerud, T. (2006). Dimensional representations of DSM-IV Cluster A personality disorders in a population-based sample of Norwegian twins: a multivariate study. *Psychol Med, 36*, 1583–1591.

Kendler, K. S., Myers, J., Torgersen, S., Neale, M. C., & Reichborn-Kjennerud, T. (2007). The heritability of Cluster A personality disorders assessed by both personal interview and questionnaire. *Psychol Med, 37*, 655–665.

Kendler, K. S., Aggen SH, Czajkowski N, Røysamb, E., Tambs, K., Torgersen, S., Neale, M. C., & Reichborn-Kjennerud, T. (2008). The structure of genetic and environmental risk factors for DSM-IV personality disorders—a multivariate twin study. *Arch Gen Psychiatry, 65*, 1438–1446.

Kendler, K. S., Aggen, S. H., Knudsen, G. P., Røysamb, E., Neale, M. C., & Reichborn-Kjennerud, T. (2011). The structure of genetic and environmental risk factors for syndromal and subsyndromal common DSM-IV axis I and all axis II disorders. *Am J Psychiatry, 168*, 29–39.

Kendler, K. S., Myers, J., & Reichborn-Kjennerud, T. (2011). Borderline personality disorder traits and their relationship with dimensions of normative personality: a web-based cohort and twin study. *Acta Psychiatr Scand, 123*, 349–359.

Kendler, K. S., Aggen, S. H., Neale, M. C., Knudsen, G. P., Krueger, R. F., Tambs, K, . . . Reichborn-Kjennerud, T. (2015). A longitudinal twin study of cluster A personality disorders. *Psychol Med, 45*, 1531–1538.

Kendler, K. S., Aggen, S. H., Gillespie, N., Neale, M. C., Knudsen, G. P., Krueger, R. F., . . . Reichborn-Kjennerud, T. (2016). The genetic and environmental sources of resemblance between normative personality and personality disorder traits. *J Personal Disord, 20*, 1–15.

Kim-Cohen, J., Caspi, A., Taylor, A., Williams, B., Newcombe, R., Craig, I. W., & Moffitt, T. E. (2006). MAOA, maltreatment, and gene-environment interaction predicting children's mental health: new evidence and a meta-analysis. *Mol Psychiatry, 11*, 903–913.

Krueger, R. F. (2005). Continuity of axes I and II: toward a unified model of personality, personality disorders, and clinical disorders. *J Personal Disord, 19*, 233–261.

Krueger, R. F. (2013). Personality disorders are the vanguard of the post-DSM-5.0 era. *Personal Disord, 4*, 355–362. doi:10.1037/per0000028

Krueger, R. F., & Markon, K. E. (2006). Reinterpreting comorbidity: a model-based approach to understanding and classifying psychopathology. *Annu Rev Clin Psychol, 2*, 111–133.

Krueger, R. F., Skodol, A. E., Livesley, W. J., Shrout, P. E., & Huang, Y. (2007). Synthesizing dimensional and categorical approaches to personality disorders: refining the research agenda for DSM-V axis II. *Int J Methods Psychiatr Res, 16*(Suppl. 1), S65–S73.

Krueger, R. F, South, S. C., Johnson, W., & Iacono, W. (2008). The heritability of personality is not always 50%: gene-environment interactions and correlations between personality and parenting. *J Per, 76*, 1485–1522.

Krueger, R. F., Derringer, J., Markon, K. E., Watson, D., & Skodol, A. E. (2012). Initial construction of a maladaptive personality trait model and inventory for DSM-5. *Psychol Med*, *42*, 1879–1890.

Light, K. J., Joyce, P. R., Luty, S. E., Mulder, R. T., Frampton, C. M., Joyce, L. R., . . . Kennedy, M. A. (2006). Preliminary evidence for an association between a dopamine D3 receptor gene variant and obsessive–compulsive personality disorder in patients with major depression. *Am J Med Genet B Neuropsychiatr Genet*, *141*, 409–413.

Long, E. C., Aggen, S. H., Neale MC, Knudsen, G. P., Krueger, R. F., South, S. C., . . . Reichborn-Kjennerud, T. (2017). The association between personality disorders with alcohol use and misuse: A population-based twin study. *Drug and Alcohol Depend*, *7*, 171–180.

Lubke, G. H., Laurin, C., Amin, N., Hottenga, J. J., Willemsen, G., van Grootheest, G., . . . Boomsma, D. I. (2014). Genome-wide analyses of borderline personality features. *Mol Psychiatry*, *19*, 923–929.

Lyons, M. J., True, W. R., Eisen, S. A., Goldberg, J., Meyer, J. M., Faraone, S. V., . . . Tsuang, M. T. (1995). Differential heritability of adult and juvenile antisocial traits. *Arch Gen Psychiatry*, *52*, 906–915.

Lyons-Ruth, K., Holmes, B. M., Sasvari-Szekely, M., Ronai, Z., Nemoda, Z., & Pauls, D. (2007). Serotonin transporter polymorphism and borderline or antisocial traits among low-income young adults. *Psychiatr Gen*, *17*, 339–343.

Morey, L. C., & Hopwood, C. J. (2013). Stability and change in personality disorders. *Annu Rev Clin Psychol*, *9*, 499–528.

Neale, M. C., Eaves, L. J., & Kendler, K. S. (1994). The power of the classical twin study to resolve variation in threshold traits. *Behav Genet*, *24*, 239–258.

Nestadt, G., Di, C., Samuels, J. F., Bienvenu, O. J., Reti, I. M., Costa, P., . . . Bandeen-Roche, K. (2010). The stability of DSM personality disorders over twelve to eighteen years. *J Psychiatr Res*, *44*, 1–7.

Ni, X., Chan, D., Chan, K., McMain, S., & Kennedy, J. L. (2009). Serotonin genes and gene-gene interactions in borderline personality disorder in a matched case-control study. *Prog Neuropharmacol Biol Psychiatry*, *33*, 128–133.

Rautiainen, M. R., Paunio, T., Repo-Tiihonen, E., Virkkunen, M., Ollila, H. M., Sulkava, S., . . . Tiihonen, J. (2016). Genome-wide association study of antisocial personality disorder. *Transl Psychiatry*, *6*, e883. doi:10.1038/tp.2016.155

Reichborn-Kjennerud, T., Czajkowski, N., Neale, M. C., Orstavik, R. E., Torgersen, S., Tambs, K., . . . Kendler, K. S. (2007a). Genetic and environmental influences on dimensional representations of DSM-IV cluster C personality disorders: a population-based multivariate twin study. *Psychol Med*, *37*, 645–653.

Reichborn-Kjennerud, T., Czajkowski, N., Torgersen, S., Neale, M. C., Ørstavik, R. E., Tambs, K., & Kendler, K. S. (2007b). The relationship between avoidant personality disorder and social phobia: a population-based twin study. *Am J Psychiatry*, *164*, 1722–1728.

Reichborn-Kjennerud, T., Czajkowski, N., Røysamb, E., Ørstavik, R. E., Neale, M. C., Torgersen, S., & Kendler, K. S. (2010). Major depression and dimensional representations of DSM-IV personality disorders: a population-based twin study. *Psychol Med*, *40*, 1475–1484

Reichborn-Kjennerud, T., Ystrom, E., Neale, M. C., Aggen, S. H., Mazzeo, S. E., Knudsen, G. P., . . . Kendler, K. S. (2013). Structure of genetic and environmental risk factors for symptoms of DSM-IV borderline personality disorder. *JAMA Psychiatry*, *70*, 1206–1214.

Reichborn-Kjennerud, T., Czajkowski, N., Ystrøm, E., Ørstavik, R., Aggen, S. H., Tambs, K., . . . Kendler, K. S. (2015). A longitudinal twin study of borderline and antisocial personality disorder traits in early to middle adulthood. *Psychol Med*, *45*, 3121–31.

Reichborn-Kjennerud, T., Krueger, R. F., Ystrom, E., Torvik, F. A., Rosenström, T. H., Aggen, S. H., . . . Czajkowski, N. O. (2017). Do DSM-5 Section II personality disorders and Section III personality trait domains reflect the same genetic and environmental risk factors? *Psychol Med*, *47*, 2205–2215.

Rhee, S. H., & Waldman, I. D. (2002). Genetic and environmental influences on antisocial behavior: a meta-analysis of twin and adoption studies. *Psychol Bull*, *128*, 490–529.

Rosmond, R., Rankinen, T., Chagnon, M., Pérusse, L., Chagnon, Y. C., Bouchard, C., & Björntorp, P. (2001). Polymorphism in exon 6 of the dopamine D-2 receptor gene (DRD2) is associated with elevated blood pressure and personality disorders in men. *J Hum Hyperten*, *15*, 553–558.

Rutter, M., Moffitt, T. E., & Caspi, A. (2006). Gene-environment interplay and psychopathology: multiple varieties but real effects. *J Child Psychol Psychiatry*, *47*, 226–261.

Schurhoff, F., Szoke, A., Chevalier, F., Roy, I., Méary, A., Bellivier, F., . . . Leboyer, M. (2007). Schizotypal dimensions: an intermediate phenotype associated with the COMT high activity allele. *Am J Med Genet B Neuropsychiatr Genet*, *144*, 64–68.

Silberg, J. L., Rutter, M., Tracy, K., Maes, H. H., & Eaves, L. (2007). Etiological heterogeneity in the development of antisocial behavior: the Virginia Twin Study of Adolescent Behavioral Development and the Young Adult Follow-Up. *Psychol Med*, *37*, 1193–1202.

Skodol, A. E. (2012). Personality disorders in DSM-5. *Annu Rev Clin Psychol*, *8*, 317–344.

South, S. C., Krueger, R. F., Elkins, I. J., Iacono, W. G., & McGue, M. (2016). Romantic relationship satisfaction moderates the etiology of adult personality. *Behav Genet*, *46*, 124–142.

South, S. C., Krueger, R. F., Knudsen, G. P., Ystrom, E., Czajkowski, N., Aggen, S. H., . . . Reichborn-Kjennerud, T. (2016). A population based twin study of DSM-5 maladaptive personality domains. *Personal Disord*. http://dx.doi.org/10.1037/per0000220

Stein, M. B., Fallin, M. D., Schork, N. J., & Gelernter, J. (2005). COMT polymorphisms and anxiety-related personality traits. *Neuropsychopharmacology*, *30*, 2092–2102.

Tielbeek, J. J., Medland, S. E., Benyamin, B., Byrne, E. M., Heath, A. C., Madden, P. A. F., . . . Verweij, K. J. H. (2012). Unraveling the genetic etiology of adult antisocial behavior: a genome-wide association study. *PLoS ONE*, *7*, e45086. doi: 10.1371/journal.pone.0045086

Torgersen, S., Czajkowski N, Jacobson K, Reichborn-Kjennerud, T., Røysamb, E., Neale, M. C., & Kendler, K. S. (2008). Dimensional representations of DSM-IV Cluster B personality disorders in a population-based sample of Norwegian twins: a multivariate study. *Psychol Med*, *38*, 1617–1625.

Torgersen, S., Lygren, S., Oien, P. A., Skre, I., Onstad, S., Edvardsen, J., Tambs, K., & Kringlen, E. (2000). A twin study of personality disorders. *Compr Psychiatry*, *41*, 416–425.

Torgersen, S., Myers, J., Reichborn-Kjennerud, T., Røysamb, E., Kubarych, T. S., & Kendler, K. S. (2012). The heritability of Cluster B personality disorders assessed both by personal interview and questionnaire. *J Personal Disord*, *26*, 848–866.

Torvik, F. A., Welander-Vatn, A., Ystrom, E., Knudsen, G. P., Czajkowski, N., Kendler, K. S., & Reichborn-Kjennerud, T. (2016). Longitudinal associations between social anxiety disorder and avoidant personality disorder: a twin study. *J Abnorm Psychol*, *125*(1), 114–124.

Vukasović, T., & Bratko, D. (2015). Heritability of personality: a meta-analysis of behavior genetic studies. *Psychol Bull*, *141*(4), 769–785.

Vinkhuyzen, A. A. E., & Wray, N. R. (2015). Novel directions for G x E analyses in psychiatry. *Epidemiol Psychiatr Sci*, *24*, 12–19.

White, C. N., Gunderson, J. G., Zanarini, M. C., & Hudson, J. I. (2003). Family studies of borderline personality disorder: a review. *Harv Rev Psychiatry, 11,*

Widiger, T. A., & Simonsen, E. (2005). Alternative dimensional models of personality disorder: finding a common ground. *J Personal Disord, 19,* 110–130. 8–19.

Widiger, T. A., & Trull, T. J. (2007). Plate tectonics in the classification of personality disorder: shifting to a dimensional model. *Am Psychol, 62,* 71–83.

Wilson, S. T., Stanley, B., Brent, D. A., Oquendo, M. A., Huang, Y. Y., & Mann, J. J. (2009). The tryptophan hydroxylase-1 A218C polymorphism is associated with diagnosis, but not suicidal behavior, in borderline personality disorder. *Am J Med Genet B, 150,* 202–208.

Zachar, P., Krueger, R. F., & Kendler, K. S. (2016). Personality disorder in DSM-5: an oral history. *Psychol Med, 46,* 1–10.

Zanarini, M. C., Barison, L. K., Frankenburg, F. R., Reich, B., & Hudson, J. I. (2009). Family history study of the familial coaggregation of borderline personality disorder with axis I and nonborderline dramatic cluster axis II disorders. *J Personal Disord, 23,* 357–369.

4 Cognitive Neuroscience Approaches to Personality Disorders

■ ANDREW POPPE AND
ANGUS W. MACDONALD III

■ RATIONALE FOR COGNITIVE NEUROSCIENCE OF PERSONALITY DISORDERS: OPENING THE BLACK BOX

Cognitive neuroscience and neuroimaging may not be the first methods researchers turn to when attempting to understand personality disorders. As other chapters in this volume demonstrate, a great deal of knowledge about personality disorders can be ascertained by examining the epidemiology of these forms of psychopathology, the covariation of symptoms, and their impact on day-to-day functioning and behavior. These techniques often treat the brain as the proverbial black box: the inputs are stimuli and events, and the outputs are adaptive or maladaptive responses. What connects these two streams of information, however, remains shrouded in mystery.

Cognitive neuroscience techniques are designed to pry open this black box and allow us to peer inside to understand the psychological and neural mechanisms that connect stimulus to response. But in so doing, this approach serves a number of additional purposes. One important role for cognitive neuroscience is to serve as a **translational link** between macroscopic and person-level variables, such as symptoms and functioning, and more molecular levels of analysis, such as genes, neurotransmitters, and small circuit functioning. If our imaging measures were sufficiently precise, then the signal of a genetic polymorphism might be more strongly related to brain functions than to a psychological symptom as symptom manifestation may depend on more extraneous factors.

In addition to bridging the molecular and macroscopic levels of analysis, cognitive neuroscience provides a **bridge between species.** Specifically, cognitive neuroscience efforts may link animal and human models of disorder. One of the great limitations of pseudo-experimental designs is the challenge of establishing causation between a particular gene or event and the onset of symptoms. To overcome this limitation in human studies, many researchers use animal models. Mice, rats, nonhuman primates, and a host of other model organisms have been recruited to examine how direct manipulations of these systems contribute to symptom development. The weakness of this approach is that animals' symptoms rarely look like human symptoms (and do not, to date, include verbal self-reports attesting to emotional turmoil or aggression). Thus this type of translational work relies upon arguing by analogy, for example this animal's behavior is *like* the isolative behavior of avoidant people, or this behavior is *analogous to* interpersonal aggression. These arguments by analogy are considerably strengthened if evidence can demonstrate similar patterns of behavior on similar tasks in human subjects. Such points are strengthened further if homologous brain regions are involved in both humans and animals during the analog behavior. Finally, showing a difference in functioning or structure in the same brain region in personality disorder patients tightens this kind of argument further.

Another advantage of cognitive neuroscience approaches is that they generally involve testing hypotheses about **mechanisms**. A psychological mechanism is a hypothetical entity that governs the response elicited from a particular class of stimuli. For example, operant conditioning stipulates a psychological mechanism whereby a conditioned stimulus will evoke a conditioned response. A more modern variant of this mechanism suggests that reward expectation builds through the application of temporal difference error learning, such that the conditioned stimulus prompts an expectation in the organism that relies on subcortical dopamine (Tobler, Fiorillo, & Schultz, 2005). Abnormal functioning of learning mechanisms such as these (or abnormalities in cognitive mechanisms underlying other processes such as maintaining context information and interpreting others' facial expressions) is an example of a mechanism that may characterize a particular personality disorder. This same dysfunction may also be present in other psychiatric or neurological disorders. As we move toward understanding the relations between mechanistic failures and personality disorders, researchers can utilize cognitive neuroscience to determine the extent to which specific mechanisms are unique (or not unique) to disorders that may appear similar on the surface.

Closely linked to the technique of identifying and isolating particular psychological and neural mechanisms is the opportunity to **detect and identify specific treatment targets**, whether those are pharmacological or psychosocial. These mechanisms represent critical spotlights in the search for more targeted, effective treatments. Although many current pharmaceuticals prescribed for personality disorders are the result of old fashioned trial-and-error pharmacology, drug development is increasingly rational. In rational drug development a treatment target is identified a priori and medicines are tailored to change functioning at the target. Similarly, psychosocial treatments are explicitly designed around a particular theory of psychological mechanisms that have led to a particular disorder. In both cases, the intermediate level of analysis provided by cognitive neuroscience techniques facilitates this work by highlighting mechanisms impaired in the target population and working to modify the brain through that mechanism. One analogous example is the development of L-Dopa as a treatment for Parkinson's disease shortly after it was discovered that patients with the disease had too little dopamine in the substantia nigra.

At the same time, it is important to keep in mind that cognitive neuroscience approaches to personality disorders are **not providing a more true** account of personality or its causes than psychosocial levels of analysis. Many students, as well as many experts in the field who should know better, have a natural reductionist bias. This bias, which some might even call a fetish, leads us to believe that understanding the constituent brain mechanisms underlying a pattern of behavior is closer to the truth of that behavior. Although this chapter discusses many techniques for understanding brain-behavior relationships, we do not claim that these are "higher" truths than those discerned by other important methods, and in most cases the findings from cognitive neuroscience remain more tentative and harder to replicate than the findings of other methodologies (e.g., behavioral). We do believe, however, that a full account of personality disorders will necessarily involve understanding the neural systems related to these dysfunctional patterns of behavior.

This chapter unpacks this claim by examining structural aspects of the brain. We then review the diversity of functional brain imaging techniques. We use the example of schizotypal personality disorder (SPD) to illustrate the application and findings from these techniques. There are a number of important orienting concepts for the cognitive neuroscience approach. Therefore, before diving into specific applications, we begin with fundamental considerations involved in choosing a lens for examining the brain.

■ **FUNDAMENTAL CONSIDERATIONS FOR THE COGNITIVE NEUROSCIENTIST**

To Activate or Not to Activate

One of the most important decisions that shapes the techniques a cognitive neuroscientist will employ is whether testing a hypothesis requires perturbing the brain or not. Many hypotheses about differences in various brain structures and circuits may not depend on activating the brain. For example, a person's brain volume is not expected to change when processing a particular stimulus or producing a particular response. However, this volume still may reflect an impairment—for example a thinner or smaller region that is insufficiently developed—or an augmentation, perhaps reflecting greater use (Maguire et al., 2000; Münte, Altenmüller, & Jäncke, 2002). Either way, the extent to which the regional volume is causally related to a disorder is thought to lie in its potential capacity, or lack of capacity, to influence thinking, affect, and behavior. In effect, its relevance to a disorder lies in its potential to engage appropriately to particular stimuli or to produce particular responses.

A number of functional techniques are also thought to measure the potential of various brain structures and do not involve activating the brain. As we describe here, techniques that measure functional connectivity using functional magnetic resonance imaging (MRI) and electroencephalography (EEG) may focus on brain activity in the *absence* of any particular stimulus. Such resting-state techniques seem to provide a number of advantages. Data collection is easier because there is not the need to develop and pilot a complicated behavioral experiment. There is also an increase in comparability of data collected by different investigators. Because the data are not collected in the context of a particular behavioral paradigm, resting-state data collection appears to justify the collection of larger samples, the importance of which is discussed later in the context of reliability and sample size. But there are also drawbacks and challenges for the collection of resting-state data. For example, the resting state is not a quiescent state. As anyone who has experimented with trying to control his or her attention for an extended period of time can attest, the unstimulated mind wanders where it will. The experimenter has surrendered control and no longer knows when or in what processes a participant's brain is engaging. If participants systematically differ in regard to where their attention goes when unstimulated—for example, neurotic individuals may worry more when left to their own devices—then correlations observed with a personality trait may reflect this tendency to think about something more or less. This flips causality on its head if the point of the experiment was to find the causes—not the effects—of a personality trait or diagnosis. In the schizophrenia literature, this problem has been discussed as a performance or causality confound (Ebmeier, Lawrie, Blackwood, Johnstone, & Goodwin, 1995; MacDonald & Chafee, 2006). In addition to this interpretive challenge, it is easier to fall asleep during resting scans, and it can be challenging for the experimenter to know when sleeping has occurred.

These considerations suggest activating the brain could be helpful. Activation studies use behavioral paradigms that are sensitive to individual differences in a personality trait or diagnosis. These behavioral paradigms can require substantial modifications to make them mechanistically interpretable, sensitive to individual differences, and appropriate for a neuroimaging modality. These can be very elegant experiments when accomplished. Nonetheless, there are a number of drawbacks. Generally, in this method examination of a brain region has been conditioned on seeing activation evoked by the task, which means a small fraction of the data collected can then be examined for group difference effects. Other regions of the brain may be relevant to the group difference, but these will not be examined because they are not related to activity during the task. In addition, the specificity of the mechanisms being examined usually allows fewer other questions to be asked of the data. In a funding environment with limited resources, this tends to lead to smaller targeted sample sizes, which can reduce the robustness of the finding.

Trade-Offs between Neuroimaging Techniques

Thus there are trade-offs to consider when determining whether to activate or not. The key is to recognize and manage these trade-offs. Table 4.1 summarizes a variety of noninvasive, human neuroimaging approaches. There are many more techniques that are invasive and used exclusively in animal experiments. Additional insights have been gained from cases of brain damage (as in the examples of Phineas Gage [Damasio, 1995 or the brain-surgery case of HM). One of the most commonly observed trade-offs among the techniques in Table 4.1 is the trade-off between spatial and temporal resolution. No neuroimaging technique provides everything; where spatial resolution is maximal (e.g., in structural MRI), there is no temporal resolution; where temporal resolution is best (e.g., in event-related potentials [ERPs] and magnetoencephalography [MEG]) spatial resolution is reduced or in other ways limited.

In addition to the trade-off between spatial and temporal resolution, these techniques differ in the various kinds of artifacts to which they are vulnerable and the preprocessing steps involved in maximizing their signal. At the end of the day, whether examining structure or function, at rest or during activation, what these techniques share is that they provide a quantitative measurement of some aspect of brain functioning. In this they are not only similar to each other but to other quantitative measurements. Therefore the same questions asked of other measures can be asked of brain-related measures. In particular, reliability undergirds all of our subsequent assumptions about a measure's validity. In contrast to other domains of the behavioral sciences where reliability has been carefully documented, here it has received less attention than warranted.

TABLE 4.1. *Prominent Neuroimaging Techniques*

Technique	Activation	Selected Advantages	Selected Disadvantages
Structural MRI (sMRI)	No	High spatial resolution (millimeters/mms)	No temporal resolution; very sensitive to motion
Diffusion tensor imaging (DTI)	No	High spatial resolution (mms)	No temporal resolution; very sensitive to motion
Functional MRI (fMRI) and functional connectivity MRI (fcMRI)	Both[a]	Safe for most people, noninvasive, and tremendously versatile (not unique to fMRI)	Low temporal resolution (seconds); sensitive to motion
Positron emission tomography (PET)	Both	Moderate spatial resolution (centimeters/cms) specific to different neurotransmitter systems	Very low temporal resolution (minutes)
Single-photon emission computed tomography (SPECT)	Yes	Moderate spatial resolution (cms); specific to different neurotransmitter systems	Very low temporal resolution (minutes); relatively uncommon technique
Electroencephalography (EEG)	Both[b]	High temporal resolution (milliseconds/ms)	Low spatial resolution; sensitive to motion
Event-related potentials (ERP)	Yes	High temporal resolution (ms)	Low spatial resolution; sensitive to motion
Functional near-infrared spectroscopy (fNIRS)	Yes	Moderately high temporal resolution (10s of ms)	Spatial resolution limited to a priori selected surface structures
Magnetoencephalography (MEG)	Both	High temporal resolution (ms); moderate spatial resolution (cms)	Gyrification of the brain causes variance in the strength of the neural signals; signal drops off strongly in deeper brain areas; sensitive to motion

[a] Functional connectivity is a fMRI technique that is commonly measured at rest; however, it can also be measured during a task. [b] EEG is commonly measured at rest; however, evoked EEG can be measured during a task.

Reliability of Neuroimaging Techniques

Reliability refers to the reproducibility or the consistency of a measurement, and, to-gether with validity, it represents a fundamental requirement for a measure's usefulness. A test must be capable of providing consistent measurements for it to generate worth-while data. The reliability of a test places an upper bound on expected correlations between its results and those of another dependent measure. From classical test theory, we know that the variance in observed scores on an instrument is composed of true score variance and variance due to noise. Low reliability can be thought of as too much noise variance in the observed score. Also from classical test theory, we know that the noise in a measurement is random, so it only acts to *reduce correlations between measurements*. Two tests or measures can only correlate with each other to the de-gree that the two measures are themselves reliable, and any correlation greater than this is the product of chance. For example, if positron emission tomography (PET) were found to have a reliability of 0.7, we could not expect measurements using that tool to have a correlation with, for instance, questionnaire symptom ratings higher than 0.7. Therefore, arriving at accurate assessments of the reliability of neuroimaging techniques is necessary to interpret brain-behavioral relationships.

Accurate assessment of the reliability of neuroimaging techniques is also important for experimental planning and evaluating statistical power. Figure 4.1 illustrates this relationship across 196 scenarios, where the reliability of measurement of the inde-pendent variable (IV) and dependent variables (DV) were varied (intraclass correla-tion coefficients [ICCs] from .3 to .9) and the true correlation between the measures ranged from .4 to .7 according to standard computations (Nunnally, 1970). Take the case of a personality variable (DV) that is measured relatively accurately, ICC = .8, and a brain measurement (IV) that is measured somewhat less accurately, ICC = .5. The personality variable is retrospective and involves reporting on the past year (or longer), whereas the brain measurement is a snapshot on a given day, and there are other sources of method variance. Thus a closely causal relationship can optimistically be expected to have a very attenuated *true* correlation, say $r = .5$. About 75 subjects would be needed to have power of .8 to test a single hypothesized activation as a sta-tistical threshold (p) of .05. However, we often collect a whole brain's worth of data. If more than two brain regions are being tested, 75 subjects is a low estimate; if a whole brain's worth of voxels are being tested, the statistical threshold is much more severe, and 75 is a very low estimate indeed. As we shall see, many neuroimaging experiments are inadequately powered, highlighting the importance of replication across studies (see also Vul, Harris, Winkielman, & Pashler, 2009) in order to focus on useful and nonspurious brain-behavior relationships.

To complicate matters, sources of noise that differentially affect experimental groups (or individuals of the same group that share characteristics with each other) can lead to erroneous interpretations. In neuroimaging, both random and systematic noise exist, and only some of their sources are known. There are some commonalities in the sources of noise for a given imaging technique, but many sources of noise are related to the method of data acquisition. An example of such a noise source would be the presence of a metallic dental prosthesis precluding an accurate image in MRI. Such a dental prosthesis would pose much less of a problem for a PET scan. A common source of noise to all imaging techniques to various extents is subject movement, which may be higher in some subject groups than others.

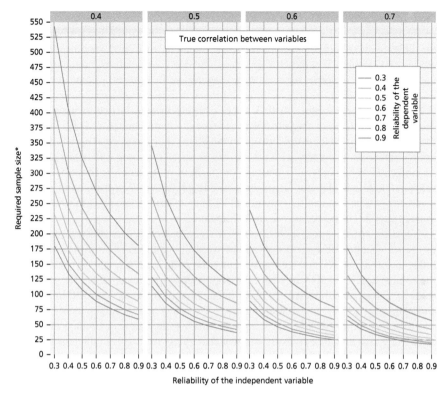

Figure 4.1 Reliability, power and sample size. Each panel represents a different true correlation between two variables, for example a personality factor and a brain activation, as if measured without error. The x-axis shows different reliabilities of one of the variables, and the color represents different reliabilities of the other variable. The y-axis shows how many subjects are required to observe the correlation (* for a=.05, b=.80).

Although most researchers know the importance of reliability in principle, there is arguably a dearth of studies assessing the reliability of neuroimaging techniques. Moreover, tools to facilitate these analyses have not been readily available nor regularly demanded. That being said, no description of cognitive neuroscience techniques can be thought to be complete without some consideration of these neurometric qualities. To this end, we have included some discussion of the neurometric properties of which we are aware for each technique. Now we are prepared to consider these techniques one by one. We begin with imaging techniques that provide a "photograph" of the brain: structural imaging techniques.

■ STRUCTURAL IMAGING TECHNIQUES

Structural MRI

Rather than a single method, MRI machines are something like a toolbox that allows for many kinds of measurements to be taken. The first kind of MRI technique we consider has come to be called structural MRI (sMRI). One of the oldest and still one of the most common, sMRI is the source of many of the pictures most associated with brain imaging. sMRI creates high-resolution, almost photo-like images optimized for differentiating between various tissues in the brain, including grey matter, white matter, and cerebrospinal fluid. One approach to sMRI data analysis is to quantify the volume of a brain region by measuring the thickness and extent of the tissue in a particular region of interest. Another popular approach is to use voxel-based morphometry (VBM, Ashburner & Friston, 2000). VBM transforms the high-resolution brain images produced by sMRI into a single template and then computes the amount of grey matter that originally existed for every location in the brain. Thus it quantifies each individual brain's features so that extent or thickness can be tested for group differences or linear relationships. While other alternatives exist, such as measuring the shape of a structure (and there exist elaborate algorithms for doing this; see Wang et al., 2006), manual measurements of thickness and extent and VBM are the two approaches that have been most utilized in the personality disorder literature.

Naturally, sMRI is most useful in cases where a trait or disease affects brain structure. Such changes must occur over and above the great number of other factors that influence brain size, even after transforming the brain onto a single template to aid the comparison of relative differences in brain volume. For example, in the 15 sMRI studies considered in the review of structural differences in people with SPD by Hazlett and colleagues (2012), the median number of subjects was 21 SPD patients and 31 controls. It is somewhat less surprising then that a wide variety of findings has been reported in this literature (see also Fervaha & Remington, 2013). In the largest study conducted in the field of which we are aware, Hazlett and colleagues (2008) used a manual tracing technique to examine the regional volume of gray and white matter across 39 Brodmann brain areas. They imaged 79 patients with SPD and used both healthy controls and patients with schizophrenia as comparison groups. The authors found a number of abnormal regions in both SPD and schizophrenia, among which was an increase in white matter volume and a decrease in grey matter volume in ventral anterior cingulate (BA 24) and dorsal posterior cingulate (BA 31). Of all the regions identified as being different in SPD patients, reduced grey matter in ventral anterior cingulate, a region implicated in cognitive control processes, was one of only two regions associated with symptoms, in this case greater interpersonal impairment ($r = -0.31, p = .007$).

Measurement Considerations

sMRI techniques can seem quite simple—what could be difficult about measuring the size of something? In fact there are several steps in making precise measurements. First, subjects' heads must remain still for a prolonged period of time. Unfortunately there are no established methods to correct for head motion during a structural scan, and such motion degrades the quality of the image like an old-fashioned daguerreotype. In addition, sMRI studies often include some manner of segmentation of the brain into grey matter, white matter, and cerebral spinal fluid and parcellation of the brain into various regions and structures. Therefore, there are two other kinds of factors that influence the reliability of measurements in sMRI studies: those that influence the data acquisition and those that influence the segmentation and parcellation. The factors influencing the acquisition of the sMRI images include subject-specific variables, such as motion and hydration status (Walters, Fox, Crum, Taube, & Thomas, 2001), as well as scanner-related factors, such as the magnetic strength of the scanner (known as the B_0 field strength) and the pulse sequence. There are other factors that may affect image quality and, consequently, reliability. In terms of reliability of segmentation and parcellation, a study of the reliability of automatic parcellation of subcortical structures used the Dice overlap measure (Dice, 1945) to quantify the spatial reliability of automatic parcellation (Jovicich et al., 2009). This metric is comparable in scale to a kappa statistic. This study also examined different scanner manufacturers, acquisition sequences, and field strength to determine their effects on reliability of segmentation. They found a range of Dice values from 0.79 to 0.94 across subcortical brain structures. The average Dice across brain regions ranged from 0.83 for the comparison of different scanner manufacturers to 0.88 for the comparison that held scanner, field strength, and pulse sequence steady. Overall, these results suggest automatic parcellation of brain structures can be robust, although rarely perfect.

Diffusion Tensor Imaging

Diffusion tensor imaging (DTI) represents a second MRI-based method for obtaining structural information. Although sMRI can provide some information about white matter organization, it does so at a macro level, without providing precise quantification of individual differences in white matter integrity. DTI measures the diffusion of molecules (typically water) in the brain, which can shed light on the organization and integrity of white matter in the brain. This is possible because the white matter fibers create a preferential direction in which water can diffuse.

Researchers use a few different analytic methods based on DTI measurements to assess white matter integrity, but fractional anisotropy (FA) is still the most common. FA measures to what extent water diffuses parallel to the main white matter tracts in the brain. Lower FA has been hypothesized to represent aberrant myelination of white matter fibers as well as fiber organization that departs from typical parallel structures. However, in addition to white matter fibers, the diffusion of water molecules can also be constrained by various pathologies, such as an accumulation of macromolecules as in Alzheimer's disease. DTI is therefore a promising tool for both the detection of and research into pathologies related to degraded or disrupted white matter organization or integrity.

One example of the use of DTI is a study conducted by Hazlett and colleagues (2011), in which they compared FA measurements in three brain regions between 30 participants diagnosed with SPD and 35 healthy controls. The regions they were interested in examining based on previous research were bilateral temporal lobes, dorsolateral prefrontal cortex (dlPFC), and anterior cingulate cortex. They expected that SPD subjects would demonstrate reduced FA in temporal and cingulate areas but not in frontal regions. They found that SPD subjects did in fact show reduced FA in temporal regions and did not observe significant differences in dlPFC. However, in the cingulate there was a group by region interaction such that subjects with SPD demonstrated lower FA in posterior and right cingulate regions but higher FA in anterior regions.

An interesting additional analysis showed significant correlations between both negative symptom severity and odd speech with lower FA in both left and right cingulate regions. The authors interpret the complex cingulate findings to largely support previous DTI findings in schizophrenia as well as gray and white matter structural volume studies in SPD. Previous research has attributed to the cingulate functions involved with emotion, cognition, and social functioning, all aspects impaired in people diagnosed with SPD. The results of this study extend previous research to both strengthen the evidence for a biological link between SPD and schizophrenia and to provide clues as to the specific nature of neural pathology in people with SPD. This latter extension would not be possible using a different imaging technique.

Measurement Considerations

The factors affecting the reliability of DTI results are largely similar to those affecting sMRI. However, the reliability of results may depend on the choice of analysis method and dependent variable. In a comprehensive study of the reliability of different DTI measures, Wang and colleagues (2012) note the four studies of DTI reliability performed up to that date found that both the variable being measured (e.g., fractional anisotropy, tract volume) and the anatomical structure being measured both influenced reliability estimates. The authors decided to estimate intra- and intersession reliability using various dependent measures and various fiber tracts. They indeed found that the degree of reliability of their measurements depended on which variable they measured as well as the fiber tract under investigation. Overall, they found that measuring DTI with 15 directions produced less reliable measurements than measuring with 30 directions and that fractional anisotropy and mean diffusivity both produced good reliability (ICCs > 0.7) for many of the nine major fiber tracts. It is likely that more subtle DTI measurements, for smaller tracts or for features relating to crossing tracts, are less reliably measured.

■ FUNCTIONAL IMAGING TECHNIQUES

Functional MRI and Functional Connectivity MRI

Functional magnetic resonance imaging (fMRI) measures brain activity indirectly by quantifying the amount of oxygenated blood flow in the brain. It is assumed that brain regions with many active neurons require more oxygenated blood than less active regions. fMRI is most often employed to examine the strength of activation in particular brain regions in response to a cognitive task. The extent of this task-related activation can be examined with respect to group differences, personality, or other clinical measures to make inferences about the brain regions and the psychological variables in question.

A strength of fMRI is the spatial resolution of the method. Although the images produced by fMRI are not as clear as those of sMRI, they are more detailed than those of EEG, MEG, PET, single-photon emission computed tomography (SPECT), and functional near-infrared spectroscopy (fNIRS). There are two large drawbacks of fMRI, however. The first is the cost associated with operating an MRI scanner. Compared with a technique like EEG, fMRI is prohibitively expensive for some applications, such as screening a large number of participants. The second drawback is the temporal resolution of the technique. This is a problem with two main causes, namely the long interval between volumes of the brain being measured (usually around 2000 to 3000 ms) and the delay of signal associated with the hemodynamic response. Briefly, researchers have to wait for blood to flow to the neurons which have activated before they can detect the activation. Individual differences in the time and shape of the hemodynamic response function can lead to inaccuracies of measurement. Compared with EEG and MEG, which more directly measure the effects of the neuronal activity, fMRI temporal resolution is rather poor. A minor drawback is that due to the high magnetic field present at all times around an MRI scanner, nonmagnetic apparatus must be carefully selected for any fMRI experiment. In some cases, this limits the questions that researchers can ask using fMRI.

One instance of this method in the psychometric schizotypy literature is a study conducted by Corlett and Fletcher (2012), in which the authors scanned 18 healthy subjects during the completion of a Kamin blocking task (Kamin, 1969). The authors also administered the Peters delusion inventory (Peters, Joseph, Day, & Garety, 2004) and the Chapman scales of physical and social anhedonia (Chapman, Chapman, & Raulin, 1976), perceptual aberrations (Chapman, Chapman, & Raulin, 1978), and magical ideation (Eckblad & Chapman, 1983) to each subject. While underpowered, the authors reported a significant negative correlation between scores on the magical ideation scale and brain activation in the striatum during the prediction errors on the Kamin blocking task.

Although task-related activation studies are the most common use for fMRI in psychological research, other experimental designs and analysis methods are becoming more common. Resting-state fMRI involves no task paradigm; instead subjects are asked to lay still for the duration of the scan without outside stimulation. Because there is no task with which to compare activation in specific brain regions, researchers measure the temporal association of disparate brain regions with each other. This method is known as functional connectivity, and it represents a wholly different approach to understanding brain dynamics compared with task-related activation. Lagioia and colleagues (2010) examined functional connectivity of a mixed sample of adolescents from the community and from an outpatient psychiatric clinic. To measure functional connectivity, the authors employed independent component analysis, a data-driven method of breaking up fMRI data into components of coherent signals that are spatially independent from each other. The subjects in the study were also administered the Schizotypal Personality Questionnaire (Raine, 1991). The negative correlation between the disorganization factor and high frequency power in a posterior cingulate network, a region associated with self-referential cognition, suggests that disrupted coherence in that region may underpin the lack of coherence in behavior observed in persons with SPD. This region may represent a target for interventions seeking to ameliorate disorganization.

Measurement Considerations

fMRI is very sensitive to subject head motion. In studies including both healthy control subjects and psychiatric patients, group differences in the amount of motion in the scanner may result in diminished data quality in one group compared with the other (i.e., reduced reliability). This can cause problems when comparing the two groups, as it may appear that the group who was measured more precisely is activating more to a given stimulus than the other group.

In addition to movement, fMRI has its own unique considerations. Because of the difference in density between air and tissue, structures near sinus cavities, such as orbitofrontal cortex (Ojemann et al., 1997), and structures in close proximity to the circle of Willis, such as the medial temporal lobes, are prone to signal loss and image distortions. There are corrections available for these distortions, but there is no correction for image loss. Furthermore, not all researchers employ the corrections for image distortion as they necessitate the collection of a separate data image.

A review of studies examining the test-retest reliability of fMRI activation studies was conducted by Bennett and Miller (2010). They separated their findings by the method by which the studies reported reliability, namely by ICC, Dice coefficient, or other. Across the 15 studies they report as employing the ICC, overall mean ICC they found to represent fMRI reliability was 0.50. Likewise, the average reported Dice overlap statistic for the studies they reviewed was 0.48. Although these values must be taken with a grain of salt, it does suggest that activation studies in fMRI may have lower reliability than some other imaging techniques.

PET and SPECT

PET and SPECT are similar imaging modalities that both rely on radioactive tracer compounds to measure blood flow/metabolic information in the brain. Briefly, both methods employ scanners that "catch" the by-products of the decay of radioactive tracers ingested/injected by the subject. Regional metabolism can be inferred by measuring the amount of radiation coming from different areas. The two methods differ in spatial resolution, with PET providing higher resolution. However, that resolution comes at higher cost and shorter half-life of the tracer compound, which makes using PET less convenient for some hospitals. Although fMRI has better spatial resolution than either PET or SPECT, these latter methods are capable of measuring the specific metabolism of certain neurotransmitters (e.g., dopamine) by varying the radioactive tracer compound. This benefit is unique among the imaging techniques, and it allows researchers to ask interesting questions not only about neural activation generally but about the role of neurotransmitters in brain function among groups with psychopathology.

One study to make use of this benefit using PET did so by testing the hypothesis that healthy people high in schizotypy would demonstrate an increased release of dopamine in the striatum when placed under emotional stress (Soliman et al., 2008). The authors scanned subjects who scored highly on the Chapman scales of physical and social anhedonia (Chapman et al., 1976) and perceptual aberrations (Chapman et al., 1978) as well control subjects twice: once during a stress-inducing task and once during a control task. They found that those in the high negative schizotypy group showed increased striatal dopamine release during the stress task but not those in the high positive schizotypy group or the controls. This study extended previous research showing increased dopamine release in schizophrenia patients when given amphetamine compared to controls; however, in schizophrenia patients this elevated dopamine response is typically more related to positive symptoms.

One study to investigate amphetamine-induced striatal dopamine release in schizotypal personality disorder using SPECT was conducted by Abi-Dargham and others (2004). Subjects diagnosed with SPD as well as healthy controls were scanned once at baseline and again an hour after amphetamine injection. The authors found that although they could not detect differences in baseline striatal dopamine between groups, the SPD group demonstrated dysregulation of dopamine following amphetamine administration.

Measurement Considerations

No review of PET reliability could be found, but individual test–retest reliability studies have been conducted. These typically involved assessing the reliability of PET data for some particular goal, for example localizing language centers (Billingsley-Marshall, Simos, & Papanicolaou, 2004). In a study of one ligand used to mark serotonin receptors, Costes and colleagues (2007) found overall acceptable reliability (mean ICC of 0.84 for most regions). Notably, though, the authors found variability in the reliability of brain regions, with the lowest ICC found in anterior cingulate cortex (ICC = 0.50) and the highest found in inferior parietal cortex (ICC = 0.93). In a six-month test–retest study of glucose metabolism in subcortical structures, Schaefer and colleagues (2000) found significant variation among structures both within hemisphere and between contralateral structures. In their study, they found that measurements from the thalamus had high reliability in both hemispheres (right ICC = 0.93, left ICC = 0.92). However, other subcortical regions showed either consistently lower (hippocampus: R ICC = 0.64, L ICC = 0.54) or inconsistently reliable measurements between hemispheres (amygdala: R ICC = 0.53, L ICC = 0.17). Another study, which examined the reliability of presynaptic dopaminergic function assessment, found a different set of results. Egerton and colleagues (2010) measured eight healthy adults twice, two years apart, and measured the test–retest reliability of PET in various brain regions. The reported bilateral median ICC values ranged from 0.24 in the amygdala to 0.94 in the caudate. The average of the reported bilateral median ICCs was 0.67, indicating generally acceptable reliability. Similarly to the Schaefer study, Egerton and others found high reliability in the thalamus (ICC = 0.89) and lower reliability in both the amygdala (ICC = 0.24) and the hippocampus (ICC = 0.46). Unlike the Costes study, Egerton and colleagues did not find that the anterior cingulate produced the lowest reliability; however, the obtained reliability value was similar in magnitude given the differences in study characteristics (0.50 in Costes vs. 0.61 in Egerton).

EEG, Evoked EEG, and ERPs

EEG involves placing electrodes on a subject's scalp and measuring neural electrical activity. Oftentimes in cognitive neuroscience the electrical activity associated with a particular stimulus is sought, so the EEG signal following many trials with that stimulus is averaged into an ERP. Because EEG deals directly with electrical signals as opposed to blood flow, its temporal resolution is on the order of milliseconds. However, the spatial resolution of the EEG signal is limited compared to other techniques, such as fMRI. Because of these strengths and weaknesses, EEG is often used to detect very fast, subtle group differences in neural responses to stimuli at particular epochs of the neural response, but these responses may not be localized to particular brain regions.

One example of this method is a study performed by Kiang and colleagues (2010), in which healthy subjects assessed using the SPQ performed a task which varied the lexical association of word stimuli. The authors were interested in the N400 amplitude, which is a "negative peak" in the ERP signal that is present approximately 400 milliseconds following a stimulus. They reported that previous research showed the N400 amplitude is stronger when the two stimuli are strongly semantically related, and it is weaker when the words are unrelated. Thus the ERP response provided an indication of the way in which participants perceived semantic relationships. The authors found that SPQ total scores were negatively correlated with N400 indirect priming effects, meaning that those with higher SPQ total scores showed a smaller difference between the N400 amplitudes when stimulus words were unrelated and when they were indirectly related. They also observed a negative correlation between higher SPQ cognitive-perceptual factor scores and N400 direct priming effects, which are differences between the N400 amplitudes when stimulus words were unrelated and when they were directly related. The authors interpreted these results to mean those with more schizotypy, especially cognitive-perceptual, demonstrated less activation in the presence of semantic relationships.

A methodology that provides data comparable to EEG and ERP is MEG. This method detects very subtle changes in the magnetic field that occur due to the electrical activity of neurons (Hämäläinen et al., 1993). Although this method is not particularly novel, the apparatus for conducting MEG studies have been slow to spread and no results in our particular domain of inquiry, schizotypy, can be reported at this time.

Measurement Considerations

Three considerations when making recordings using EEG are high impedances, uneven impedances and eye-blinks. If the impedance between the electrodes and the brain is too high it can appear as spurious signal. This false signal is difficult to distinguish from true signal. This problem can also result from the impedance differing too much between electrodes. Additionally, noise can be introduced by the blinking of a subject's eyes as well as electromuscular effects produced by clenched jaws and "stiff necks." Movement artifacts are also a concern with EEG, as they are with other imaging techniques mentioned previously. One other problem with the analysis of EEG data is that of the reference point. Because the signal detected by EEG electrodes is relative, a reference signal must be chosen by the experimenter. There are several options for this reference point, and results can differ significantly based on the experimenter's decision.

As with the other types of neuroimaging, the question of the reliability of EEG requires defining exactly what is measured and how it is quantified. Thatcher (2010) made this point explicitly in a review of the reliability and validity of quantitative EEG (qEEG) as opposed to qualitative ("eyeball") EEG. Across various methods and populations, Thatcher reports very high test–retest reliability values for qEEG in the studies he included in his review (most around 0.9). This is notable because some of these studies recorded for only 20 seconds. Other, less quantitative methods of EEG produced less reliable results. However, this review was in reference to the method of identifying features of an EEG recording as opposed to reliability of the data themselves, so it is unclear how comparable these results are to those of reliability studies of other methodologies, and it certainly says nothing about the reliability of ERP data as currently practiced.

fNIRS

fNIRS is a technique designed to collect similar information to that of fMRI. However, instead of using the magnetic properties of oxygenated blood to form images, fNIRS relies on the distinctive difference between oxygenated and nonoxygenated hemoglobin in absorption of near-infrared light. The outcome is that fNIRS generates information about the changes in oxygenated blood flow in the brain. A benefit compared with fMRI is that the technology required for most fNIRS applications is relatively inexpensive and portable compared with an MRI scanner. Additionally the temporal resolution is much better than fMRI, with a resolution on the level of 10 ms. Some significant drawbacks exist compared with fMRI. First, the light absorption method only allows images to be taken on the surface of the brain, whereas fMRI allows for whole brain images. Second, the spatial resolution of fNIRS is limited compared with fMRI. Third, information about the depth of the signal is difficult to distinguish using fNIRS, unlike fMRI.

Hori and colleagues (2008) employed fNIRS to examine schizotypy and whether people high in schizotypy demonstrated increased hemispheric laterality in frontal regions during a verbal fluency task. They assessed 32 healthy subjects using the SPQ and imaged them during the performance of both a letter and a sematic category version of a verbal fluency task. The sample was divided into high- and low-schizotypy groups. The authors observed an interaction in frontal hemispheric activation between groups, where the high-schizotypy group showed more activation in the right frontal regions and less activation in the left frontal region during both fluency tasks. These results mirrored those of schizophrenia patients, who also show a right-greater-than-left pattern of activation during verbal fluency tasks.

Measurement Considerations

Previous studies have examined the reliability of activations as measured by fNIRS. One study involved presenting a periodic checkerboard pattern to participants and measuring activation in the occipital cortex (Plichta et al., 2006). For this very robust signal, the average cluster-level results had ICCs in the 0.7 to 0.8 range, whereas single-channel results were somewhat lower in the 0.5 to 0.6 range. Another study examining both short- and long-term reliability found similar results. Schecklmann and colleagues (2008) examined the reliability of activation during a verbal fluency task in a region of interest representing aspects of inferior, ventro-, and dorsolateral prefrontal cortex as well as part of superior temporal lobe across two time periods: 3 weeks and 53 weeks. Like the Plichta study, the authors found higher ICCs in the cluster-level results (ICCs ≥ 0.7 between times 1 and 3) compared with single channel results (ICCs in the 0.5 to 0.6 range); however, these results were not as strong when comparing times 1 and 2 or times 2 and 3, which suggests they may be somewhat inflated than what would be expected on average. The test–retest reliability of event-related fNIRS in prefrontal regions during a cognitive risk-taking task, the Balloon Analogue Risk Task, has also been found to be good ICCs (≥.72; Li et al., 2013).

■ CONCLUSION

The understanding of personality disorders can certainly be broadened by the use of cognitive neuroscience and neuroimaging techniques. Although these methods may not be any closer to "ground truth" than traditional quantitative behavioral research paradigms, they do allow researchers to ask and answer different kinds of questions. By elucidating the relationship between brain systems and psychological systems and simultaneously acting as a bridge between molecular (genetic) data and macroscopic, symptom-based data, neuroimaging techniques may assist researchers in more fully understanding the nature and manifestation of personality disorders.

There is an assumption that effect sizes closer to the infrastructure supporting behavior (i.e. the brain) would be larger than the effect sizes for behavioral or symptom indices. However, there is increasing reason to doubt this optimistic claim, suggesting early promises about neuroimaging technique may have been simply misleading. Instead we are coming to a place in our understanding of personality disorders that suggests replicable effects will begin to emerge when sample sizes appropriately power hypothesis tests about the brain and also take into consideration the number of tests that are being conducted.

There are several different methodologies that fall under the umbrella of neuroimaging, each with a myriad flavors housed within it. Each category has its own strengths and its own weaknesses, but they also have common virtues as well as common pitfalls. Some methods excel in allowing the researcher to "see" what is happening in the brain on a miniscule timescale. Others produce incredibly detailed three-dimensional images that rival photographs in their detail. Each method represents a noninvasive attempt to assign a number to a physical, biological process or attribute. Inherent in that attempt are limitations introduced by biology and physics. Incremental increases in the signal-to-noise ratios of these techniques have produced amazing advances in signal quality. It is up to the researchers employing these tools to do so with knowledge of their limitations so that they may be used to their full potential. The potential of these tools will remain just that until sample sizes increase to account for the relatively modest reliability currently achievable using these methods.

■ REFERENCES

Abi-Dargham, A., Kegeles, L. S., Zea-Ponce, Y., Mawlawi, O., Martinez, D., Mitropoulou, V., . . . Siever, L. J. (2004). Striatal amphetamine-induced dopamine release in patients with schizotypal personality disorder studied with single photon emission computed tomography and [123I]iodobenzamide. *Biol Psychiatry, 55*(10), 1001–1006. doi:10.1016/j.biopsych.2004.01.018

Ashburner, J., & Friston, K. J. (2000). Voxel-based morphometry—the methods. *NeuroImage, 11*(6 Pt 1), 805–821. doi:10.1006/nimg.2000.0582

Bennett, C. M., & Miller, M. B. (2010). How reliable are the results from functional magnetic resonance imaging? *Ann N Y Acad Sci, 1191,* 133–155. doi:10.1111/j.1749-6632.2010.05446.x

Billingsley-Marshall, R. L., Simos, P. G., & Papanicolaou, A. C. (2004). Reliability and validity of functional neuroimaging techniques for identifying language-critical areas in children and adults. *Dev Neuropsychol, 26,* 541–563. doi:10.1207/s15326942dn2602_1

Chapman, L. J., Chapman, J. P., & Raulin, M. L. (1976). Scales for physical and social anhedonia. *J Abnorm Psychol, 85,* 374–382. doi:10.1037/0021-843X.85.4.374

Chapman, L. J., Chapman, J. P., & Raulin, M. L. (1978). Body-image aberration in schizophrenia. *J Abnorm Psychol, 87,* 399–407. doi:10.1037/0021-843X.87.4.399

Corlett, P. R., & Fletcher, P. C. (2012). The neurobiology of schizotypy: fronto-striatal prediction error signal correlates with delusion-like beliefs in healthy people. *Neuropsychologia, 50,* 3612–3620. doi:10.1016/j.neuropsychologia.2012.09.045

Costes, N., Zimmer, L., Reilhac, A., Lavenne, F., Ryvlin, P., & Le Bars, D. (2007). Test-retest reproducibility of 18F-MPPF PET in healthy humans: a reliability study. *J Nucl Med*, *48*, 1279–1288. doi:10.2967/jnumed.107.041905

Dice, L. R. (1945). Measures of the amount of ecologic association between species. *Ecology*, *26*, 297–302. doi:10.2307/1932409

Ebmeier, K. P., Lawrie, S. M., Blackwood, D. H., Johnstone, E. C., & Goodwin, G. M. (1995) Hypofrontality revisited: a high resolution single photon emission computed tomography study in schizophrenia. *J Neurol Neurosurg Psychiatry*, *58*(4), 452–456. PMID: 7738553.

Eckblad, M., & Chapman, L. J. (1983). Magical ideation as an indicator of schizotypy. *J Consult Clin Psychol*, *51*, 215–225. doi:10.1037/0022-006X.51.2.215

Egerton, A., Demjaha, A., McGuire, P., Mehta, M. A., & Howes, O. D. (2010). The test-retest reliability of 18F-DOPA {PET} in assessing striatal and extrastriatal presynaptic dopaminergic function. *NeuroImage*, *50*(2), 524–531. http://dx.doi.org/10.1016/j.neuroimage.2009.12.058

Fervaha, G., & Remington, G. (2013). Neuroimaging findings in schizotypal personality disorder: a systematic review. *Prog Neuropsychopharmacol Biol Psychiatry*, *43*, 96–107. doi:10.1016/j.pnpbp.2012.11.014

Hämäläinen, M., Hari, R., Ilmoniemi, R. J., Knuutila, J., & Lounasmaa, O. V. (1993). Magnetoencephalography: theory, instrumentation, and applications to noninvasive studies of the working human brain. *Rev Mod Phys*, *65*(2), 413–497.

Hazlett, E., Goldstein, K. E., & Kolaitis, J. C. (2012). A review of structural MRI and diffusion tensor imaging in schizotypal personality disorder. *Curr Psychiatry Rep*, *14*(1), 70–78. doi:10.1007/s11920-011-0241-z

Hazlett, E. A., Buchsbaum, M. S., Haznedar, M. M., Newmark, R., Goldstein, K. E., Zelmanova, Y., . . . Siever, L. J. (2008). Cortical gray and white matter volume in unmedicated schizotypal and schizophrenia patients. *Schizophr Res*, *101*(1–3), 111–123. doi:10.1016/j.schres.2007.12.472

Hazlett, E. A., Goldstein, K. E., Tajima-Pozo, K., Speidel, E. R., Zelmanova, Y., Entis, J. J., . . . Siever, L. J. (2011). Cingulate and temporal lobe fractional anisotropy in schizotypal personality disorder. *NeuroImage*, *55*, 900–908. doi:10.1016/j.neuroimage.2010.12.082

Hori, H., Ozeki, Y., Terada, S., & Kunugi, H. (2008). Functional near-infrared spectroscopy reveals altered hemispheric laterality in relation to schizotypy during verbal fluency task. *Prog Neuropsychopharmacol Biol Psychiatry*, *32*, 1944–1951. doi:10.1016/j.pnpbp.2008.09.019

Jovicich, J., Czanner, S., Han, X., Salat, D., van der Kouwe, A., Quinn, B., . . . Fischl, B. (2009). MRI-derived measurements of human subcortical, ventricular and intracranial brain volumes: reliability effects of scan sessions, acquisition sequences, data analyses, scanner upgrade, scanner vendors and field strengths. *NeuroImage*, *46*, 177–192. doi:10.1016/j.neuroimage.2009.02.010

Kamin, L. J. (1969). Predictability, surprise, attention, and conditioning. In B. A. Campbell & R. M. Church (Eds.), *Punishment and aversive behavior* (pp. 279–296). New York: Appleton-Century-Crofts. Retrieved from http://scholar.google.com/scholar?hl=en&q=Predictability,+surprise,+attention,+and+conditioning&btnG=Search&as_sdt=0,5&as_ylo=&as_vis=0#0

Kiang, M., Prugh, J., & Kutas, M. (2010). An event-related brain potential study of schizotypal personality and associative semantic processing. *Int J Psychophysiol*, *75*, 119–126. doi:10.1016/j.ijpsycho.2009.10.005

Lagioia, A., Van De Ville, D., Debbané, M., Lazeyras, F., & Eliez, S. (2010). Adolescent resting state networks and their associations with schizotypal trait expression. *Front Syst Neurosci, 4.* doi:10.3389/fnsys.2010.00035

Li, L., Lin, Z., Cazzell, M., & Liu, H. (2013). Test-retest assessment of functional near-infrared spectroscopy to measure risk decision making in young adults. *Prog Biomed Opt Imag—Proceed SPIE, 8565.* doi:10.1117/12.2005552

MacDonald, A. W., 3rd, Chafee, M. V. (2006). Translational and developmental perspective on N-methyl-D-aspartate synaptic deficits in schizophrenia. *Dev Psychopathol, 18*(3), 853–876. Review.

Maguire, E. A., Gadian, D. G., Johnsrude, I. S., Good, C. D., Ashburner, J., Frackowiak, R. S., & Frith, C. D. (2000). Navigation-related structural change in the hippocampi of taxi drivers. *PNAS, 97*(8), 4398–4403. doi:10.1073/pnas.070039597

Münte, T. F., Altenmüller, E., & Jäncke, L. (2002). The musician's brain as a model of neuroplasticity. *Nature Rev Neurosci, 3*(6), 473–478. doi:10.1038/nrn843

Nunnally, J. C. (1970). *Introduction to psychological measurement.* New York: McGraw-Hill.

Ojemann, J. G., Akbudak, E., Snyder, A. Z., McKinstry, R. C., Raichle, M. E., & Conturo, T. E. (1997). Anatomic localization and quantitative analysis of gradient refocused echo-planar fMRI susceptibility artifacts. *NeuroImage, 6,* 156–167. doi:10.1006/nimg.1997.0289

Peters, E., Joseph, S., Day, S., & Garety, P. (2004). Measuring delusional ideation: the 21-item Peters et al. Delusions Inventory (PDI). *Schizophr Bull, 30,* 1005–1022.

Plichta, M. M., Herrmann, M. J., Baehne, C. G., Ehlis, A. C., Richter, M. M., Pauli, P., & Fallgatter, A. J. (2006). Event-related functional near-infrared spectroscopy (fNIRS): are the measurements reliable? *NeuroImage, 31,* 116–124. doi:10.1016/j.neuroimage.2005.12.008

Raine, A. (1991). The SPQ: a scale for the assessment of schizotypal personality based on DSM-III-R criteria. *Schizophr Bulletin, 17,* 555–564.

Schaefer, S. M., Abercrombie, H. C., Lindgren, K. A., Larson, C. L., Ward, R. T., Oakes, T. R., . . . Davidson, R. J. (2000). Six-month test–retest reliability of MRI-defined PET measures of regional cerebral glucose metabolic rate in selected subcortical structures. *Hum Brain Mapp, 10*(1), 1–9. doi:10.1002/(SICI)1097-0193(200005)10:1<1::AID-HBM10>3.0.CO;2-O

Schecklmann, M., Ehlis, A. C., Plichta, M. M., & Fallgatter, A. J. (2008). Functional near-infrared spectroscopy: a long-term reliable tool for measuring brain activity during verbal fluency. *NeuroImage, 43,* 147–155. doi:10.1016/j.neuroimage.2008.06.032

Soliman, A., O'Driscoll, G. A., Pruessner, J., Holahan, A.-L. V, Boileau, I., Gagnon, D., & Dagher, A. (2008). Stress-induced dopamine release in humans at risk of psychosis: a [11C]raclopride PET study. *Neuropsychopharmacol, 33,* 2033–2041. doi:10.1038/sj.npp.1301597

Thatcher, R. W. (2010). Validity and reliability of quantitative electroencephalography. *J Neurotherapy, 14*(2), 122–152.

Tobler, P. N., Fiorillo, C. D., & Schultz, W. (2005). Adaptive coding of reward value by dopamine neurons. *Science, 307,* 1642–1645.

Vul, E., Harris, C., Winkielman, P., & Pashler, H. (2009). Puzzlingly high correlations in fMRI studies of emotion, personality, and social cognition. *Perspect Psychol Sci, 4*(3), 274–290. doi: 10.1111/j.1745-6924.2009.01125.x. PMID: 26158964.

Walters, R. J., Fox, N. C., Crum, W. R., Taube, D., & Thomas, D. J. (2001). Haemodialysis and cerebral oedema. *Nephron, 87,* 143–147. doi:10.1159/000045903

Wang, J. Y., Abdi, H., Bakhadirov, K., Diaz-Arrastia, R., & Devous, M. D. (2012). A comprehensive reliability assessment of quantitative diffusion tensor tractography. *NeuroImage, 60,* 1127–1138. doi:10.1016/j.neuroimage.2011.12.062

Wang, L., Miller, J. P., Gado, M. H., McKeel, D. W., Rothermich, M., Miller, M. I., . . . Csernansky, J. G. (2006). Abnormalities of hippocampal surface structure in very mild dementia of the Alzheimer type. *NeuroImage, 30*(1), 52–60. doi:10.1016/j.neuroimage.2005.09.017

5 Minding the Emotional Thermostat

Integrating Social Cognitive and Affective Neuroscience Evidence to Form a Model of the Cognitive Control of Emotion

■ BRYAN T. DENNY AND
KEVIN N. OCHSNER

Every day brings with it some inevitable variation in emotional temperature: the rising heat of anger in response to an insult; the coolness of detached, analytical reflection on how such a situation may be de-escalated, and the temperate quotidian moments in between. Like we are able to adjust the thermostat of a room in an attempt to change its temperature, we are also able to attempt to adjust our own emotional temperature through a variety of means. However, unlike adjusting a thermostat on a wall, our internal emotional adjustments may be conscious or unconscious, may require persistent effort over time, and may or may not be successful in changing how we feel.

Despite how perplexing these changes in temperature may seem, the rapidly burgeoning field of affective neuroscience has begun to provide critical insight into the functional neural architecture and mechanisms that subserve these ubiquitous emotional states. The goal of this chapter is to provide a brief overview of the literature on the neural bases of the generation and regulation of emotion, and, in so doing, substantiate and elaborate a model of the cognitive control of emotion that has been given previously (Ochsner & Gross, 2005, 2008; Ochsner, Silvers, & Buhle, 2012).

Given the plethora of means of regulating emotion, both implicit (i.e., not requiring conscious attention) and explicit (i.e., requiring conscious effort); the model organisms in which these processes may be examined (e.g., humans, nonhuman primates, rodents), the developmental as well as psychopathological state of the target population, and the substantial extant literatures on each, given space limitations this chapter will necessarily be circumscribed in its scope. In particular, our aim is to integrate evidence from basic social cognitive and affective neuroscience research involving healthy adult humans in order to establish a model of the neural mechanisms that underlie and guide both the generation and regulation of emotion—a model that may provide a point of reference when considering the neural mechanisms underlying various forms of psychopathology, a striking number of which involve some deficit in generating, experiencing, and/or regulating emotion (Berking, Ebert, Cuijpers, & Hofmann, 2013; Berking et al., 2008; Denny, Silvers, & Ochsner, 2009; Gross, 2013; Gross & Munoz, 1995).

We devote particular focus to one explicit emotion regulation strategy, reappraisal, given that it has been particularly informative theoretically as well as relatively well studied (Buhle et al., 2014; Ochsner & Gross, 2008; Ochsner et al., 2012). To that end, after briefly reviewing the theoretical framework that underlies social cognitive and affective neuroscience research, the first two parts of this chapter present evidence for a model of cognitive control of emotion with a focus on processes and neural systems involved in emotion generation and regulation, respectively. The final part of the chapter highlights the relevance of this model to psychopathology and other future directions.

■ THEORETICAL FRAMEWORK

Prior to presenting evidence for a model of the cognitive control of emotion, it is important to establish the overarching framework on which this evidence rests. In order to make inferences about the affective and cognitive processes, a multilevel approach is employed involving measurement of both behavior and neural activity. Measuring behavior involves analyzing self-reports of emotional experience (whether under the instruction to regulate or not) and measuring neural activity involves using a functional neuroimaging modality (typically functional magnetic resonance imaging [fMRI]) in order to establish which brain regions and systems are involved in subserving emotion generation and/or emotion regulation. In this way, by examining the interrelationship and patterns of converging evidence between the empirical data at hand across multiple levels of analysis (e.g., behavior; fMRI), one may make inferences about the underlying affective and cognitive processes involved (see Ochsner, 2007; Ochsner et al., 2012 for a more in-depth discussion).

■ PROCESSES AND SYSTEMS INVOLVED IN EMOTION GENERATION

A useful framework for understanding the generation of an emotion can be found in the process model described by James Gross (Gross, 1998b; Gross & Thompson, 2007). Therein, emotions are taken to be response tendencies that arise in characteristic patterns during the evaluation (i.e., appraisal) of emotional stimuli in one's environment (Gross, 1998a, 1998b). As described in the framework previously, these response tendencies occur at several levels of analysis, including behavior, experience, and physiology. As the name implies, these response tendencies are likely to be expressed as emotional responses in the absence of any intervening conscious or unconscious regulation. Indeed, as we discuss later in the section on emotion regulation, this appraisal process inherent to the generation of an emotion may be modulated prior to the full expression of an emotional response.

But how is this process of emotion generation subserved by the healthy adult brain? The extraordinary volume of human functional neuroimaging studies that have been published in the last 20 years (>5,000) has shed considerable light on this question. However, in synthesizing a model of emotion generation from this rich corpus of neuroscience data, it is essential to consider two theoretical accounts of the linkage between neuroimaging data and different emotional states: namely, whether discrete emotions (e.g., happiness, sadness, anger, fear) are each linked to discrete anatomical regions (or discrete networks of regions) in the brain that cannot be further reduced, or rather, whether such discrete emotional states arise from common progenitor regions and networks and achieve differentiation via variation in neuronal communication among the nodes of the network (Lindquist, Wager, Kober, Bliss-Moreau, & Barrett, 2012).

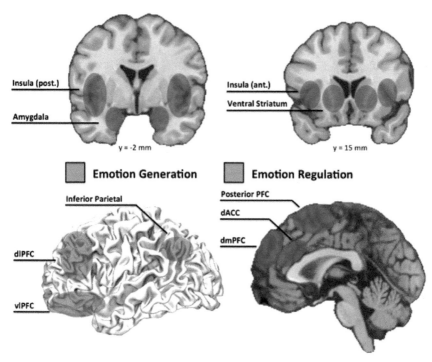

Figure 5.1 Model of the principal brain regions involved in emotion generation.

The former account, termed a *locationist* view, has intuitive appeal, and it was consistent with the results of many studies of the neural basis of emotional experience that connected discrete regions (e.g., the insula) with the processing of specific emotions (e.g., disgust). However, recent quantitative meta-analyses have provided support for the latter account, termed a *psychological constructionist* view, showing that the neural mechanisms underlying the generation and expression of diverse discrete emotions largely rely on common neural architecture (Kober et al., 2008; Lindquist et al., 2012).

These quantitative meta-analyses have informed our model of the principal brain regions involved in emotion generation. This model is summarized in Figure 5.1, highlighting brain regions that have been principally associated with emotion generation and experience (shown in red): the amygdala, the insula, and the ventral striatum. Critically, as discussed later, these regions each subserve generalized affective processes that contribute to the expression of diverse specific emotions in a manner consistent with the psychological constructionist viewpoint. We next consider each of these regions in more detail.

Amygdala

The amygdalae, located bilaterally in the anterior portion of the ventral medial temporal lobes, have long been known from experimental work in animals to play a key role in emotion, attention, and memory (LeDoux, 1995, 2000). Early work in rodents on the functional contribution of the amygdala emphasized its critical role in the acquisition and expression of conditioned fear (Maren, Aharonov, & Fanselow, 1996; Quirk, Repa, & LeDoux, 1995). Extensive work in humans has further substantiated the role of the amygdala in facilitating conditioned fear responses (LaBar, Gatenby, Gore, LeDoux, & Phelps, 1998; LaBar, LeDoux, Spencer, & Phelps, 1995; Phelps, 2006; Phelps et al., 2001). Indeed, a vast human neuroimaging literature on the amygdala has evolved, with clear evidence for the amygdala being likewise involved in the appraisal of fearful expressions (Hariri, Tessitore, Mattay, Fera, & Weinberger, 2002; Whalen et al., 1998; Whalen et al., 2001) as well as threatening and unpleasant scenes (Hariri, Mattay, Tessitore, Fera, & Weinberger, 2003; Ochsner, Bunge, Gross, & Gabrieli, 2002; Ochsner et al., 2004). Moreover, amygdala activity has also been observed during the observation of sadness as well as appraisal of fearful and threatening information (Levesque et al., 2003; Wang, McCarthy, Song, & Labar, 2005).

While these results initially suggested that the amygdala may serve a specialized role in the detection of negative emotion, additional work has clarified that the amygdala is also significantly attuned to the appraisal of positively valenced stimuli as well, including pleasant faces and scenes (Kim & Hamann, 2007; Yang et al., 2002) as well as sexually arousing stimuli (Beauregard, Levesque, & Bourgouin, 2001; Hamann, Ely, Hoffman, & Kilts, 2002). Indeed, a quantitative meta-analysis of 148 functional neuroimaging studies of emotion has substantiated the amygdala's role in appraising both negatively and positively valenced information (Sergerie, Chochol, & Armony, 2008). Amygdala activity has further been shown to predict the magnitude of self-reported emotional responses (Ochsner, Ray, et al., 2009; Wager, Davidson, Hughes, Lindquist, & Ochsner, 2008) and is the most reliably modulated target of cognitive control (Buhle et al., 2014; Ochsner & Gross, 2008). Thus our model holds the predominant, contemporary view that the amygdala is involved in a more generalized assessment of the arousal and salience of a stimulus (Ochsner et al., 2012).

Insula

The insula, located deep within the lateral sulcus of the cortex, is associated with diverse psychological and physiological phenomena, including somatosensation, motor association, and language, as well a key role in emotional awareness and integration (Augustine, 1996; Craig, 2003, 2009; Wager & Barrett, 2004) and thus represents a key node in our model. Indeed, the insula and amygdala frequently coactivate in response to emotional stimuli (Etkin & Wager, 2010; Kober et al., 2008; Stein et al., 2007) and share substantial structural connectivity as well (Flynn, Benson, & Ardila, 1999; Mesulam & Mufson, 1982b; Mufson, Mesulam, & Pandya, 1981).

Early functional neuroimaging studies highlighted the role of insula in processing disgust experiences in particular (Damasio et al., 2000; Phillips et al., 2004; Phillips et al., 1997; Wicker et al., 2003), suggesting again a more specialized, locationist account of its involvement in emotion. However, as with the amygdala, more recent research has indicated that the insula is also involved in appraising positive stimuli, including pleasant music, voices, and faces (Craig, 2009; Hennenlotter et al., 2005; Johnstone, van Reekum, Oakes, & Davidson, 2006; Koelsch, Fritz, v. Cramon, Muller, & Friederici, 2006), and in integrating affective information (Menon & Uddin, 2010; Singer, Critchley, & Preuschoff, 2009).

Evidence for some functional specialization within insula has been provided by structural (Mesulam & Mufson, 1982a, 1982b) and functional (Deen, Pitskel, &

Pelphrey, 2011) connectivity work as well as neuroimaging meta-analyses (Wager & Barrett, 2004). This work has suggested an anterior–posterior distinction, with posterior insula being particularly attuned to processing primary visceral somatosensations from the body, while the more anterior portion has been particularly associated with interoceptive awareness and emotional and motivational states (Craig, 2009; Wager & Barrett, 2004). Functionally, the anterior–posterior distinction is not absolute, however (Denny et al., 2014; Flynn et al., 1999) and may be best thought of as a gradient (Ochsner et al., 2012). Thus in our model the insula is associated with affective and somatosensory integration.

Ventral Striatum

A final region consistently recruited during emotion generation is the ventral striatum, including the nucleus accumbens, which has been consistently linked to processing the anticipation of reward (Abler, Walter, Erk, Kammerer, & Spitzer, 2006; Knutson, Adams, Fong, & Hommer, 2001; Knutson & Cooper, 2005; O'Doherty et al., 2004). This representation of future reward is elicited by predictive cues, which are often abstract, that one learns to associate with a rewarding outcome (Knutson & Cooper, 2005; O'Doherty et al., 2004). Thus the ventral striatum is taken to represent the reward value of a stimulus in our model.

■ PROCESSES AND SYSTEMS INVOLVED IN EMOTION REGULATION

In the next section we turn our attention to mechanisms by which emotional responses may be modified once the emotion generative process is underway. Returning to the process model of Gross (1998b), once an emotional stimulus has been appraised (i.e., evaluated) as salient, the emotional response tendencies that determine the final shape of the emotional response may be modulated in various ways through the application of different emotion regulation strategies. As described, the initial determination of salience value draws upon the integrated functioning of the brain regions involved in emotion generation, including amygdala, insula, and the ventral striatum.

How then can emotional responses be modified once the appraisal process is underway? In Gross's model (Gross, 1998b; Gross & Thompson, 2007), an important distinction is made between antecedent-focused strategies (i.e., reshaping emotional response tendencies prior to the onset of an emotional response) versus response-focused strategies. Five main strategies are considered and briefly described here. As an example, imagine that you happen to see the aftermath of a gruesome car accident just ahead of you while driving down the highway. While your appraisal of this situation need not necessarily be conscious in order to engage the systems described previously in generating an emotional response, imagine that you are conscious of the upcoming scene. As such, you could take several routes to successful emotion regulation. Two antecedent-focused regulatory strategies include *situation selection* and *situation modification*; for this example, you may thus choose to take the next exit immediately and entirely change your surroundings (situation selection) or continue down the road but drive by the scene as fast as possible (situation modification). Alternatively, another antecedent-focused strategy is *attentional deployment*, whereby you could change what aspects of the situation you allow to flow through your attentional gates. For example, you might selectively attend to certain aspects of the situation, such as the highway and the overhead signs, rather than the emergency along the side of the road. Another means of attentional deployment is via distraction, whereby you continue to appraise an emotional situation while bearing other information in mind as well. In the example, to distract yourself, you may continue to observe the car wreck while at the same time considering your upcoming meeting (in addition to maintaining focus on the road).

A fourth and final antecedent-focused emotion regulation strategy is *cognitive change*, which involves changing the meaning of an emotion-eliciting stimulus. One well-studied exemplar is reappraisal, which involves cognitively reframing an emotional event in a way that modulates one's emotional response to it. Thus one could use reappraisal to upregulate or to downregulate either positive or negative emotion, though the majority of the reappraisal literature to date has focused on down-regulation of negative emotion (Ochsner & Gross, 2008; Ochsner et al., 2012). Two principal tactics one could use to implement the reappraisal strategy are reinterpretation and psychological distancing (Denny & Ochsner, 2014; McRae, Ciesielski, & Gross, 2012; Ochsner & Gross, 2008). Reinterpretation involves mentally changing the meaning of the actions, context, or outcomes of an emotion-eliciting situation, whereas psychological distancing involves changing one's construal of an event to be more distant (e.g., by appraising an event as an objective, impartial observer). Thus, for the car wreck example, if you were reinterpreting the situation you may think to yourself about how highly skilled the paramedics on the scene are and how it is very possible that the victims will survive. If you were employing psychological distancing, you would also be employing reappraisal, but in that case you may choose to focus on viewing the scene as a news reporter might, simply gathering information about how many cars were involved, how many people appear to have been involved, and whether anyone appears hurt. Last, a fifth emotion regulation strategy you might employ is a response-focused strategy, *response modulation*, meaning a strategy that targets the behavioral expression of emotion, rather than modifying the antecedents to an emotional response (i.e., modifying the situations, aspects, or meanings of an event, as described earlier; Gross, 1998a; Gross, 1998b; Gross & Thompson, 2007). A quintessential response-focused strategy is expressive suppression (Gross, 1998a); in our example, this would entail focusing on "keeping a poker face" and not showing any outward emotion while passing the car accident.

In this chapter, in describing the neural systems involved in emotion regulation, we give particular attention to describing the neural mechanisms that support reappraisal. Reappraisal is examined in depth as a paradigm case of emotion regulation for several reasons. First, reappraisal is the best-studied strategy in the emotion regulation literature (Buhle et al., 2014; Ochsner et al., 2012), with over 50 functional neuroimaging studies of reappraisal completed to date. Second, part of the reason for this investigational interest stems from reappraisal's relative advantages as a strategy. Reappraisal has been shown to reliably modulate emotional experience without increasing sympathetic arousal, in contrast to expressive suppression, which has been associated with increased sympathetic arousal, poorer memory for emotional events, and reduced well-being relative to reappraisal (Gross, 1998a, 2002; Gross & John, 2003; Richards & Gross, 2000). Further, reappraisal effects on behavior and neural activity have been shown to endure beyond initial regulation (Denny, Inhoff, Zerubavel, Davachi, & Ochsner, 2015; Denny & Ochsner, 2014; Kross & Ayduk, 2008; Walter et al., 2009) in contrast to other strategies like distraction (Kross & Ayduk, 2008; Thiruchselvam, Blechert, Sheppes, Rydstrom, & Gross, 2011). Finally, improving emotion regulation efficacy is a crucial target of many clinical therapies for mood, anxiety, and personality disorders (Berking et al., 2013; Berking et al., 2008; Denny et al., 2009; Ochsner et al., 2012). Reappraisal, in particular, is a key ingredient of several forms of cognitive-behavioral therapy, and understanding the neural mechanisms and trainability of reappraisal may assist in the development and refinement of novel cognitive therapies (Denny & Ochsner, 2014), as discussed in the "Conclusion and Future Directions" section of this chapter.

Thus what follows is our model of the principal brain regions involved in emotion regulation via reappraisal. This model has been informed by recent meta-analyses of functional neuroimaging studies of reappraisal (Buhle et al., 2014; Ochsner et al., 2012) and is summarized in Figure 5.1, with regulation-related regions highlighted in blue. These include several regions in the prefrontal cortex (PFC), including the ventrolateral PFC, dorsolateral PFC, posterior PFC, dorsomedial PFC, as well as the inferior parietal cortex and dorsal anterior cingulate cortex (dACC). We next discuss these regions associated with implementing reappraisal in more detail according to their grouping into four subsystems based on patterns of coactivation during cognitive control tasks (Ochsner & Gross, 2005; Ochsner et al., 2012).

Ventrolateral PFC

Ventrolateral PFC has been particularly implicated in the selection of goal-appropriate responses and the inhibition of goal-inappropriate responses during cognitive control and semantic memory retrieval (Aron, Robbins, & Poldrack, 2004, 2014; Badre, Poldrack, Pare-Blagoev, Insler, & Wagner, 2005), thus functioning as an important mental "brake" (Aron et al., 2014). Thus one would expect ventrolateral PFC to be reliably active during reappraisal implementation, where choosing a relevant and effective reconstrual of an emotional stimulus—and inhibiting the appraisal to which one is predisposed as well as many unhelpful or irrelevant reappraisals—would be of great importance. Indeed, this is the case, as ventrolateral PFC activity has been consistently observed in reappraisal tasks (Buhle et al., 2014; Ochsner et al., 2012).

Moreover, ventrolateral PFC activity during reappraisal implementation has been shown to predict the magnitude of amygdala activity attenuation (Johnstone, van Reekum, Urry, Kalin, & Davidson, 2007; Ochsner et al., 2002) as well as increases in self-reported reappraisal success (Wager et al., 2008). Wager and colleagues unpacked this positive relationship between ventrolateral PFC activity and reappraisal success further, showing the existence of two separable mediation pathways underlying this effect, each incorporating a mediator region that has been highlighted earlier as being involved in emotion generation. In one pathway, right ventrolateral PFC activity predicted greater reappraisal success in a relationship mediated by ventral striatum activity; right ventrolateral PFC activity predicted greater ventral striatum activity during reappraisal to downregulate negative emotion, and greater ventral striatum activity predicted greater reappraisal success. In another pathway, right ventrolateral PFC activity predicted reduced reappraisal success in a relationship mediated by amygdala activity; right ventrolateral PFC activity predicted greater amygdala activity during reappraisal to downregulate negative emotion, and greater amygdala activity predicted poorer reappraisal success (Wager et al., 2008). Thus, while there has not been a universally consistent association between ventrolateral PFC activity and amygdala activity during reappraisal implementation (which may due to variance in reappraisal tactics and stimuli), there has been a consistent association between ventrolateral PFC and both the selection of appropriate regulation responses as well as the inhibition of potentially unhelpful, negative thoughts, leading to overall reappraisal success. Thus in our model ventrolateral PFC plays a key role in appropriate response selection and inhibition.

Dorsolateral PFC, Posterior PFC, and Inferior Parietal Cortex

In the cognitive control literature, dorsolateral PFC, posterior PFC around Brodmann area 8, and inferior parietal cortex have all been implicated in selective attention and maintenance of information in working memory (Miller, 2000; Owen, McMillan, Laird, & Bullmore, 2005; Wager, Jonides, & Reading, 2004; Wager & Smith, 2003). These areas are all likewise reliably activated in reappraisal tasks (Buhle et al., 2014), consistent with the idea that reappraisal involves focusing attention on reappraisal-relevant aspects of a stimulus and holding relevant information in mind about the stimulus itself as well as information about the particular tactic or tactics to be used.

Further, in a manner similar to ventrolateral PFC, dorsolateral PFC has been shown to predict reappraisal success in a relationship mediated by an emotion generation region mentioned earlier. In a recent study by Kober and colleagues (2010), dorsolateral PFC activity when attempting to downregulate responses to appetitive cues (for either enticing food or for cigarettes among cigarette smokers) was associated with greater reappraisal success (i.e., less reported craving) in a relationship mediated by ventral striatum activity. In particular, greater dorsolateral PFC activity during reappraisal predicted less ventral striatum activity, and less ventral striatum activity predicted greater reappraisal success. The direction of these effects make sense in this context, given the presence of an appetitive rather than an aversive stimulus, and are thus consistent with the mediation study reviewed earlier involving ventrolateral PFC, ventral striatum, and reappraisal success (Wager et al., 2008). The existence of analogous mediated relationships involving posterior PFC and inferior parietal cortex is unclear, although we would make similar predictions for each. Thus, in our model, dorsolateral PFC, posterior PFC, and inferior parietal cortex are associated with selective attention and working memory.

Dorsomedial PFC

One of the functions most consistently associated with medial PFC is mentalizing, which refers to thoughts and inferences about one's own or someone else's mental state. In a recent meta-analysis of 107 functional neuroimaging studies, we have shown that in addition to medial PFC being robustly associated with mentalizing, a functional gradient exists such that relatively ventral aspects of medial PFC process self-focused mentalizing, while relatively dorsal aspects of medial PFC process other-focused mentalizing (Denny, Kober, Wager, & Ochsner, 2012). In the context of reappraisal, where dorsomedial PFC activity is often observed (Buhle et al., 2014), such a relationship makes sense, for both the association with mentalizing in general and for mentalizing about others in particular. Indeed, reappraisals—particularly using the reinterpretation tactic—involve mentalizing about how someone else may feel, or will feel, after a reconstrual of a situation that involves changing the actions, context, or outcomes. Therefore, in our model dorsomedial PFC plays an important role in supporting mentalizing about oneself and, especially, about others.

dACC

Finally, we review the role of the dACC. Across cognitive, affective, and social domains, dACC activity has consistently been associated with conflict monitoring (Botvinick, Cohen, & Carter, 2004; Botvinick, Nystrom, Fissell, Carter, & Cohen, 1999; Ochsner, Hughes, Robertson, Cooper, & Gabrieli, 2009; Zaki, Hennigan, Weber, & Ochsner, 2010). Conflict monitoring refers to the process of attending to and selecting among competing environmental inputs and the appropriate responses that are associated with each. In the context of reappraisal, where dACC activity is frequently observed (Buhle et al., 2014), this could involve evaluating multiple, potentially mutually exclusive reconstruals in the process of selecting the most appropriate one, and then ensuring that one's reappraisal is indeed efficacious in changing one's emotional response. Thus dACC is taken to facilitate conflict monitoring in our model.

■ CONCLUSION AND FUTURE DIRECTIONS

We have provided evidence for a model of the cognitive control of emotion that integrates evidence from the burgeoning social, cognitive, and affective neuroscience literature on the neural bases of emotion generation and emotion regulation. In this final section, we briefly outline several future directions that follow from the discussion of our model. First, as the pace of research into emotion regulation has greatly accelerated in recent years (Gross, 2013; Ochsner et al., 2012), it is becoming possible to refine models of emotion regulation to differentiate among different goals (i.e., to downregulate or upregulate emotion), strategies (e.g., reappraisal or attentional deployment), tactics (e.g., reinterpretation or distancing), and valences (i.e., regulating negative or positive emotion). Further, additional work is beginning to elucidate the temporal dynamics of emotion regulation, including reappraisal; thus, while there has been recent evidence for the longitudinal trainability of reappraisal in an experimental context (Denny & Ochsner, 2014), an exciting host of questions persist, including the optimal delivery methods for emotion regulation training (e.g., massed versus temporally distributed practice; repeated versus novel stimuli); the relative trainability of different strategies; examination of how long emotion regulation effects endure beyond training across multiple levels of analysis (e.g., behavior, psychophysiology, neurobiology); and, crucially, the adaptive translational impacts that may be observed in daily life (Berkman & Falk, 2013; Denny & Ochsner, 2014). Further, understanding how emotion regulation changes across the lifespan is likewise essential, providing an opportunity to understand the critical periods during which interventions might be most effectively initiated (Charles & Carstensen, 2014; Riediger & Klipker, 2014; Silvers, Buhle, & Ochsner, 2014).

However, the future directions most relevant to the aims of this book involve extending this model, derived from healthy adult data, to psychopathological populations, including personality disorder patients. Indeed, emotion regulation is a signal deficit in many forms of psychopathology (Denny et al., 2009; Gross & Munoz,

1995; Werner & Gross, 2009), and the refinement of cognitive-behavioral interventions aimed at improving emotion regulation skills represents a promising and ongoing project (Berking et al., 2013; Berking et al., 2008). In testing the applicability of this model to psychopathological populations, it will be fascinating to examine whether the neural mechanisms supporting emotion regulation in many forms of psychopathology are fundamentally the same as those in healthy adults, though involving gradiential differences in the activity of key nodes in a manner suggesting dimensional boundaries between groups, or rather whether the nodes most central to the phenomenology of certain mental disorders are fundamentally distinct from other mental disorders and from healthy populations in a manner supporting categorically distinct neurobiological models. For personality disorders in particular, preliminary evidence of at least partial mechanistic overlap exists, with hyperactivation of amygdala activity reported as an important component of the neurobiological basis of emotion generation and regulation in several disorders, including borderline personality disorder (Herpertz et al., 2001; Koenigsberg et al., 2009; Schulze et al., 2011) and avoidant personality disorder (Denny et al., 2015).

Ultimately, gaining a robust understanding of the neurobiological bases of emotion generation and regulation across healthy and psychopathological populations offers myriad potential benefits. Certainly, the implications for treatment could be substantial. With this knowledge, we may be able to better target certain interventions to certain individuals at critical times and in ways that are most likely to improve health and well-being. And, of course, most fundamentally, we may be better able to characterize the nature of the disorders themselves.

■ REFERENCES

Abler, B., Walter, H., Erk, S., Kammerer, H., & Spitzer, M. (2006). Prediction error as a linear function of reward probability is coded in human nucleus accumbens. *Neuroimage*, *31*(2), 790–795.

Aron, A. R., Robbins, T. W., & Poldrack, R. A. (2004). Inhibition and the right inferior frontal cortex. *Trends Cogn Sci*, *8*(4), 170–177.

Aron, A. R., Robbins, T. W., & Poldrack, R. A. (2014). Inhibition and the right inferior frontal cortex: one decade on. *Trends Cogn Sci*, *18*(4), 177–185.

Augustine, J. R. (1996). Circuitry and functional aspects of the insular lobe in primates including humans. *Brain Res Brain Res Rev*, *22*(3), 229–244.

Badre, D., Poldrack, R. A., Pare-Blagoev, E. J., Insler, R. Z., & Wagner, A. D. (2005). Dissociable controlled retrieval and generalized selection mechanisms in ventrolateral prefrontal cortex. *Neuron*, *47*(6), 907–918.

Beauregard, M., Levesque, J., & Bourgouin, P. (2001). Neural correlates of conscious self-regulation of emotion. *J Neurosci*, *21*(18), RC165.

Berking, M., Ebert, D., Cuijpers, P., & Hofmann, S. G. (2013). Emotion regulation skills training enhances the efficacy of inpatient cognitive behavioral therapy for major depressive disorder: a randomized controlled trial. *Psychother Psychosom*, *82*(4), 234–245.

Berking, M., Wupperman, P., Reichardt, A., Pejic, T., Dippel, A., & Znoj, H. (2008). Emotion-regulation skills as a treatment target in psychotherapy. *Behav Res Ther*, *46*(11), 1230–1237.

Berkman, E. T., & Falk, E. B. (2013). Beyond brain mapping: using neural measures to predict real-world outcomes. *Curr Dir Psychol Sci*, *22*(1), 45–50.

Botvinick, M. M., Cohen, J. D., & Carter, C. S. (2004). Conflict monitoring and anterior cingulate cortex: an update. *Trends Cogn Sci, 8*(12), 539–546.

Botvinick, M. M., Nystrom, L. E., Fissell, K., Carter, C. S., & Cohen, J. D. (1999). Conflict monitoring versus selection-for-action in anterior cingulate cortex. *Nature, 402*(6758), 179–181.

Buhle, J. T., Silvers, J. A., Wager, T. D., Lopez, R., Onyemekwu, C., Kober, H., et al. (2014). Cognitive reappraisal of emotion: a meta-analysis of human neuroimaging studies. *Cereb Cortex, 24*(11), 2981–2990.

Charles, S. T., & Carstensen, L. L. (2014). Emotion regulation and aging. In J. J. Gross (Ed.), *Handbook of emotion regulation* (2nd ed., pp. 203–220). New York: Guilford Press.

Craig, A. D. (2003). Interoception: the sense of the physiological condition of the body. *Curr Opin Neurobiol, 13*(4), 500–505.

Craig, A. D. (2009). How do you feel—now? The anterior insula and human awareness. *Nat Rev Neurosci, 10*(1), 59–70.

Damasio, A. R., Grabowski, T. J., Bechara, A., Damasio, H., Ponto, L. L., Parvizi, J., et al. (2000). Subcortical and cortical brain activity during the feeling of self-generated emotions. *Nat Neurosci, 3*(10), 1049–1056.

Deen, B., Pitskel, N. B., & Pelphrey, K. A. (2011). Three systems of insular functional connectivity identified with cluster analysis. *Cereb Cortex, 21*(7), 1498–1506.

Denny, B. T., Fan, J., Liu, X., Guerreri, S., Mayson, S. J., Rimsky, L., et al. (2014). Insula-amygdala functional connectivity is correlated with habituation to repeated negative images. *Soc Cogn Affect Neurosci, 9*(11), 1660–1667.

Denny, B. T., Fan, J., Liu, X., Ochsner, K. N., Guerreri, S., Mayson, S. J., et al. (2015). Elevated amygdala activity during reappraisal anticipation predicts anxiety in avoidant personality disorder. *J Affect Disord, 172*, 1–7.

Denny, B. T., Inhoff, M. C., Zerubavel, N., Davachi, L., & Ochsner, K. N. (2015). Getting over it: Long-lasting effects of emotion regulation on amygdala response. *Psychol Sci, 26*(9), 1377–1388.

Denny, B. T., Kober, H., Wager, T. D., & Ochsner, K. N. (2012). A meta-analysis of functional neuroimaging studies of self- and other judgments reveals a spatial gradient for mentalizing in medial prefrontal cortex. *J Cogn Neurosci, 24*(8), 1742–1752.

Denny, B. T., & Ochsner, K. N. (2014). Behavioral effects of longitudinal training in cognitive reappraisal. *Emotion, 14*(2), 425–433.

Denny, B. T., Silvers, J. A., & Ochsner, K. N. (2009). How we heal what we don't want to feel: the functional neural architecture of emotion regulation. In A. M. Kring & D. M. Sloan (Eds.), *Emotion regulation and psychopathology: a transdiagnostic approach to etiology and treatment* (pp. 59–87). New York: Guilford Press.

Etkin, A., & Wager, T. D. (2010). Brain systems underlying anxiety disorders: a view from neuroimaging. In H. B. Simpson, F. Schneier, Y. Neria, & R. Lewis-Fernandez (Eds.), *Anxiety disorders: theory, research and clinical perspectives* (pp. 192–203). Cambridge, UK: Cambridge University Press.

Flynn, F. G., Benson, D. F., & Ardila, A. (1999). Anatomy of the insula—functional and clinical correlates. *Aphasiology, 13*(1), 55–78.

Gross, J. J. (1998a). Antecedent- and response-focused emotion regulation: divergent consequences for experience, expression, and physiology. *J Pers Soc Psychol, 74*(1), 224–237.

Gross, J. J. (1998b). The emerging field of emotion regulation: an integrative review. *Rev Gener Psychol, 2*(3), 271–299.

Gross, J. J. (2002). Emotion regulation: affective, cognitive, and social consequences. *Psychophysiology, 39*(3), 281–291.

Gross, J. J. (2013). Emotion regulation: taking stock and moving forward. *Emotion, 13*(3), 359–365.

Gross, J. J., & John, O. P. (2003). Individual differences in two emotion regulation processes: implications for affect, relationships, and well-being. *J Pers Soc Psychol, 85*(2), 348–362.

Gross, J. J., & Munoz, R. F. (1995). Emotion regulation and mental health. *Clin Psychol Sci Pract, 2*(2), 151–164.

Gross, J. J., & Thompson, R. A. (2007). Emotion regulation: conceptual foundations. In J. J. Gross (Ed.), *Handbook of emotion regulation* (pp. 3–24). New York: Guilford Press.

Hamann, S. B., Ely, T. D., Hoffman, J. M., & Kilts, C. D. (2002). Ecstasy and agony: activation of the human amygdala in positive and negative emotion. *Psychol Sci, 13*(2), 135–141.

Hariri, A. R., Mattay, V. S., Tessitore, A., Fera, F., & Weinberger, D. R. (2003). Neocortical modulation of the amygdala response to fearful stimuli. *Biol Psychiatry, 53*(6), 494–501.

Hariri, A. R., Tessitore, A., Mattay, V. S., Fera, F., & Weinberger, D. R. (2002). The amygdala response to emotional stimuli: a comparison of faces and scenes. *Neuroimage, 17*(1), 317–323.

Hennenlotter, A., Schroeder, U., Erhard, P., Castrop, F., Haslinger, B., Stoecker, D., et al. (2005). A common neural basis for receptive and expressive communication of pleasant facial affect. *Neuroimage, 26*(2), 581–591.

Herpertz, S. C., Dietrich, T. M., Wenning, B., Krings, T., Erberich, S. G., Willmes, K., et al. (2001). Evidence of abnormal amygdala functioning in borderline personality disorder: a functional MRI study. *Biol Psychiatry, 50*(4), 292–298.

Johnstone, T., van Reekum, C. M., Oakes, T. R., & Davidson, R. J. (2006). The voice of emotion: an FMRI study of neural responses to angry and happy vocal expressions. *Soc Cogn Affect Neurosci, 1*(3), 242–249.

Johnstone, T., van Reekum, C. M., Urry, H. L., Kalin, N. H., & Davidson, R. J. (2007). Failure to regulate: counterproductive recruitment of top-down prefrontal-subcortical circuitry in major depression. *J Neurosci, 27*(33), 8877–8884.

Kim, S. H., & Hamann, S. (2007). Neural correlates of positive and negative emotion regulation. *J Cogn Neurosci, 19*(5), 776–798.

Knutson, B., Adams, C. M., Fong, G. W., & Hommer, D. (2001). Anticipation of increasing monetary reward selectively recruits nucleus accumbens. *J Neurosci, 21*(16), RC159.

Knutson, B., & Cooper, J. C. (2005). Functional magnetic resonance imaging of reward prediction. *Curr Opin Neurol, 18*(4), 411–417.

Kober, H., Barrett, L. F., Joseph, J., Bliss-Moreau, E., Lindquist, K., & Wager, T. D. (2008). Functional grouping and cortical-subcortical interactions in emotion: a meta-analysis of neuroimaging studies. *Neuroimage, 42*(2), 998–1031.

Kober, H., Mende-Siedlecki, P., Kross, E. F., Weber, J., Mischel, W., Hart, C. L., et al. (2010). Prefrontal-striatal pathway underlies cognitive regulation of craving. *Proc Natl Acad Sci U S A, 107*(33), 14811–14816.

Koelsch, S., Fritz, T., v. Cramon, D. Y., Muller, K., & Friederici, A. D. (2006). Investigating emotion with music: an fMRI study. *Hum Brain Mapp, 27*(3), 239–250.

Koenigsberg, H. W., Fan, J., Ochsner, K. N., Liu, X., Guise, K. G., Pizzarello, S., et al. (2009). Neural correlates of the use of psychological distancing to regulate responses to negative social cues: a study of patients with borderline personality disorder. *Biol Psychiatry, 66*(9), 854–863.

Kross, E., & Ayduk, O. (2008). Facilitating adaptive emotional analysis: distinguishing distanced-analysis of depressive experiences from immersed-analysis and distraction. *Pers Soc Psychol Bull, 34*(7), 924–938.

LaBar, K. S., Gatenby, J. C., Gore, J. C., LeDoux, J. E., & Phelps, E. A. (1998). Human amygdala activation during conditioned fear acquisition and extinction: a mixed-trial fMRI study. *Neuron, 20*(5), 937–945.

LaBar, K. S., LeDoux, J. E., Spencer, D. D., & Phelps, E. A. (1995). Impaired fear conditioning following unilateral temporal lobectomy in humans. *J Neurosci, 15*(10), 6846–6855.

LeDoux, J. E. (1995). Emotion: clues from the brain. *Annu Rev Psychol, 46*, 209–235.

LeDoux, J. E. (2000). Emotion circuits in the brain. *Annu Rev Neurosci, 23*, 155–184.

Levesque, J., Eugene, F., Joanette, Y., Paquette, V., Mensour, B., Beaudoin, G., et al. (2003). Neural circuitry underlying voluntary suppression of sadness. *Biol Psychiatry, 53*(6), 502–510.

Lindquist, K. A., Wager, T. D., Kober, H., Bliss-Moreau, E., & Barrett, L. F. (2012). The brain basis of emotion: a meta-analytic review. *Behav Brain Sci, 35*(3), 121–143.

Maren, S., Aharonov, G., & Fanselow, M. S. (1996). Retrograde abolition of conditional fear after excitotoxic lesions in the basolateral amygdala of rats: absence of a temporal gradient. *Behav Neurosci, 110*(4), 718–726.

McRae, K., Ciesielski, B., & Gross, J. J. (2012). Unpacking cognitive reappraisal: goals, tactics, and outcomes. *Emotion, 12*(2), 250–255.

Menon, V., & Uddin, L. Q. (2010). Saliency, switching, attention and control: a network model of insula function. *Brain Struct Funct, 214*(5-6), 655–667.

Mesulam, M. M., & Mufson, E. J. (1982a). Insula of the old world monkey. I. Architectonics in the insulo-orbito-temporal component of the paralimbic brain. *J Comp Neurol, 212*(1), 1–22.

Mesulam, M. M., & Mufson, E. J. (1982b). Insula of the old world monkey. III: Efferent cortical output and comments on function. *J Comp Neurol, 212*(1), 38–52.

Miller, E. K. (2000). The prefrontal cortex and cognitive control. *Nat Rev Neurosci, 1*(1), 59–65.

Mufson, E. J., Mesulam, M. M., & Pandya, D. N. (1981). Insular interconnections with the amygdala in the rhesus monkey. *Neuroscience, 6*(7), 1231–1248.

O'Doherty, J., Dayan, P., Schultz, J., Deichmann, R., Friston, K., & Dolan, R. J. (2004). Dissociable roles of ventral and dorsal striatum in instrumental conditioning. *Science, 304*(5669), 452–454.

Ochsner, K. N. (2007). Social cognitive neuroscience: Historical development, core principles, and future promise. In A. Kruglankski & E. T. Higgins (Eds.), *Social psychology: a handbook of basic principles* (2nd ed., pp. 39–66). New York: Guilford Press.

Ochsner, K. N., Bunge, S. A., Gross, J. J., & Gabrieli, J. D. (2002). Rethinking feelings: an FMRI study of the cognitive regulation of emotion. *J Cogn Neurosci, 14*(8), 1215–1229.

Ochsner, K. N., & Gross, J. J. (2005). The cognitive control of emotion. *Trends Cogn Sci, 9*(5), 242–249.

Ochsner, K. N., & Gross, J. J. (2008). Cognitive emotion regulation: Insights from social cognitive and affective neuroscience. *Curr Dir Psychol Sci, 17*(2), 153–158.

Ochsner, K. N., Hughes, B., Robertson, E. R., Cooper, J. C., & Gabrieli, J. D. (2009). Neural systems supporting the control of affective and cognitive conflicts. *J Cogn Neurosci, 21*(9), 1842–1855.

Ochsner, K. N., Ray, R. D., Cooper, J. C., Robertson, E. R., Chopra, S., Gabrieli, J. D., et al. (2004). For better or for worse: neural systems supporting the cognitive down- and up-regulation of negative emotion. *Neuroimage, 23*(2), 483–499.

Ochsner, K. N., Ray, R. R., Hughes, B., McRae, K., Cooper, J. C., Weber, J., et al. (2009). Bottom-up and top-down processes in emotion generation: common and distinct neural mechanisms. *Psychol Sci, 20*(11), 1322–1331.

Ochsner, K. N., Silvers, J. A., & Buhle, J. T. (2012). Functional imaging studies of emotion regulation: a synthetic review and evolving model of the cognitive control of emotion. *Ann N Y Acad Sci, 1251,* E1–E24.

Owen, A. M., McMillan, K. M., Laird, A. R., & Bullmore, E. (2005). N-back working memory paradigm: a meta-analysis of normative functional neuroimaging studies. *Hum Brain Mapp, 25*(1), 46–59.

Phelps, E. A. (2006). Emotion and cognition: insights from studies of the human amygdala. *Annu Rev Psychol, 57,* 27–53.

Phelps, E. A., O'Connor, K. J., Gatenby, J. C., Gore, J. C., Grillon, C., & Davis, M. (2001). Activation of the left amygdala to a cognitive representation of fear. *Nat Neurosci, 4*(4), 437–441.

Phillips, M. L., Williams, L. M., Heining, M., Herba, C. M., Russell, T., Andrew, C., et al. (2004). Differential neural responses to overt and covert presentations of facial expressions of fear and disgust. *Neuroimage, 21*(4), 1484–1496.

Phillips, M. L., Young, A. W., Senior, C., Brammer, M., Andrew, C., Calder, A. J., et al. (1997). A specific neural substrate for perceiving facial expressions of disgust. *Nature, 389*(6650), 495–498.

Quirk, G. J., Repa, C., & LeDoux, J. E. (1995). Fear conditioning enhances short-latency auditory responses of lateral amygdala neurons: parallel recordings in the freely behaving rat. *Neuron, 15*(5), 1029–1039.

Richards, J. M., & Gross, J. J. (2000). Emotion regulation and memory: the cognitive costs of keeping one's cool. *J Pers Soc Psychol, 79*(3), 410–424.

Riediger, M., & Klipker, K. (2014). Emotion regulation in adolescence. In J. J. Gross (Ed.), *Handbook of emotion regulation* (2nd ed., pp. 187–202). New York: Guilford Press.

Schulze, L., Domes, G., Kruger, A., Berger, C., Fleischer, M., Prehn, K., et al. (2011). Neuronal correlates of cognitive reappraisal in borderline patients with affective instability. *Biol Psychiatry, 69*(6), 564–573.

Sergerie, K., Chochol, C., & Armony, J. L. (2008). The role of the amygdala in emotional processing: a quantitative meta-analysis of functional neuroimaging studies. *Neurosci Biobehav Rev, 32*(4), 811–830.

Silvers, J. A., Buhle, J. T., & Ochsner, K. N. (2014). The neuroscience of emotion regulation: Basic mechanisms and their role in development, aging and psychopathology. In K. N. Ochsner & S. M. Kosslyn (Eds.), *The Oxford handbook of cognitive neuroscience,* Vol. 2: *The cutting edges* (pp. 52–78). New York: Oxford University Press.

Singer, T., Critchley, H. D., & Preuschoff, K. (2009). A common role of insula in feelings, empathy and uncertainty. *Trends Cogn Sci, 13*(8), 334–340.

Stein, J. L., Wiedholz, L. M., Bassett, D. S., Weinberger, D. R., Zink, C. F., Mattay, V. S., et al. (2007). A validated network of effective amygdala connectivity. *Neuroimage, 36*(3), 736–745.

Thiruchselvam, R., Blechert, J., Sheppes, G., Rydstrom, A., & Gross, J. J. (2011). The temporal dynamics of emotion regulation: an EEG study of distraction and reappraisal. *Biol Psychol, 87*(1), 84–92.

Wager, T. D., & Barrett, L. F. (2004). From affect to control: functional specialization of the insula in motivation and regulation. https://www.biorxiv.org/content/early/2017/01/23/102368

Wager, T. D., Davidson, M. L., Hughes, B. L., Lindquist, M. A., & Ochsner, K. N. (2008). Prefrontal-subcortical pathways mediating successful emotion regulation. *Neuron, 59*(6), 1037–1050.

Wager, T. D., Jonides, J., & Reading, S. (2004). Neuroimaging studies of shifting attention: a meta-analysis. *Neuroimage, 22*(4), 1679–1693.

Wager, T. D., & Smith, E. E. (2003). Neuroimaging studies of working memory: a meta-analysis. *Cogn Affect Behav Neurosci*, *3*(4), 255–274.

Walter, H., von Kalckreuth, A., Schardt, D., Stephan, A., Goschke, T., & Erk, S. (2009). The temporal dynamics of voluntary emotion regulation. *PLoS One*, *4*(8), e6726.

Wang, L., McCarthy, G., Song, A. W., & Labar, K. S. (2005). Amygdala activation to sad pictures during high-field (4 tesla) functional magnetic resonance imaging. *Emotion*, *5*(1), 12–22.

Werner, K., & Gross, J. J. (2009). Emotion regulation and psychopathology: a conceptual framework. In A. M. Kring & D. M. Sloan (Eds.), *Emotion regulation and psychopathology: a transdiagnostic approach to etiology and treatment* (pp. 13–37). New York: Guilford Press.

Whalen, P. J., Rauch, S. L., Etcoff, N. L., McInerney, S. C., Lee, M. B., & Jenike, M. A. (1998). Masked presentations of emotional facial expressions modulate amygdala activity without explicit knowledge. *J Neurosci*, *18*(1), 411–418.

Whalen, P. J., Shin, L. M., McInerney, S. C., Fischer, H., Wright, C. I., & Rauch, S. L. (2001). A functional MRI study of human amygdala responses to facial expressions of fear versus anger. *Emotion*, *1*(1), 70–83.

Wicker, B., Keysers, C., Plailly, J., Royet, J. P., Gallese, V., & Rizzolatti, G. (2003). Both of us disgusted in My insula: the common neural basis of seeing and feeling disgust. *Neuron*, *40*(3), 655–664.

Yang, T. T., Menon, V., Eliez, S., Blasey, C., White, C. D., Reid, A. J., et al. (2002). Amygdalar activation associated with positive and negative facial expressions. *Neuroreport*, *13*(14), 1737–1741.

Zaki, J., Hennigan, K., Weber, J., & Ochsner, K. N. (2010). Social cognitive conflict resolution: contributions of domain-general and domain-specific neural systems. *J Neurosci*, *30*(25), 8481–8488.

6 The Neurobiology of Attachment and Mentalizing

A Neurodevelopmental Perspective

■ PATRICK LUYTEN AND PETER FONAGY

■ INTRODUCTION

This chapter addresses the neurobiology of attachment and mentalizing from a developmental psychopathology perspective. *Attachment* refers to an evolutionarily prewired, basic biobehavioral system that is activated in situations of stress and threat (Bowlby, 1973; Ein-Dor, Mikulincer, Doron, & Shaver, 2010; Mikulincer & Shaver, 2007; Panksepp, 1998). Developmentally, the attachment system plays a key role in the modulation of the stress response, another key biobehavioral system, and thus in survival (Gunnar & Quevedo, 2007; Hostinar, Sullivan, & Gunnar, 2014; Lupien, McEwen, Gunnar, & Heim, 2009; Panksepp & Watt, 2011; Watt & Panksepp, 2009). It does so because activation of the attachment system normatively leads to the seeking of proximity of attachment figures, either in reality, or by means of activating representations of secure attachment experiences, or both. This leads to (a) the downregulation of stress at the subjective and neurobiological level and (b) renewed energy and motivation to explore the world, leading to the so-called broaden-and-build cycles (Fredrickson, 2001) associated with attachment security (Mikulincer & Shaver, 2007). In individuals with a secure attachment history, this pattern gradually becomes generalized to different situations and circumstances. From a biological perspective, the attachment system is underpinned by a mesocorticolimbic dopaminergic reward system that is involved in the rewarding features of infant–parent, parent–infant, pair-bonding, and other attachment relationships (Insel & Young, 2001; Panksepp & Watt, 2011; Rutherford, Williams, Moy, Mayes, & Johns, 2011; Strathearn, Fonagy, Amico, & Montague, 2009; Swain, Lorberbaum, Kose, & Strathearn, 2007).

The attachment system is also closely related to the *mentalizing* or *social cognition* system, which subserves the human capacity to understand oneself and others in terms of intentional mental states (e.g., feelings, desires, wishes, attitudes, and values). This system has most likely evolved out of the need for human beings to develop the needed computational power to navigate a complex social world (Fonagy, Luyten, & Allison, 2015; Tomasello & Vaish, 2013). From a biological perspective, as we describe in more detail in this chapter, different capacities or features of mentalizing are underpinned by relatively different neural circuits (Lieberman, 2007; Luyten & Fonagy, 2015).

Both attachment disruptions and mentalizing impairments, and their links with impairments in stress and arousal regulation, have been amply demonstrated in individuals vulnerable for psychopathology, particularly in individuals with personality disorder (Fonagy & Luyten, 2016; Levy, Meehan, Weber, Reynoso, & Clarkin, 2005). Knowledge of the normal development of neurobiological systems underlying attachment and mentalizing, and disruptions in these normal developmental trajectories, may therefore directly inform our understanding of psychopathology and of personality disorders specifically.

In this chapter, we first consider the neurobiology of attachment. We then discuss the neurobiological underpinning of mentalizing in relation to attachment and stress regulation. We focus on the early development of both capacities in relation to stress regulation and discuss the relationship to the development of psychopathology and personality disorder in particular across the lifespan, with a focus on early childhood and adolescence.

■ ATTACHMENT AND REWARD

The Roots of Attachment in Rewarding Experiences

That social and attachment relationships should be one of the most rewarding experiences is predicted by both evolutionary (Gilbert, 2006) and psychological (Beck, 2009; Blatt, 2008) theories. Research in both animals and human beings has suggested that attachment, particularly in normal development, is underpinned by a powerful neurobiological reward system (Champagne et al., 2004; Ferris et al., 2005; Insel & Young, 2001; Strathearn, Li, Fonagy, & Montague, 2008). This reward system has been relatively well described in the literature as comprising various mesolimbic and mesocortical pathways. The ventral tegmental area is the origin of mesolimbic pathways, which mainly project to ventral striatal regions, in particular the nucleus accumbens, hippocampus, and amygdala. Meanwhile the mesocortical pathways mainly project to the prefrontal cortex (PFC) and anterior cingulate cortex (ACC; Nestler & Carlezon, 2006; Pizzagalli, 2014; Russo & Nestler, 2013; Spear, 2000). Dopamine and oxytocin have been regarded as the key biological mediators involved in this system. However, opioid and cannabinoid systems are also of considerable interest because they are associated with the sensation of pain arising from rejection and social loss, a response that is heightened in adolescence, particularly in females (Hsu et al., 2015; Panksepp & Watt, 2011; Spear, 2000).

Studies in animals (including higher primates) and a growing body of research in human beings (Hostinar et al., 2014; Strathearn, 2011; Swain et al., 2014) suggest that this attachment/reward system plays a key developmental role in the emergence and ongoing regulation of the stress system. Typically, secure attachment experiences serve to cushion the effects of stress in early development; this results in "adaptive hypoactivity" of the hypothalamic–pituitary–adrenal (HPA) axis in early development (Gunnar & Quevedo, 2007). For securely attached individuals, relationships become increasingly rewarding, and experiences of effective downregulation lead to feelings of autonomy and confidence in one's capacity to deal with adversity (i.e., *resilience*). By contrast, insecure attachment experiences can lead to increased susceptibility to stress, indicated by dysfunctions of both the HPA axis and the reward system (Auerbach, Admon, & Pizzagalli, 2014; Pizzagalli, 2014; Strathearn, 2011). In these individuals, attachment experiences become increasingly aversive, which also undermines these individuals' ability to deal with adversity and their confidence in their ability to do so.

Neuropeptides such as oxytocin and vasopressin are key modulators of the relationship between attachment and stress regulation. Oxytocin seems to increase affiliative behavior in the face of distress, particularly in securely attached individuals and in relation to in-group members. Such behavior serves to optimize opportunities for the effective coregulation of stress with others, reducing behavioral and neuroendocrinological stress responses (Neumann, 2008). Oxytocin also has anxiolytic and antistress effects by acting to downregulate the HPA axis system. Furthermore, it fosters mentalizing and trust in others, again increasing opportunities for the effective downregulation of distress and the use of exploration (Bartz, Zaki, Bolger, & Ochsner, 2011; Neumann, 2008) and leading to broaden-and-build cycles (Fredrickson, 2001; Mikulincer & Shaver, 2007). However, even in community samples these effects seem mainly limited to in-group members. Research has shown that in relation to out-group members, the administration of oxytocin leads to increased distrust, more bias in attributing intentions, and decreases in cooperative behavior (Bartz, Simeon, et al., 2011).

Further, in individuals with an insecure attachment history, decreased basal oxytocin levels have been observed, and the administration of oxytocin can have negative effects on social behavior, leading to disruption of the stress response (Bartz, Simeon, et al., 2011; Bertsch, Schmidinger, Neumann, & Herpertz, 2013; Cyranowski et al., 2008; Fries, Hesse, Hellhammer, & Hellhammer, 2005; Heim, Newport, Mletzko, Miller, & Hemeroff, 2008; Meinlschmidt & Heim, 2007; Stanley & Siever, 2010). The effect of oxytocin therefore seems to be that it increases the salience of attachment issues in either a positive or a negative direction. This may be a particular problem in individuals with personality disorders, who often have a marked history of early adversity, particularly attachment trauma. For such individuals, attachment experiences lack rewarding features and are, at best, associated with both reward and anxiety, anger, and/or frustration.

Adolescence and Reward: A Critical Juncture?

During adolescence, the attachment/reward system undergoes marked reorganization (Auerbach et al., 2014; Davey, Yücel, & Allen, 2008; Forbes & Dahl, 2012; Luciana, 2013; Spear, 2000). One of the primary shifts lies in the area of relatedness, which occurs alongside entry into the complex world of peer and romantic relationships (expressed in increased rejection sensitivity) and greater expectations in relation to achievement (reflected in increased sensitivity to failure). At the same time, adolescence is also characterized by the lowest levels of dopamine in striatal regions and the highest levels of dopamine in prefrontal regions; these changes have been suggested to lead to a "mini-reward deficiency syndrome" typical of adolescence (Spear, 2007). This may encourage compensatory behaviors, including risk-taking and drug abuse, as are typically found in individuals with personality disorders (Davey et al., 2008; Spear, 2000).

These findings may also explain why disappointment and/or frustration of needs for relationships and struggles with feelings of belongingness and achievement/status (which are closely intertwined, particularly in adolescence) may lead to a downward spiral characterized by suppression of the reward system, higher levels of stress, and resulting impairments in mentalizing. It has been speculated that the decrease in the incentive value of rewards in adolescence is evolutionarily adaptive, as it serves to encourage novelty and sensation-seeking behavior, which in turn supports adolescents in accomplishing important developmental tasks (e.g., developing feelings of autonomy and achievement and establishing complex relationships with others).

Two explanations have been formulated to explain the mini-reward deficiency syndrome in adolescence. Low levels of tonic dopamine in combination with high levels of phasic dopamine release in response to rewards might explain why adolescents are particularly keen to seek out novel and highly rewarding stimuli (Davey et al., 2008; Luciana, 2013). On the other hand, excessive downregulation of the PFC, as a result of high levels of dopamine in the PFC resulting from increased stress, might lead to impairments in reward sensitivity in adolescence (Pizzagalli, 2014; Spear, 2000). Specifically, high levels of mesocortical dopamine impair mentalizing and representational capacities more generally and thus may also make the incentive value of rewards seem diminished: there is a heightened perception that the important rewards in adolescence (i.e., love and status) are abstract and temporally distant (Davey et al., 2008).

■ MENTALIZING, ATTACHMENT, AND STRESS REGULATION

Origins of the Capacity for Mentalizing in Attachment Relationships

Higher social cognition, in particular the ability to mentalize, is considered to be the factor that underpins humanity's capacity to live in very large social groups. In primate species, including *Homo sapiens*, the size of the social group typically tolerated correlates with the size of the neocortex (the prefrontal and temporoparietal areas that support the large-scale social interactions characteristic of human beings; Dunbar & Shultz, 2007; Kanai, Bahrami, Roylance, & Rees, 2012; Sallet et al., 2011). With the emergence of this heightened social cognitive capacity in human beings, new and complex ways of collaborating, teaching, and learning—which go far beyond conditioning and emulative learning—were made possible (Csibra & Gergely, 2009; Humphrey, 1988; Tomasello & Vaish, 2013). This form of social cognition made possible (a) the capacity for self-awareness and self-consciousness, (b) the human striving to transcend physical reality, and (c) the human capacity for complex forms of collaboration and relatedness (see Allen, Fonagy, & Bateman, 2008). At the same time, however, these new capacities also resulted in an increased risk for psychopathology (Luyten, Fonagy, Lemma, & Target, 2012).

This vulnerability arising from the capacity for higher social cognition speaks to the fact that mentalizing is not a constitutional given but is largely a developmental achievement. The precise nature of any individual's mentalizing profile—his or her strengths and weaknesses in relation to mentalizing across the dimensions (see section on "Mentalizing Dimensions")—is shaped in the first instance by the cumulative nature of the interactions that take place with the individual's attachment relationships, in particular early attachments during infancy (Fonagy & Luyten, 2016; Kovacs, Teglas, & Endress, 2010). Attachment figures' capacity to respond with contingent and marked affective displays of their own experience in response to the infant's subjective experience positively influences the child's ability to develop mentalizing capacities (see Figure 6.1). Subsequently, contact with other human beings (e.g., peers, teachers,

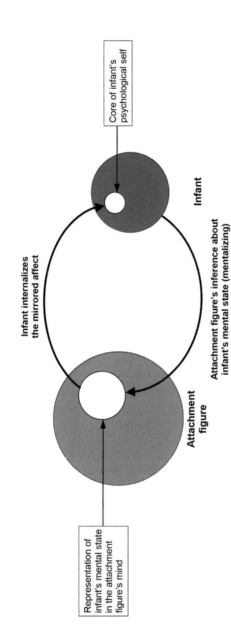

Core of infant's
psychological self

Infant

Attachment figure's inference about
infant's mental state (mentalizing)

Infant internalizes
the mirrored affect

Attachment
figure

Representation of
infant's mental state
in the attachment
figure's mind

Figure 6.1 The role of marked mirroring in the development of mentalizing.

and friends) broadens and strengthens the development of mentalizing (Fonagy & Luyten, 2016).

Conversely, consistent or serious failures in marked mirroring by early attachment figures lead to impairments in the capacity to reflect on the self and others, as they lead to unmentalized self-experiences (also called *alien self-experiences*). These experiences are subjectively felt as invalidating the individual's experience and thus are felt as alien to the self (see Figure 6.2). Such failures are to an extent a part of the fabric of everyday life: some misattunements in marked mirroring are an inevitable experience, as the caregiver may not be constantly available or inclined to engage sensitively with the infant's subjective state at all times. Consequently, all people will have unmentalized self-states. However, in various forms of psychopathology—most paradigmatically, in the case of borderline personality disorder (BPD) and most often as the result of a combination of biological vulnerability and environmental circumstances—these alien self-experiences are so marked that they almost completely dominate the feelings and thoughts of the individual. This leads to a constant pressure to externalize such unmentalized, alien self-experiences, which can manifest itself in the tendency to dominate the mind of others and/or in various types of self-harming behavior (Fonagy & Luyten, 2016).

Mentalizing Dimensions

Studies concerning the neurobiology of mentalizing have shown that this capacity is organized around at least four dimensions, with each dimension involving relatively distinct neural circuits (see Table 6.1; Fonagy & Luyten, 2009; Luyten, Fonagy, Lowyck, & Vermote, 2012). These dimensions cover a broad range of related constructs from social cognition research, including empathy, mindfulness, and Theory of Mind (ToM; Choi-Kain & Gunderson, 2008). Mindfulness, for instance, focuses on a core component of mentalizing about the self (e.g., the ability to attend to one's own internal mental states), while empathy and ToM respectively focus on more affective and more cognitive mentalizing about others.

Solid mentalizing reflects a balance between these four dimensions. Psychopathology (particularly personality disorder) is thought to reflect imbalances between the dimensions. For instance, individuals with BPD are typically overly sensitive to the emotional states of others while showing marked impairments in the capacity to reflect on their own mental states.

Neurobiology of Mentalizing Dimensions

Automatic or *implicit* mentalizing involves relatively parallel and fast processing, which requires little effort, focused attention, or intention (Satpute & Lieberman, 2006). Studies suggest that an elementary capacity for implicit mentalizing is present in infants from as young as seven months of age (Kovacs et al., 2010). Automatic mentalizing clearly facilitates survival (Lieberman, 2007; Mayes, 2006), as the fast processing of social information best serves the fight/flight response in threatening situations. However, in more complex social situations, automatic mentalizing is far less adaptive, as it is typically based on biased assumptions. Hence, human beings need *controlled or explicit* mentalizing to understand both one's own mind and the mind of others, particularly in complex social situations. Controlled mentalizing is verbal, reflective, and

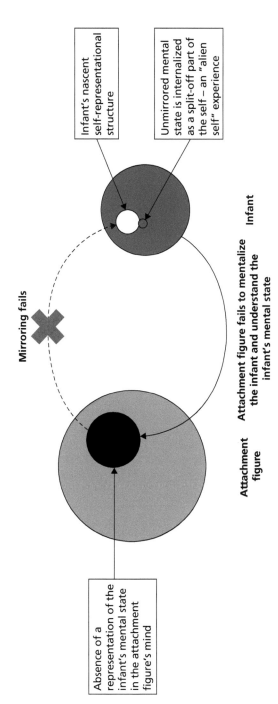

Infant's nascent self-representational structure

Unmirrored mental state is internalized as a split-off part of the self – an "alien self" experience

Mirroring fails

Infant

Attachment figure fails to mentalize the infant and understand the infant's mental state

Attachment figure

Absence of a representation of the infant's mental state in the attachment figure's mind

Figure 6.2 Failure to adequately mirror mental states, problems with mentalizing, and the emergence of alien self-parts.

TABLE 6.1. *Dimensions of Mentalizing*

Dimension	Defining Features	Hypothesized Neural Circuits
Automatic	Unconscious, parallel, fast processing of social information	Amygdala, basal ganglia, ventromedial prefrontal cortex (VMPFC), lateral temporal cortex (LTC), dorsal anterior cingulate cortex (dACC)
Controlled	Conscious, verbal, and reflective processing of social information that relies on effortful control and language	Lateral prefrontal cortex (LPFC), medial prefrontal cortex (MPFC), lateral parietal cortex (LPAC), medial parietal cortex (MPAC), medial temporal lobe (MTL), rostral anterior cingulate cortex (rACC)
Internal	Understanding one's own mind and that of others through direct focus on the mental interiors	Medial frontoparietal network (more controlled)
External	or through a focus on external features (such as facial expressions, posture, and prosody)	Lateral frontotemporoparietal (more automatic)
Self–Other	Capacity to reflect about both the self and others in terms of inner mental states	Shared representation system (more automatic) versus mental state attribution system (more controlled)
Cognitive–Affective	Focus on cognitive (more controlled), such as belief-desire reasoning and perspective-taking, versus affective features (more automatic), including affective empathy and mentalized affectivity (the feeling and thinking-about-the-feeling), of mental states of self and others	Prefrontal cortex (cognitive mentalizing) versus VMPFC (affectively oriented mentalizing)

conscious, and therefore involves much slower serial processing of social information. Extant research suggests that phylogenetically older brain circuits underlie automatic mentalizing, while controlled mentalizing is underpinned by phylogenetically newer neural circuits. Automatic mentalizing tends to involve the amygdala, basal ganglia, ventromedial prefrontal cortex (VMPFC), lateral temporal cortex (LTC), and dorsal ACC (dACC; Satpute & Lieberman, 2006). The relation of these brain circuits to threat detection and the fight/flight response is clear. The amygdala, for instance, has been suggested to play a key role in the processing of the biological "value" of information. The VMPFC modulates both the amygdala and basal ganglia, and the VMPFC and basal ganglia have been linked to automatic intuition. Importantly, the basal ganglia have also been linked to reward-related implicit emotion processing, while areas such as the dACC seem to play a central role in the nonreflective processing of emotional distress and pain. The LTC has been linked to the automatic processing of faces, biological motion, and attribution of intentions to others.

Controlled mentalizing relies more on the lateral PFC, medial PFC (MPFC), the lateral and medial parietal cortices, medial temporal lobe, and rostral ACC (Lieberman, 2007; Satpute & Lieberman, 2006; Uddin, Iacoboni, Lange, & Keenan, 2007). The lateral PFC and lateral parietal cortex have been related to complex causal reasoning, while the medial parietal cortex has been linked to explicit perspective-taking. The rostral ACC has been implicated in tasks involving explicit conflict processing and the medial temporal lobe in explicit, declarative memory. Importantly, the MPFC, one of the brain areas that has been most consistently linked to mentalizing, may play a central role in both automatic and controlled mentalizing. Yet, because this structure is larger in human beings than in other primates, and because increasing cognitive load leads to decreasing performance of this structure, it has been suggested that the MPFC is more closely linked to the controlled system (Lieberman, 2007; Satpute & Lieberman, 2006; Uddin et al., 2007).

Mentalizing based on external features of self and others (e.g., facial expressions, posture, movements, and prosody) involves a more lateral frontotemporoparietal network (e.g., the posterior superior temporal sulcus and temporal poles; indicative of more automatic processing), while mentalizing based on internal features of self and others tends to recruit a medial frontoparietal network (e.g., MPFC; indicative of more controlled reflective processes; Lieberman, 2007).

With regard to the self-other dimension, the same core network tends to be activated whenever we reflect on ourselves and others involving the medial prefrontal cortex, temporal poles, and the posterior superior temporal sulcus/temporoparietal junction in the LTC (Frith & Frith, 2006; Lieberman, 2007; Uddin et al., 2007; Van Overwalle, 2009; Van Overwalle & Baetens, 2009).

The finding of a common network underlying mentalizing with regard to both self and others sheds light on interesting findings concerning the centrality of both identity problems and problems with mentalizing about others in most individuals with personality disorders. This may be related to an imbalance in two neural systems involved in self-knowing and knowing others (Dimaggio, Lysaker, Carcione, Nicolo, & Semerari, 2008; Lieberman, 2007; Lombardo, Barnes, Wheelwright, & Baron-Cohen, 2007; Shamay-Tsoory, 2011; Uddin et al., 2007). Ripoll et al. (2013) have called these systems the *shared representation* (SR) system and the *mental state attribution* (MSA) system. The SR system involves a rapid, automatic "visceral recognition" of the experience of others (Lombardo et al., 2010), involving a more body-based, frontoparietal (mirror-neuron) system (Gallese, Keysers, & Rizzolatti, 2004; Rizzolatti & Craighero, 2004; Van Overwalle & Baetens, 2009). Neural areas that have been linked to the SR system include the amygdala, inferior frontal gyrus, inferior parietal lobule, anterior insula, and (dorsal) ACC.

A more controlled, cortical midline system consisting of the ventromedial and dorsomedial PFC, the temporoparietal junction and the medial temporal pole (Lieberman, 2007; Uddin et al., 2007) underlies explicit perspective-taking and both cognitive ToM (dorsomedial PFC) and affective ToM (VMPFC). The MSA plays a central role in the inhibition of the SR system, that is, of automatic mimicry or identification with the mental states of others (Brass & Haggard, 2008; Brass, Ruby, & Spengler, 2009; Brass, Schmitt, Spengler, & Gergely, 2007). For instance, people with BPD seem to be particularly prone to such automatic identification processes, which suggests the existence of impairments in the MSA system (Fonagy & Luyten, 2016). As a result, these individuals are particularly prone to emotional contagion and identity diffusion.

The capacity for mentalizing involves the integration of cognition and affect. Mentalizing has a clear cognitive component, such as perspective-taking and belief-desire reasoning. It depends on several areas of the PFC (Sabbagh, 2004; Shamay-Tsoory & Aharon-Peretz, 2007; Shamay-Tsoory, Aharon-Peretz, & Levkovitz, 2007). The affective components include affective empathy and mentalized affectivity (Fonagy,

Gergely, Jurist, & Target, 2002; Jurist, 2005). The VMPFC appears to play a central role in affective mentalizing, that is, in "marking" mental representations with affect (Rochat & Striano, 1999). This dissociation between the neural systems involved in cognitive and affective mentalizing may also explain, at least in part, the distinction between affective and cognitive empathy. Affective empathy involves a more basic "emotional contagion" system, whereas cognitive empathy involves a cognitive perspective-taking system (Shamay-Tsoory, Aharon-Peretz, & Perry, 2009). Again, these findings concerning the dissociable capacities involved in cognitive versus affective mentalizing have immediate relevance for understanding of personality disorders. Individuals with antisocial personality disorder, particularly those with psychopathic features, show normal cognitive mentalizing but gross impairments in affective mentalizing (Blair, 2013; Viding & McCrory, 2012).

A Developmental Perspective on the Relationships among Arousal, Attachment, and Mentalizing

With increasing stress or arousal, controlled, slow, and reflective mentalizing is replaced by automatic, fast, and typically biased automatic mentalizing, or *prementalizing* modes of experiencing oneself and others (see Table 6.2 and Figure 6.3).

Both noradrenergic and dopaminergic systems have been shown to be involved in this switch from controlled to automatic mentalizing, which has been hypothesized to protect the PFC from excessive stimulation and to facilitate coordination among the attentional, executive, and sensory systems in response to threat (Arnsten, Mathew, Ubriani, Taylor, & Li, 1999). Norepinephrine enhances the activation of the PFC, while α_1 postsynaptic receptor stimulation impairs its functioning. The D1 dopamine receptor family also enhances PFC functioning, but when amygdala activation leads to catecholamine release, D1 impairs PFC functioning.

Individuals' attachment history plays an important role in modulating three key parameters involved in this switch: (a) the point at which an individual switches from controlled to automatic mentalizing, (b) the extent of the loss of the capacity for controlled mentalizing, and (c) the duration of the loss of controlled mentalizing until it is re-established (Fonagy & Luyten, 2009; Fonagy & Luyten, 2016; Luyten, Fonagy, Lowyck, et al., 2012).

TABLE 6.2. *Automatic Nonmentalizing Modes That Emerge with the Loss of Controlled Mentalizing*

Nonmentalizing Mode	Features
Psychic equivalence mode	• Equation of inner reality with outer reality: "What I think is real"
	• Overly concrete/literal understanding
Teleological mode	• Focus on directly observable goals or actions
	• Only observable changes or actions can be true indicators of the intentions of others
Pretend mode	• Thoughts and feelings are decoupled from external reality
	• May lead to "dissociation" of thought (hypermentalizing or pseudomentalizing)

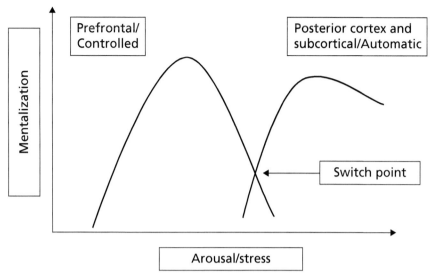

Figure 6.3 A biobehavioral switch model of the relationship between arousal/stress and controlled versus automatic mentalizing.

Secure Attachment

Individuals who predominantly use *secure attachment strategies* in response to stress seem to be able to keep controlled mentalizing on-line longer and more effectively compared with individuals who tend to rely on insecure attachment strategies. They also seem to be able to recover from losses of controlled mentalizing faster and more effectively. In securely attached individuals, studies suggest that activation of the attachment system actually fosters controlled mentalizing in combination with a relaxation of epistemic hypervigilance, leading to effective downregulation of stress and the development of broaden-and-build cycles (Fredrickson, 2001).

The neuropeptides oxytocin, vasopressin, and opioids appear to play an important role here, leading to deactivation of behavioral mechanisms involved in social avoidance and attenuating both behavioral and neuroendocrine stress responses (Heinrichs & Domes, 2008; Insel & Young, 2001; Panksepp & Watt, 2011). Oxytocin release has also been found to foster mentalizing in securely attached individuals, as apparent in improvements in social memory (and memory of facial expressions in particular) and the recognition of mental states based on facial expressions, as well as increasing trust in others (Bartz, Zaki, et al., 2011; Neumann, 2008). These findings may have important implications for our understanding of the neurobiology of resilience (Fonagy, Steele, Steele, Higgitt, & Target, 1994). Yet, even in securely attached individuals, mentalizing is not always solid, as contextual factors play an important role in determining both the quality and quantity of mentalizing (Bartz, Zaki, et al., 2011). With increasing arousal, the capacity for controlled mentalizing is easily lost, particularly in relation to out-group members (Bartz, Zaki, et al., 2011). For instance, research has consistently shown that, even in normal community samples, the majority of whose members are securely attached, oxytocin administration leads to increased distrust, increased bias in attributing intentions to others, and decreases in cooperative behavior with regard to out-group members (Bartz, Zaki, et al., 2011). From a neurobiological perspective, increasing arousal and the neurobiological cascade of events that follows seems to make attachment issues more salient, which increases the likelihood of a deactivation of controlled mentalizing.

Attachment Hyperactivating Strategies

Some individuals tend to use attachment hyperactivating strategies in response to stress because of their developmental history or because of contextual factors. These strategies reflect attempts to find security and to coregulate stress with others, based on the underlying belief that others are not able to provide security and support, despite these individuals' strong wishes for care, support, and love. Attachment hyperactivating strategies have been shown to be characterized by a low threshold for switching to nonmentalizing modes, more extensive lapses in controlled mentalizing, and a longer time to recovery from such lapses, compared with individuals whose attachment strategies are secure. This may lead, in the extreme, to hyperactivation of the attachment system, with resulting impairments in stress regulation and mentalizing as a result of a failure to benefit from broaden-and-build experiences. This is particularly the case in traumatized individuals, who often show marked hypersensitivity to stress, hyperactivation of the attachment system, and profound impairments in mentalizing. For example, studies have shown that early trauma is associated with kindling of the amygdala (Botterill et al., 2014), leading to an exaggerated response to threats. Similarly, research clearly suggests both structural and functional changes in the amygdala (and the stress response more generally) in individuals with a history of early adversity. Dysfunction of the HPA axis has been demonstrated in a wide variety of conditions characterized by marked early adversity, ranging from depression to functional somatic disorders to personality disorders (Jogems-Kosterman, de Knijff, Kusters, & van Hoof, 2007; Nater et al., 2010; Scott, Levy, & Granger, 2013; Wingenfeld, Spitzer, Rullkotter, & Lowe, 2010). In BPD patients with an explicit trauma history, for instance, a reduction in pituitary volume (Garner et al., 2007), elevated levels of corticotropin-releasing factor in cerebrospinal fluid (Lee, Geracioti, Kasckow, & Coccaro, 2005), dysfunctions of cortisol responsivity (Jogems-Kosterman et al., 2007; Minzenberg et al., 2006; Walter et al., 2008), and disturbed dexamethasone suppression test responses (Wingenfeld et al., 2007) have been observed.

Impaired stress regulation as a result of continued stress has been shown to negatively influence brain areas involved in mentalizing, as is, for instance, demonstrated by findings that chronic stress disrupts amygdala–VMPFC connectivity (Tottenham & Sheridan, 2009).

Attachment Deactivating Strategies

Attachment deactivating strategies involve denying attachment needs and asserting one's own autonomy and independence when faced with adversity, in an attempt to downregulate stress. Developmentally, attachment deactivating strategies develop on the basis of repeated experiences that others are unavailable to provide security, support, and comfort. In response, these individuals tend to de-emphasize the importance of attachment relationships, which becomes a habitual response associated with rapid deactivation of the attachment system and social information processing of threat cues. Yet, at the same time, these individuals are often able to keep the neural systems involved in controlled mentalizing online even when under considerable stress because they have had to learn to rely on their own capacity for affect regulation (Vrticka, Andersson, Grandjean, Sander, & Vuilleumier, 2008). Experimental studies have shown that these deactivating strategies are likely to fail under increasing stress, leading to a "rebound" of suppressed feelings of insecurity and lack of self-worth (Mikulincer & Shaver, 2007; Vrticka et al., 2008).

A series of studies by Strathearn and colleagues (Strathearn et al., 2009; Strathearn et al., 2008) provides a good example of the influence of attachment deactivating strategies on stress regulation and mentalizing. Strathearn and colleagues first assessed attachment security in 30 first-time mothers using the Adult Attachment Interview before the birth of their child. About 10 months after birth of their child, the same mothers were asked to view images of their own or other infants' smiling and crying faces. Mothers who were classified as securely attached showed greater activation in brain regions of the reward system, such as the ventral striatum, and the oxytocin-associated hypothalamus/pituitary region. They also showed higher and increasing peripheral oxytocin release while playing with their infant, which was positively correlated with brain activation to their own infant in the reward system. By contrast, mothers who were categorized as having insecure/dismissing attachment (who would tend to rely predominantly on attachment deactivating) showed less activation of the reward system and greater activation of the insula in response to seeing their own infant's sad face. Studies have suggested that the insula plays a key role in generating feelings of unfairness, pain, and disgust (see review by Montague & Lohrenz, 2007) and is involved in automatic mentalizing. Thus these mothers appeared to be less able to regulate the sad feelings evoked in them by viewing their infant's crying face. These findings are consistent with findings in adults showing that attachment deactivating strategies are associated with downregulation of activity in reward-related brain regions and, at the same time, activation of the MPFC and the ventral ACC, brain areas that have been implicated in controlled mentalizing as well as social rejection and emotion suppression (Vrticka et al., 2008).

■ GENETICS OF ATTACHMENT AND MENTALIZING: ARE ATTACHMENT STYLES EVOLUTIONARY AND CULTURALLY DETERMINED ADAPTIVE STRATEGIES?

Although the genetic loading of attachment in childhood is probably very small, this may change over the course of life. Indeed, a recent twin study found that by adolescence approximately 40% of individual differences in attachment security may be genetically determined (Fearon, Shmueli-Goetz, Viding, Fonagy, & Plomin, 2014), again pointing to adolescence as a critical juncture in the development of attachment and associated capacities such as mentalizing and stress/affect regulation. Specifically, adolescence may involve a resetting of the attachment system, for better or for worse, that is determined in part by genetic factors.

If further replicated, these findings shed an important light on the potential evolutionary functions of insecure attachment. Indeed, if attachment is an evolutionarily rooted capacity that enhances the survival of the human species, why would insecure attachment strategies still exist in the human behavioral repertoire? Building on the work of Ein-Dor and colleagues (2010), we argue that insecure attachment styles represent a strategy to adapt to the environment, but one that may come with a high cost, as is evidenced most clearly by individuals with personality disorder (Fonagy &

Luyten, 2016; Tottenham & Sheridan, 2009). From this perspective, secure attachment is accompanied by a relative relaxation of threat processing as a result of repeated experiences of security in relation to attachment figures, which leads to a relaxation of interpersonal distrust and avoidance. These individuals show appropriate openness and flexibility in new relationships and novel situations, which increases opportunities for salutogenesis (Antonovsky, 1987).

By contrast, insecure attachment experiences give rise to hypersensitivity to threat. A pattern of attachment hyperactivation may follow, characterized by hypersensitivity to threat that is expressed as an emphasis on externally focused mentalizing, to the neglect of more internally focused mentalizing. Although this is adaptive to some extent in an environment characterized by attachment figures who are unreliable, the cost associated with this adaptation strategy is that these individuals show constant hypervigilance to threat, leading to chronic stress and, as a consequence of the wear and tear of chronic stress, dysregulation of the reward and stress regulation systems. Hypervigilance is also related to problems with epistemic trust, that is, the capacity to trust others as a source of knowledge about the world; impairments in epistemic trust seriously limit opportunities for salutogenesis (Fonagy et al., 2015). BPD might be considered the disorder par excellence of this pattern. However, insecure attachment experiences have also been shown to give rise to the excessive use of attachment deactivating strategies, downplaying the importance of attachment relationships and subjective distress. Although these strategies are also adaptive in the short term, the compulsive autonomy and often marked distrust of others (as is, for instance, observed in paranoid personality disorder) that they entail is associated with considerable intra- and interpersonal costs.

■ CONCLUSIONS AND FUTURE DIRECTIONS

This chapter summarizes extant research and thinking concerning the relationships among attachment, stress/affect regulation, and social cognition/mentalizing in relation to the development of personality disorders.

Although research in these areas has considerably improved our insight into the nature of personality disorders, and their underlying neurobiology in particular, much remains to be explored. Many of the research findings summarized in this chapter rest on cross-sectional and small sample size studies. The generalization of findings from research in animals to humans continues to be a major challenge, although research over the past two decades has generally confirmed findings from studies of animals in humans. Future research should employ more ecologically valid paradigms to study the interplay between attachment, stress regulation, and mentalizing over time in both normative development and clinical populations. In addition, rather than relying on consensus-based descriptive diagnoses as the basis for research, future research should investigate the neurobiology of attachment-related processes from a developmental psychopathology perspective, focusing on the role of these systems across different types of psychopathology. The study of major transitions in life, such as from childhood to adolescence and from adolescence to adulthood, as illustrated in this chapter, may be particularly productive.

■ REFERENCES

Allen, J. G., Fonagy, P., & Bateman, A. W. (2008). *Mentalizing in clinical practice*. Washington, DC: American Psychiatric Publishing.

Antonovsky, A. (1987). *Unraveling the mystery of health: how people manage stress and stay well.* San Francisco, CA: Jossey-Bass.

Arnsten, A. F., Mathew, R., Ubriani, R., Taylor, J. R., & Li, B. M. (1999). α-1 noradrenergic receptor stimulation impairs prefrontal cortical cognitive function. *Biol Psychiatry, 45,* 26–31. doi: 10.1016/S0006-3223(98)00296-0

Auerbach, R. P., Admon, R., & Pizzagalli, D. A. (2014). Adolescent depression: stress and reward dysfunction. *Harv Rev Psychiatry, 22,* 139–148. doi: 10.1097/hrp.0000000000000034

Bartz, J., Simeon, D., Hamilton, H., Kim, S., Crystal, S., Braun, A., . . . Hollander, E. (2011). Oxytocin can hinder trust and cooperation in borderline personality disorder. *Soc Cogn Affect Neurosci, 6,* 556–563. doi: 10.1093/scan/nsq085

Bartz, J. A., Zaki, J., Bolger, N., & Ochsner, K. N. (2011). Social effects of oxytocin in humans: context and person matter. *Trends Cogn Sci, 15,* 301–309. doi: 10.1016/j.tics.2011.05.002

Beck, A. T. (2009). Cognitive aspects of personality disorders and their relation to syndromal disorders: a psychoevolutionary approach. In C. R. Cloninger (Ed.), *Personality and psychopathology* (pp. 411–429). Washington, DC: American Psychiatric Press.

Bertsch, K., Schmidinger, I., Neumann, I. D., & Herpertz, S. C. (2013). Reduced plasma oxytocin levels in female patients with borderline personality disorder. *Horm Behav, 63,* 424–429. doi: 10.1016/j.yhbeh.2012.11.013

Blair, R. J. R. (2013). The neurobiology of psychopathic traits in youths. *Nature Rev Neurosci, 14,* 786–799. doi: 10.1038/nrn3577

Blatt, S. J. (2008). *Polarities of experience: relatedness and self definition in personality development, psychopathology, and the therapeutic process.* Washington, DC: American Psychological Association.

Botterill, J. J., Fournier, N. M., Guskjolen, A. J., Lussier, A. L., Marks, W. N., & Kalynchuk, L. E. (2014). Amygdala kindling disrupts trace and delay fear conditioning with parallel changes in Fos protein expression throughout the limbic brain. *Neuroscience, 265,* 158–171. doi: 10.1016/j.neuroscience.2014.01.040

Bowlby, J. (1973). *Attachment and loss. Vol. 2: Separation: anxiety and anger.* New York: Basic Books.

Brass, M., & Haggard, P. (2008). The what, when, whether model of intentional action. *Neuroscientist, 14,* 319–325. doi: 10.1177/1073858408317417

Brass, M., Ruby, P., & Spengler, S. (2009). Inhibition of imitative behaviour and social cognition. *Philos Trans R Soc Lond B Biol Sci, 364,* 2359–2367. doi: 10.1098/rstb.2009.0066

Brass, M., Schmitt, R. M., Spengler, S., & Gergely, G. (2007). Investigating action understanding: inferential processes versus action simulation. *Curr Biol, 17,* 2117–2121. doi: 10.1016/j.cub.2007.11.057

Champagne, F. A., Chretien, P., Stevenson, C. W., Zhang, T. Y., Gratton, A., & Meaney, M. J. (2004). Variations in nucleus accumbens dopamine associated with individual differences in maternal behavior in the rat. *J Neurosci, 24,* 4113–4123. doi: 10.1523/JNEUROSCI.5322-03.2004

Choi-Kain, L. W., & Gunderson, J. G. (2008). Mentalization: ontogeny, assessment, and application in the treatment of borderline personality disorder. *Am J Psychiatry, 165,* 1127–1135. doi: 10.1176/appi.ajp.2008.07081360

Csibra, G., & Gergely, G. (2009). Natural pedagogy. *Trends Cogn Sci, 13,* 148–153. doi: 10.1016/j.tics.2009.01.005

Cyranowski, J. M., Hofkens, T. L., Frank, E., Seltman, H., Cai, H. M., & Amico, J. A. (2008). Evidence of dysregulated peripheral oxytocin release among depressed women. *Psychosom Med, 70,* 967–975. doi: 10.1097/PSY.0b013e318188ade4

Davey, C. G., Yücel, M., & Allen, N. B. (2008). The emergence of depression in adolescence: development of the prefrontal cortex and the representation of reward. *Neurosci Biobehav Rev, 32,* 1–19. doi: 10.1016/j.neubiorev.2007.04.016

Dimaggio, G., Lysaker, P. H., Carcione, A., Nicolo, G., & Semerari, A. (2008). Know yourself and you shall know the other . . . to a certain extent: multiple paths of influence of self-reflection on mindreading. *Conscious Cogn, 17,* 778–789. doi: 10.1016/j.concog.2008.02.005

Dunbar, R. I. M., & Shultz, S. (2007). Evolution in the social brain. *Science, 317,* 1344–1347. doi: 10.1126/science.1145463

Ein-Dor, T., Mikulincer, M., Doron, G., & Shaver, P. R. (2010). The attachment paradox: how can so many of us (the insecure ones) have no adaptive advantages? *Perspect Psychol Sci, 5,* 123–141. doi: 10.1177/1745691610362349

Fearon, P., Shmueli-Goetz, Y., Viding, E., Fonagy, P., & Plomin, R. (2014). Genetic and environmental influences on adolescent attachment. *J Child Psychol Psychiatry, 55,* 1033–1041. doi: 10.1111/jcpp.12171

Ferris, C. F., Kulkarni, P., Sullivan, J. M., Harder, J. A., Messenger, T. L., & Febo, M. (2005). Pup suckling is more rewarding than cocaine: evidence from functional magnetic resonance imaging and three-dimensional computational analysis. *J Neurosci, 25,* 149–156. doi: 10.1523/Jneurosci.3156-04.2005

Fonagy, P., Gergely, G., Jurist, E., & Target, M. (2002). *Affect regulation, mentalization, and the development of the self.* New York: Other Press.

Fonagy, P., & Luyten, P. (2009). A developmental, mentalization-based approach to the understanding and treatment of borderline personality disorder. *Dev Psychopathol, 21,* 1355–1381. doi: 10.1017/s0954579409990198

Fonagy, P., & Luyten, P. (2016). A multilevel perspective on the development of borderline personality disorder. In D. Cicchetti (Ed.), *Dev Psychopathol* (3rd ed., pp. 726–792). New York: Wiley.

Fonagy, P., Luyten, P., & Allison, E. (2015). Epistemic petrification and the restoration of epistemic trust: a new conceptualization of borderline personality disorder and its psychosocial treatment. *J Pers Disord, 29,* 575–609. doi: 10.1521/pedi.2015.29.5.575

Fonagy, P., Steele, M., Steele, H., Higgitt, A., & Target, M. (1994). The Emanuel Miller Memorial Lecture 1992. The theory and practice of resilience. *J Child Psychol Psychiatry, 35,* 231–257.

Forbes, E. E., & Dahl, R. E. (2012). Research review: altered reward function in adolescent depression: what, when and how? *J Child Psychol Psychiatry, 53,* 3–15. doi: 10.1111/j.1469-7610.2011.02477.x

Fredrickson, B. L. (2001). The role of positive emotions in positive psychology. The broaden-and-build theory of positive emotions. *Am Psychol, 56,* 218–226.

Fries, E., Hesse, J., Hellhammer, J., & Hellhammer, D. H. (2005). A new view on hypocortisolism. *Psychoneuroendocrinology, 30,* 1010–1016. doi: 10.1016/j.psyneuen.2005.04.006

Frith, C. D., & Frith, U. (2006). The neural basis of mentalizing. *Neuron, 50,* 531–534. doi: 10.1016/j.neuron.2006.05.001

Gallese, V., Keysers, C., & Rizzolatti, G. (2004). A unifying view of the basis of social cognition. *Trends Cogn Sci, 8,* 396–403. doi: 10.1016/j.tics.2004.07.002

Garner, B., Chanen, A. M., Phillips, L., Velakoulis, D., Wood, S. J., Jackson, H. J., . . . McGorry, P. D. (2007). Pituitary volume in teenagers with first-presentation borderline personality disorder. *Psychiatry Res, 156,* 257–261. doi: 10.1016/j.pscychresns.2007.05.001

Gilbert, P. (2006). Evolution and depression: issues and implications. *Psychol Med, 36,* 287–297. doi: 10.1017/s0033291705006112

Gunnar, M., & Quevedo, K. (2007). The neurobiology of stress and development. *Annu Rev Psychol, 58,* 145–173. doi: 10.1146/annurev.psych.58.110405.085605

Heim, C., Newport, D. J., Mletzko, T., Miller, A. H., & Hemeroff, C. B. (2008). The link between childhood trauma and depression: insights from HPA axis studies in humans. *Psychoneuroendocrinology*, *33*, 693–710. doi: 10.1016/j.psyneuen.2008.03.008

Heinrichs, M., & Domes, G. (2008). Neuropeptides and social behaviour: effects of oxytocin and vasopressin in humans. *Prog Brain Res*, *170*, 337–350. doi: 10.1016/S0079-6123(08)00428-7

Hostinar, C. E., Sullivan, R. M., & Gunnar, M. R. (2014). Psychobiological mechanisms underlying the social buffering of the hypothalamic-pituitary-adrenocortical axis: a review of animal models and human studies across development. *Psychol Bull*, *140*, 256–282. doi: 10.1037/a0032671

Hsu, D. T., Sanford, B. J., Meyers, K. K., Love, T. M., Hazlett, K. E., Walker, S. J., . . . Zubieta, J. K. (2015). It still hurts: altered endogenous opioid activity in the brain during social rejection and acceptance in major depressive disorder. *Mol Psychiatry*, *20*, 193–200. doi: 10.1038/mp.2014.185

Humphrey, N. K. (1988). The social function of intellect. In R. W. Byrne & A. Whiten (Eds.), *Machiavellian intelligence: social expertise and the evolution of intellect in monkeys, apes, and humans* (pp. 13–26). New York: Oxford University Press.

Insel, T. R., & Young, L. J. (2001). The neurobiology of attachment. *Nature Rev Neurosci*, *2*, 129–136. doi: 10.1038/35053579

Jogems-Kosterman, B. J., de Knijff, D. W., Kusters, R., & van Hoof, J. J. (2007). Basal cortisol and DHEA levels in women with borderline personality disorder. *J Psychiatr Res*, *41*, 1019–1026. doi: 10.1016/j.jpsychires.2006.07.019

Jurist, E. L. (2005). Mentalized affectivity. *Psychoanal Psychol*, *22*, 426–444. doi: 10.1037/0736-9735.22.3.426

Kanai, R., Bahrami, B., Roylance, R., & Rees, G. (2012). Online social network size is reflected in human brain structure. *Proc Biol Sci*, *279*, 1327–1334. doi: 10.1098/rspb.2011.1959

Kovacs, A. M., Teglas, E., & Endress, A. D. (2010). The social sense: susceptibility to others' beliefs in human infants and adults. *Science*, *330*, 1830–1834. doi: 10.1126/science.1190792

Lee, R., Geracioti, T. D. Jr., Kasckow, J. W., & Coccaro, E. F. (2005). Childhood trauma and personality disorder: positive correlation with adult CSF corticotropin-releasing factor concentrations. *Am J Psychiatry*, *162*, 995–997. doi: 10.1176/appi.ajp.162.5.995

Levy, K. N., Meehan, K. B., Weber, M., Reynoso, J., & Clarkin, J. F. (2005). Attachment and borderline personality disorder: implications for psychotherapy. *Psychopathology*, *38*, 64–74. doi: 10.1159/000084813

Lieberman, M. D. (2007). Social cognitive neuroscience: a review of core processes. *Annu Rev Psychol*, *58*, 259–289. doi: 10.1146/annurev.psych.58.110405.085654

Lombardo, M. V., Barnes, J. L., Wheelwright, S. J., & Baron-Cohen, S. (2007). Self-referential cognition and empathy in autism. *PLoS One*, *2*, e883. doi: 10.1371/journal.pone.0000883

Lombardo, M. V., Chakrabarti, B., Bullmore, E. T., Wheelwright, S. J., Sadek, S. A., Suckling, J., . . . Baron-Cohen, S. (2010). Shared neural circuits for mentalizing about the self and others. *J Cogn Neurosci*, *22*, 1623–1635. doi: 10.1162/jocn.2009.21287

Luciana, M. (2013). Adolescent brain development in normality and psychopathology. *Dev Psychopathol*, *25*, 1325–1345. doi: 10.1017/s0954579413000643

Lupien, S. J., McEwen, B. S., Gunnar, M. R., & Heim, C. (2009). Effects of stress throughout the lifespan on the brain, behaviour and cognition. *Nature Rev Neurosci*, *10*, 434–445. doi: 10.1038/nrn2639

Luyten, P., & Fonagy, P. (2015). The neurobiology of mentalizing. *Person Disord, 6*, 366–379. doi: 10.1037/per0000117

Luyten, P., Fonagy, P., Lemma, A., & Target, M. (2012). Depression. In A. Bateman & P. Fonagy (Eds.), *Handbook of mentalizing in mental health practice* (pp. 385–417). Washington, DC: American Psychiatric Association.

Luyten, P., Fonagy, P., Lowyck, B., & Vermote, R. (2012). Assessment of mentalization. In A. W. Bateman & P. Fonagy (Eds.), *Handbook of mentalizing in mental health practice* (pp. 43–65). Washington, DC: American Psychiatric Publishing.

Mayes, L. C. (2006). Arousal regulation, emotional flexibility, medial amygdala function, and the impact of early experience: comments on the paper of Lewis et al. *Ann N Y Acad Sci, 1094*, 178–192. doi: 10.1196/annals.1376.018

Meinlschmidt, G., & Heim, C. (2007). Sensitivity to intranasal oxytocin in adult men with early parental separation. *Biol Psychiatry, 61*, 1109–1111. doi: 10.1016/j.biopsych.2006.09.007

Mikulincer, M., & Shaver, P. R. (2007). *Attachment in adulthood: structure, dynamics and change.* New York: Guilford Press.

Minzenberg, M. J., Grossman, R., New, A. S., Mitropoulou, V., Yehuda, R., Goodman, M., . . . Siever, L. J. (2006). Blunted hormone responses to ipsapirone are associated with trait impulsivity in personality disorder patients. *Neuropsychopharmacology, 31*, 197–203. doi: 10.1038/sj.npp.1300853

Montague, P. R., & Lohrenz, T. (2007). To detect and correct: norm violations and their enforcement. *Neuron, 56*, 14–18. doi: 10.1016/j.neuron.2007.09.020

Nater, U. M., Bohus, M., Abbruzzese, E., Ditzen, B., Gaab, J., Kleindienst, N., . . . Ehlert, U. (2010). Increased psychological and attenuated cortisol and alpha-amylase responses to acute psychosocial stress in female patients with borderline personality disorder. *Psychoneuroendocrinology, 35*, 1565–1572. doi: 10.1016/j.psyneuen.2010.06.002

Nestler, E. J., & Carlezon, W. A. Jr. (2006). The mesolimbic dopamine reward circuit in depression. *Biol Psychiatry, 59*, 1151–1159. doi: 10.1016/j.biopsych.2005.09.018

Neumann, I. D. (2008). Brain oxytocin: a key regulator of emotional and social behaviours in both females and males. *J Neuroendocrinol, 20*, 858–865. doi: 10.1111/j.1365-2826.2008.01726.x

Panksepp, J. (1998). *Affective neuroscience: the foundations of human and animal emotions.* Oxford: Oxford University Press.

Panksepp, J., & Watt, D. (2011). Why does depression hurt? Ancestral primary-process separation-distress (PANIC/GRIEF) and diminished brain reward (SEEKING) processes in the genesis of depressive affect. *Psychiatry, 74*, 5–13. doi: 10.1521/psyc.2011.74.1.5

Pizzagalli, D. A. (2014). Depression, stress, and anhedonia: toward a synthesis and integrated model. *Annu Rev Clin Psychol, 10*, 393–423. doi: 10.1146/annurev-clinpsy-050212-185606

Ripoll, L. H., Snyder, R., Steele, H., & Siever, L. J. (2013). The neurobiology of empathy in borderline personality disorder. *Curr Psychiatry Rep, 15*, 344. doi: 10.1007/s11920-012-0344-1

Rizzolatti, G., & Craighero, L. (2004). The mirror-neuron system. *Annu Rev Neurosci, 27*, 169–192. doi: 10.1146/annurev.neuro.27.070203.144230

Rochat, P., & Striano, T. (1999). Social-cognitive development in the first year. In P. Rochat (Ed.), *Early social cognition* (pp. 3–34). Mahwah, NJ: Lawrence Erlbaum Associates.

Russo, S. J., & Nestler, E. J. (2013). The brain reward circuitry in mood disorders. *Nature Rev Neurosci, 14*, 609–625. doi: 10.1038/nrn3381

Rutherford, H. J., Williams, S. K., Moy, S., Mayes, L. C., & Johns, J. M. (2011). Disruption of maternal parenting circuitry by addictive process: rewiring of reward and stress systems. *Front Psychiatry, 2*, 37. doi: 10.3389/fpsyt.2011.00037

Sabbagh, M. A. (2004). Understanding orbitofrontal contributions to theory-of-mind reasoning: implications for autism. *Brain and Cogn, 55*, 209–219. doi: 10.1016/j.bandc.2003.04.002

Sallet, J., Mars, R. B., Noonan, M. P., Andersson, J. L., O'Reilly, J. X., Jbabdi, S., . . . Rushworth, M. F. (2011). Social network size affects neural circuits in macaques. *Science, 334*, 697–700. doi: 10.1126/science.1210027

Satpute, A. B., & Lieberman, M. D. (2006). Integrating automatic and controlled processes into neurocognitive models of social cognition. *Brain Res, 1079*, 86–97. doi: 10.1016/j.brainres.2006.01.005

Scott, L. N., Levy, K. N., & Granger, D. A. (2013). Biobehavioral reactivity to social evaluative stress in women with borderline personality disorder. *Person Disord, 4*, 91–100. doi: 10.1037/a0030117

Shamay-Tsoory, S. G. (2011). The neural bases for empathy. *Neuroscientist, 17*, 18–24. doi: 10.1177/1073858410379268

Shamay-Tsoory, S. G., & Aharon-Peretz, J. (2007). Dissociable prefrontal networks for cognitive and affective theory of mind: a lesion study. *Neuropsychologia, 45*, 3054–3067. doi: 10.1016/j.neuropsychologia.2007.05.021

Shamay-Tsoory, S. G., Aharon-Peretz, J., & Levkovitz, Y. (2007). The neuroanatomical basis of affective mentalizing in schizophrenia: comparison of patients with schizophrenia and patients with localized prefrontal lesions. *Schizophr Res, 90*, 274–283. doi: 10.1016/j.schres.2006.09.020

Shamay-Tsoory, S. G., Aharon-Peretz, J., & Perry, D. (2009). Two systems for empathy: a double dissociation between emotional and cognitive empathy in inferior frontal gyrus versus ventromedial prefrontal lesions. *Brain, 132*, 617–627. doi: 10.1093/brain/awn279

Spear, L. (2007). The developing brain and adolescent-typical behavior patterns: an evolutionary approach. In D. Romer & E. F. Walker (Eds.), *Adolescent psychopathology and the adolescent brain* (pp. 9–30). New York: Oxford University Press.

Spear, L. P. (2000). The adolescent brain and age-related behavioral manifestations. *Neurosci Biobehav Rev, 24*, 417–463. doi: 10.1016/S0149-7634(00)00014-2

Stanley, B., & Siever, L. J. (2010). The interpersonal dimension of borderline personality disorder: toward a neuropeptide model. *Am J Psychiatry, 167*, 24–39. doi: 10.1176/appi.ajp.2009.09050744

Strathearn, L. (2011). Maternal neglect: oxytocin, dopamine and the neurobiology of attachment. *J Neuroendocrinol, 23*, 1054–1065. doi: 10.1111/j.1365-2826.2011.02228.x

Strathearn, L., Fonagy, P., Amico, J., & Montague, P. R. (2009). Adult attachment predicts maternal brain and oxytocin response to infant cues. *Neuropsychopharmacology, 34*, 2655–2666. doi: 10.1038/npp.2009.103

Strathearn, L., Li, J., Fonagy, P., & Montague, P. R. (2008). What's in a smile? Maternal brain responses to infant facial cues. *Pediatrics, 122*, 40–51. doi: 10.1542/peds.2007-1566

Swain, J. E., Kim, P., Spicer, J., Ho, S. S., Dayton, C. J., Elmadih, A., & Abel, K. M. (2014). Approaching the biology of human parental attachment: brain imaging, oxytocin and coordinated assessments of mothers and fathers. *Brain Res, 1580*, 78–101. doi: 10.1016/j.brainres.2014.03.007

Swain, J. E., Lorberbaum, J. P., Kose, S., & Strathearn, L. (2007). Brain basis of early parent-infant interactions: psychology, physiology, and in vivo functional neuroimaging studies. *J Child Psychol Psychiatry, 48*, 262–287. doi: 10.1111/j.1469-7610.2007.01731.x

Tomasello, M., & Vaish, A. (2013). Origins of human cooperation and morality. *Annu Rev Psychol, 64*, 231–255. doi: 10.1146/annurev-psych-113011-143812

Tottenham, N., & Sheridan, M. A. (2009). A review of adversity, the amygdala and the hippocampus: a consideration of developmental timing. *Front Hum Neurosci, 3*, 68. doi: 10.3389/neuro.09.068.2009

Uddin, L. Q., Iacoboni, M., Lange, C., & Keenan, J. P. (2007). The self and social cognition: the role of cortical midline structures and mirror neurons. *Trend Cogn Sci, 11*, 153–157. doi: 10.1016/j.tics.2007.01.001

Van Overwalle, F. (2009). Social cognition and the brain: a meta-analysis. *Hum Brain Mapp, 30*, 829–858. doi: 10.1002/hbm.20547

Van Overwalle, F., & Baetens, K. (2009). Understanding others' actions and goals by mirror and mentalizing systems: a meta-analysis. *Neuroimage, 48*, 564–584. doi: 10.1016/j.neuroimage.2009.06.009

Viding, E., & McCrory, E. J. (2012). Genetic and neurocognitive contributions to the development of psychopathy. *Dev Psychopathol, 24*, 969–983. doi: 10.1017/s095457941200048x

Vrticka, P., Andersson, F., Grandjean, D., Sander, D., & Vuilleumier, P. (2008). Individual attachment style modulates human amygdala and striatum activation during social appraisal. *PLoS One, 3*, e2868. doi: 10.1371/journal.pone.0002868

Walter, M., Bureau, J. F., Holmes, B. M., Bertha, E. A., Hollander, M., Wheelis, J., . . . Lyons-Ruth, K. (2008). Cortisol response to interpersonal stress in young adults with borderline personality disorder: a pilot study. *Eur Psychiatry, 23*, 201–204. doi: 10.1016/j.eurpsy.2007.12.003

Watt, D. F., & Panksepp, J. (2009). Depression: an evolutionarily conserved mechanism to terminate separation distress? A review of aminergic, peptidergic, and neural network perspectives. *Neuro-Psychoanalysis, 11*, 7–51.

Wingenfeld, K., Lange, W., Wulff, H., Berea, C., Beblo, T., Saavedra, A. S., . . . Driessen, M. (2007). Stability of the dexamethasone suppression test in borderline personality disorder with and without comorbid PTSD: a one-year follow-up study. *J Clin Psychol, 63*, 843–850. doi: 10.1002/jclp.20396

Wingenfeld, K., Spitzer, C., Rullkotter, N., & Lowe, B. (2010). Borderline personality disorder: hypothalamus pituitary adrenal axis and findings from neuroimaging studies. *Psychoneuroendocrinology, 35*, 154–170. doi: 10.1016/j.psyneuen.2009.09.014

Critical Domains/Dimensions
of Brain Function/Circuits
for Personality and Its Disorders

7 Emotion Regulation

■ KATJA BERTSCH, HAROLD KOENIGSBERG,
INGA NIEDTFELD, AND
CHRISTIAN SCHMAHL

■ INTRODUCTION

Emotions can be defined as complex and evolved patterns of response to both external and internal stimuli, providing a fast situational interpretation along with a corresponding action tendency. Emotion processing involves automatic and intentional processes that influence the occurrence, intensity, duration, and expression of emotions. There is a wide spectrum of theories on how emotions can influence self-theory, identity, decision-making, social interaction, and even policy (for an overview, see Lewis et al. 2008).

Among others, Gross and colleagues (Gross 2002, Ochsner and Gross 2014) have proposed a model of emotion regulation, which emphasizes the explicit or implicit appraisal of external or internal emotional cues that trigger a set of experiential, physiological, and behavioral response tendencies. According to this model, emotions can be modulated automatically or by either manipulating the input to the system (*antecedent-focused emotion regulation strategies*) or by manipulating the output of the regulation process (*response-focused emotion regulation strategies*). Antecedent-focused strategies include both implicit and explicit strategies, such as situation selection or modification and cognitive techniques (e.g., reappraisal, attention deployment, or reframing of the situation), while response-focused strategies include both implicit and explicit strategies that can be subdivided into physiological, cognitive, and behavioral processes.

Neuroanatomically, the central areas involved in emotion regulation are the dorsolateral and ventral areas of the prefrontal cortex (including the anterior cingulate cortex [ACC]), as well as the amygdala, the hippocampus, and the insula (Ochsner and Gross 2014). These authors suggest a psychobiological circular model of emotion processing where emotions are generated and modulated by interplaying macro- and micro-circuits of "bottom-up" and "top-down" processes. According to this model, central areas such as the amygdala and the insula are involved in the evaluation of external and internal stimuli regarding their emotional valence. These stimuli are further processed in the hypothalamus and in brainstem regions in order to activate autonomic and behavioral responses. In parallel, prefrontal and parietal cortical areas serve to allocate attention and to activate potential behavioral responses. Regulatory processes associated with areas of the lateral and medial prefrontal cortex (MPFC) act to control and modulate emotional activation, thereby covering typical response-focused regulation strategies. Studies suggest a regulatory hierarchy, whereby the dorsolateral prefrontal cortex (DLPFC) and areas of the anterior medio-prefrontal cortex modulate the cingulate, which in turn modulates the amygdala and further subcortical areas (Meyer-Lindenberg et al. 2005, Buckholtz et al. 2007; see Figure 7.1).

A. Strategies and Processes

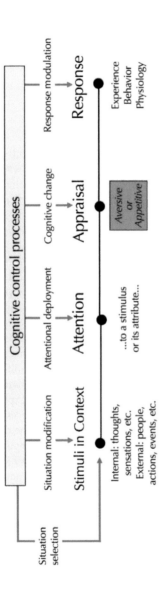

B. Neural Systems

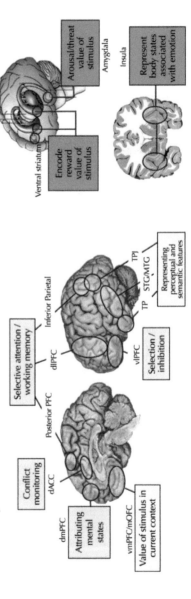

Figure 7.1 Strategies and processes (A) and neural systems (B) involved in emotion regulation. *Source:* Reprinted with permission from Ochsner et al. 2012.

Regulatory processes can also be activated by cognitive reappraisal, by changing attention, or by activating memories (Ochsner and Gross 2005). These cognitive strategies result in an activation of lateral and medial prefrontal areas which, in turn, involve the ACC and ultimately dampen emotional arousal by attenuating the activity of the amygdala, the medial cingulate, and areas of the insula. It should be stressed here that mechanisms of emotion regulation are subject to genetic variation, to maturing processes, and to interindividual variation, as well as to environmental risk factors such as early adversity or poverty.

In this chapter, we delineate the current state of knowledge regarding emotion regulation in personality disorders. We follow the Gross model of emotion regulation and first describe *antecedent-focused emotion regulation strategies* with attentional processes and cognitive regulation of emotions. In addition to the "classical" aspects as delineated in the Gross model, we have added two sections on aspects, which in our view are of importance in the understanding of special aspects of emotion regulation in personality disorders, namely habituation processes and problem behaviors such as self-injury, which are associated with dysfunction of several aspects of emotion regulation. The final section is devoted to *response-focused emotion regulation strategies*.

■ ANTECEDENT-FOCUSED EMOTION REGULATION STRATEGIES

Attentional Processes

Within the process of emotion generation and regulation, as described in the emotion regulation model, an early possibility of emotion control is attentional deployment. Since the brain has a limited processing capacity, external and internal stimuli compete for neural resources (e.g., Desimone and Duncan 1995). Therefore, it is possible to influence emotion generation by *attentional distraction* or *attentional bias*, denoting the attentional direction toward or away from aspects of a situation.

For example, *attentional distraction* resulting from engagement in a secondary task (e.g., Stroop task, working memory task) was shown to reduce emotional reactions (e.g., Raymond et al. 2003). At the neural level, attentional distraction from emotional pictures resulted in reduced amygdala activity in healthy subjects, as well as increased activation in anterior cingulate and prefrontal regions (McRae et al. 2010). Pessoa and colleagues (2002) also found deactivation of the amygdala within an attentional distraction condition when subjects were viewing emotional faces. In another line of research, attentional distraction from painful stimuli was shown to be associated with deactivation of prefrontal cortex and anterior cingulate cortex, both involved in secondary appraisal (Valet et al. 2004).

In contrast to attentional distraction, *attentional biases* can lead to the focusing of attention to several aspects of a stimulus. For example, the negativity bias is a well-established psychological phenomenon by which subjects pay more attention to, remember better, and more frequently recall negative information (Baumeister et al. 2001; Rozin and Royzman 2001). At the neural level, it has been shown that salient stimuli are processed by a brain network comprised of amygdala, insula, and dorsal anterior cingulate cortex (dACC; Seeley et al. 2007, Menon and Uddin 2010). Regarding social stimuli, an attentional bias to potential threat in preattentive processing may be facilitated by a direct subcortical pathway from the thalamus to the amygdala (Vuilleumier et al. 2001, Dolan and Vuilleumier 2003).

Finally, both mechanisms, *attentional distraction* and *attentional bias* were repeatedly shown to be relevant for the majority of emotional disorders (Koster et al. 2009). In the following, evidence for alterations of these basic emotion regulation mechanisms for different personality disorders are summarized.

Attentional Distraction

There is evidence that patients with borderline personality disorder (BPD) use attentional distraction as means of emotional regulation, but unfortunately there is often a high functional cost to this approach to emotion regulation (Schramm et al. 2013). It was argued that BPD patients use problem behavior to direct their attention away from emotional contents. Within the experiential avoidance model, self-injurious or high-risk behavior serve to escape from aversive internal stimuli like emotions, thoughts, tension, or somatic sensations (Chapman et al. 2006). Accordingly, several studies emphasized the important role of self-injury in the regulation of negative affect (Nock and Prinstein 2004, Klonsky 2007, Kleindienst et al. 2008). Studies on neural correlates of pain processing in BPD suggested that painful stimuli serve as a possibility to reduce limbic arousal (Schmahl et al. 2006) and to distract attention from emotional contents (Niedtfeld et al. 2012). Experiential avoidance and self-injurious behavior also show aspects of a response-focused emotion regulation strategy and will be depicted there in greater detail.

In addition to serving as an emotion regulation strategy, attentional distraction may interfere with cognitive processes, and there is evidence that BPD patients have a particular vulnerability to certain types of distraction. Attentional distraction by negative stimuli was found to be more pronounced in BPD patients. In two studies using a Sternberg item recognition task, Krause-Utz et al. (2012, 2014) investigated working memory performance in BPD while subjects were distracted by negative pictures or emotional faces. After distraction by negatively arousing stimuli and also by neutral facial expressions, BPD patients showed decreased working memory performance and slower reaction times (Krause-Utz et al. 2014). Regarding neural correlates, emotional distraction in BPD was accompanied by higher activation in the amygdala and decreased activity in DLPFC (Krause-Utz et al. 2012). These results suggest that BPD patients were more distracted by emotional pictures during the working memory task. In a similar vein, Prehn and colleagues (2013) used an n-back task and presented negative pictures as emotional distraction. Male patients with BPD and antisocial personality disorder showed slower reaction times and higher activation of the left amygdala during the presentation of negative pictures. Furthermore, BPD patients showed more pronounced distraction by fearful faces during a modified flanker task, which was accompanied by higher ACC activation and increased amygdala activation (Holtmann et al. 2013). Attentional avoidance of threatening faces was found in a visual dot probe task in subjects with high rejection sensitivity and borderline features (Berenson et al. 2009). Regarding the emotional Stroop task (EST), the evidence in BPD is rather inconclusive. Three studies found more interference by emotional words in BPD (Sieswerda et al. 2007), but the effect was also found in patients with other (Cluster C) personality disorders (Arntz et al. 2000) or could be attributed to comorbid posttraumatic stress disorder (Wingenfeld et al. 2009). Two other studies could not demonstrate an enhanced Stroop effect in BPD (Domes et al. 2006, Jacob et al. 2010). At the neural level, BPD patients showed increased activation of the ACC and prefrontal regions when working on the EST (Wingenfeld et al. 2009).

Dissociation constitutes an emotional overmodulation mode that responds to the experience of (traumatic) stress (Lanius et al. 2010) and is closely related to disturbed attentional processes (Winter et al. 2014). In particular, overactivity of medial prefrontal brain regions with concomitant limbic downregulation was hypothesized to underlie dissociative psychopathology. Corroboration of these assumptions comes from several sources. In one study, patients with high levels of dissociation were found to have significantly lower startle responses compared to those with low levels of dissociation (Ebner-Priemer et al. 2005), while another study found that dissociation scores were negatively correlated with activity in the amygdala, insula, and ACC during emotional distraction that took place while the participants were performing a working memory task (Krause-Utz et al. 2012). Dissociation was also related to longer reaction times and alterations in DLPFC activation in an EST study in BPD patients (Winter et al., 2015).

A number of studies investigated attentional processes in schizotypal personality disorder (SPD) or in subjects with high versus low schizotypal personality traits. Working on an EST, subjects with high schizotypy showed more interference, pointing to poorer attentional performance (Mohanty et al. 2008, Volter et al. 2012) and larger switching costs, supposedly caused by difficulties selecting task-relevant information (Cimino and Haywood 2008). Poor performance in the EST was more pronounced for words presented to the left visual field (Van Strien and Van Kampen 2009), and in a neuroimaging study it was accompanied by decreased activity in left DLPFC and higher activity in hippocampus and amygdala (Mohanty et al. 2005). In two studies on latent inhibition, subjects had to work on a primary task demanding attentional resources (e.g., judgment whether a pair of upright letters are the same vs. different), while they were presented with geographical forms (task-irrelevant stimuli). Subjects with high SPD traits were found to be more distracted by task-irrelevant stimuli (Braunstein-Bercovitz and Lubow 1998). Another study concludes that the difficulties in attention direction were driven by an anxiety-related component of schizotypy (Braunstein-Bercovitz 2000).

Finally, attentional processes were also shown to deviate in psychopathy/antisocial personality disorder (AsPD). Three studies showed reduced interference in the Stroop task in offenders with high psychopathy (Hiatt et al. 2004), in adolescents with high psychopathy and low anxiety (Vitale et al. 2005), and in psychopathic female offenders (Vitale et al. 2007). In offenders with AsPD, an attentional bias toward violence-related words in the Stroop task was found (Domes et al. 2013). In two neuroimaging studies, subjects with psychopathy and antisocial behavior were found to recruit the ACC and regions in the temporal cortex to a lesser extent (Sadeh et al. 2013) and show more activation in the amygdala (Schiffer et al. 2014).

In conclusion, attentional processes appear to be more easily disrupted by irrelevant information in BPD and SPD, especially when the distraction is of negative valence. On the other hand, subjects with psychopathy or AsPD seem less distracted by task-irrelevant stimuli.

Attentional Bias

Apart from specific personality disorders, it was shown that the detection sensitivity for fearful faces is related to trait anxiety (Japee et al. 2009; Surcinelli et al. 2006) as well as personality traits such as neuroticism and harm avoidance (Doty et al. 2013). As an example for a personality disorder with high trait anxiety, neuroticism, and harm avoidance, BPD patients were shown to process faces displaying negative emotions differently from neutral or positive ones (Daros et al. 2013), resulting in enhanced processing and higher false alarm rates for negative faces. Interestingly, the most pronounced differences compared to healthy controls were found when BPD patients had to label neutral facial expressions, because they overreported anger and fear (Dyck et al. 2009), suggesting that BPD patients tend to direct their attention toward facial cues of anger and fear. Although studies on labeling (i.e., appraisal processes) of facial expressions point to deficiencies in BPD when stimuli are ambiguous (Meyer et al. 2004, Domes et al. 2008), it is not clear whether BPD patients show a negativity bias in early stages of emotion processing (i.e., attentional processes).

When BPD patients had to detect emotions in a neutral face that gradually changes into an emotional one, one study found they recognize emotions earlier than the control group (Lynch et al. 2006), whereas Robin et al. (2012) found that adolescent BPD patients recognized expressions later. Finally, Domes and coworkers (2008) as well as Jovev and coworkers (2011) did not observe a different sensitivity in their BPD groups. A recent study (Veague and Hooley 2014) found an enhanced sensitivity and response bias for anger, but this was specific for male faces.

Investigating fast emotion detection in BPD, Hagenoff et al. (2013) assessed how sensitive BPD patients are in detecting happy and angry faces in a crowd of neutral faces, using the well-established face-in-the-crowd paradigm (Hansen and Hansen 1988). Although angry faces were detected faster than positive ones by both groups, patients did not show a greater anger superiority effect than healthy controls (Hagenoff et al. 2013). In a series of laboratory and web-based studies with a similar design, Hepp and coworkers (2016) accumulated evidence against the existence of a BPD-specific negativity bias at the attentional level.

Reduced sensitivity for emotional facial displays was repeatedly found in AsPD (for an overview, see Marsh and Blair 2008) and also in psychopathy (for an overview, see Dawel et al. 2012). In a recent study by Schönenberg and coworkers (2013), subjects with AsPD had to label facial expressions that were gradually morphed from neutral to angry, fearful, or happy. While subjects with AsPD required higher emotional intensity to correctly identify anger, no differences to healthy controls were found regarding fearful or happy facial expressions. In an EEG-study, it was highlighted that differences in the processing of emotional expressions can be observed during early stages of attention allocation, concluding that participants with high AsPD traits attended less to facial emotional stimuli (Pfabigan et al. 2012). Subjects with low AsPD traits showed larger P1 amplitudes than subjects with high AsPD traits within 100 ms after both happy and angry facial feedback presentation.

Subjects with SPD appear to have difficulties detecting happy emotional expressions. Overall poorer emotion recognition, which was most pronounced regarding happy expressions, was found in subjects with high schizotypal traits (Abbott and Byrne 2013) when they were asked to label emotion displays in short video clips. In another study, the appearance of happy facial expressions led to less deactivation of the ACC and more deactivation in the posterior cingulate cortex and superior temporal gyrus in subjects with high SPD traits compared to subjects with low SPD traits (Huang et al. 2013).

A recent study by Denny et al. (2015) demonstrated increased amygdala activity in avoidant personality disorder (AvPD) patients compared to healthy controls during the anticipation of an emotional task. There are few other neuroimaging studies of AvPD (see Koenigsberg et al. 2014), and results from research in social phobia suggest that subjects with high social anxiety show an attentional bias toward potentially threatening social stimuli and an interpretational bias toward self-relevant social information (Heinrichs and Hofmann 2001, Machado-de-Sousa et al. 2010). In the first study on emotion recognition in AvPD, Rosenthal et al. (2011) showed that AvPD subjects made more errors when they had to classify a fearful expression, but no differences in the speed to classify emotional expressions were found in AvPD.

In narcissistic personality disorder (NPD), a recent study also showed less accuracy in the recognition of emotional expressions, which was most pronounced in faces representing fear and disgust (Marissen et al. 2012). Another study by Ritter and coworkers (2011) found no differences in emotion recognition in subjects with NPD but difficulties in emotional empathy. In a neuroimaging study, subjects high in narcissism showed less activation in the right anterior insula, a brain region typically associated with empathy, suggesting that narcissism is linked to empathic functioning (Fan et al. 2011).

To summarize the studies outlined, most personality disorders show attentional biases in the processing of facial expressions. While subjects with BPD and AvPD show enhanced activity regarding the detection of negative emotional expressions, subjects with AsPD, SPD, and NPD show reduced sensitivity regarding different emotional expressions.

Habituation of Emotions

Habituation of emotions can be considered a mechanism of implicit regulation separate from those included in Gross's process model, which entails a reduction in subjective distress upon repeated exposure to an aversive stimulus. Habituation is an implicit, highly adaptive, and widely employed emotion regulatory mechanism. It underlies the common experience of "getting used to" something disturbing by repeated exposure to it. Studies of healthy subjects have shown decreases in amygdala BOLD activation upon repeated exposure to negative faces or emotional pictures (Breiter et al. 1996, Wright et al. 2001, Fischer et al. 2003). Decreases in activation to repeated presentations have also been reported in the hippocampus, the ventrolateral prefrontal cortex (VLPFC), the fusiform gyrus, the medial and inferior temporal cortex, and in regions associated with working memory and control and allocation of attentional resources such as the DLPFC, the MPFC, and the ACC (Feinstein et al. 2002, Fischer et al. 2003, Phan et al. 2003, Denny et al. 2013). Increases in insula, posterior cingulate cortex, precuneus, and DLPFC activation have also been identified with repeated viewing of emotional pictures (Feinstein et al. 2002, Denny et al. 2013). Moreover, the degree to which healthy individuals increase insula-amygdala functional connectivity with repeated viewing is directly correlated with the degree to which they decrease their negative reactions to aversive pictures (Denny et al. 2013).

The high emotional reactivity of BPD patients could be a consequence, in part, of impairment in the capacity to habituate to negative stimuli. Two studies have looked at this question. Koenigsberg and colleagues (2014) found that BPD patients did not increase activity in the dACC, left superior/middle temporal gyri, and right transverse temporal gyrus to the extent that healthy subjects did when viewing aversive pictures of social interactions a second time compared to novel viewing, demonstrating anomalous neural functioning when habituating. Furthermore, consistent with the hypothesis that impairment in neural habituation underlies affective instability in BPD, these authors found that the less BPD subjects activated the dACC when viewing repeated images, the greater their self-reported affective instability. In addition, BPD patients did not show the increase in insula-amygdala functional connectivity seen in healthy subjects when viewing repeated versus novel pictures.

A study examining habituation to negative, positive, and neutral valence pictures (Hazlett et al. 2012) found that BPD subjects showed greater amygdala activation to repeated, compared to novel, presentation of negative and positive pictures, whereas healthy subjects showed a decrease in activation to repeated positive pictures and little change to negative pictures, suggesting that BPD patients actually sensitize rather than habituate neurally to emotional pictures. These two studies converge to indicate anomalies in neural processing when BPD patients habituate to repeated emotional stimuli and support the hypothesis that impairments in the implicit emotional regulatory mechanism of habituation play a role in the emotional dysregulation seen in BPD.

Few studies of habituation in personality disorders other than BPD have been carried out. Koenigsberg et al. (2014) examined habituation in AvPD, a disorder sharing with BPD high emotional reactivity to interpersonal situations. Like the BPD patients, the AvPD patients did not increase dACC activity when viewing repeat pictures as healthy subjects did, but for the AvPD patients there was no correlation between dACC activity and self-reported affective instability, a finding consistent with the absence of affective instability as a key symptom of AvPD. A neural finding distinct to the AvPD patients is that, relative to healthy subjects, they show less of an increase in connectivity between the insula and a broad region of the middle frontal gyrus (including the DLPFC and MPFC). Since the MPFC is implicated in fear extinction learning (Phelps et al. 2004), the failure to increase insula-MPFC connectivity during repeated exposure may interfere with fear extinction, contributing to the persistence of fear of social settings.

The habituation response in SPD patients was examined by Hazlett and coworkers (2012). Unlike BPD patients, the SPD patients increased amygdala activation to repeated viewing of neutral pictures and decreased activation to repeated viewing of negative and positive pictures. This interesting finding suggests that SPD patients may show greater reactivity to ambiguous or subtle (i.e., less clearly positive or negative) emotional stimuli than the other groups.

Cognitive Regulation of Emotions

An individual's emotional reaction to a particular situation is strongly determined by the meaning attributed to the situation. Thus, one approach to emotion regulation is for the individual to cognitively alter the meaning of a situation in such a way as to change its emotional valence. One well-studied and highly adaptive strategy for emotion regulation is cognitive reappraisal, a method in which one reconceptualizes an emotion-eliciting situation to alter the emotional reaction to it (Gross 1998). Cognitive reappraisal is most often employed to reduce the intensity of negative feelings engendered by aversive situations or to increase positive feelings to neutral or positive cues. However, the strategy is quite versatile and may be used to increase negative feelings or decrease positive feelings. For example, as an important exam approaches, one might elect to imagine severe consequences of poor performance to heighten one's anxiety level in order to increase motivation to study. Cognitive reappraisal has been shown to be a highly adaptive regulation strategy (John and Gross 2004), reducing the subjective experience, behavioral expression, and physiological concomitants of negative feeling states. Moreover, it has been demonstrated that healthy volunteers can be trained through focused practice to improve their reappraisal skills, and this in turn has been associated with reduced levels of overall perceived stress in daily life (Denny and Ochsner 2014).

Two distinct reappraisal tactics have been studied in detail, a situation-directed reinterpretation tactic and a distancing tactic (Gross and John, 2003, Ochsner et al. 2004, Kross and Ayduk 2008, McRae et al. 2012). In the former a narrative is created for a situation to alter its affective valence. Thus, for example, the hospitalization of a relative for a serious illness can be reconceptualized as an opportunity for that person to get expert medical care and attention, leading to rapid improvement. In the distancing tactic, the subject assumes an emotionally distant stance from the situation (i.e., views the situation as a detached, objective, impartial observer). This tactic is employed, for example, when the emergency room physician assumes a clinical distance in attending to a severely injured person to reduce emotionality that could interfere with his or her effectiveness.

The neural systems that participate in cognitive reappraisal have been well studied in healthy subjects (Buhle et al. 2013). During cognitive reappraisal, regions involved in working memory and selective attention (DLPFC, posterior parietal cortex, and ACC), mental state attribution (DMPFC), and response selection and inhibition (VLPFC) are recruited and activity of target limbic emotional appraisal regions, most notably the amygdala, is modulated.

Cognitive Regulation of Emotion in Personality Disorders

Dysfunction of normal emotion regulatory systems could explain some or all of the emotion dysregulation seen in personality disorders. Impairment in cognitive reappraisal is one candidate. Koenigsberg and colleagues (2009) suggested that BPD patients' vulnerability to oscillation between intense overinvolvement and withdrawal in interpersonal situations could reflect an underlying impairment in the ability to employ the reappraisal-by-distancing tactic. Consistent with this hypothesis, they found that when instructed to emotionally distance from scenes of negative interpersonal interaction, BPD subjects showed anomalous neural activity, engaging the dACC or the intraparietal sulcus less than healthy subjects did (Koenigsberg et al. 2009). These regions, which participate in attention allocation and working memory, are engaged when healthy individuals reappraise. In addition, when reappraising, BPD patients, unlike healthy subjects, did not show a decrease in activity in the amygdala, a structure whose activity reflects arousal and threat detection. Employing a slightly different reappraisal task in which subjects were given the option of either distancing or imagining that the scene was make-believe, Schulze et al. (2011) also reported BPD subjects, compared to healthy volunteers, showed anomalous reappraisal activity, particularly diminished activity in the left orbitofrontal cortex, middle frontal gyrus, left precuneus, left middle temporal gyrus, right superior temporal gyrus, and right pallidum, and did not downregulate the insula, a region reflecting negative affective appraisal (Denny et al. 2013). Thus, although the methodologies were slightly different, both studies converge to indicate disturbances in the neural substrates of cognitive reappraisal in BPD.

Interestingly, neither study showed group differences in behavioral reappraisal success, as measured by subjects' valence rating of pictures following reappraisal compared to a just looking condition. Several models have been proposed to explain this difference between behavioral and neural findings, a pattern identified in other studies of BPD as well. These include the possibilities that alexithymia (New et al. 2012), characteristic of BPD patients, interferes with their ability to accurately report affective experience; that BPD subjects were strongly influenced by the demand characteristics of the task; or that neural effects simply have a greater sensitivity to show change than behavioral reports. This phenomenon merits further study. Of further interest is also the effect of psychotherapy on these described neural alterations. In a study on BPD patients before and after a three-month intensive dialectical behavioral therapy (DBT) treatment, responders showed reduced amygdala activation and stronger amygdala-VLPFC connectivity than nonresponders during a reappraisal paradigm (Schmitt et al. 2014).

Cognitive regulation of emotion has been examined in only one personality disorder other than BPD, AvPD (Denny et al., 2015). Here, no difference in behavioral ratings of picture valence was observed between AvPD patients and heathy volunteers when reappraising by distancing versus looking at negative interpersonal scenes. During reappraisal, the AvPD subjects as well as the healthy volunteers recruited medial, dorsolateral, and ventral prefrontatal cortex as well as dACC and reduced activity of the amygdala. However, there were no group differences in activation during reappraisal by distancing compared to looking. Thus, unlike BPD patients, AvPD patients do not show evidence of impaired cognitive reappraisal. This finding needs to be replicated.

Further work is called for to examine cognitive regulatory processes in other personality disorders. Of particular interest in this regard is antisocial personality disorder (AsPD). AsPD patients, scoring high in psychopathy, can be callous and emotionally unresponsive to fear and pain in others (Brook et al. 2013). While the neuroimaging findings in AsPD remain mixed, there is a convergence of studies suggesting diminished amygdala or associated limbic activity in AsPD patients (Blair 2010, Brook et al. 2013). Thus it is possible that AsPD patients could show the opposite dysregulation in emotional distancing to that seen in BPD (i.e., an excessive activation of reappraisal-by-distancing networks).

■ RESPONSE-FOCUSED EMOTION REGULATION STRATEGIES

These strategies, also called response modulation, refer to a common form of regulation strategies that intervenes rather late in the emotion process, after an emotional response tendency has been generated (Gross 2014). Response modulation occurs when an individual directly changes the way he or she responds in an emotional situation and involves direct influencing of physiological, experiential, or behavioral responding (Gross 2014). Hence, response modulation can serve to either upregulate (exaggeration) or downregulate (suppression) the emotional intensity and may also change the experienced emotion itself. Examples of response-focused strategies are exercise, anxiolytic drugs, or the suppression of expressive (facial) or physiological reactions.

So far, response-focused strategies have not received much scientific attention, and researchers have only started to investigate and compare the effects of different response-focused strategies in healthy individuals (Dan-Glauser and Gross 2011).

First results indicate differences in response-focused emotion regulation between patients with personality disorders and healthy controls. In patients with BPD, who are characterized by enhanced emotional sensitivity and show deficits in the attentional and cognitive regulation of emotions as delineated (e.g., Schulze et al. 2011, Prehn et al. 2013), dysfunctional behaviors, such as nonsuicidal self-injury, bingeing, or drug and alcohol abuse, may be regarded as—albeit maladaptive—response-focused emotion regulation strategies (e.g., see In-Albon et al. 2013, McKenzie and Gross 2014). In addition, response-modulation strategies have long been used and proven effective in psychotherapeutic treatment of patients with personality disorders and in particular of those with BPD (see, e.g., Linehan 1993). Although emotion dysregulation also plays a prominent role in other personality disorders, such as AsPD, SPD, or histrionic personality disorder, only very few experimental studies have investigated alterations in response-focused emotion regulation. Examples are a reduced ability to exaggerate expressive behaviors in SPD patients (Henry et al. 2009) or enhanced prevalence of self-harming behaviors, such as restricted or binge eating, nonsuicidal self-injury, or drug and alcohol abuse in patients with various personality disorders (see, e.g., Chapman et al. 2006, Davis et al. 2013, Reas et al. 2013, Sansone and Sansone 2013).

In the following section we therefore first review the literature on the role of response modulation in personality disorders and discuss dysfunctional behaviors of patients with personality disorders in light of attempted emotional response modulation. We then review response-focused interventions that have been effectively used in psychotherapeutic treatment of patients with personality disorders.

Facial and Bodily Responses to Emotional Stimuli

Several studies have investigated facial and bodily reactions to emotional pictures or faces in patients with BPD. Although the results from studies on BPD patients' physiological reactions to emotional or social stimuli have been rather mixed, they indicate exaggerated psychophysiological responses including heart rate and skin conductance level to negative social stimuli related to experiences of abandonment, rejection, neglect, or social stress (Limberg et al. 2011, Lobbestael and Arntz 2010, Sieswerda et al. 2007). Consistent with this, patients with BPD showed more mixed and fewer positive emotional facial expressions during social interactions (Staebler et al. 2011). Studying facial reactions in female BPD patients, Matzke et al. (2014) found increased electromyographic activity in frowning muscle (i.e., the corrugator supercilia) while processing angry, sad, or disgusted facial expressions and decreased activity in the smiling muscle (i.e., the levator labii superioris) in response to happy and surprised faces compared to healthy women. According to the afferent facial feedback hypothesis, the pattern of exaggerated expression of frowning-related muscle activity to negative facial expressions and of suppression of smiling-associated muscle activity to positive facial expression may at least partly explain the enhanced frequency and levels of negative emotional and stressful daily experiences reported by patients with BPD (Ebner-Priemer et al. 2007, Ebner-Priemer et al. 2008, Stiglmayr et al. 2001, Stiglmayr et al. 2005).

In individuals with AsPD or psychopathy, blunted physiological, in particular cardiovascular and electrodermal, responses to emotionally negative stimuli or situations have consistently been reported (e.g., Herpertz et al. 2001, Lobbestael et al. 2009). However, facial or bodily expressive behavior has not yet been investigated in AsPD or psychopathy. Deficits in the conscious modulation of expressive behavior have been reported in highly schizotypal individuals (Henry et al. 2009). While there was no difference between the high and low schizotypal group in suppression, highly schizotypal individuals were less able to exaggerate their expression of positive emotions. In addition, difficulties in exaggerating emotional expressive behavior was associated with blunted affect. Although conscious modulation of expressive facial or bodily responses in emotion-eliciting or social situations is an important skill taught in DBT (Linehan 1993; see following section), its effects have not been experimentally investigated in BPD patients. In healthy males, Dan-Glauser and Gross (2011) found that both instructed expressive and physiological suppression could produce rapid response modulation and change subjective experience, facial expressivity, as well as autonomic responses to emotional pictures. Interestingly, both response-modulation strategies produced very similar effects, indicating that consciously influencing (suppressing or exaggerating) facial or bodily emotional responses could be an effective therapeutic intervention for patients with deficits in attentional and/or cognitive emotion regulation.

Experiential Avoidance

Experiential avoidance (i.e., an unwillingness to remain in contact with uncomfortable sensations, thoughts, memories, or emotions) is another dysfunctional response-focused strategy often used by patients with personality disorders, in particular BPD, to avoid or escape negative affective states. In a recent study, Iverson et al. (2012) found a positive association between experiential avoidance and BPD symptomatology as well as emotion dysregulation in young outpatients with BPD symptoms. Experiential avoidance has also been shown to be positively associated with depression and reductions in experiential avoidance during psychotherapy-predicted subsequent reductions in depression in patients with BPD (Berking et al. 2009). This is in line with the results of a recent path-analytical study, which showed that experiential avoidance maintains the lack of positive emotions in BPD (Jacob et al. 2013). Dissociative symptoms such as depersonalization and derealization are highly prevalent in patients with BPD and may be regarded as an extreme form of experiential avoidance. Thus, experiential avoidance and dissociation may serve to suppress aversive emotional experiences but also hinder functional emotion regulation and coping strategies.

Self-Harming Behavior

Non-suicidal self-injury (NSSI) is highly prevalent in patients with BPD and has been conceptualized as a behavior that reduces or eliminates unwanted emotional responses, and in particular the physiological aspects of emotional responses (Chapman et al. 2006). Self-harming behavior not only NSSI, such as cutting, burning, scratching the skin, or self-hitting and head banging, but also bingeing or starving; abusing alcohol, drugs, or prescribed medication; and being promiscuous (Sansone et al. 2010). Several studies have found enhanced prevalence for alcohol and/or drug abuse as well as eating disorders in various personality disorders, such as AsPD (substance abuse), BPD (substance abuse, binge eating, bulimia), obsessive-compulsive personality disorder (anorexia nervosa), or schizotypal personality disorder (cannabis abuse; see, e.g., Chapman et al. 2006, Davis et al. 2013, Reas et al. 2013, Sansone and Sansone 2013).

BPD patients report a multitude of motives for the use of self-harming behaviors with relieving aversive inner tension (Brown et al. 2002, Kleindienst et al. 2008) and decreasing negative affective states (Chapman et al. 2006, Sadeh et al. 2014) being reported by the majority of patients. In fact, high levels of negative affect, particularly feelings of rejection, anger, or guilt prior to self-harming behavior, and a reduction of negative affect and inner tension as well as increased calmness and relief during and after self-injury have been reported by self-injuring patients across studies (for review, see In-Albon et al. 2013).

Individuals who use NSSI also showed reduced psychophysiological activation after experimentally induced pain or script-driven imagery of self-injurious behavior (Brainet al. 1998, Haines et al. 1995, Reitz et al. 2012). In a study that tested the aspect of emotion regulation by sensory stimulation, pain that was experimentally induced by thermal stimuli was found to result in the attenuation of amygdala hyperactivity induced by affective pictures (Niedtfeld et al. 2010). Functional connectivity analyses revealed normal inhibitory connectivity between the left amygdala and MPFC and between the right anterior insula and DLPFC when negative pictures were combined with painfully hot stimulation but not when they were combined with nonpainfully warm stimulation (Niedtfeld et al. 2012), suggesting that there may be a specificity of painful stimuli in the context of sensory emotion regulation in BPD. Using incision-induced pain, which takes into account tissue damage and thus provides a more valid model for nonsuicidal self-injury, a stress-reducing effect of an incision in the forearm in terms of reduced subjective arousal and increased heart rate variability could be demonstrated (Reitz et al. 2012). These findings were recently replicated in a functional magnetic resonance imaging study in which an additional restitution of poststress amygdala-MPFC coupling following incision was shown (Reitz et al. 2015).

Self-harming behavior may thus be regarded as a maladaptive response-focused emotion regulation strategy that provides an escape from emotional arousal and suppresses inner tension and uncontrollable and intense negative emotions, particularly feelings of anger or rejection (Favazza and Conterio 1989, Linehan 1993, Paris 2005) and is used because other attentional and/or cognitive regulation strategies seem insufficient (Prehn et al. 2013, Schulze et al. 2011). In a study on BPD patients before and after a three-month intensive DBT treatment, patients showed reduced amygdala activation in response to negative pictures after psychotherapy, and painful stimuli did also not result in the attenuation of amygdala response anymore (Niedtfeld et al. 2017).

Response Modulation in Psychotherapy

In DBT, patients learn to use a range of distress tolerance skills with the aim to downregulate the extreme physiological arousal that often accompanies intense emotions and to inhibit maladaptive behaviors, such as NSSI or dissociation (Linehan 1993). The skills are designed to quickly reduce high arousal without requiring a high level of cognitive involvement (Neacsiu, Eberle, et al. 2014). DBT distress tolerance skills are designed to regulate the expressive and physiological response subjective experience of emotions and comprise strong physical distractors, such as ice water, intense exercise, strong sensory stimuli as well as paced breathing and progressive relaxation and opposite action (physiological and expressive suppression). The latter involves facial and bodily expressions and actions that oppose or are inconsistent to the emotional state in order to prevent impulsive emotional actions.

Studies have proven DBT skills efficient in reducing self-injurious and suicidal behavior, BPD symptomatology, experiential avoidance, dissociation, and depression and in increasing anger control of (suicidal) patients with BPD, patients with BPD and substance abuse, and patients with (complex) posttraumatic stress disorder (e.g., Berking et al. 2009, Bohus et al. 2013, Harned et al. 2014, Neacsiu, Rizvi, et al. 2010, Neacsiu, Lungu, et al. 2014).

Taken together, patients with BPD who have deficits in attentional and cognitive emotion regulation have been shown to use several albeit dysfunctional response-focused attempts to regulate intense and aversive negative emotions. Studies have shown that exaggerated expressive and physiological responses to negative and suppressed expressive responses to positive emotional situations could at least partly explain the enhanced frequency and intensity of subjectively experienced negative affective states and increased inner tension. In addition, blunted affect of schizotypal individuals could be related to deficits in exaggerating the expression of positive emotions. However, despite the relevance of emotional dysregulation, little is still known about facial and bodily responses in patients with other personality disorders. Experiential avoidance, dissociation, and self-harming behavior may be regarded as frequently used strategies to regulate these emotional states. Again, the core of the literature is based on studies in patients with BPD, although the prevalence for self-harming behaviors including eating disorders and substance abuse is enhanced in various personality disorders. DBT stress tolerance skills offer alternative response-focused emotion regulation strategies and have been shown to efficiently reduce dysfunctional behaviors and psychopathology.

■ SUMMARY AND CONCLUSIONS

Although the data base on emotion regulation in personality disorders, particularly those in personality disorders other than BPD, is still thin, a few aspects have been consistently shown in the literature and a few tentative conclusions can be drawn.

Regarding attentional processes, these appear to be more easily disrupted by irrelevant information in BPD and SPD, especially when the distraction is of negative valence. On the other hand, subjects with psychopathy or AsPD seem less distracted by task-irrelevant stimuli. Most personality disorders show attentional biases in the processing of facial expressions. While subjects with BPD and AsPD show enhanced activity regarding the detection of negative emotional expressions, subjects with AsPD, SPD, and NPD show reduced sensitivity regarding different emotional expressions. Habituating to aversive situations is an implicit emotion regulation process that reduces the intensity of the negative experience in healthy subjects via engagement of the ACC and other regions. BPD and AvPD subjects do not engage the ACC as BPD subjects do when habituating and do not show the decrease in negative experience to repeated exposures seen in healthy individuals. Moreover, the degree to which BPD subjects do not engage the ACC during habituation is correlated with their levels of affective instability. When explicitly employing distancing as a cognitive reappraisal tactic to reduce negative emotional responses to aversive cues, BPD subjects show an anomalous pattern of neural activity compared to healthy individuals. Anomalies in neural engagement in cognitive reappraisal, however, is not a characteristic of personality disorder patients in general as is not seen in AvPD subjects.

Patients with BPD often reveal response-focused attempts to regulate intense and aversive negative emotions, such as non-suicial self-injury or dissociation. These strategies can be subsumed under the phenomenon of experiential avoidance. Successful treatment strategies, such as in DBT skills training, particularly focus on these dysfunctional strategies.

■ REFERENCES

Abbott, G., & Byrne L. K. (2013). Schizotypal traits are associated with poorer identification of emotions from dynamic stimuli. *Psychiatry Res, 207*(1–2), 40–44.

Arntz, A., C. Appels, & Sieswerda S. (2000). Hypervigilance in borderline disorder: a test with the emotional Stroop paradigm. *J Pers Disord, 14*(4), 366–373.

Baumeister, R. F., Bratslavsky, E., Finkenauer, C., & Vohs, K. D. (2001). Bad is stronger than good. *Rev Gen Psychol, 5*(4), 323–370.

Berenson, K. R., Gyurak, A., Ayduk, O., Downey, G., Garner, M. J., Mogg, K., Bradley, B. P., & Pine, D. S. (2009). Rejection sensitivity and disruption of attention by social threat cues. *J Res Personal, 43*(6), 1064–1072.

Berking, M., Neacsiu, A., Comtois, K. A., & Linehan, M. M. (2009). The impact of experiential avoidance on the reduction of depression in treatment for borderline personality disorder. *Behav Res Ther, 47*(8), 663–670.

Blair, R. J. R. (2010). Neuroimaging of psychopathy and antisocial behavior: a targeted review. *Curr Psychiatry Rep, 12*(1), 76–82.

Bohus, M., Dyer, A. S., Priebe, K., Kruger, A., Kleindienst, N., Schmahl, C., Niedtfeld, I., & Steil, R. (2013). Dialectical behaviour therapy for post-traumatic stress disorder after childhood sexual abuse in patients with and without borderline personality disorder: a randomised controlled trial. *Psychother Psychosom, 82*(4), 221–233.

Brain, K. L., Haines, J., & Williams, C. L. (1998). The psychophysiology of self-mutilation: evidence of tension reduction. *Arch Suicide Res, 4*, 227–242.

Braunstein-Bercovitz, H. (2000). Is the attentional dysfunction in schizotypy related to anxiety? *Schizophr Res, 46*(2–3), 255–267.

Braunstein-Bercovitz, H., & Lubow, R. E. (1998). Are high-schizotypal normal participants distractible or limited in attentional resources? A study of latent inhibition as a function of masking task load and schizotypy level. *J Abnorm Psychol, 107*(4), 659–670.

Breiter, H. C., Etcoff, N. L., Whalen, P. J., Kennedy, W. A., Rauch, S. L., Buckner, R. L., Strauss, M. M., Hyman, S. E., & Rosen, B. R. (1996). Response and habituation of the human amygdala during visual processing of facial expression. *Neuron, 17*(5), 875–887.

Brook, M., Brieman, C. L., & Kosson, D. S. (2013). Emotion processing in Psychopathy Checklist-assessed psychopathy: a review of the literature. *Clin Psychol Rev, 33*(8), 979–995.

Brown, M. Z., Comtois, K. A., & Linehan, M. M. (2002). Reasons for suicide attempts and nonsuicidal self-injury in women with borderline personality disorder. *J Abnorm Child Psychol, 111*(1), 198–202.

Buckholtz, J. W., Sust, S., Tan, H. Y., Mattay, V. S., Straub, R. E., Meyer-Lindenberg, A., Weinberger, D. R., & Callicott, J. H. (2007). fMRI evidence for functional epistasis between COMT and RGS4. *Mol Psychiatry, 12*(10), 893–895, 885.

Buhle, J. T., Silvers, J. A., Wager, T. D., Lopez, R., Onyemekwu, C., Kober, H., Weber, J., & Ochsner, K. N. (2013). Cognitive reappraisal of emotion: a meta-analysis of human neuroimaging studies. *Cereb Cortex, 24*(11), 2981–2990.

Chapman, A. L., Gratz, K. L., & Brown, M. Z. (2006). Solving the puzzle of deliberate self-harm: the experiential avoidance model. *Behav Res Ther, 44*(3), 371–394.

Cimino, M., & Haywood, M. (2008). Inhibition and facilitation in schizotypy. *J Clin Exp Neuropsychol, 30*(2), 187–198.

Dan-Glauser, E. S., & Gross, J. J. (2011). The temporal dynamics of two response-focused forms of emotion regulation: experiential, expressive, and autonomic consequences. *Psychophysiology, 48*(9), 1309–1322.

Daros, A. R., Zakzanis, K. K., & Ruocco, A. C. (2013). Facial emotion recognition in borderline personality disorder. *Psychol Med, 43*(9), 1953–1963.

Davis, G. P., Compton, M. T., Wang, S., Levin, F. R., & Blanco, C. (2013). Association between cannabis use, psychosis, and schizotypal personality disorder: findings from the National Epidemiologic Survey on Alcohol and Related Conditions. *Schizophr Res, 151*(1–3), 197–202.

Dawel, A., O'Kearney, R., McKone, E., & Palermo, R. (2012). Not just fear and sadness: meta-analytic evidence of pervasive emotion recognition deficits for facial and vocal expressions in psychopathy. *Neurosci Biobehav Rev, 36*(10), 2288–2304.

Denny, B. T., Fan, J., Liu, X., Guerreri, S., Mayson, S. J., Rimsky, L., New, A. S., Siever, L. J., & Koenigsberg, H. W. (2013). Insula-amygdala functional connectivity is correlated with habituation to repeated negative images. *Soc Cogn Affect Neurosci.*

Denny, B. T., Fan, J., Liu, X., Ochsner, K. N., Guerreri, S., Mayson, S. J., Rimsky, L., McMaster, A., New, A. S., Goodman, M., Siever, L. J., & Koenigsberg, H. W. (2015). Elevated amygdala activity during reappraisal anticipation predicts anxiety in avoidant personality disorder. *J Affect Disord, 172*, 1–7.

Denny, B. T., & Ochsner, K. N. (2014). Behavioral effects of longitudinal training in cognitive reappraisal. *Emotion, 14*(2), 425–433.

Desimone, R., & Duncan, J. (1995). Neural mechanisms of selective attention. *Annu Rev Neurosci, 18*, 193–222.

Dolan, R. J., & Vuilleumier, P. (2003). Amygdala automaticity in emotional processing. *Ann N Y Acad Sci, 985*, 348–355.

Domes, G., Czieschnek, D., Weidler, F., Berger, C., Fast, K., & Herpertz, S. C. (2008). Recognition of facial affect in borderline personality disorder. *J Pers Disord, 22*(2), 135–147.

Domes, G., Mense, J., Vohs, K., & Habermeyer, E. (2013). Offenders with antisocial personality disorder show attentional bias for violence-related stimuli. *Psychiatry Res, 209*(1), 78–84.

Domes, G., Winter, B., Schnell, K., Vohs, K., Fast, K., & Herpertz, S. C. (2006). The influence of emotions on inhibitory functioning in borderline personality disorder. *Psychol Med, 36*(8), 1163–1172.

Doty, T. J., Japee, S., Ingvar, M., & Ungerleider, L. G. (2013). Fearful face detection sensitivity in healthy adults correlates with anxiety-related traits. *Emotion, 13*(2), 183–188.

Dyck, M., Habel, U., Slodczyk, J., Schlummer, J., Backes, V., Schneider, F., & Reske, M. (2009). Negative bias in fast emotion discrimination in borderline personality disorder. *Psychol Med, 39*(5), 855–864.

Ebner-Priemer, U. W., Badeck, S., Beckmann, C., Wagner, A., Feige, B., Weiss, I., Lieb, K., & Bohus, M. (2005). Affective dysregulation and dissociative experience in female patients with borderline personality disorder: a startle response study. *J Psychiatr Res, 39*(1), 85–92.

Ebner-Priemer, U. W., Kuo, J., Schlotz, W., Kleindienst, N., Rosenthal, M. Z., Detterer, L., Linehan, M. M., & Bohus, M. (2008). Distress and affective dysregulation in patients with borderline personality disorder: a psychophysiological ambulatory monitoring study. *J Nerv Ment Dis*, *196*(4), 314–320.

Ebner-Priemer, U. W., Welch, S. S., Grossman, P., Reisch, T., Linehan, M. M., & Bohus, M. (2007). Psychophysiological ambulatory assessment of affective dysregulation in borderline personality disorder. *Psychiatry Res*, *150*(3), 265–275.

Fan, Y., Wonneberger, C., Enzi, B., de Greck, M,. Ulrich, C., Tempelmann, C., Bogerts, B., Doering, S., & Northoff, G. (2011). The narcissistic self and its psychological and neural correlates: an exploratory fMRI study. *Psychol Med*, *41*(8), 1641–1650.

Favazza, A. R., & Conterio, K. (1989). Female habitual self-mutilators. *Acta Psychiatr Scand*, *79*(3), 283–289.

Feinstein, J. S., Goldin, P. R., Stein, M. B., Brown, G. G., & Paulus, M. P. (2002). Habituation Habituation of attentional networks during emotion processing. *Neuroreport*, *13*(10), 1255–1258.

Fischer, H., Wright, C. I., Whalen, P. J., McInerney, S. C., Shin, L. M., & Rauch, S. L. (2003). Brain habituation during repeated exposure to fearful and neutral faces: a functional MRI study. *Brain Res Bull*, *59*(5), 387–392.

Gross, J. J. (1998). Antecedent- and response-focused emotion regulation: divergent consequences for experience, expression, and physiology. *J Pers Soc Psychol*, *74*(1), 224–237.

Gross, J. J. (2002). Emotion regulation: affective, cognitive, and social consequences. *Psychophysiology*, *39*(3), 281–291.

Gross, J. J. (2014). Emotion regulation: Conceptual and empirical foundations. In *Handbook of emotion regulation*. J. J. Gross. New York: Guilford Press: 3–22.

Gross, J. J., & John, O. P. (2003). Individual differences in two emotion regulation processes: implications for affect, relationships, and well-being. *J Pers Soc Psychol*, *85*(2), 348–362.

Hagenhoff, M., Franzen, N., Gerstner, L., Koppe, G., Sammer, G., Netter, P., Gallhofer, B., & Lis, S. (2013). Reduced sensitivity to emotional facial expressions in borderline personality disorder: effects of emotional valence and intensity. *J Personal Disord*, *27*(1), 19–35.

Haines, J., Williams, C. L., Brain, K. L., & Wilson, G. V. (1995). The psychophysiology of self-mutilation. *J Abnorm Psychology*, *104*(3), 471–489.

Hansen, C. H., & Hansen, R. D. (1988). Finding the face in the crowd: an anger superiority effect. *J Pers Soc Psychol*, *54*(6), 917–924.

Harned, M. S., Korslund, K. E., & Linehan, M. M. (2014). A pilot randomized controlled trial of dialectical behavior therapy with and without the dialectical behavior therapy prolonged exposure protocol for suicidal and self-injuring women with borderline personality disorder and PTSD. *Behav Res Ther*, *55*, 7–17.

Hazlett, E. A., Zhang, J., New, A. S., Zelmanova, Y., Goldstein, K. E., Haznedar, M. M., Meyerson, D., Goodman, M., Siever, L. J., & Chu, K. W. (2012). Potentiated amygdala response to repeated emotional pictures in borderline personality disorder. *Biol Psychiatry*, *72*(6), 448–456.

Heinrichs, N., & Hofmann, S. G. (2001). Information processing in social phobia: a critical review. *Clin Psychol Rev*, *21*(5), 751–770.

Henry, J. D., Green, M. J., Restuccia, C., de Lucia, A., Rendell, P. G., McDonald, S., & Grisham, J. R. (2009). Emotion dysregulation and schizotypy. *Psychiatry Res*, *166*(2–3), 116–124.

Hepp, J., Hilbig, B., Kieslich, P., Herzog, J., Lis, S., Schmahl, C., & Niedtfeld, I. (2016). Borderline Personality and the Detection of Angry Faces". *PLoS ONE*, *11*(3),e0152947.

Herpertz, S. C., Werth, U., Lukas, G., Qunaibi, M., Schuerkens, A., Kunert, H. J., Freese, R., Flesch, M., Mueller-Isberner, R., Osterheider, M., & Sass, H. (2001). Emotion in criminal offenders with psychopathy and borderline personality disorder. *Arch Gen Psychiatry, 58*(8), 737–745.

Hiatt, K. D., Schmitt, W. A., & Newman, J. P. (2004). Stroop tasks reveal abnormal selective attention among psychopathic offenders." *Neuropsychology, 18*(1), 50–59.

Holtmann, J., Herbort, M. C., Wustenberg, T., Soch, J., Richter, S., Walter, H., Roepke, S., & Schott, B. H. (2013). Trait anxiety modulates fronto-limbic processing of emotional interference in borderline personality disorder. *Front Hum Neurosci, 7*, 54.

Huang, J., Wang, Y., Jin, Z., Di, X., Yang, T., Gur, R. C., Gur, R. E., Shum, D. H., Cheung, E. F., & Chan, R. C. (2013). Happy facial expression processing with different social interaction cues: an fMRI study of individuals with schizotypal personality traits. *Prog Neuropsychopharmacol Biol Psychiatry, 44*, 108–117.

In-Albon, T., Burli, M., Ruf, C., & Schmid, M. (2013). Non-suicidal self-injury and emotion regulation: a review on facial emotion recognition and facial mimicry. *Child Adolesc Psychiatry Ment Health, 7*(1), 5.

Iverson, K. M., Follette, V. M., Pistorello, J., & Fruzzetti, A. E. (2012). An investigation of experiential avoidance, emotion dysregulation, and distress tolerance in young adult outpatients with borderline personality disorder symptoms. *Personal Disord, 3*(4), 415–422.

Jacob, G. A., Gutz, L., Bader, K., Lieb, K., Tuscher, O., & Stahl, C. (2010). Impulsivity in borderline personality disorder: impairment in self-report measures, but not behavioral inhibition. *Psychopathology, 43*(3), 180–188.

Jacob, G. A., Ower, N., & Buchholz, A. (2013). The role of experiential avoidance, psychopathology, and borderline personality features in experiencing positive emotions: a path analysis. *J Behav Ther Exp Psychiatry, 44*(1), 61–68.

Japee, S., Crocker, L., Carver, F., Pessoa, L., & Ungerleider, L. G. (2009). Individual differences in valence modulation of face-selective M170 response. *Emotion, 9*(1), 59–69.

John, O. P., & Gross, J. J. (2004). Healthy and unhealthy emotion regulation: personality processes, individual differences, and life span development. *J Pers, 72*(6), 1301–1333.

Jovev, M., Chanen, A., Green, M., Cotton, S., Proffitt, T., Coltheart, M., & Jackson, H. (2011). Emotional sensitivity in youth with borderline personality pathology. *Psychiatry Res, 187*(1-2), 234–240.

Kleindienst, N., Bohus, M., Ludascher, P., Limberger, M. F., Kuenkele, K., Ebner-Priemer, U. W., Chapman, A. L., Reicherzer, M., Stieglitz, R. D., & Schmahl, C. (2008). Motives for nonsuicidal self-injury among women with borderline personality disorder. *J Nerv Ment Dis, 196*(3), 230–236.

Klonsky, E. D. (2007). The functions of deliberate self-injury: a review of the evidence. *Clin Psychol Rev, 27*(2), 226–239.

Koenigsberg, H. W., Denny, B. T., Fan, J., Liu, X., Guerreri, S., Mayson, S. J., Rimsky, L., New, A. S., Goodman, M., & Siever L. J., (2014). The neural correlates of anomalous habituation to negative emotional pictures in borderline and avoidant personality disorder patients. *Am J Psychiatry, 171*(1), 82–90.

Koenigsberg, H. W., Fan, J., Ochsner, K. N., Liu, X., Guise, K. G., Pizzarello, S., Dorantes, C., Guerreri, S., Tecuta, L., Goodman, M., New, A., & Siever, L. J. (2009). Neural correlates of the use of psychological distancing to regulate responses to negative social cues: a study of patients with borderline personality disorder. *Biol Psychiatry, 66*(9), 854–863.

Koster, E. H., Fox, E., & MacLeod, C. (2009). Introduction to the special section on cognitive bias modification in emotional disorders. *J Abnorm Psychol, 118*(1), 1–4.

Krause-Utz, A., Elzinga, B. M., Oei, N. Y., Spinhoven, P., Bohus, M., & Schmahl, C. (2014). Susceptibility to distraction by social cues in borderline personality disorder. *Psychopathology, 47*(3), 148–157.

Krause-Utz, A., Oei, N. Y., Niedtfeld, I., Bohus, M., Spinhoven, P., Schmahl, C., & Elzinga, B. M. (2012). Influence of emotional distraction on working memory performance in borderline personality disorder. *Psychol Med, 42*(10), 2181–2192.

Kross, E., & Ayduk, O. (2008). Facilitating adaptive emotional analysis: distinguishing distanced-analysis of depressive experiences from immersed-analysis and distraction. *Pers Soc Psychol Bull, 34*(7), 924–938.

Lanius, R. A., Vermetten, E., Loewenstein, R. J., Brand, B., Schmahl, C., Bremner, J. D., & Spiegel, D. (2010). Emotion modulation in PTSD: Clinical and neurobiological evidence for a dissociative subtype. *Am J Psychiatry, 167*(6), 640–647.

Lewis, M., Haviland-Jones, J. M., & Barrett, L. E. (2008). *Handbook of emotions.* New York: Guilford Press.

Limberg, A., Barnow, S., Freyberger, H. J., & Hamm, A. O. (2011). Emotional vulnerability in borderline personality disorder is cue specific and modulated by traumatization. *Biol Psychiatry, 69*(6), 574–582.

Linehan, M. M. (1993). Dialectical behavior therapy for treatment of borderline personality disorder: implications for the treatment of substance abuse. [Review]. NIDA Res Monogr, *137*, 201–216.

Lobbestael, J., & Arntz, A. (2010). Emotional, cognitive and physiological correlates of abuse-related stress in borderline and antisocial personality disorder. *Behav Res Ther, 48*(2), 116–124.

Lobbestael, J., Arntz, A., Cima, M., & Chakhssi, F. (2009). Effects of induced anger in patients with antisocial personality disorder. *Psychol Med, 39*(4), 557–568.

Lynch, T. R., Rosenthal, M. Z., Kosson, D. S., Cheavens, J. S., Lejuez, C. W., & Blair, R. J. (2006). Heightened sensitivity to facial expressions of emotion in borderline personality disorder. *Emotion, 6*(4), 647–655.

Machado-de-Sousa, J. P., Arrais, K. C., Alves, N. T., Chagas, M. H., de Meneses-Gaya, C., Crippa, J. A., & Hallak, J. E. (2010). Facial affect processing in social anxiety: tasks and stimuli. *J Neurosci Methods, 193*(1), 1–6.

Marissen, M. A., Deen, M. L., & Franken, I. H. (2012). Disturbed emotion recognition in patients with narcissistic personality disorder. *Psychiatry Res, 198*(2), 269–273.

Marsh, A. A., & Blair, R. J. (2008). Deficits in facial affect recognition among antisocial populations: a meta-analysis. *Neurosci Biobehav Rev, 32*(3), 454–465.

Matzke, B., Herpertz, S. C., Berger, C., Fleischer, M., & Domes, G. (2014). Facial reactions during emotion recognition in borderline personality disorder: a facial electromyography study. *Psychopathology, 47*(2), 101–110.

McKenzie, K. C., & Gross, J. J. (2014). Nonsuicidal self-injury: an emotion regulation perspective. *Psychopathology, 47*(4), 207–219.

McRae, K., Ciesielski, B., & Gross, J. J. (2012). Unpacking cognitive reappraisal: goals, tactics, and outcomes. *Emotion, 12*(2), 250–255.

McRae, K., Hughes, B., Chopra, S., Gabrieli, J. D., Gross, J. J., & Ochsner, K. N. (2010). The neural bases of distraction and reappraisal. *J Cogn Neurosci, 22*(2), 248–262.

Menon, V., & Uddin, L. Q. (2010). Saliency, switching, attention and control: a network model of insula function. *Brain Struct Funct, 214*(5-6), 655–667.

Meyer-Lindenberg, A., Kohn, P. D., Kolachana, B., Kippenhan, S., McInerney-Leo, A., Nussbaum, R., Weinberger, D. R., & Berman, K. F. (2005). Midbrain dopamine and prefrontal function in humans: interaction and modulation by COMT genotype. *Nat Neurosci, 8*(5), 594–596.

Meyer, B., Pilkonis, P. A., & Beevers, C. G. (2004). What's in a (neutral) face? Personality disorders, attachment styles, and the appraisal of ambiguous social cues. *J Pers Disord*, 18(4), 320–336.

Mohanty, A., Heller, W., Koven, N. S., Fisher, J. E., Herrington, J. D., & Miller, G. A. (2008). Specificity of emotion-related effects on attentional processing in schizotypy. *Schizophr Res*, 103(1-3), 129–137.

Mohanty, A., Herrington, J. D., Koven, N. S., Fisher, J. E., Wenzel, E. A., Webb, A. G., Heller, W. Banich, M. T., & Miller, G. A. (2005). Neural mechanisms of affective interference in schizotypy. *J Abnorm Psychol*, 114(1), 16–27.

Neacsiu, A. D., Eberle, J. W., Kramer, R., Wiesmann, T., & Linehan, M. M. (2014). Dialectical behavior therapy skills for transdiagnostic emotion dysregulation: a pilot randomized controlled trial. *Behav Res Ther*, 59, 40–51.

Neacsiu, A. D., Lungu, A., Harned, M. S., Rizvi, S. L., & Linehan, M. M. (2014). Impact of dialectical behavior therapy versus community treatment by experts on emotional experience, expression, and acceptance in borderline personality disorder. *Behav Res Ther*, 53, 47–54.

Neacsiu, A. D., Rizvi, S. L., & Linehan, M. M. (2010). Dialectical behavior therapy skills use as a mediator and outcome of treatment for borderline personality disorder." *Behav Res Ther*, 48(9), 832–839.

New, A. S., Aan Het Rot, M., Ripoll, L. H., Perez-Rodriguez, M. M., Lazarus, S., Zipursky, E. Weinstein, S. R., Koenigsberg, H. W., Hazlett, E. A., Goodman, M., & Siever, L. J. (2012). Empathy and alexithymia in borderline personality disorder: clinical and laboratory measures. *J Pers Disord*, 26(5), 660–675.

Niedtfeld, I., Kirsch, P., Schulze, L., Herpertz, S. C., Bohus, M., & Schmahl, C. (2012). Functional connectivity of pain-mediated affect regulation in borderline personality disorder. *PLoS One*, 7(3), e33293.

Niedtfeld, I., Schulze, L., Kirsch, P., Herpertz, S. C., Bohus, M., & Schmahl, C. (2010). Affect regulation and pain in borderline personality disorder: a possible link to the understanding of self-injury. *Biol Psychiatry*, 68(4), 383–391.

Niedtfeld, I., Winter, D., Schmitt, R., Bohus, M., Schmahl, C., & Herpertz, S. C. (2017). Pain-mediated affect regulation is reduced after dialectical behavior therapy in borderline personality disorder: a longitudinal fMRI study. *Soc Cogn Affect Neurosci*, 12(5), 739–747.

Nock, M. K., & Prinstein, M. J. (2004). A functional approach to the assessment of self-mutilative behavior. *J Consult Clin Psychol*, 72(5), 885–890.

Ochsner, K. N., & Gross, J. J. (2005). The cognitive control of emotion. *Trends Cogn Sci*, 9(5), 242–249.

Ochsner, K. N., & Gross, J. J. (2014). The neural bases of emotion and emotion regulation: a valuation perspective. In J. J. Gross (Ed.), *Handbook of emotion regulation* (pp. 23–42). New York: Guilford Press.

Ochsner, K. N., Knierim, K., Ludlow, D. H., Hanelin, J., Ramachandran, T., Glover, G., & Mackey, S. C. (2004). Reflecting upon feelings: an fMRI study of neural systems supporting the attribution of emotion to self and other. *J Cogn Neurosci*, 16(10), 1746–1772.

Ochsner K. N., Silvers, J. A., & Buhle, J. T. (2012). Functional imaging studies of emotion regulation: a synthetic review and evolving model of the cognitive control of emotion. *Ann N Y Acad Sci*, 1251, E1–24.

Paris, J. (2005). Understanding self-mutilation in borderline personality disorder. *Harvard Rev Psychiatry*, 13(3), 179–185.

Pessoa, L., McKenna, M., Gutierrez, E., & Ungerleider, L. G. (2002). Neural processing of emotional faces requires attention. *Proc Natl Acad Sci U S A*, 99(17), 11458–11463.

Pfabigan, D. M., Alexopoulos, J., & Sailer, U. (2012). Exploring the effects of antiso-cial personality traits on brain potentials during face processing. *PLoS One*, 7(11), e50283.

Phan, K. L., Liberzon, I., Welsh, R. C., Britton, J. C., & Taylor, S. F. (2003). Habituation of rostral anterior cingulate cortex to repeated emotionally salient pictures. *Neuropsychopharmacology*, 28(7), 1344–1350.

Phelps, E. A., Delgado, M. R., Nearing, K. I., & LeDoux, J. E. (2004). Extinction learning in humans: role of the amygdala and vmPFC. *Neuron*, 43(6), 897–905.

Prehn, K., Schulze, L., Rossmann, S., Berger, C., Vohs, K., Fleischer, M., Hauenstein, K., Keiper, P., Domes, G., & Herpertz, S. C. (2013). Effects of emotional stimuli on working memory processes in male criminal offenders with borderline and antisocial personality disorder. *World J Biol Psychiatry*, 14(1), 71–78.

Raymond, J. E., Fenske, M. J., & Tavassoli, N. T. (2003). Selective attention determines emo-tional responses to novel visual stimuli. *Psychol Sci*, 14(6), 537–542.

Reas, D. L., Ro, O., Karterud, S., Hummelen, B., & Pedersen, G. (2013). Eating disorders in a large clinical sample of men and women with personality disorders. *Int J Eat Disord*, 46(8), 801–809.

Reitz, S., Kluetsch, R., Niedtfeld, I., Knorz, T., Lis, S., Paret, C., Kirsch, P., Meyer-Lindenberg, A., Treede, R. D., Baumgaertner, U., Bohus, M., & Schmahl, C. (2015). Incision and stress regulation in borderline personality disorder: neurobiological mechanisms of self-injurious behavior. *Br J Psychiatry*, 207(2), 165–172.

Reitz, S., Krause-Utz, A., Pogatzki-Zahn, E. M., Ebner-Priemer, U., Bohus, M., & Schmahl, C. (2012). Stress regulation and incision in borderline personality disorder--a pilot study modeling cutting behavior. *J Pers Disord*, 26(4), 605–615.

Ritter, K., Dziobek, I., Preissler, S. Ruter, A., Vater, A., Fydrich, T., Lammers, C. H., Heekeren, H. R., & Roepke, S. (2011). Lack of empathy in patients with narcissistic personality dis-order. *Psychiatry Res*, 187(1-2), 241–247.

Robin, M., Pham-Scottez, A., Curt, F., Dugre-Le Bigre, C., Speranza, M., Sapinho, D., Corcos, M., Berthoz, S., & Kedia, G. (2012). Decreased sensitivity to facial emotions in adolescents with borderline personality disorder. *Psychiatry Res*, 200(2-3), 417–421.

Rosenthal, M. Z., Kim, K., Herr, N. R., Smoski, M. J., Cheavens, J. S., Lynch, T. R., & Kosson, D. S. (2011). Speed and accuracy of facial expression classification in avoidant person-ality disorder: a preliminary study. *Personal Disord*, 2(4), 327–334.

Rozin, P., & Royzman, E. B. (2001). Negativity bias, negativity dominance, and contagion. *Person Social Psychol Rev*, 5(4), 296–320.

Sadeh, N., Londahl-Shaller, E. A., Piatigorsky, A., Fordwood, S., Stuart, B. K., McNiel, D. E., Klonsky, E. D., Ozer, E. M., & Yaeger, A. M. (2014). Functions of non-suicidal self-injury in adolescents and young adults with borderline personality disorder symptoms. *Psychiatry Res*, 216(2), 217–222.

Sadeh, N., Spielberg, J. M., Heller, W., Herrington, J. D., Engels, A. S., Warren, S. L., Crocker, L. D., Sutton, B. P., & Miller, G. A. (2013). Emotion disrupts neural activity during selec-tive attention in psychopathy. *Soc Cogn Affect Neurosci*, 8(3), 235–246.

Sansone, R. A., Lam, C., & Wiederman, M. W. (2010). Self-harm behaviors in borderline personality: an analysis by gender. *J Nerv Ment Dis*, 198(12), 914–915.

Sansone, R. A., & Sansone, L. A. (2013). The relationship between borderline personality and obesity. *Innov Clin Neurosci*, 10, 36–40.

Schiffer, B., Pawliczek, C., Mu Ller, B., Forsting, M., Gizewski, E., Leygraf, N., & Hodgins, S. (2014). Neural mechanisms underlying cognitive control of men with lifelong antisocial behavior. *Psychiatry Res*, 222(1-2), 43–51.

Schmahl, C., Bohus, M., Esposito, F., Treede, R. D., Di Salle, F., Greffrath, W., Ludaescher, P., Jochims, A., Lieb, K., Scheffler, K., Hennig, J., & Seifritz, E. (2006). Neural correlates of antinociception in borderline personality disorder. *Arch Gen Psychiatry, 63*(6), 659–667.

Schmitt, R., Winter, D., Niedtfeld, I., Herpertz, S. C., & Schmahl, C. (2016). Effects of of psychotherapy on neuronal correlates of reappraisal in female patients with borderline personality disorder. *Biological Psychiatry: Cognitive Neuroscience and Neuroimaging, 1*, 548–557.

Schonenberg, M., Louis, K., Mayer, S., & Jusyte, A. (2013). Impaired identification of threat-related social information in male delinquents with antisocial personality disorder. *J Pers Disord, 27*(4), 496–505.

Schramm, A. T., Venta, A., & Sharp, C. (2013) The role of experiential avoidance in the association between borderline features and emotion regulation in adolescents, *Personal Disord Theory Res Treat, 4*, 138–144.

Schulze, L., Domes, G., Kruger, A., Berger, C., Fleischer, M., Prehn, K., Schmahl, C., Grossmann, A., Hauenstein, K., & Herpertz, S. C. (2011). Neuronal correlates of cognitive reappraisal in borderline patients with affective instability. *Biol Psychiatry, 69*(6), 564–573.

Seeley, W. W., Menon, V., Schatzberg, A. F., Keller, J., Glover, G. H., Kenna, H., Reiss, A. L., & Greicius, M. D. (2007). Dissociable intrinsic connectivity networks for salience processing and executive control. *J Neurosci, 27*(9), 2349–2356.

Sieswerda, S., Arntz, A., Mertens, I., & Vertommen, S. (2007). Hypervigilance in patients with borderline personality disorder: specificity, automaticity, and predictors. *Behav Res Ther, 45*(5), 1011–1024.

Staebler, K., Renneberg, B., Stopsack, M., Fiedler, P., Weiler, M., & Roepke, S. (2011). Facial emotional expression in reaction to social exclusion in borderline personality disorder. *Psychol Med*, 1–10.

Stiglmayr, C. E., Grathwol, T., Linehan, M. M., Ihorst, G., Fahrenberg, J., & Bohus, M. (2005). Aversive tension in patients with borderline personality disorder: a computer-based controlled field study. *Acta Psychiatr Scand, 111*(5), 372–379.

Stiglmayr, C. E., Shapiro, D. A., Stieglitz, R. D., Limberger, M. F., & Bohus, M. (2001). Experience of aversive tension and dissociation in female patients with borderline personality disorder—a controlled study. *J Psychiatr Res, 35*(2), 111–118.

Surcinelli, P., Codispoti, M., Montebarocci, O., Rossi, N., & Baldaro, B. (2006). Facial emotion recognition in trait anxiety. *J Anxiety Disord, 20*(1), 110–117.

Valet, M., Sprenger, T., Boecker, H., Willoch, F., Rummeny, E., Conrad, B., Erhard, P., & Tolle, T. R. (2004). Distraction modulates connectivity of the cingulo-frontal cortex and the midbrain during pain--an fMRI analysis. *Pain, 109*(3), 399–408.

Van Strien, J. W., & Van Kampen, D. (2009). Positive schizotypy scores correlate with left visual field interference for negatively valenced emotional words: A lateralized emotional Stroop study. *Psychiatry Res, 169*(3), 229–234.

Veague, H. B., & Hooley, J. M. (2014). Enhanced sensitivity and response bias for male anger in women with borderline personality disorder. *Psychiatry Res, 215*(3), 687–693.

Vitale, J. E., Brinkley, C. A., Hiatt, K. D., & Newman, J. P. (2007). Abnormal selective attention in psychopathic female offenders. *Neuropsychology, 21*(3), 301–312.

Vitale, J. E., Newman, J. P., Bates, J. E., Goodnight, J., Dodge, K. A., & Pettit, G. S. (2005). Deficient behavioral inhibition and anomalous selective attention in a community sample of adolescents with psychopathic traits and low-anxiety traits. *J Abnorm Child Psychol, 33*(4), 461–470.

Volter, C., Strobach, T., Aichert, D. S., Wostmann, N., Costa, A., Moller, H. J., Schubert, T., & Ettinger, U. (2012). Schizotypy and behavioural adjustment and the role of neuroticism. *PLoS One*, *7*(2), e30078.

Vuilleumier, P., Armony, J., Driver, J., & Dolan, R. (2001). Effects of attention and emotion on face processing in the human brain: an event-related fMRI study. *Neuron*, *30*, 829–841.

Wingenfeld, K., Mensebach, C., Rullkoetter, N., Schlosser, N., Schaffrath, C., Woermann, F. G., Driessen, M., & Beblo, T. (2009). Attentional Bias to Personally Relevant Words in Borderline Personality Disorder is strongly Related to Comorbid Posttraumatic Stress Disorder. *J Personal Disord*, *23*(2), 141–155.

Winter, D., Elzinga, B., & Schmahl, C. (2014). Emotions and memory in borderline personality disorder. *Psychopathology*, *47*(2), 71–85.

Winter, D., Krause-Utz, A., Lis, S., Chiu, C. D., Lanius, R. A., Schriner, F., Bohus M., & Schmahl, C. (2015). Dissociation in borderline personality disorder: disturbed cognitive and emotional inhibition and its neural correlates. *Psychiatry Res*, *233*(3), 339–351.

Wright, C. I., Fischer, H., Whalen, P. J., McInerney, S. C., Shin, L. M., & Rauch, S. L. (2001). Differential prefrontal cortex and amygdala habituation to repeatedly presented emotional stimuli. *Neuroreport*, *12*(2), 379–383.

8 The Clinical Neuroscience of Impulsive Aggression

■ ROYCE LEE, JENNIFER R. FANNING,
AND EMIL F. COCCARO

■ INTRODUCTION

Aggressive behavior is usually adaptive, and so it preserves, and leaves a biological footprint. When this genetically encoded but epigenetically regulated trait is predominantly maladaptive and causes suffering, it is pathological. These two facts have respectively enabled and motivated a translational neuroscience of aggressive behavior in humans. Aggression can be categorized into three subtypes. Premeditated aggression is a behavior calculated to provide at least temporary advantage to the individual. Its pathological and extreme form is studied in the context of psychopathic and antisocial behavior. Nonpathological examples of this include socially sanctioned forms of aggression, as is encountered in military and sports-related contexts. Pure frustration-related aggressive behavior is generally sporadic and motivated by primary rewards and punishments. It is encountered in developmental disorders such as autism, neuropsychiatric conditions such as dementia, and medical conditions such as delirium and encephalopathy. Impulsive aggression, which is the focus of this chapter, is generally a trait-like pattern of behavior. It has little adaptive value to the individual and more often than not leads to severely deleterious effects on social function. It is generally impulsive, characterized by intense affect, and triggered by social stimuli. It, too, has a close relationship with frustration.

In the *Diagnostic and Statistical Manual of Mental Disorders* (fifth edition [DSM-5]), impulsive aggression, when it occurs in a persistent pattern of dysfunctional behavior, is codified as intermittent explosive disorder (IED). *DSM-5* IED requires the presence of either frequent (no less than twice weekly for at least three months), though low-intensity, aggressive outbursts or infrequent (at least three times a year) but high-intensity aggressive outbursts. In both cases, the outbursts are out of proportion to the circumstances, impulsive/angry in nature, without obvious gain, and associated with significant distress and/or impairment. While several other psychiatric disorders may be seen in individuals with IED, the diagnosis of IED can be made in the presence of other disorders if aggressive outbursts also occur in the absence of these disorders. IED has a 3.9% annual prevalence (Kessler et al., 2006) An estimated 7.3% of adults (Kessler et al., 2006) and 7.8% of adolescents develop IED (McLaughlin et al., 2012).

IED is a categorical description of maladaptive impulsive aggression. The dimensional perspective on impulsive aggression is arguably more compatible with biological findings. The proposed National Institute of Mental Health Research Domain Criteria (RDoC) description of impulsive aggression is frustrative non-reward, a negatively valenced but positively motivated state with a specific neural circuit topology. Other neural circuits and RDoC are relevant to impulsive aggression, such as those associated with fear conditioning and understanding the mental states of others.

The approach taken in this chapter to clinical neuroscience of impulsive aggression is based on a model of social cognition, social information processing. This is related to brain correlates of impulsive aggression, according to a view of the brain as a predictive encoding engine.

▪ THE SOCIAL INFORMATION PROCESSING MODEL OF IMPULSIVE AGGRESSION

In the clinic, it becomes clear that most episodes of impulsive aggression are triggered by social provocation. Social conflict evokes strong emotional reactions, such as anger, shame, disgust, or fear. In the laboratory, these processes have been studied scientifically under the conceptual framework of social-emotional information processing (SEIP; Dodge & Price, 1994; Crick & Dodge, 1994; Dodge, 1993). The SEIP model has heuristic, descriptive, and explanatory applications. It describes six stages leading to the commission of the aggressive or nonaggressive response (Crick & Dodge, 1996; Fontaine, Burks, & Dodge, 2002): (1) social information encoding, (2) attribution of the intent of the behavior of the other participant in the social interaction, (3) clarification of goals, (4) response generation, (5) response evaluation, and (6) response enactment. Research in children and adolescents confirms that impulsive-aggressive children and adolescents, particularly those with a history of abuse, demonstrate a reduction in the mental encoding of socially relevant information *and* the presence of a hostile attribution bias (Dodge & Price, 1994; Crick & Dodge, 1996). A series of empirical studies has shown that adults with IED have reduced encoding of social cues (Coccaro, Noblett, & McCloskey, 2009), heightened hostile attribution, intensified negative emotional response (Coccaro, Fanning, & Lee, 2016), and a bias to choose directly, or relationally, aggressive responses to socially ambiguous cues. Simultaneous analysis of each of these SEIP steps reveals the critical importance of negative emotional response to socially ambiguous cues as well as the bias to choose aggressive responses to such cues.

Because SEIP theory is based on a biopsychosocial framework, each stage can be related to brain-based processes relevant to the understanding of impulsive aggression. In the next sections of this chapter, we describe the neurobiological correlates of relevant SEIP stages and relate them to findings in impulsive-aggressive patients. Toward this end, we propose that impulsive aggression is related to dysfunction in three circuits. These three circuits contribute in varying degrees to encoding (stage 1), attribution (stage 2), and response selection (stages 3–6). The psychological processes described in SEIP theory is translated into a predictive encoding model of brain function.

▪ THE THREE-CIRCUIT MODEL

The dominant contemporary theoretical account of human brain function is the predictive encoding model (Friston, Stephan, Montague, & Dolan, 2014). Rather than viewing the brain as an information filter, which can result in conceptual cul-de-sacs such as the homunculus fallacy, the predictive coding model views brain circuits as "inference generators" that are updated through the process of temporal difference learning. This process is related to Bayesian inference, whereby statistical inferences are made based on the prior probability of a prediction being true. Brain circuits will by default generate fantasies in the form of statistical models, which are refined in iterative fashion with updates of sensory, proprioceptive, or cognitive data. Generating the statistical models are neural networks, formed through unsupervised, temporal difference learning.

For impulsive-aggressive behavior, evidence points to dysfunction in three brain circuits: (a) ventral prefrontal-amygdala circuits involved in fear learning, (b) fronto-striatal circuits involved in reinforcement learning and cognitive control, and (c) fronto-parietal circuits involved in embodied and social cognition.

Ventral Prefrontal-Amygdala Circuits and Fear Learning

The first major psychological theory of emotions by William James and Carl Lange (Cannon, 1987) hypothesized that emotional awareness is interoceptive awareness. A predictive coding model posits something very similar: summed interoceptive inputs create a statistical model of the internal state of an organism. For example, self-perceived increases in heart rate, breathing rate, muscle tension, and perspiration can create a model of the internal motivational state of fear. When considering stimuli outside of the self, the bottom-up awareness of a visceral response to emotionally relevant stimuli, for example of a feared object like a snake, will result in a top-down inference that the object is to be feared because it induces a fearful state. But beyond the subjective experience, from a computational perspective, states of fear are related to associative conditioning and/or aversive temporal difference learning. Associative conditioning refers to the Pavlovian process by which a conditioned stimulus (CS) is associated with an unconditioned stimulus (US). When it is aversive, it is known as aversive conditioning. Aversive conditioning is mediated by long-term potentiation in the basolateral amygdala between inputs representing the CS and US. The basolateral amygdala has outputs to the central nucleus of the amygdala, which sends the excitatory connections to the hypothalamus that characterize the fear response. Fear extinction, a form of inhibitory learning, is mediated by the hippocampus and ventromedial prefrontal cortex. Beyond associative conditioning, the amygdala also plays a role in temporally dependent learning. In aversive temporal difference learning, neural activity related to aversive stimuli predicts future outcomes based on past outcomes. Recent research has confirmed that neural activity in the amygdala and connected structures is predictive of aversive outcome: increasing with worse-than-expected outcomes and decreasing with better-than-expected outcomes (Cole & McNally, 2009; McHugh et al., 2014).

A critically important modulator of amygdala activity and emotional behavior is the orbitofrontal cortex (OFC). The OFC is extensively interconnected with the amygdala (Ongür & Price, 2000) via a thick, white matter bundle, the uncinate fasciculus. The analogous region in rodents, the ventromedial prefrontal cortex, suppresses fear-related amygdala activity via connections to the basomedial amygdala. This is the basis of lasting fear extinction (Adhikari et al., 2015). The medial OFC receives extensive sensory input, enabling its delay activity to represent complex object reward associations, even when reward associations change or reverse over time (Elliott et al., 2000). To do this, the OFC is reliant on its connectivity with the amygdala (Ongür & Price, 2000). OFC-amygdala connectivity is the neural circuit basis of reversal learning. Reversal learning is a form of temporal difference learning whereby stimulus associations change in valence over time. It is generally adaptive and promotes behavioral and cognitive flexibility. OFC-amygdala connectivity and its mediation of aversive learning correspond to *encoding* in the SEIP model of impulsive aggression.

Frontostriatal Circuits and Reinforcement

Polysynaptic neural loops connect the cortex to the striatum, subthalamic nucleus, globus pallidus, thalamus, and back to the cortex again. The neural circuits connecting the orbitofrontal and cingulate cortex to the striatum play an important role in action selection and reinforcement learning (Schönberg, Daw, Joel, & O'Doherty, 2007; Seo, Lee, & Averbeck, 2012).

Theoretical work in the area of Pavlovian conditioning resulted in a highly influential formal model of associative conditioning by Rescorla and Wagner (Rescorla, 1971). In this model, change in the associative strength of a conditioned stimulus is represented by $\Delta V^{n+1} = \alpha \times \beta\ (\lambda - V_{total})$; where α is the salience of the CS, β is the rate parameter, λ is the maximum conditioning value of the US, and V_{total} is the total associative strength of all CS. The Rescorla-Wagner model was later modified to account for trial-by-trial changes in associative strength, resulting in the temporal difference model. Temporal difference reinforcement learning describes an iterative decision making process that updates a value function of associative strength (V) for each trial (t) (Sutton, 1988), such that the predictive response on sequential trials ($V_{next\ trial}$) is: $V_{next\ trial} = V_{last\ trial} + \alpha\ (R_{current\ trial} - V_{last\ trial})$, given "associative strength," learning rate (α), and the error term ($R_{current\ trial} - V_{last\ trial}$).

One of the most valuable predictions of the Rescorla-Wagner and temporal difference learning models is regarding the role of brain dopamine signaling in computing error, or the difference between actual and expected reward. In the striatum (caudate, putamen) and connected structures (ventral tegmental area, nucleus accumbens, substantia nigra), phasic dopamine firing increases to unexpected rewards and silences to unexpected omissions of reward (Bayer & Glimcher, 2005; Saddoris, Cacciapaglia, & Wightman, 2015). The phasic drop in dopamine to error, or worse-than-expected outcomes, triggers a response in the anterior cingulate, which may further propagate a corrective signal to the premotor cortex (Cohen, Botvinick, & Carter, 2000). An important frontostriatal function is cognitive control, a working memory-based cognitive process that relies on the dorsolateral prefrontal cortex (DLPFC) to suppress prepotent but undesired responses. The DLPFC is a neural hub for circuits involved in decision-making, response inhibition, and attention (Gourley & Taylor, 2016). In the SEIP model, functions of the frontostriatal circuit would correspond to *response evaluation* and *selection*.

Frontoparietal Circuits and Social Cognition

Long-distance networks between the frontal and parietal lobes, connected by the superior longitudinal fasciculus, have long been recognized to be important in working memory, focused attention, and visual reorientation. These domain-general functions are thought to underlie a more specific role in cognitive empathy, or mentalizing. Cognitive empathy is the ability to take another person's perspective to make inferences about mental and emotional state (Decety & Lamm, 2007).

A recent meta-analysis of functional magnetic resonance imaging (fMRI) studies, including 3,150 subjects, confirmed the role of the frontoparietal network in cognitive empathy (Molenberghs, Johnson, Henry, & Mattingley, 2016). The network includes the medial prefrontal cortex, precunues, and temporo-parietal junction (TPJ). Neural activity in the TPJ appears to be necessary for this ability (Otti et al., 2015), and discrete TPJ lesions of it have been found to cause deficits in theory of mind while sparing most other cognitive abilities (Samson et al., 2004).

Another aspect of social cognition that is linked to posterior parietal function is motoric and affective imitation. When a person observes an action by another person, activations in the subject's premotor and sensorimotor cortex, nearly identical to that seen in self-movement, strongly suggest that we perceive and understand another person's action through vicarious brain activity. Vicarious activation of motor planning and proprioceptive circuits has been called "mirror neuron" activity and can be indexed by desynchronization of alpha and low beta frequency electrophysiological activity (mu suppression; Hoenen, Schain, & Pause, 2013). Motor imitation also involves error-related activity in the striatum and basal ganglia, as joint action requires fine-tuning of motor output to match what is perceived. For example, an ensemble of musicians must coordinate their motor activity despite a 200-ms delay between action initiation in the premotor cortex and action perception in the sensory motor cortex; the time delays would require a highly fine-tuned error-monitoring response from the basal ganglia and mirror neuron system (Keysers & Gazzola, 2014). In the SEIP model, the frontoparietal functions described would correspond to *attribution*. Attribution, through top-down processes, would also affect *encoding*.

The Special Case of Anger and Frustration

As an emotion, anger has long been recognized to have *both* aversive valence *and* approach-related motivational qualities (Carver & Harmon-Jones, 2009). Frustrative non-reward, whereby unexpected non-reward leads to increased drive, rather than passive learned helplessness, accounts for the approach-avoidance conflict that underlies anger and aggression. There is some evidence of a U-shaped curve, whereby moderate or brief frustration increases drive, while chronic or severe frustration decreases it (Pittman & Pittman, 1979). Interesting linkages have been found between positive incentive motivation and anger. Approach-based motivation (Drive/BAS) predicts increased attention to angry faces (Putman, Hermans, & van Honk, 2004) as well as increased brain activity in the amygdala and decreased activity in the ventral anterior cingulate and ventral striatum (Beaver, Lawrence, Passamonti, & Calder, 2008). Recently, the RDoC has proposed to classify problems of impulsive aggression in the frustrative non-reward subconstruct under negatively valenced emotion. Although not much recent work has formalized frustrative non-reward, an intriguing example comes from a computational study of motor learning. The authors adapted the Rescorla-Wagner learning rule to account for a biologically modelled frustration function (E_f) that modulates prediction error (P_e; Grzyb, Boedecker, Asada, Pobil, & Smith, 2011): $P_e(t + 1) = P_e(t) + (P_e(t) - A_o)*E_f$. Recognizing the dynamic nature of frustration, frustration (f) was modeled as a leaky integrator ($df/dt = -L * f + A_o$), accounting for current frustration (f), outcome of action (A_o), and a fixed leak rate (L). In this model, frustration levels can rise rapidly with an adverse outcome and fall rapidly with no adverse outcome. In the SEIP model, frustration would correspond to response selection but also encoding and attribution. These three aspects of SEIP in impulsive aggression are intercorrelated (Coccaro et al., 2016).

Impulsive Aggression and Ventral Prefrontal-Amygdala Circuits

The aversive quality of anger and findings that impulsive-aggressive individuals have a bias in interpreting social and emotional stimuli suggest a mechanistic role for associative conditioning and/or aversive temporal difference learning in impulsive aggression. Accordingly, destructive OFC lesions can result in highly dysfunctional, unrestrained anger and aggression (Grafman et al., 1996).

Research in normal subjects has found that experimentally evoked anger and anger-related stimuli increase metabolic activity in the medial OFC (Kimbrell et al., 1999; Northoff et al., 2000; Marsh, Dougherty, Moeller, Swann, & Spiga, 2002). Other research suggests that the OFC may regulate the outward expression of anger, as decreased metabolic activity of the OFC has been found when volunteers imagine unrestrained physical aggression (Pietrini, Guazzelli, Basso, Jaffe, & Grafman, 2000).

Structural brain imaging studies in IED have recently been conducted. Morphometric analysis of high resolution structural brain magnetic resonance images reveal that IED is associated with inward deformation of the superior and medial-anterior amygdala. Interestingly, these deformations may include the basomedial amygdala, previously identified to be the targets of modulation by the ventral prefrontal cortex (Adhikari et al., 2015) Additionally, IED is associated with inward deformation of the hippocampus head and inferior aspect of the hippocampus tail compared with healthy controls (Coccaro et al., 2015). Although the etiology of these shape differences are not known, they are generally consistent with structural neuroimaging work conducted in borderline personality disorder (BPD), also associated with dysregulated anger. BPD has been repeatedly found to be associated with smaller volumes of the amygdala (Schulze, Schmahl, & Niedtfeld, 2016) and hippocampus (Wenzel, Borges, Porto, Caminha, & de Oliveira, 2009). Thus, structural neuroimaging results indicate that the amygdala is deformed, if not reduced in overall volume, in impulsive-aggressive individuals. These results could suggest deficiencies in aversive conditioning in impulsive aggression.

In contrast, evidence to date suggests that, functionally, the amygdala is hyperreactive to emotional stimuli. Two studies have now shown that individuals with IED display greater amygdala response to exposure to angry faces relative to healthy controls. This finding is true for implicit (Coccaro et al., 2007) and explicit emotional processing (McCloskey et al., 2016). In both studies, life history of aggression measures correlate directly with amygdala response to the angry faces. In addition, both studies found reduced functional connectivity between the amygdala, and prefrontal regions are disrupted in IED compared with healthy controls. In McCloskey et al. (2016), the ventral medial prefrontal cortex showed positive coupling between the amygdala and ventral prefrontal cortex, rather than the expected inverse coupling that was seen in controls. In Coccaro et al. (2007), healthy control subjects showed inverse coupling between the medial OFC and amygdala that was diminished in IED subjects. The areas of the ventral prefrontal cortex failing to show expected inverse coupling during viewing of angry faces are associated with emotion regulation and fear extinction. The second study, using an explicit paradigm, also found evidence for sensitization of the amygdala to angry faces in IED subjects (McCloskey et al., 2016). Comparison of amygdala BOLD response in the first versus second half of stimuli presentations in IED subjects found that amygdala metabolic response increased, while no such difference was found in controls. This finding could be explained by deficient OFC-mediated extinction of amygdala response to angry faces in impulsive-aggressive individuals. Another possibility could be increased frustration with persistent exposure to "non-rewarding" or disapproving angry faces. Supporting this second interpretation, a positron emission tomography (PET) study of BPD-IED patients performing the Point Subtraction Paradigm (PSAP) found increased regional glucose metabolic rate in the amygdala *and* OFC when subjects were provoked, while controls did not show this pattern (New et al., 2009).

Impulsive Aggression and Frontostriatal Circuits

The error-related negativity (ERN) is a classic EEG/event-related potential (ERP) measure of performance monitoring that is elicited by errors. It is thought to originate from the anterior cingulate region of the brain. The ERN is triggered by a phasic decrease in dopamine with worse-than-expected outcomes. As such, it is a physical manifestation of the error term in temporal difference learning. Diminished ERN, reflecting deficient error detection by the striatum and anterior cingulate, has been found in association with externalizing psychopathology (Hall, Bernat, & Patrick, 2007) and in violent offenders (Vila-Ballo, Hdez-Lafuente, Rostan, Cunillera, & Rodriguez-Fornells, 2014). Diminished ERN is more closely related to impulsive antisocial behavior as opposed to fearless dominance, suggesting it may be more relevant to impulsive rather than premeditated aggression (Heritage & Benning, 2012). BPD has been associated with decreased feedback-related negativity, a stimulus-locked ERP, and to positive and negative outcomes (Endrass, Schuermann, Roepke, & Kessler-Scheil, 2016). Further work needs to be done to characterize performance monitoring in impulsive-aggressive subjects.

Given the proposed role of striatal dopamine activity in temporal difference learning and reward-related behavior, studies have been conducted examining striatal metabolism. Low dopamine transmission, as measured by 6-[18F]-fluoro L-DOPA PET imaging during a modified PSAP session has been found to be associated with aggressive responding after provocation (Schlüter et al., 2013). Another PET study, also conducted during the PSAP, showed that male patients with comorbid BPD-IED showed lower striatal glucose metabolism as measured by (18)-flouro-deoxyglucose (FDG) PET imaging (Mercedes Perez-Rodriguez et al., 2012). An fMRI study of the PSAP in aggressive children with attention deficit hyperactivity disorder and control children found that aggressive children failed to show normative activation of the anterior cingulate region during aggressive responding (Bubenzer-Busch et al., 2016). A separate study in normal subjects found a similar normative result: aggressive responding, this time during the Taylor Aggression Paradigm, was associated with anterior cingulate activation (Beyer, Münte, Göttlich, & Krämer, 2014). In summary, impulsive aggression is associated with diminished reactivity of the frontostriatal circuit. From the temporal-difference learning perspective, these results would be consistent with a diminished capacity to compute errors and thus a proneness to errors of commission. Further work would be needed to confirm if committing an inappropriate aggressive act would be an example of such an error.

Impulsive Aggression and Frontoparietal Circuits

The role of brain circuits involved in mentalizing is relatively understudied in impulsive aggression. Mentalizing has been conceptualized as a top-down, executive function. As such, it is likely vulnerable to disruption by bottom-up processes. Evidence for this comes from studies finding that emotional arousal appears to suppress it. Enhanced sensitivity to fear conditioning has been associated with relative deactivation of the mentalizing brain network (medial prefrontal, precuneus, TPJ) as measured by fMRI (Beyer, Münte, Erdmann, & Krämer, 2013).

Previous work in BPD, a disorder which also exhibits interpersonal dysfunction, has found evidence of reduced size of the parietal lobes, with decreased rightward symmetry and decreased volume (Irle, Lange, & Sachsse, 2005). Decreased resting metabolism of the parietal lobes, including the TPJ, as measured by FDG PET brain imaging, has also been found in BPD (Lange, Kracht, Herholz, Sachsse, & Irle, 2005). A diffusion tensor imaging study in a sample of IED, psychiatric controls and healthy controls revealed lower fractional anisotropy (FA) in IED subjects in two clusters located in the superior longitudinal fasciculus (SLF; Lee et al., 2016). Exploratory analyses found that BPD subjects also had lower FA in this region. The SLF is a long-range, white matter track connecting the frontal lobes to the posterior parietal lobes, as well as connecting the superior temporal and inferior parietal lobes. Disruption in these connections would be expected to affect brain circuits mediating social cognitive functions such as theory of mind and perspective-taking.

An fMRI study incorporating a social exclusion task and the Taylor Aggression Paradigm finds evidence for a role for predictive encoding in the mentalizing network. Exclusion was associated with activation of the mentalizing, mirror neuron network (superior and inferior temporal gyrus, precuneus, precentral gyrus). The effects of exclusion on aggressive responding were predicted by exclusion-related left inferior temporal and right precentral activation. The authors concluded that increased mentalization, as indexed by activation of the mirror neuron network during exclusion, could enhance aggressive responding (Beyer, Münte, & Krämer, 2014). These results would suggest that the mentalizing network could affect the motivation context of a social interaction, perhaps increasing the effect of frustration on the computation of an error, or thwarted expectation of cooperation.

■ NEUROMODULATORS AND NEUROTRANSMITTERS IN IMPULSIVE AGGRESSION

A large body of basic and clinical research has examined the role of neurotransmitters (glutamate, GABA) and neuromodulators (monoamines and neuropeptides) in impulsive aggression. A useful conceptual framework for understanding their role in predictive encoding of the brain was put forth by Doya (2002). It proposes that (a) dopamine signals the temporal difference error; (b) serotonin (5-HT) controls delay discounting; (c) norepinephrine controls surprise, or arousal; and (d) acetylcholine controls memory encoding, or learning rate.

Of the monoamine neuromodulators, serotonin is the most consistently linked to impulsive aggression and receives the bulk of attention in this section. Afterwards, we discuss noradrenergic findings in aggression. The small body of work concerning dopamine function has been covered in the discussion on frontostriatal function and aggression. Very little work has been done regarding cholinergic function and aggression, and so this will not be reviewed here.

5-HT and Impulsive Aggression

5-HT neurons in the prefrontal cortex arise from the rostral 5-HT system, whose cell bodies in the midbrain and rostral pons ascend to the forebrain (Piñeyro & Blier, 1999). In the prefrontal cortex, the majority of neurons, even non-serotonergic neurons, contain 5-HT receptors. 5-HT$_{1A}$ and 5-HT$_{2A}$ receptor mRNA is found in approximately 60% of prefrontal cortical cells, including pyramidal cell neurons. The two receptor subtypes are frequently colocalized (Amargós-Bosch et al., 2004); 5-HT$_{1A}$ receptors are predominantly inhibitory while 5-HT$_2$ receptors are mixed (Amargòs-Bosch et al., 2004). Together, the two can shape the transmission of neural information to the prefrontal cortex (Aghajanian & Marek, 1997; Jakab & Goldman-Rakic, 1998). Disruptions of 5-HT spare working memory and attention but lead to specific impairments in OFC-related functions such as preference for immediate versus time-delayed reinforcers, or delay discounting (Mobini, Chiang, Ho, Bradshaw, & Szabadi, 2000) and the closely related associative learning phenomena of reversal learning (Clarke et al., 2005; Clarke, Walker, Dalley, Robbins, & Roberts, 2007).

The first studies of the serotonin system in humans involved measurement of the 5-HT metabolite, 5-hydroxyinoleacetic acid (5-HIAA). 5-HIAA levels in the cerebrospinal fluid (CSF) were first related to suicidal behavior (Åsberg, 1997). Then studies began to explore the role of 5-HT in aggression and violence, finding that low 5-HIAA was associated with impulsive aggression (Brown, Goodwin, Ballenger, Goyer, & Major, 1979; Linnoila et al., 1983; Virkkunen, Nuutila, Goodwin, & Linnoila, 1987). To characterize the receptor pharmacology, serotonin receptors were probed in living humans using receptor-specific pharmacological probes. Using neuroendocrine response as a readout, these studies found that 5-HT$_{2A/C}$ receptor sensitivity, but not 5-HT$_{1A}$, is blunted in impulsive aggression (Coccaro, Kavoussi, Cooper, & Hauger, 1997; reviewed in Yanowitch & Coccaro, 2011). In a meta-analytic study, pooled results from 171 studies of the serotonin aggression relationship found a small ($r = -0.12$), but significant, inverse relationship overall between measures of 5-HT functioning and aggression, with pharmaco-challenge studies yielding the largest ($r = -0.21$) and CSF 5-HIAA concentrations yielding the smallest ($r = -0.06$) effect size (Duke, Bègue, Bell, & Eisenlohr-Moul, 2013).

In humans, depletion of the molecular precursor to serotonin, tryptophan, affects brain function in fronto-amygdala circuits. Tryptophan depletion enhances amygdala activation to fearful face stimuli in subjects (Cools et al., 2005), enhances recognition of fearful faces in healthy controls (Harmer, Rogers, Tunbridge, Cowen, & Goodwin, 2003), and causes more severe mood induction following a stressor (Richell, Deakin, & Anderson, 2005). Mixed results have been seen regarding the effects of serotonergic depletion on response inhibition, a subtype of impulsivity (Dougherty, Richard, James, & Mathias, 2010; Rubia et al., 2005). Instead, serotonergic depletion appears to affect another aspect of impulsivity: delay discounting, or consequence sensitivity (Dougherty et al., 2010). These alterations in emotion processing and behavioral inhibition explain how tryptophan depletion increases aggressive responding in simulated social provocations (Bond, Wingrove, & Critchlow, 2001; Cleare & Bond, 1995; Bjork, Dougherty, Moeller, & Swann, 2000; Marsh et al., 2002). We have found that individuals diagnosed with IED are particularly susceptible to the effects of trypto-phan depletion on mood and affective reactivity, with increased anger and perception of increased angry emotional intensity when viewing angry faces relative to controls (Lee, Gill, Chen, McCloskey, & Coccaro, 2012). Thus, serotonin affects limbic function by modulating connectivity between the prefrontal cortex and amygdala during asso-ciative learning, as has been confirmed in an fMRI study of the effects of tryptophan depletion on brain processing of angry faces (Passamonti et al., 2012).

5-HT Function in Ventral Prefrontal-Amygdala Circuits and Impulsive Aggression

Recent work using in vivo neuroimaging techniques have localized 5-HT dysfunc-tion to brain regions relevant to aggressive behavior, further validating the work using peripheral and CSF measures of 5-HT function. Because 5-HT is synthesized in the brain, reduced brain synthesis could theoretically alter brain 5-HT activity and hence lead to impulsive or impulsive-aggressive behavior. Leyton and others (2001), using a PET radioligand for the 5-HT precursor tryptophan, found reduced 5-HT synthesis in corticostriatal pathways to be inversely correlated with impulsivity in a sample of BPD subjects. These findings would be consistent with a model of 5-HT dysfunction affecting aversive and reinforcement learning in impulsive aggression.

Fenfluramine, which causes synaptic release of serotonin, is associated with met-abolic activation of the prefrontal cortex (Mann et al., 1996). Impulsive-aggressive personality-disordered patients show blunted metabolic response in the prefrontal cortex when challenged with fenfluramine during PET scanning (Siever et al., 1999), results that were largely replicated by Soloff, Meltzer, Greer, Constantine, and Kelly (1999). These findings were refined by work using a 5-HT$_{2A/C}$ agonist, meta-chlorophenylpiperizine, revealing blunted prefrontal cortex activation in impulsive-aggressive personality-disordered subjects (New et al., 2002). Consistent with this, OFC 5-HT$_{2A}$ receptor availability, as measured with [(11)C]MDL100907, is decreased in impulsive-aggressive adults (Rosell et al., 2010). Downregulation of serotonergic receptors may extend to the 5-HT$_{1A}$ subtype as well, as radioactive tracer binding to the 5-HT$_{1A}$ receptor with [c-11] WAY-100635 has been found to be inversely related to impulsive aggression (Parsey et al., 2002).

Augmenting Serotonergic Function Alters Frontal Limbic Brain Metabolism and Decreases Impulsive Aggression

Given the large body of data indicating serotonergic dysfunction in aggression, the effect of manipulating serotonergic function for therapeutic purposes is of great clin-ical and scientific interest. Chronic administration of the serotonin precursor mole-cule tryptophan has been found to decrease aggressive behavior in healthy controls (Moskowitz, Pinard, Zuroff, Annable, & Young, 2003). Blocking the degradation of serotonin with serotonin reuptake inhibitors (SSRI) is another intervention that has been tested. The mechanism of action in depression is complex, as SSRIs have multiple biological time-dependent effects. However, it is known that chronic SSRI administration leads to OFC 5-HT terminal autoreceptor desensitization in the rat, which would permit an eventual increase in OFC 5-HT activity (Mansari, Bouchard, & Blier, 1995). Randomized, double-blind, placebo-controlled trials of SSRI for the treatment of impulsive aggression in personality-disordered subjects have found mostly positive effects. In a study of the SSRI fluoxetine, fluoxetine was more effective than placebo at reducing verbal aggression in IED patients (Coccaro, Lee, & Kavoussi, 2009). The effective dose appeared to be higher, and the time needed to separate from placebo appeared to be longer, in comparison to treatment studies of major depressive disorder, suggesting parallels between the treatment of aggression and treatment of anxiety. Analysis of the results of this trial suggested that more severely aggressive subjects, who were also more likely to have blunted 5-HT receptor sensitivity to d-fenfluramine, were less likely to improve with fluoxetine treatment. Fluoxetine was similarly found to reduce aggressive behavior in depressed patients with anger attacks (Fava et al., 1993). However, a randomized, placebo-controlled study of fluvoxamine for the treatment of affective and impulsive symptoms in females with BPD did not find that fluvoxamine was superior to placebo in reducing impulsive aggression (Rinne, van den Brink, Wouters, & van Dyck, 2002). It is possible the study was too short, at six weeks, to detect an effect. The therapeutic effect of SSRI treatment of aggression may be by increasing OFC activity. An innovative PET-imaging/treatment study, before and after scanning with PET imaging in 10 BPD-IED patients, found that treatment with fluoxetine caused increased OFC metabolism (New et al., 2004). Improvement in aggression was correlated with an increase in OFC and anterior cingulate metabolic activity, suggesting that the therapeutic effect of SSRI treatment on impulsive aggression is mediated by increased OFC function. Increased OFC activity may be due to 5-HT_{2A} desensitization, as preclinical research has found that chronic treatment with citalopram reduces cortical 5-HT_{2A} binding (Peremans et al., 2005), and 5-HT_{2A} has inhibitory effects on OFC electrophysiology (Bergqvist, Dong, & Blier, 1999). Consistent with these findings, treatment of BPD patients with olanzapine, which is an antagonist of the 5-HT_{2A} receptor, has been found to reduce impulsive aggression (Zanarini, Frankenburg, & Parachini, 2004). Because olanzapine has other pharmacological actions outside of 5-HT_{2A} receptor antagonism, follow-up research with a specific 5-HT_{2A} receptor antagonist in impulsive aggression would be of interest to confirm the importance of this receptor subtype.

Finally, the effects of SSRI administration may not be restricted to the prefrontal cortex. A recent study of the effects of acute administration of the SSRI citalopram on the neural response to emotional face stimuli found that citalopram dosing was associated with increased activity in the left TPJ in IED compared with healthy control individuals (Cremers, Lee, Keedy, Phan, & Coccaro, 2015). Such effects could indicate that SSRI treatment may reduce aggression by increasing mentalizing ability. Serotonergic modulation of the top-down process of mentalizing, if confirmed, would mirror the role for serotonin in modulating another top-down process, delay discounting.

Norepinephrine and Impulsive Aggression

As norepinephrine is released in acute stress (Berridge & Waterhouse, 2003), it is plausibly linked to aggressive behavior. Preclinical work has confirmed that frustration causes norepinephrine release in the right amygdala (Young & Williams, 2010), consistent with a role for norepinephrine in mediating the effects of surprise and arousal on decision-making (Doya, 2002). Clinical findings have not been supportive of a link for alpha-2 receptor involvement (Coccaro & Kavoussi, 2010), although there is some support for other aspects of noradrenergic signaling (Haden & Scarpa, 2007). In the CSF, levels of the norepinephrine metabolite 3-methoxy-5-hydroxyphenylglycol are positively correlated with aggression in adult males with personality disorders (Brown et al., 1979) and adults with depression (Placidi et al., 2001; Prochazka & Ågren, 2003). Aggressive individuals show higher plasma norepinephrine release during aggressive responding, albeit without baseline differences, suggesting that norepinephrine release is either causally related to the expression of aggression or triggered by frustration (Gerra et al., 1997). Not surprisingly, then, treatment with antidepressant medications that increase norepinephrine worsens aggression in personality-disordered patients (Soloff, George, Nathan, Schulz, & Perel, 1986).

Neuropeptides and Impulsive Aggression

Preclinical work with the social neuropeptides has linked the expression of oxytocin and vasopressin to prosocial behaviors (Caldwell & Albers, 2015). The effects can be complex and may be context-dependent, as is seen with social modulation of oxytocin effects on fear conditioning (Guzmán et al., 2013). In humans, CSF oxytocin levels are inversely correlated with life history of aggression measures in adults with impulsive aggression (Lee, Ferris, Van de Kar, & Coccaro, 2009), while vasopressin levels are positively correlated with life history of aggression (Coccaro, Kavoussi, Hauger, Cooper, & Ferris, 1998). However, intranasal administration of oxytocin has been found to increase, rather than decrease, aggressive responding (Ne'eman, Perach-Barzilay, Fischer-Shofty, Atias, & Shamay-Tsoory, 2016). We found that intranasal oxytocin had neither pro- or anti-aggressive effects when tested in a group of controls and IED individuals. However, an indirect "cybernetic" effect of oxytocin was found in decreasing computer confederate aggression, likely via a tendency of subjects when given oxytocin to increase defensive "C" button presses that was not statistically significant (Lee, 2014). These results reveal that the role on the social neuropeptides in human aggressive behavior is far from simple. The fact that augmentation of oxytocin does not reduce or eliminate aggressive behavior indicates that increasing social motivation may not be sufficient to reduce aggression. In reality, social interaction is characterized by frustration. If so, then perhaps decreasing frustration indirectly, by reducing social motivation, would be fruitful. Blocking vasopressin receptor signaling with vasopressin receptor antagonists may represent a reasonable approach in impulsive-aggressive individuals. Preliminary evidence from work demonstrating that a novel vasopressin V1a-receptor antagonist can reduce response of the social brain to emotional face stimuli suggests that this is a plausible approach (Lee et al., 2013).

■ ETIOLOGICAL FACTORS

Aggression is heritable (Coccaro, Bergeman, Kavoussi, & Seroczynski, 1997), but genetic factors are still under investigation. Leading candidates are the 30 base pair variable number of tandem repeats of the monoamine oxidase A gene (*MAOA-uVNTR*) and the serotonin transporter linked polymorphic region of the serotonin transporter gene (*5HTTLPR*; Courtney & Waldman, 2014). Both of these encode for proteins that affect serotonin signaling, as well as other neuromodulators. Environmental factors, such as history of childhood trauma, also likely play a role in the development of impulsive aggression (Fanning, Meyerhoff, Lee, & Coccaro, 2014). How genetic and environmental factors interact is under investigation, but involvement of serotonin signaling raises the intriguing possibility that genes may control the impact of environment on the development and function of the neural circuits described. One possible molecular mechanism by which neural circuit function is affected by stress is via inflammation. Impulsive aggression is associated with increased peripheral expression of interleukin-6 and both peripheral and central C-reactive protein (Coccaro, Lee, & Coussons-Read, 2014; Coccaro, Lee, & Coussons-Read, 2015). Impulsive aggression has also been associated with increased oxidative stress, as evidenced by elevated 8-hydroxy-2'-deoxyguanosine and 8-isoprostane in impulsive aggression (Coccaro, Lee, & Gozal, 2016). How inflammatory factors associated with impulsive aggression affect the development of the brain is an important topic of further study.

■ CONCLUSION

Impulsive aggression remains a major public health problem. Progress has been made in the scientific understanding of its neurobiological mechanisms as well as how it may be manifesting in the clinic in the form of IED. The phenomenology and behavioral manifestation of impulsive aggression can be understood in the framework of the SEIP model. Work thus far indicates IED is associated with deficits in encoding of social and emotional information, a bias toward hostile attribution, and a tendency toward responding aggressively. A prominent role for an angry emotional response is found in multiple steps. Clinical neuroscience work provides biological validation of the SEIP framework in impulsive aggression. For purposes of this review, a predictive encoding model of brain function was adopted. Research findings for the most part fit into this model, finding evidence that impulsive aggression is related to abnormal aversive learning, mentalizing ability, and performance monitoring. These functions are mediated, respectively, by ventral prefrontal-amygdala, frontoparietal, and frontostriatal circuits. A large body of work links serotonin signalling in these circuits to aggressive behavior generally and impulsive aggression specifically. Rather than pointing to a "chemical imbalance" or absolute deficit in serotonin production, in total the evidence points to a disruption in serotonin dynamic range. Molecular genetic determinants of impulsive aggression are still under investigation, and so the field awaits resolution of this important question. In the interim, a fascinating link to states of inflammation and oxidative stress provide hope that a causal biological mechanism for disrupted neural function in IED will be found in the near future. Existing evidence points toward clinical interventions that address deficits in SEIP, such as cognitive-behavioral therapy and pharmacological interventions impacting the three circuits described in this chapter.

■ REFERENCES

Adhikari, A., Lerner, T. N., Finkelstein, J., Pak, S., Jennings, J. H., Davidson, T. J., . . . Deisseroth, K. (2015). Basomedial amygdala mediates top-down control of anxiety and fear. *Nature, 527*, 179–185. http://doi.org/10.1038/nature15698

Aghajanian, G. K., & Marek, G. J. (1997). Serotonin induces excitatory postsynaptic potentials in apical dendrites of neocortical pyramidal cells. *Neuropharmacology, 36*(4–5), 589–599. http://doi.org/10.1016/S0028-3908(97)00051-8

Amargós-Bosch, M., Bortolozzi, A., Puig, M. V., Serrats, J., Adell, A., Celada, P., . . . Artigas, F. (2004). Co-expression and in vivo interaction of serotonin1a and serotonin2a receptors in pyramidal neurons of pre-frontal cortex. *Cerebr Cortex, 14*(3), 281–299. http://doi.org/10.1093/cercor/bhg128

Åsberg, M. (1997). Neurotransmitters and suicidal behavior. The evidence from cerebrospinal fluid studies. *Ann N Y Acad Sci, 836*, 158–181. http://doi.org/10.1111/j.1749-6632.1997.tb52359.x

Bayer, H. M., & Glimcher, P. W. (2005). Midbrain dopamine neurons encode a quantitative reward prediction error signal. *Neuron, 47*(1), 129–141. http://doi.org/10.1016/j.neuron.2005.05.020

Beaver, J. D., Lawrence, A. D., Passamonti, L., & Calder, A. J. (2008). Appetitive motivation predicts the neural response to facial signals of aggression. *J Neurosci, 28*(11), 2719–2725. http://doi.org/10.1523/jneurosci.0033-08.2008

Bergqvist, P. B., Dong, J., & Blier, P. (1999). Effect of atypical antipsychotic drugs on 5-HT2 receptors in the rat orbito-frontal cortex: an in vivo electrophysiological study. *Psychopharmacology, 143*(1), 89–96. http://www.ncbi.nlm.nih.gov/entrez/query.fcgi?cmd=Retrieve&db=PubMed&dopt=Citation&list_uids=10227084

Berridge, C. W., & Waterhouse, B. D. (2003). The locus coeruleus-noradrenergic system: modulation of behavioral state and state-dependent cognitive processes. *Brain Res Rev, 42*(1), 33–84. http://doi.org/10.1016/S0165-0173(03)00143-7

Beyer, F., Münte, T. F., Erdmann, C., & Krämer, U. M. (2013). Emotional reactivity to threat modulates activity in mentalizing network during aggression. *Soc Cogn Affect Neurosci, 9*(10), 1552–1560. http://doi.org/10.1093/scan/nst146

Beyer, F., Münte, T. F., Göttlich, M., & Krämer, U. M. (2014). Orbitofrontal cortex reactivity to angry facial expression in a social interaction correlates with aggressive behavior. *Cerebr Cortex, 25*(9), 3057–3063. http://doi.org/10.1093/cercor/bhu101

Beyer, F., Münte, T. F., & Krämer, U. M. (2014). Increased neural reactivity to socio-emotional stimuli links social exclusion and aggression. *Biol Psychol, 96*(1), 102–110. http://doi.org/10.1016/j.biopsycho.2013.12.008

Bjork, J. M., Dougherty, D. M., Moeller, F. G., & Swann, A. C. (2000). Differential behavioral effects of plasma tryptophan depletion and loading in aggressive and nonaggressive men. *Neuropsychopharmacology, 22*(4), 357–369. http://doi.org/10.1016/S0893-133X(99)00136-0

Bond, A. J., Wingrove, J., & Critchlow, D. G. (2001). Tryptophan depletion increases aggression in women during the premenstrual phase. *Psychopharmacology, 156*(4), 477–480. http://doi.org/10.1007/s002130100795

Brown, G. L., Goodwin, F. K., Ballenger, J. C., Goyer, P. F., & Major, L. F. (1979). Aggression in humans correlates with cerebrospinal fluid amine metabolites. *Psychiatry Res, 1*(2), 131–139. http://doi.org/10.1016/0165-1781(79)90053-2

Bubenzer-Busch, S., Herpertz-Dahlmann, B., Kuzmanovic, B., Gaber, T. J., Helmbold, K., Ullisch, M. G., . . . Zepf, F. D. (2016). Neural correlates of reactive aggression in children with attention-deficit/hyperactivity disorder and comorbid disruptive behaviour disorders. *Acta Psychiatr Scand, 133*(4), 310–323. http://doi.org/10.1111/acps.12475

Caldwell, H. K., & Albers, H. E. (2015). Oxytocin, vasopressin, and the motivational forces that drive social behaviors. *Curr Top Behav Neurosci, 27*, 51–103. http://doi.org/10.1007/7854_2015_390

Cannon, W. B. (1987). The James-Lange theory of emotions: a critical examination and an alternative theory. By Walter B. Cannon, 1927. *Am J Psychol, 100*(3–4), 567–586. http://doi.org/10.2307/1415404

Carver, C. S., & Harmon-Jones, E. (2009). Anger is an approach-related affect: evidence and implications. *Psychol Bull*, *135*(2), 183–204. http://doi.org/10.1037/a0013965

Clarke, H. F., Walker, S. C., Crofts, H. S., Dalley, J. W., Robbins, T. W., & Roberts, A. C. (2005). Prefrontal serotonin depletion affects reversal learning but not attentional set shifting. *J Neurosci*, *25*(2), 532–538. http://doi.org/10.1523/JNEUROSCI.3690-04.2005

Clarke, H. F., Walker, S. C., Dalley, J. W., Robbins, T. W., & Roberts, A. C. (2007). Cognitive inflexibility after prefrontal serotonin depletion is behaviorally and neurochemically specific. *Cerebr Cortex*, *17*(1), 18–27. http://doi.org/10.1093/cercor/bhj120

Cleare, A. J., & Bond, A. J. (1995). The effect of tryptophan depletion and enhancement on subjective and behavioural aggression in normal male subjects. *Psychopharmacology*, *118*(1), 72–81. http://doi.org/10.1007/BF02245252

Coccaro, E. F., Bergeman, C. S., Kavoussi, R. J., & Seroczynski, A. D. (1997). Heritability of aggression and irritability: a twin study of the Buss-Durkee aggression scales in adult male subjects. *Biol Psychiatry*, *41*(3), 273–284. http://doi.org/10.1016/S0006-3223(96)00257-0

Coccaro, E. F., & Kavoussi, R. J. (2010). GH response to intravenous clonidine challenge: absence of relationship with behavioral irritability, aggression, or impulsivity in human subjects. *Psychiatry Res*, *178*(2), 443–445. http://doi.org/10.1016/j.psychres.2010.03.018

Coccaro, E. F., Kavoussi, R. J., Cooper, T. B., & Hauger, R. L. (1997). Central serotonin activity and aggression: inverse relationship with prolactin response to d-fenfluramine, but not CSF 5-HIAA concentration, in human subjects. *Am J Psychiatry*, *154*(10), 1430–1435. http://doi.org/10.1176/ajp.154.10.1430

Coccaro, E. F., Kavoussi, R. J., Hauger, R. L., Cooper, T. B., & Ferris, C. F. (1998). Cerebrospinal fluid vasopressin levels: correlates with aggression and serotonin function in personality-disordered subjects. *Arch Gen Psychiatry*, *55*(8), 708–714. http://doi.org/10.1001/archpsyc.55.8.708

Coccaro, E. F., Lee, R., & Coussons-Read, M. (2014). Elevated plasma inflammatory markers in individuals with intermittent explosive disorder and correlation with aggression in humans. *JAMA Psychiatry*, *71*, 158–165.

Coccaro, E. F., Lee, R., & Coussons-Read, M. (2015). Cerebrospinal fluid and plasma C-reactive protein and aggression in personality-disordered subjects: a pilot study. *J Neural Transm*, *122*(2), 321–326. http://doi.org/10.1007/s00702-014-1263-6

Coccaro, E. F., Lee, R., & Gozal, D. (2014). Elevated plasma oxidative stress markers in individuals with intermittent explosive disorder and correlation with aggression in humans. *Biol Psychiatry*, *79*(2), 127–135.

Coccaro, E. F., Lee, R. J., & Kavoussi, R. J. (2009). A double-blind, randomized, placebo-controlled trial of fluoxetine in patients with intermittent explosive disorder. *J Clin Psychiatry*, *70*(5), 653–662. http://doi.org/10.4088/JCP.08m04150

Coccaro, E. F., McCloskey, M. S., Fitzgerald, D. A., & Phan, K. L. (2007). Amygdala and orbitofrontal reactivity to social threat in individuals with impulsive aggression. *Biol Psychiatry*, *62*(2), 168–178.

Coccaro, E. F., Noblett, K. L., & McCloskey, M. S. (2009). Attributional and emotional responses to socially ambiguous cues: validation of a new assessment of social/emotional information processing in healthy adults and impulsive aggressive patients. *J Psychiatr Res*, *43*(10), 915–925. http://doi.org/10.1016/j.jpsychires.2009.01.012

Coccaro, E., Fanning, J., & Lee, R. (2016). Development of a social emotional information processing assessment for adults (SEIP-Q). *Aggress Behav*, *43*(1). https://doi.org/10.1002/ab.21661

Cohen, J. D., Botvinick, M., & Carter, C. S. (2000). Anterior cingulate and prefrontal cortex: who's in control? *Nature Neurosci*, *3*(5), 421–423. http://doi.org/10.1038/74783

Cole, S., & McNally, G. P. (2009). Complementary roles for amygdala and periaqueductal gray in temporal-difference fear learning. *Learn Mem*, *16*(1), 1–7. http://doi.org/10.1101/lm.1120509

Cools, R., Calder, A. J., Lawrence, A. D., Clark, L., Bullmore, E., & Robbins, T. W. (2005). Individual differences in threat sensitivity predict serotonergic modulation of amygdala response to fearful faces. *Psychopharmacology*, *180*(4), 670–679. http://doi.org/10.1007/s00213-005-2215-5

Courtney, A. F., & Waldman, I. D. (2014). Candidate genes for aggression and antisocial behavior: a meta-analysis of association studies of the 5HTTLPR and MAOA-uVNTR. Title. *Behav Genet*, *44*(5), 427–444.

Cremers, H., Lee, R., Keedy, S., Phan, K. L., & Coccaro, E. (2015). Effects of escitalopram administration on face processing in intermittent explosive disorder: an fMRI study. *Neuropsychopharmacology*, *41*(2), 590–597. http://doi.org/10.1038/npp.2015.187

Crick, N. R., & Dodge, K. A. (1994). A review and reformulation of social information-processing mechanisms in children's social adjustment. *Psychol Bull*, *115*(1), 74–101. http://doi.org/10.1037/0033-2909.115.1.74

Crick, N. R., & Dodge, K. A. (1996). Social information-processing mechanisms in reactive and proactive aggression. *Child Dev*, *67*(3), 993–1002. http://doi.org/10.1111/j.1467-8624.1996.tb01778.x

Decety, J., & Lamm, C. (2007). The role of the right temporoparietal junction in social interaction: how low-level computational processes contribute to meta-cognition. *Neuroscientist*, *13*(6), 580–593. http://doi.org/10.1177/1073858407304654

Dodge, K. A. (1993). Social-cognitive mechanisms in the development of conduct disorder and depression. *Annu Rev Psychol*, *44*, 559–584. http://doi.org/10.1146/annurev.ps.44.020193.003015

Dodge, K., & Price, J. (1994). On the relation between social information processing and socially competent behavior in early school-aged children. *Child Dev*, *65*, 1385–1397. http://doi.org/10.2307/1131505

Dougherty, D. M., Richard, D. M., James, L. M., & Mathias, C. W. (2010). Effects of acute tryptophan depletion on three different types of behavioral impulsivity. *Int J Tryptophan Res*, *3*, 99–111. http://doi.org/10.1210/jc.76.5.1160

Doya, K. (2002). Metalearning and neuromodulation. *Neural Netw*, *15*(4–6), 495–506. http://doi.org/10.1016/S0893-6080(02)00044-8

Duke, A. A., Bègue, L., Bell, R., & Eisenlohr-Moul, T. (2013). Revisiting the serotonin-aggression relation in humans: a meta-analysis. *Psychol Bull*, *139*(5), 1148–1172. http://doi.org/10.1037/a0031544

Elliott, R., Dolan, R. J., & Frith, C. D. (2000). Dissociable functions in the medial and lateral orbitofrontal cortex: evidence from human neuroimaging studies. *Cerebr Cortex*, *10*(3), 308–317.

el Mansari, M., Bouchard, C., & Blier, P. (1995). Alteration of serotonin release in the guinea pig orbito-frontal cortex by selective serotonin reuptake inhibitors. Relevance to treatment of obsessive-compulsive disorder. *Neuropsychopharmacology*, *13*(2), 117–127. http://doi.org/0893-133X(95)00045-F [pii]\r10.1016/0893-133X(95)00045-F

Endrass T, Schuermann B, Roepke S, Kessler-Scheil S, K. N. (2016). Reduced risk avoidance and altered neural correlates of feedback processing in patients with borderline personality disorder. *Psychiatry Res*, *243*, 14–22.

Fanning, J. R., Meyerhoff, J. J., Lee, R., & Coccaro, E. F. (2014). History of childhood maltreatment in Intermittent Explosive Disorder and suicidal behavior. *J Psychiatr Res*, *56*(1), 10–17. http://doi.org/10.1016/j.jpsychires.2014.04.012

Fava, M., Rosenbaum, J. F., Pava, J. A., McCarthy, M. K., Steingard, R. J., & Bouffides, E. (1993). Anger attacks in unipolar depression, Part 1: clinical correlates and response to fluoxetine treatment. *Am J Psychiatry, 150*(8), 1158–1163. http://doi.org/10.1176/ajp.150.8.1158

Fontaine, R. G., Burks, V. S., & Dodge, K. A. (2002). Response decision processes and externalizing behavior problems in adolescents. *Dev Psychopathol, 14,* 107–122. http://doi.org/http://dx.doi.org/10.1017/S0954579402001062

Friston, K. J., Stephan, K. E., Montague, R., & Dolan, R. J. (2014). Computational psychiatry: the brain as a phantastic organ. *Lancet Psychiatry, 1*(2), 148–158. http://doi.org/10.1016/S2215-0366(14)70275-5

Gerra, G., Zaimovic, A., Avanzini, P., Chittolini, B., Giucastro, G., Caccavari, R., . . . Brambilla, F. (1997). Neurotransmitter-neuroendocrine responses to experimentally induced aggression in humans: influence of personality variable. *Psychiatry Res, 66*(1), 33–43. http://doi.org/10.1016/S0165-1781(96)02965-4

Gourley, S. L., & Taylor, J. R. (2016). Going and stopping: dichotomies in behavioral control by the prefrontal cortex. *Nature Neurosci, 19*(5), 656–664. http://doi.org/10.1038/nn.4275

Grafman, J., Schwab, K., Warden, D., Pridgen, A., Brown, H. R., & Salazar, A. M. (1996). Frontal lobe injuries, violence, and aggression: a report of the Vietnam Head Injury Study. *Neurology, 46*(5), 1231–1238. http://doi.org/10.1212/WNL.46.5.1231

Grzyb, B., Boedecker, J., Asada, M., Pobil, A. del, & Smith, L. (2011). Between frustration and elation: sense of control regulates the intrinsic motivation for motor learning. In *Workshops at the Twenty-Fifth AAAI Conference on Artificial Intelligence* (pp. 10–15). Palo Alto, CA: Association for the Advancement of Artificial Intelligence.

Guzmán, Y. F., Tronson, N. C., Jovasevic, V., Sato, K., Guedea, A. L., Mizukami, H., . . . Radulovic, J. (2013). Fear-enhancing effects of septal oxytocin receptors. *Nature Neurosci, 16*(9), 1185–1187. http://doi.org/10.1038/nn.3465

Haden, S. C., & Scarpa, A. (2007). The noradrenergic system and its involvement in aggressive behaviors. *Aggress Viol Behav, 12*(1), 1–15. http://doi.org/10.1016/j.avb.2006.01.012

Hall, J. R., Bernat, E. M., & Patrick, C. J. (2007). Externalizing psychopathology and the error-related negativity. *Psychol Sci, 18*(4), 326–333. http://doi.org/10.1111/j.1467-9280.2007.01899.x

Harmer, C. J., Rogers, R. D., Tunbridge, E., Cowen, P. J., & Goodwin, G. M. (2003). Tryptophan depletion decreases the recognition of fear in female volunteers. *Psychopharmacology, 167*(4), 411–7. http://doi.org/10.1007/s00213-003-1401-6

Heritage, A. J., & Benning, S. D. (2012). Impulsivity and response modulation deficits in psychopathy: evidence from the ERN and N1. *J Abnorm Psychol, 122*(1), 215–222. http://doi.org/10.1037/a0030039

Hoenen, M., Schain, C., & Pause, B. M. (2013). Down-modulation of mu-activity through empathic top-down processes. *Soc Neurosci, 8*(5), 515–24. http://doi.org/10.1080/17470919.2013.833550

Irle, E., Lange, C., & Sachsse, U. (2005). Reduced size and abnormal asymmetry of parietal cortex in women with borderline personality disorder. *Biol Psychiatry, 57,* 173–182. http://doi.org/10.1016/j.biopsych.2004.10.004

Jakab, R. L., & Goldman-Rakic, P. S. (1998). 5-Hydroxytryptamine2A serotonin receptors in the primate cerebral cortex: possible site of action of hallucinogenic and antipsychotic drugs in pyramidal cell apical dendrites. *Proc Natl Acad Sci U S A, 95*(2), 735–740. http://doi.org/10.1073/pnas.95.2.735

Kessler, R. C., Coccaro, E. F., Fava, M., Jaeger, S., Jin, R., & Walters, E. (2006). The prevalence and correlates of DSM-IV intermittent explosive disorder in the National Comorbidity Survey Replication. *Arch Gen Psychiatry, 63*(6), 669–78. http://doi.org/10.1001/archpsyc.63.6.669

Keysers, C., & Gazzola, V. (2014). Hebbian learning and predictive mirror neurons for actions, sensations and emotions. *Philos Trans R Soc B, 369*, 20130175. http://doi.org/10.1098/rstb.2013.0175

Kimbrell, T. A., George, M. S., Parekh, P. I., Ketter, T. A., Podell, D. M., Danielson, A. L., . . . Post, R. M. (1999). Regional brain activity during transient self-induced anxiety and anger in healthy adults. *Biol Psychiatry, 46*(4), 454–465. http://doi.org/10.1016/S0006-3223(99)00103-1

Lange, C., Kracht, L., Herholz, K., Sachsse, U., & Irle, E. (2005). Reduced glucose metabolism in temporo-parietal cortices of women with borderline personality disorder. *Psychiatry Res, 139*(2), 115–126. http://doi.org/10.1016/j.pscychresns.2005.05.003

Lee, R. (2014). The psychopharmacology of criminality and oxytocin modulation of social behavior in aggressive individuals. In M. DeLisi & M. G. Vaughn (Eds.), *The Routledge international handbook of biosocial criminology* (pp. 236–250). London and New York: Routledge.

Lee, R., Arfanakis, K., Evia, A. M., Fanning, J., Keedy, S., Coccaro, E. F. (2016). White matter integrity reductions in intermittent explosive disorder. *Neuropsychopharmacology, 41*(11), 2697–2703.

Lee, R., Ferris, C., Van de Kar, L. D., & Coccaro, E. F. (2009). Cerebrospinal fluid oxytocin, life history of aggression, and personality disorder. *Psychoneuroendocrinology, 34*(10), 1567–1573.

Lee, R. J., Coccaro, E. F., Cremers, H., McCarron, R., Lu, S.-F., Brownstein, M. J., & Simon, N. G. (2013). A novel V1a receptor antagonist blocks vasopressin-induced changes in the CNS response to emotional stimuli: an fMRI study. *Front Syst Neurosci, 7*, 100. http://doi.org/10.3389/fnsys.2013.00100

Leyton, M., Okazawa, H., Diksic, M., Paris, J., Rosa, P., Mzengeza, S., . . . Benkelfat, C. (2001). Brain regional alpha-[11C]methyl-L-tryptophan trapping in impulsive subjects with borderline personality disorder. *Am J Psychiatry, 158*(5), 775–782. http://doi.org/10.1176/appi.ajp.158.5.775

Linnoila, M., Virkkunen, M., Scheinin, M., Nuutila, A., Rimon, R., & Goodwin, F. K. (1983). Low cerebrospinal fluid 5-hydroxyindoleacetic acid concentration differentiates impulsive from nonimpulsive violent behavior. *Life Sci, 33*(26), 2609–2614. http://doi.org/10.1016/0024-3205(83)90344-2

Mann, J. J., Malone, K. M., Diehl, D. J., Perel, J., Nichols, T. E., & Mintun, M. A. (1996). Positron emission tomographic imaging of serotonin activation effects on prefrontal cortex in healthy volunteers. *J Cerebr Blood Flow Metab, 16*, 418–426. http://doi.org/10.1097/00004647-199605000-00008

Marsh, D. M., Dougherty, D. M., Moeller, F. G., Swann, A. C., & Spiga, R. (2002). Laboratory-measured aggressive behavior of women: acute tryptophan depletion and augmentation. *Neuropsychopharmacology, 26*(5), 660–671. http://doi.org/10.1016/S0893-133X(01)00369-4

McCloskey, M. S., Phan, K. L., Angstadt, M., Fettich, K. C., Keedy, S., & Coccaro, E. F. (2016). Amygdala hyperactivation to angry faces in intermittent explosive disorder. *J Psychiatr Res, 79*, 34–41.

McHugh, S. B., Barkus, C., Huber, A., Capitão, L., Lima, J., Lowry, J. P., & Bannerman, D. M. (2014). Aversive prediction error signals in the amygdala. *J Neurosci, 34*(27), 9024–33. http://doi.org/10.1523/JNEUROSCI.4465-13.2014

McLaughlin, K. A., Green, J. G., Hwang, I., Sampson, N. A., Zaslavsky, A. M., & Kessler, R. C. (2012). Intermittent explosive disorder in the National Comorbidity Survey Replication Adolescent Supplement. *Arch Gen Psychiatry, 69*(11), 1131–1139. http://doi.org/doi:10.1001/archgenpsychiatry.2012.592

Mercedes Perez-Rodriguez, M., Hazlett, E. A., Rich, E. L., Ripoll, L. H., Weiner, D. M., Spence, N., . . . New, A. S. (2012). Striatal activity in borderline personality disorder with comorbid intermittent explosive disorder: sex differences. *J Psychiatr Res*, *46*(6), 797–804. http://doi.org/10.1016/j.jpsychires.2012.02.014

Mobini, S., Chiang, T. J., Ho, M. Y., Bradshaw, C. M., & Szabadi, E. (2000). Effects of central 5-hydroxytryptamine depletion on sensitivity to delayed and probabilistic reinforcement. *Psychopharmacology*, *152*(4), 390–397. http://doi.org/10.1007/s002130000542

Molenberghs, P., Johnson, H., Henry, J. D., & Mattingley, J. B. (2016). Understanding the minds of others: a neuroimaging meta-analysis. *Neurosci Biobehav Rev*, *65*, 276–291. http://doi.org/10.1016/j.neubiorev.2016.03.020

Moskowitz, D. S., Pinard, G., Zuroff, D. C., Annable, L., & Young, S. N. (2003). Tryptophan, serotonin and human social behavior. *Adv Exp Med Biol*, *527*. http://doi.org/10.1007/978-1-4615-0135-0

National Institute of Mental Health. (2011). Negative valence systems: workshop proceedings. Research Domain Criteria. http://www.nimh.nih.gov/research–priorities/rdoc/n

Ne'eman, R., Perach-Barzilay, N., Fischer-Shofty, M., Atias, A., & Shamay-Tsoory, S. G. (2016). Intranasal administration of oxytocin increases human aggressive behavior. *Horm Behav*, *80*, 125–131. http://doi.org/10.1016/j.yhbeh.2016.01.015

New, A. S., Buchsbaum, M. S., Hazlett, E. A., Goodman, M., Koenigsberg, H. W., Lo, J., . . . Siever, L. J. (2004). Fluoxetine increases relative metabolic rate in prefrontal cortex in impulsive aggression. *Psychopharmacology*, *176*(3–4), 451–458. http://doi.org/10.1007/s00213-004-1913-8

New, A. S., Hazlett, E. A., Buchsbaum, M. S., Goodman, M., Reynolds, D., Mitropoulou, V., . . . Siever, L. J. (2002). Blunted prefrontal cortical 18fluorodeoxyglucose positron emission tomography response to meta-chlorophenylpiperazine in impulsive aggression. *Arch Gen Psychiatry*, *59*(7), 621–629. http://doi.org/10.1001/archpsyc.59.7.621

New, A. S., Hazlett, E. A., Newmark, R. E., Zhang, J., Triebwasser, J., Meyerson, D., . . . Buchsbaum, M. S. (2009). Laboratory induced aggression: a positron emission tomography study of aggressive individuals with borderline personality disorder. *Biol Psychiatry*, *66*(12), 1107–1114. http://doi.org/10.1016/j.biopsych.2009.07.015

Northoff, G., Richter, A., Gessner, M., Schlagenhauf, F., Fell, J., Baumgart, F., . . . Heinze, H. J. (2000). Functional dissociation between medial and lateral prefrontal cortical spatiotemporal activation in negative and positive emotions: a combined fMRI/MEG study. *Cerebr Cortex*, *10*(1), 93–107. http://doi.org/10.1093/cercor/10.1.93

Ongür, D., & Price, J. L. (2000). The organization of networks within the orbital and medial prefrontal cortex of rats, monkeys and humans. *Cerebr Cortex*, *10*(3), 206–219.

Otti, A., Wohlschlaeger, A. M., Noll-Hussong, M. (2015). Is the medial prefrontal cortex necessary for theory of mind? *PLoS One*, *10*(8):e0135912.

Parsey, R. V., Oquendo, M. A., Simpson, N. R., Ogden, R. T., Van Heertum, R., Arango, V., & Mann, J. J. (2002). Effects of sex, age, and aggressive traits in man on brain serotonin 5-HT1A receptor binding potential measured by PET using [C-11]WAY-100635. *Brain Res*, *954*(2), 173–182. http://doi.org/10.1016/S0006-8993(02)03243-2

Passamonti, L., Crockett, M. J., Apergis-Schoute, A. M., Clark, L., Rowe, J. B., Calder, A. J., & Robbins, T. W. (2012). Effects of acute tryptophan depletion on prefrontal-amygdala connectivity while viewing facial signals of aggression. *Biol Psychiatry*, *71*(1), 36–43. http://doi.org/10.1016/j.biopsych.2011.07.033

Peremans, K., Audenaert, K., Hoybergs, Y., Otte, A., Goethals, I., Gielen, I., . . . Dierckx, R. (2005). The effect of citalopram hydrobromide on 5-HT2A receptors in the impulsive-aggressive dog, as measured with 123I-5-I-R91150 SPECT. *Eur J Nucl Med Mol Imaging*, *32*, 708–716.

Pietrini, P., Guazzelli, M., Basso, G., Jaffe, K., & Grafman, J. (2000). Neural correlates of imaginal aggressive behavior assessed by positron emission tomography in healthy subjects. *Am J Psychiatry, 157*(11), 1772–1781. http://doi.org/10.1176/appi.ajp.157.11.1772

Piñeyro, G., & Blier, P. (1999). Autoregulation of serotonin neurons: role in antidepressant drug action. *Pharmacol Rev, 51*(3), 533–591.

Pittman, N. L., & Pittman, T. S. (1979). Effects of amount of helplessness training and internal-external locus of control on mood and performance. *J Person Soc Psychol, 37*(1), 39–47. http://doi.org/10.1037/0022-3514.37.1.39

Placidi, G. P. A., Oquendo, M. A., Malone, K. M., Huang, Y. Y., Ellis, S. P., & Mann, J. J. (2001). Aggressivity, suicide attempts, and depression: relationship to cerebrospinal fluid monoamine metabolite levels. *Biol Psychiatry, 50*(10), 783–791. http://doi.org/10.1016/S0006-3223(01)01170-2

Prochazka, H., & Ågren, H. (2003). Self-rated aggression and cerebral monoaminergic turnover: sex differences in patients with persistent depressive disorder. *Eur Arch Psychiatry Clin Neurosci, 253*(4), 185–192. http://doi.org/10.1007/s00406-003-0423-8

Putman, P., Hermans, E., & van Honk, J. (2004). Emotional Stroop performance for masked angry faces: it's BAS, not BIS. *Emotion, 4*(3), 305–311. http://doi.org/10.1037/1528-3542.4.3.305

Rescorla, R. A. (1971). Variation in the effectiveness of reinforcement and nonreinforcement following prior inhibitory conditioning. *Learn Motiv, 2*(2), 113–123. http://doi.org/10.1016/0023-9690(71)90002-6

Richell, R. A., Deakin, J. F. W., & Anderson, I. M. (2005). Effect of acute tryptophan depletion on the response to controllable and uncontrollable noise stress. *Biol Psychiatry, 57*(3), 295–300. http://doi.org/10.1016/j.biopsych.2004.10.010

Rinne, T., van den Brink, W., Wouters, L., & van Dyck, R. (2002). SSRI treatment of borderline personality disorder: a randomized, placebo-controlled clinical trial for female patients with borderline personality disorder. *Am J Psychiatry, 159*(12), 2048–2054. http://doi.org/10.1176/appi.ajp.159.12.2048

Rosell, D. R., Thompson, J. L., Slifstein, M., Xu, X., Frankle, W. G., New, A. S., . . . Siever, L. J. (2010). Increased serotonin 2A receptor availability in the orbitofrontal cortex of physically aggressive personality disordered patients. *Biol Psychiatry, 67*(12), 1154–1162. http://doi.org/10.1016/j.biopsych.2010.03.013

Rubia, K., Lee, F., Cleare, A. J., Tunstall, N., Fu, C. H. Y., Brammer, M., & McGuire, P. (2005). Tryptophan depletion reduces right inferior prefrontal activation during response inhibition in fast, event-related fMRI. *Psychopharmacology, 179*(4), 791–803. http://doi.org/10.1007/s00213-004-2116-z

Saddoris, M. P., Cacciapaglia, F., Wightman, R., & Carelli, R. M. (2015). Differential dopamine release dynamics in the nucleus accumbens core and shell reveal complementary signals for error prediction and incentive motivation. *J Neurosci, 35*, 11572–11582.

Samson, D., Apperly, I. A., Chiavarino, C., & Humphreys, G. W. (2004). Left temporoparietal junction is necessary for representing someone else's belief. *Nature Neurosci, 7*(5), 499–500.

Schlüter, T., Winz, O., Henkel, K., Prinz, S., Rademacher, L., Schmaljohann, J., . . . Vernaleken, I. (2013). The impact of dopamine on aggression: an [18F]-FDOPA PET Study in healthy males. *J Neurosci, 33*(43), 16889–16896. http://doi.org/10.1523/JNEUROSCI.1398-13.2013

Schönberg, T., Daw, N. D., Joel, D., & O'Doherty, J. P. (2007). Reinforcement learning signals in the human striatum distinguish learners from nonlearners during reward-based decision making. *J Neurosci, 27*(47), 12860–12867. http://doi.org/10.1523/JNEUROSCI.2496-07.2007

Schulze, L., Schmahl, C., & Niedtfeld, I. (2016). Neural correlates of disturbed emotion processing in borderline personality disorder: a multimodal meta-analysis. *Biol Psychiatry*, *79*(2), 97–106. http://doi.org/10.1016/j.biopsych.2015.03.027

Seo, M., Lee, E., & Averbeck, B. B. (2012). Action selection and action value in frontal-striatal circuits. *Neuron*, *74*(5), 947–960. http://doi.org/10.1016/j.neuron.2012.03.037

Siever, L. J., Buchsbaum, M. S., New, A. S., Spiegel-Cohen, J., Wei, T., Hazlett, E. A., . . . Mitropoulou, V. (1999). d,l-Fenfluramine response in impulsive personality disorder assessed with [18F]fluorodeoxyglucose positron emission tomography. *Neuropsychopharmacology*, *20*(5), 413–423. http://doi.org/10.1016/S0893-133X(98)00111-0

Soloff, P. H., George, A., Nathan, R. S., Schulz, P. M., & Perel, J. M. (1986). Paradoxical effects of amitriptyline on borderline patients. *Am J Psychiatry*, *143*(12), 1603–1605. http://doi.org/10.1176/ajp.143.12.1603

Soloff, P. H., Meltzer, C. C., Greer, P. J., Constantine, D., & Kelly, T. M. (1999). A fenfluramine-activated FDG-PET study of borderline personality disorder. *Biol Psychiatry*, *47*(6), 540–547. http://doi.org/10.1016/S0006-3223(99)00202-4

Sutton, R. S. (1988). Learning to predict by the method of temporal differences. *Mach Learn*, *3*(1), 9–44. http://doi.org/10.1023/A:1018056104778

Vila-Ballo, A., Hdez-Lafuente, P., Rostan, C., Cunillera, T., & Rodriguez-Fornells, A. (2014). Neurophysiological correlates of error monitoring and inhibitory processing in juvenile violent offenders. *Biol Psychol*, *102*(1), 141–152. http://doi.org/10.1016/j.biopsycho.2014.07.021

Virkkunen, M., Nuutila, A., Goodwin, F. K., & Linnoila, M. (1987). Cerebrospinal fluid monoamine metabolite levels in male arsonists. *Arch Gen Psychiatry*, *44*(3), 241–7. http://doi.org/10.1001/archpsyc.1987.01800150053007

Wenzel, A., Borges, K. T., Porto, C. R., Caminha, R. M., & de Oliveira, I. R. (2009). Volumes of the hippocampus and amygdala in patients with borderline personality disorder: a meta-analysis. *J Personal Disord*, *23*(4), 333–345. http://doi.org/10.1521/pedi.2009.23.4.333

Yanowitch, R., & Coccaro, E. F. (2011). The neurochemistry of human aggression. *Adv Genet*, *75*, 151–169. http://doi.org/10.1016/B978-0-12-380858-5.00005-8

Young, E. J., & Williams, C. L. (2010). Valence dependent asymmetric release of norepinephrine in the basolateral amygdala. *Behav Neurosci*, *124*(5), 633–644. http://doi.org/10.1037/a0020885

Zanarini, M. C., Frankenburg, F. R., & Parachini, E. A. (2004). A preliminary, randomized trial of fluoxetine, olanzapine, and the olanzapine-fluoxetine combination in women with borderline personality disorder. *J Clin Psychiatry*, *65*(7), 903–907. http://doi.org/10.4088/JCP.v65n0704

9 Social Cognition in Personality Disorders

■ STEFANIE LIS, NICOLE E. DERISH,
AND M. MERCEDES PEREZ-RODRIGUEZ

■ INTRODUCTION

Although personality disorders are characterized by interpersonal dysfunction and altered cognitions related to perception of the self and understanding of others (American Psychiatric Association, 1994, 2013; Jeung & Herpertz, 2014), dysfunctions in social cognitive processes have only recently been recognized as a core feature of personality disorders (Bertsch, Gamer, Schmidt, Schmidinger, & Herpertz, 2012; Herpertz, Lischke, Berger, & Gamer, 2012; Meyer-Lindenberg, Domes, Kirsch, & Heinrichs, 2011; Meyer-Lindenberg & Tost, 2012; Stanley & Siever, 2010).

Indeed, most of our knowledge about dysfunctions of social cognition in personality disorder, their underlying neurobiology and treatment options, stems from studies in nonhuman animals, healthy volunteers, or psychiatric disorders such as autism spectrum, mood/anxiety or psychotic disorders (Billeke & Aboitiz, 2013; Cusi, Nazarov, Macqueen, & McKinnon, 2013; Meyer-Lindenberg et al., 2011; Meyer-Lindenberg & Tost, 2012; Millan & Bales, 2013; Perez-Rodriguez, Mahon, Russo, Ungar, & Burdick, 2014; Wolkenstein, Schonenberg, Schirm, & Hautzinger, 2011). Only during the last decade has there been a growing number of studies of social cognition in patients with personality disorders; most of them have focused on patients with borderline (Schmahl et al., 2014), schizotypal (Ripoll et al., 2013), or antisocial personality disorder (Blair & Mitchell, 2009).

Social cognitive impairments are increasingly appreciated as responsible for much of the functional disability of psychiatric disorders (Brune, Abdel-Hamid, Lehmkamper, & Sonntag, 2007; Couture, Penn, & Roberts, 2006; Harvey & Bowie, 2012; Roncone et al., 2002). For example, social cognitive deficits in patients with schizophrenia cause more disability than psychosis (Doop & Park, 2009; Hooker & Park, 2002; Malaspina & Coleman, 2003; Perlick, Stastny, Mattis, & Teresi, 1992), respond only modestly to currently available medications (Goldberg et al., 2007; Green, 2006; Harvey & Bowie, 2012; Maat et al., 2014), and are independent from broader cognitive and perceptual deficits (Billeke & Aboitiz, 2013; Harvey & Bowie, 2012; Lee, Harkness, Sabbagh, & Jacobson, 2005; Montag et al., 2010).

Intact social cognitive abilities are required for optimal social functioning and navigating interpersonal relationships (Tomasello, Carpenter, Call, Behne, & Moll, 2005). Importantly, social cognitive abnormalities are a critical obstacle for successful engagement in psychological interventions (Inoue, Tonooka, Yamada, & Kanba, 2004; Jeung & Herpertz, 2014). Thus, the social cognitive impairments that characterize personality disorders may contribute to treatment failure, stigma, and discriminatory clinical practices toward individuals with these disorders (Jeung & Herpertz, 2014).

Despite the clinical significance of social cognitive impairments, treatment trials targeting this symptom domain are still sparse not only in personality disorders but even in psychiatric disorders in general. Only during the last decade has an increasing effort been made in the development of psychotherapeutic interventions that target social cognitive processes. These approaches range from social skills modules as part of broader psychotherapeutic interventions such as dialectic behavioral therapy (Stoffers et al., 2012) and social cognitive remediation paradigms that aim directly at improving social cognition (Hooker et al., 2012; Lindenmayer et al., 2012). Most of this work has been done in patients with schizophrenia. Although preliminary attempts are currently underway to apply social cognitive remediation interventions to other disorders such as autism or depression, no evidence-based data yet supports the benefits of this approach in enhancing social cognition and social functioning in personality disorders.

Pharmacological treatment of social cognitive impairments is currently not available. Nevertheless, pharmacological treatments have been shown to affect not only psychopathological symptoms in psychiatric disorders but also social cognitive functioning. Studies aiming at targeting social cognitive deficits more directly are sparse, although the neuropeptide oxytocin may be a promising substance for beneficially influencing social cognitive impairments across disorders (Bakermans-Kranenburg & van IJzendoorn, 2013; Gumley, Braehler, & Macbeth, 2014).

Definitions and Components of Social Cognition

Social cognition can broadly be defined as the "psychological processes that enable individuals to take advantage of being part of a social group" (Frith, 2008), being crucial to developing and maintaining interpersonal relationships (Eisenberg & Miller, 1987).

Social cognition is a broad concept and covers a wide range of mental processes. It may be understood as a level of analysis which deals with all those mental processes that underlie social phenomena (Gawronski & Bodenhausen, 2014). Crick and Dodge (1994) systematized these processes in their social information processing model of social adjustment. According to this model, social cognition encompasses the processes of the encoding of both internal and external cues, their interpretation, and the selection of responses based on specific goals relying on the subject's "database" (i.e., the gathered knowledge of acquired rules, social schemas, and social knowledge). Lemerise and Arsenio (2000) revised this model by integrating the modulating effects of emotion processes such as emphatic responsiveness and the affective relationship with a social partner. Thereby, it is emphasized that the final goal of social cognition is the adjustment and fine-tuning of behavior while interacting with social partners. Social interactions are dynamic sequences of social actions; that is, not only does the subject's behavior have to be adjusted to the partner's current emotions and intentions, but the effect of an individual's own behavior on the social partner has to be anticipated in order to achieve a successful social encounter (Schilbach et al., 2013).

A heuristically useful approach may be to conceptualize the multidimensional construct of social cognition as encompassing different subcomponents which can be broadly summarized into five domains: emotion recognition, theory of mind (ToM), social perception, social knowledge, and causal attribution style (Green et al., 2008; Mancuso, Horan, Kern, & Green, 2011; Ochsner, 2008; Mercedes Perez-Rodriguez,

Derish, & New, 2014). However, it has to be mentioned that this distinction is only one approach to conceptualize social cognition. It is based on the attempt to systematize research on this topic in schizophrenia and provides domains which are partially overlapping (for alternative concepts see, e.g., Green et al., 2008; Ochsner, 2008).

Emotion recognition indicates the ability to perceive and identify emotion by facial expression, body movements, and/or vocal prosody. Emotion recognition closely overlaps with the Research Domain Criteria (RDoC; Insel et al., 2010) subconstruct "Reception of Facial Communication," within the social communication construct in the social processes domain.

Theory of mind (ToM), also termed mentalizing or mentalization, refers to the broad ability to represent others' mental states and to make inferences about others' intentions, feelings, beliefs, and metaphors (Premack & Woodruff, 1978). Intact emotion recognition ability is a prerequisite for optimal ToM, which requires subjects to make inferences about the emotional state of others. ToM is closely related to the RDoC (Insel et al., 2010) subconstruct "Understanding Mental States" within the "Perception and Understanding of Others" construct in the social processes domain. ToM bears a close similarity to the construct of "empathy," which encompasses both "cognitive" and "affective" empathy, depending on whether subjects have to take the perspective of another subject or become emotionally engaged (Decety & Jackson, 2004). Shamay-Tsoory and Aharon-Peretz (2007) proposed that cognitive ToM and cognitive empathy are very similar, while affective ToM is related to cognitive and affective empathy.

Social perception refers to the ability to infer social roles, as well as rules, in complex and/or ambiguous social situations by reading nonverbal and paraverbal social cues. It also includes the capacity to determine the nature of the relationship between individuals (e.g., as professional, friendly, or romantic). Partially overlapping with social perception, *social knowledge* or *social schema* refers to the awareness of rules, roles, goals, and the corresponding behaviors that are expected in social situations and/or interactions. Social perception and social knowledge are closely linked, as a correct perception of social rules is necessary in order to determine what rules to adhere to in different social contexts (Green et al., 2008).

Attributional style refers to the tendency of an individual to assign internal or external causality to events in his or her life (Weiner, 1986). Healthy people usually have a self-serving bias in which they tend to attribute positive events to personal, internal factors and negative events to external causes (Miller & Ross, 1975).

Examples of Instruments and Tasks Commonly Used to Assess Social Cognition

With the increasing interest in social cognition, a multitude of different approaches to measure social cognitive processes have been developed during the last decades. They involve self-report questionnaires and behavioral paradigms that respectively allow for the assessment of the subjective perception of functioning and the objective measurement of behavior such as reaction times, error rates, and brain activity within standardized task settings.

In the domain of cognitive functioning, there are many well-established psychometric instruments available that have shown adequate validity, reliability, and objectivity and which provide normative data to assess performance of individual subjects. In contrast, well-validated psychometric tests rarely exist in the domain of social cognitive functioning. Most of the applied tools are experimental approaches tailored to the specific needs of research questions, which results in a high heterogeneity of assessments for each social cognitive process. However, it can be assumed that this may change in the near future. Nevertheless, there are some approaches which are used frequently, and we describe some of these in more detail shortly.

It seems worth noting that the examination of single social cognitive processes is nearly impossible since tasks always involve many (social-) cognitive and processes that have to be integrated for a successful task solution. Thus the interpretation of findings must be done with caution since dysfunctions in various processes may result in impairments in the same task. For example, ToM tasks, claiming to measure the recognition of intentions, may also require the recognition of emotions and social knowledge for successful task solution. Similarly, the recognition of an emotion relies on the accurate perception of basic features of a complex stimulus (i.e., a face). Developing tasks that allow fractionating the individual social cognitive processes involved is a prerequisite to identify deficits in single social cognitive functions linked to a specific mental disorder. However, most of the available paradigms do not provide a control condition to ensure the adequate functioning of broader cognitive processes—besides the target social cognitive function—required for performing the task.

Most measurement instruments are more or less complex versions of stimulus-response tasks; that is, in separate trials, subjects have to respond to a stimulus such as a face or a movie with a specific response such as the selection of the corresponding emotion label. During the past few years, the relevance of investigating social cognitive processes in interactive contexts has increasingly gained attention. A new set of tools has been developed that directly measure the participant's interaction behavior with real or virtual partners during standardized situations. Examples are ball-tossing games such as the cyberball paradigm (Williams & Jarvis, 2006) to investigate effects of social exclusion and exchange games from behavioral economy such as the trust game or the dictator game that focus on fairness, trust, and cooperative behavior (Baumert, Schlösser, & Schmitt, 2014). When these paradigms are combined with experimental approaches, they allow us to study specific social cognitive processes embedded in a more complex context and enable the measurement of how they affect interaction behavior. Dinsdale and Crespi (2013) suggest that such approaches are more sensitive for uncovering impairments in social cognition in personality disorders.

Emotion Recognition

The recognition of emotions is mostly investigated by multiple-choice emotion recognition tasks presenting facial stimuli with an emotional expression and asking subjects to select the appropriate emotion label from a set of response alternatives (for examples of this type of task, see Daros, Zakzanis, & Ruocco, 2013; Mitchell, Dickens, & Picchioni, 2014). Alternative approaches target the ability to detect emotional expressions. One example is the "finding the face in the crowd" paradigm that is a visual search task requiring subjects to identify a target face with an emotional expression that differs from those displayed in a surrounding crowd of distractor faces (Hansen & Hansen, 1988). Other studies present sequences of faces with increasing intensity of the expressed emotion and subjects have to indicate when they are able to identify the emotion (morphing tasks; Schonenberg et al., 2014). Tasks that focus on the discrimination of emotional expressions ask subjects to decide whether two faces depict a similar emotion or not, or to match a target face with other faces in regard to their emotional expression. Other tasks focus on the ability of subjects to assess the intensity of a specific emotion displayed in a face. While all of these approaches require subjects to focus on the expressed emotion, implicit emotion recognition tasks present emotional stimuli as distractors to analyze their effects on cognitive processing such as working memory.

Beyond this multitude of different task types, there are many task features that vary across studies, such as the intensity of the expressed emotion, the selection of types of emotions used as stimuli and response options, the duration of the presentation of the stimuli, and the use of one or several sensory channels. While most studies present facial stimuli, a few have used body movements or prosody with and without semantic content as stimuli.

Examples of tests available are the Penn Emotional Acuity Test (Erwin et al., 1992), a subtest of the University of Pennsylvania Computerized Neurocognitive Test Battery measuring emotion recognition and discrimination; the Mayer-Salovey-Caruso Emotional Intelligence Test (Mayer, Salovey, & Caruso, 2002), implemented as a subtest in the Measurement and Treatment Research to Improve Cognition in Schizophrenia (MATRICS) battery (Nuechterlein & Green, 2006), a questionnaire that assesses perceiving and understanding emotions together with facilitating thought and managing emotions; and the emotion recognition test, included in the Cambridge Neuropsychological Test Automated Battery. A recently developed test, the Geneva Emotion Recognition Test (Schlegel, Grandjean, & Scherer, 2014), extends prior approaches by using dynamic, multimodal stimulus material that depict a wider range of 14 different emotions. One of the advantages of this test is that it assesses recognition of a broader range of positive-valence emotions—in contrast to a single one (happiness), out of a total of six basic emotions included in most tests.

ToM

The Reading the Mind in the Eyes Test (RMET; Baron-Cohen, Wheelwright, Hill, Raste, & Plumb, 2001) has frequently been used to assess ToM, although the distinction between ToM and emotion recognition/perception when assessed using this measure is unclear. Other tools require subjects to interpret stories such as in the Mental State Attribution Test (Ghiassi, Dimaggio, & Brune, 2010) or the Happe's Strange Stories Test (Happe, 1994). While the first measures first- and second-order ToM, the latter uses stories with ambiguous endings that test the understanding of phenomena such as false beliefs, white lies, jokes, or irony. Another tool is the "The Movie for the Assessment of Social Cognition" (MASC; Dziobek et al., 2006). This task measures mentalizing capacity, social perception, and knowledge by requiring participants to watch short video sequences featuring several actors in social interactions and then to answer questions based on what they have seen. This naturalistic social cognition task has several strengths, including closely mimicking the demands of real life and providing some control items that measure the accuracy of judgments for neutral nonsocial information. Moreover, in addition to providing a quantitative measure of the accuracy of mentalizing, this task allows to assess the quality of the ToM impairment by identifying different types of mentalizing errors (i.e., hypermentalizing errors, such as excessive ToM, or distorted overreading of social cues), hypomentalizing errors (deficient ToM, or underreading of social cues), and errors suggesting a lack of the ability to mentalize (Sharp et al., 2011).

Empathy

Empathy is mostly assessed by self-report questionnaires. Several studies have used the Interpersonal Reactivity Index (Davis, 1983) to assess empathy. This self-report measure quantifies the degree to which one tends to feel empathically concerned (i.e., a general feeling of compassion for those who are helpless or less fortunate) and empathically distressed (i.e., feeling upset when specific negative events happen to others). Another well-established questionnaire is the Empathy Quotient Test by Baron-Cohen and Wheelwright (2004). An empathy test that uses pictures as stimuli is the Multifaceted Empathy Test (MET; Dziobek et al., 2008). It measures both implicit as well as explicit empathy by asking subjects to judge their arousal (implicit) and emphatic concern (explicit) in response to scenes displaying persons experiencing an emotion within a specific context. Additional measurements of the context as well as nonsocial stimuli serve as a control condition to differentiate emphatic responses from phenomena such as a generally increased arousal level.

Social Perception and Knowledge

In contrast to ToM, fewer tools to investigate these functions are available. One may consider the MASC to be a test of social perception which bears a close similarity to the Social Cue Recognition Test (Corrigan & Nelson, 1998) used in schizophrenia research. However, decreased performance is difficult to relate particularly to impairments in social cue perception instead of deficits in emotion or intention recognition. Once again, the overlap between the different constructs of social cognitive domains hampers clear assignments of measurement tools to a specific function. Other tasks are available, such as the Magdeburg Test of Social Intelligence (Baumgarten, Süß, & Weis, 2014), that aim more directly at measuring distinct contributions of social cues and context information to emotion recognition performance. Social schema and knowledge are mostly assessed by questionnaires. In research on personality disorders, one of the most often used questionnaires is the research version of the Early Maladaptive Schema Questionnaire (Ball & Young, 2001; Samuel & Ball, 2013). It measures stable and negative beliefs about oneself, others, or the environment that are assumed to be formed early in life and affect social cognition during subsequent life. It involves 15 subscales such as social isolation, failure, and mistrust.

Attributional Style

"Attribution" refers to how people explain the causes of events. Most models of attribution distinguish three dimensions (e.g., Heider, 1982; Weiner, 1992). "Internality" refers to whether subjects attribute events to themselves or to the environment, while "stability" and "globality" describe whether a subject assumes that the causes are stable or variable over time and situations, respectively. Causal attributions along these three dimensions vary depending on the valence of the events. Attributional styles can be assessed by self-report questionnaire such as the Internal, Personal, and Situational Attributions Questionnaire (Kinderman & Bentall, 1997) or the Attributional Style Questionnaire (Peterson et al., 1982). For further information see Hessling, Anderson, and Russell (2002).

As an alternative approach to study social cognition, exchange games from behavioral economy have been introduced during the last years to measure social cognitive impairments in mental disorders (Kishida, King-Casas, & Montague, 2010; Hasler, 2012; Kishida & Montague, 2012; Sharp, Monterosso, & Montague, 2012). They focus on concepts such as trust, cooperation, and fairness. These paradigms have the advantage to study social cognition directly during social interactions and allow for measuring interaction behavior itself, thereby providing a new perspective in the analyses of social cognitive processes and functioning. Well-established paradigms include the trust game, the ultimatum, and the dictator game. Although these games are often used to measure social interaction between two or more participants, a recent study suggests that behavior observed during such games may not correspond directly to the behavior in everyday life but rather overestimate the frequency of prosocial behavior (Winking & Mizer, 2013) and should therefore be interpreted with caution.

▪ NEUROBIOLOGY OF SOCIAL COGNITION

The Social Brain

Overlapping neural structures and systems subserve social cognitive processes. It is important to note that high-level social cognitive processes, such as mentalizing, require adequate function of more basic cognitive and social cognitive processes. For example, there is robust evidence suggesting that visual attention and eye gaze orientation to social stimuli are required for adequate social cognition. When viewing faces, eye gaze is automatically oriented to the "diagnostic" facial features (i.e., eyes and mouth regions; Adolphs et al., 2005; Benuzzi et al., 2007). This mechanism is crucial for the identification of facial emotions (Kliemann, Dziobek, Hatri, Baudewig, & Heekeren, 2012; Loughland, Williams, & Gordon, 2002a) and more broadly for social cognition (Adolphs et al., 2005). The automatic orienting of eye gaze toward emotionally diagnostic facial features is impaired in patients with amygdala lesions (Adolphs et al., 2005) and across psychiatric disorders (Bertsch et al., 2013; Itier & Batty, 2009). The social gaze orienting network (Adolphs et al., 2005; Benuzzi et al., 2007; Gamer, Zurowski, & Buchel, 2010) includes superior colliculi, thalamus, and striate visual cortex, involved in early perceptual processing of facial stimuli. The posterior amygdala (i.e., basal nucleus) is a key node (Adolphs, 2002).

Primary sensory areas and more specialized structures (e.g., the fusiform face area) are involved in *social perceptual processes* (e.g., Sabatinelli et al., 2011). *Emotion processing* is regulated in part by the amygdala which, in turn, interacts with the insula and with the anterior cingulate cortex and the orbitofrontal cortex (e.g., Meyer-Lindenberg & Tost, 2012). *Social attribution processes* are partly mediated by the ventral premotor cortex, the superior temporal sulcus, the amygdala, and the insula, whereas *ToM abilities* are subserved by the anterior medial prefrontal cortex and the temporoparietal junction (Meyer-Lindenberg & Tost, 2012). In addition to these somewhat distinct features, there are many more common structures and circuits that are involved in each domain of social cognition, and the ways in which these circuits interact are a focus of current research.

■ SOCIAL COGNITION ABNORMALITIES ACROSS PERSONALITY DISORDERS

Social Cognition Abnormalities in Schizotypal Personality Disorder and the Schizophrenia Spectrum

Schizotypal personality disorder (SPD) is a personality disorder that is part of the schizophrenia spectrum. SPD is characterized by attenuated, schizophrenia-like traits and shares many of the genetic, psychophysiological, and neural abnormalities found in schizophrenia (Siever & Davis, 2004).

Although neurocognitive impairment and poor social functioning are core features of schizophrenia, until recently little attention has been paid to the study of social cognition abnormalities in the schizophrenia spectrum (Green et al., 2008). The recent inclusion of a social cognitive domain in the MATRICS (Nuechterlein & Green, 2006)—a neurocognitive battery developed for clinical trials in schizophrenia—supports the importance of social cognition as a key symptom domain to be considered in clinical and research settings. The Cognitive Neuroscience Treatment Research to Improve Cognition in Schizophrenia initiative also has identified social cognition research as one of its priorities (Millan & Bales, 2013).

Patient populations within the schizophrenia spectrum—including SPD (Ripoll et al., 2013) and psychometric schizotypy (Gooding & Pflum, 2011; Pflum, Gooding, & White, 2013; Shean, Bell, & Cameron, 2007)—have social cognitive abnormalities that significantly impair functioning and may cause more disability than psychosis and negative symptoms (Mancuso et al., 2011). Moreover, these social cognitive impairments are independent from broader cognitive deficits (Billeke & Aboitiz, 2013; Harvey & Bowie, 2012; Lee et al., 2005; Montag et al., 2010) and do not respond well to medications (Goldberg et al., 2007; Green, 2006; Harvey & Bowie, 2012; Maat et al., 2014).

Converging multimodal social cognitive data in the schizophrenia spectrum broadly support a deficit model of social/emotional information processing—that is, an insensitivity to social cues (Corrigan & Green, 1993), which might be an endophenotype of the disorder (van 't Wout, van Rijn, Jellema, Kahn, & Aleman, 2009).

According to this model, patients with schizophrenia spectrum disorders have deficient emotional information processing due to lower than normal recruitment of brain regions usually involved in emotion processing—such as the amygdala, fusiform gyrus, basal ganglia, and prefrontal cortex (Li, Chan, McAlonan, & Gong, 2010)—while performing social cognition tasks. Also consistent with this model is the finding of impaired emotional modulation of amygdala reactivity (Pinkham et al., 2011) in patients with schizophrenia.

A hypoactivation in the extended emotion processing networks—the "social brain" (Li et al., 2010)—may result in low attention toward social stimuli, which may be regarded as less salient in patients within the schizophrenia spectrum compared to healthy controls. For example, low recruitment of attention networks when viewing social emotional stimuli may result in abnormal eye gaze patterns—for example, abnormally restricted scanpaths toward emotionally relevant features such as the eyes or the mouth, which are critical areas for recognizing emotions (Loughland et al., 2002a; Loughland, Williams, & Gordon, 2002b; Loughland, Williams, & Harris, 2004). In fact, data suggest that patients with schizophrenia and their unaffected relatives spend less time looking at the eyes and mouth of faces, which correlates with poor performance in emotion recognition tasks (Loughland et al., 2002a, 2002b; Loughland et al., 2004).

These emotion processing deficits in the schizophrenia spectrum result in broad and severe social cognitive impairments at the behavioral level (Kohler, Walker, Martin, Healey, & Moberg, 2010; Abbott & Green, 2012). For example, the impaired processing of basic social cues (Corrigan & Green, 1993)—such as gaze direction and biological motion (van 't Wout et al., 2009)—in schizophrenia spectrum patients likely contributes to poor performance in higher-order social cognitive tasks.

It should be noted that some data suggest that there is some degree of social cognitive heterogeneity in schizophrenia (Montag et al., 2011), which might also exist among schizotypal patients. Indeed, in samples with schizophrenia it has been reported that social cognitive deficits such as hypomentalizing errors are correlated with higher levels of negative symptoms, while positive symptoms correlate with hypermentalizing errors (Montag et al., 2011). This suggests that social cognition in schizophrenia may be deficient (among those with predominantly negative symptoms) or excessive/distorted (among those with predominantly positive symptoms).

While a fast-growing number of studies have examined social cognition in patients with schizophrenia (Pinkham, 2014), few studies have focused on patients with SPD. Interestingly, social cognitive deficits across the schizophrenia spectrum appear to be trait-like and independent from psychosis, as suggested by their correlation with dimensional schizotypy (Fyfe, Williams, Mason, & Pickup, 2008; Gooding & Pflum, 2011; Pflum et al., 2013).

What follows is a brief summary of the few studies that have examined social cognition in patients with SPD, which have found deficits in emotion recognition and understanding of mental states that broadly mimic the ones reported in schizophrenia (Dickey et al., 2011; Dickey et al., 2012; Huang et al., 2013; Mikhailova, Vladimirova, Iznak, Tsusulkovskaya, & Sushko, 1996; Ripoll et al., 2013; Waldeck & Miller, 2000) and are broadly related to those found in autism (Perez-Rodriguez et al., 2014) including decreased emotion recognition (Kohler et al., 2010; Abbott & Green, 2012; Averbeck, Bobin, Evans, & Shergill, 2011; Fischer-Shofty, Shamay-Tsoory, & Levkovitz, 2013; Goldman, Gomes, Carter, & Lee, 2011) and poor mentalizing (Davis et al., 2013; Fischer-Shofty, Brune, et al., 2013; Pedersen et al., 2011) due to hypomentalizing errors (Montag et al., 2011).

Dickey et al. (2011) reported that SPD patients were slower and less accurate in identifying facial emotional expressions. Mikhailova et al. (1996) found poor recognition of sad and happy expressions in depressed patients with SPD. Waldeck and Miller (2000) only found difficulties in labeling positive emotions such as joy. Neural abnormalities in emotion processing networks have also been reported in SPD patients (Huang et al., 2013). Even fewer studies have examined higher-order social cognitive processes such as mentalizing in SPD. We used a naturalistic video task (the empathic accuracy paradigm) to assess the ability to understand emotional mental states of others in patients with SPD. We found that SPD patients had lower accuracy in attributing negative mental states to others, which was correlated with social support (Ripoll et al., 2013).

■ SOCIAL COGNITION ABNORMALITIES IN BORDERLINE PERSONALITY DISORDER

During the last decade, the available data on social cognitive dysfunction in borderline personality disorder (BPD) has increased tremendously (Roepke, Vater, Preissler, Heekeren, & Dziobek, 2013; Herpertz & Bertsch, 2014; Schmahl et al., 2014). However, social cognitive findings in this population are quite heterogeneous. Possible causes include the previously mentioned variability in the tasks used to test different subprocesses of social cognition (see earlier discussion), the heterogeneity of the BPD population, and the characteristic affective instability in BPD, which may confound results of studies assessing patients across different emotional states. Moreover, studies rarely control for other factors including illness severity, age, ethnicity, neurocognition, comorbid disorders, and psychotropic medications (Mitchell et al., 2014). Common comorbid conditions in BPD cover a wide range of disorders involving depression, eating disorders, substance dependence and abuse, as well as posttraumatic stress disorders (Zanarini, Frankenburg, Hennen, Reich, & Silk, 2004; Zanarini, Frankenburg, Vujanovic, et al., 2004). The applied psychotropic medications include, among others, antipsychotics, antidepressants, and benzodiazepines. Both comorbid disorders and psychotropic substances have been shown to influence cognitive and social cognitive functioning, and they may result in partly opposite effects confounding findings on impairments linked to BPD (Lazarus, Cheavens, Festa, & Zachary Rosenthal, 2014). Various modulating factors linked genuinely to BPD such as childhood trauma, suicidality, emotion regulation deficits, rejection sensitivity, and negative mood during testing have been discussed, but further studies have to investigate whether and how these influence different social cognitive functions in BPD and may contribute to heterogeneity of findings.

Emotion Recognition

Most studies on social cognitive dysfunction in BPD have focused on emotion recognition, and several recent reviews have summarized the findings (Lazarus et al., 2014; Mitchell et al., 2014; Dinsdale & Crespi, 2013; Daros et al., 2013). Daros et al. focused in their meta-analysis on findings from multiple-choice emotion recognition tasks presenting neutral faces or prototypic expressions, that is, faces with a high intensity of one of the basic emotions. This analysis revealed reduced accuracy in the recognition of disgust and anger while recognition for sadness, fear, surprise, and happiness was preserved. A special role for anger and disgust may be plausibly derived from BPD psychopathology that describes anger as an often observed reaction in these patients and may link disgust to the perception of social rejection for which BPD patients have been described as particularly sensitive (Staebler, Helbing, Rosenbach, & Renneberg, 2011; Renneberg et al., 2012; Domsalla et al., 2013; Bungert et al., 2015). However, it contradicts studies that suggested a particularly high sensitivity for anger in facial expression with low intensity as well as in ambiguous expressions that were blends of anger with other emotions such as happiness and sadness (Domes et al., 2008). Daros et al. (2013) proposed that this contradiction may be resolved by taking the level of arousal during task -solving into account: assuming a higher level of arousal in BPD patients, they suggest a beneficial effect when identifying low-intensity emotional expressions while the increased arousal level may hamper the recognition of full-intensity faces. So far, this model has still to be confirmed by studies which combine emotion recognition tasks with self-reports and psychophysiological measures of the arousal level.

The most marked impairment in BPD consistently reported across studies is a misinterpretation of neutral faces as showing emotional expressions (Daros et al., 2013; Daros, Uliaszek, & Ruocco, 2014; Unoka, Fogd, Seres, Kéri, & Csukly, 2014); indeed, neutral faces were the most potent distractors in implicit emotion processing tasks (Krause-Utz, Elzinga, et al., 2014). The underlying causes have yet to be clarified. A predominantly emotional processing style as suggested by Mier et al. (2013) may be responsible and agrees with the fact that neutral faces are quite unusual in everyday life and might thus easily induce fear, as it was shown in the still-face paradigm already in toddlers (Tronick, Als, Adamson, Wise, & Brazelton, 1978) as well as in emotion recognition tasks in anxious individuals (Vrana & Gross, 2004). Nevertheless, it has to be investigated whether neutral faces are linked to a misattribution of specific emotions in BPD.

Findings of superior recognition performance for negative emotions in low-intensity facial expressions have led to the assumption of a negativity bias in BPD. This is consistent with the higher rejection sensitivity that is characteristic of BPD, that is, a cognitive-affective disposition that predisposes subjects to anxiously expect, readily perceive, and react more intensely to social rejection as a threat-related event (Downey & Feldman, 1996). Whether a negativity bias is actually due to an increased sensitivity to negative-valence stimuli is still under discussion. Using a visual search task with emotional facial expressions (i.e., finding the face in the crowd paradigm; Hansen & Hansen, 1988) Hagenhoff et al. (2013) found no hypersensitivity for either angry or happy faces but a slowing of detection processes that were particularly pronounced for positive-valence stimuli. Several studies suggest that the experience of positive stimuli is impaired in BPD (Matzke, Herpertz, Berger, Fleischer, & Domes, 2014; Robin et al., 2012; Unoka et al., 2014) and that this is linked to a reduced confidence of the patients in their own judgments (Thome et al., 2015). On the other hand, several studies revealed superior performance when negative emotions have to be recognized (e.g., in morphing tasks; Domes et al., 2008; Herpertz & Bertsch, 2014). In sum, research suggests so far that a combination of hypersensitivity to threat and hyposensitivity for positive emotions may underlie the emotion recognition impairments in BPD. Similar alterations have also been observed in psychophysiological measurement of basal imitation behavior in BPD: Matzke et al. (2014) showed that facial mimicry (i.e., the imitation of the emotional expression of a stimulus face) is stronger in response to negative but attenuated in response to positive facial expressions compared to healthy subjects. Taking into account that social cognitive processing serves the adjustment of behavior during a social interaction, these findings suggest that interpersonal functioning might be hampered in BPD not only by deficits in receiving social cues from social partners but also in sending social signals (see also Roepke et al., 2013) and that this holds true for both negative and positive-valence information.

ToM

Several studies have aimed to investigate the abilities of BPD patients to infer the mental states of others. Some studies used the RMET that has already been discussed to tap primarily emotion recognition processes without relating these to intentions of others, with mixed results. On the one hand, superior performance in terms of a higher accuracy and faster responses in this task has been described in BPD, linked to stronger activation in several cerebral structures such as the amygdala and the medial frontal gyrus (Fertuck et al., 2009; Frick et al., 2012). Several studies failed to find alterations in RMET performance in BPD (Preissler, Dziobek, Ritter, Heekeren, & Roepke, 2010; Schilling et al., 2012). Based on their findings, Unoka et al. (2014) proposed that altered RMET performance in BPD may result from two independent mechanisms that affect performance in a distinguishable manner: comorbid depression enhanced performance for negative stimuli, while maladaptive schemas were linked to impairments in recognizing positive and neutral stimuli. These findings emphasize that an understanding of social cognitive function in BPD requires disentangling improved, impaired, and unaffected subfunctions involved in solving a specific task and analyzing which of these are linked to specific features of this heterogenous disorder.

Alternative approaches to investigate ToM in BPD aimed at differentiating impairments in cognitive and affective ToM. While applying the Happe Test, BPD patients performed better in affective ToM (Arntz, Bernstein, Oorschot, & Schobre, 2009; Harari, Shamay-Tsoory, Ravid, & Levkovitz, 2010) compared to healthy participants. In contrast, findings on cognitive ToM (i.e., the ability to infer other people's beliefs) were more inconsistent in these studies, revealing both superior as well as impaired performance. Using cartoon picture stories, Ghiassi et al. (2010) found no alterations of ToM in BPD. However, maternal punishment, rejection, and separation were linked to reduced ToM in the BPD group.

The MASC—a naturalistic social cognition task—allows elucidation of the type of ToM errors that characterize BPD patients. Interestingly, rather than lacking the ability to mentalize, BPD patients often make mentalizing errors due to using unusual ToM strategies, characterized by excessive and distorted overreading of social cues—termed hypermentalizing (Sharp et al., 2013; Sharp et al., 2011). These findings have been supported by a recent functional magnetic resonance imaging (fMRI) study on effects of social rejection in BPD (Domsalla et al., 2013). While playing a ball-tossing game with a virtual partner, brain imaging data suggest a lack in the disengagement of structures of the "social brain" when the behavior of the players was determined by predefined rules of the game in contrast to situations during which the behavior of the co-players reflected their intentions.

Several studies have addressed ToM using exchange games such as the trust game or the ultimatum game (for a review, see Lis & Bohus, 2013; see also Jeung, Schwieren, & Herpertz, 2016; Lis & Kirsch, 2016). In order to maximize the gain during such games, subjects have to infer the intentions of their partners to adjust their stakes depending on the anticipated behavior of the co-player. The study that received the most attention was done by King-Casas et al. (2008). During a multiround trust game, the cooperation between partners failed when BPD patients participated as trustees in these dyadic interactions. The authors explained this by alterations in BPD patients' understanding of social norms during the perception of social signals. Moreover, BPD patients showed a lack of modulation of insula activation in response to the varying fairness of the investors' offers as was observed in the healthy subjects. So far, alterations in understanding of social norms have not been confirmed in BPD by subsequent studies. In contrast, both findings of Wischniewski and Brüne (2013) as well as Franzen et al. (2011) suggest that at least social judgments of fairness of others in social exchange games are comparable in BPD patients and healthy subjects. For example,

Wischniewski and Brüne (2013) used a variation of the dictator game during which the participants took the role of a third party to study "costly punishment" in BPD. While observing the exchange between two other players, subjects could punish unfair offers of the proposer at their own cost; that is, they could invest a specific amount of their own monetary units to cause a reduction of comparable size of the account of the proposer. They found no altered punishment behavior in these patients, suggesting the application of similar social norms. However, the extent of punishment was related in BPD patients and healthy controls to different dimensions of personality traits such as extraversion, neuroticism, openness, and agreeableness, suggesting different motivations for a similar behavior. One may argue that the patients were not part of these interactions and social norms may only be altered in case of self-related expectations (i.e., BPD patients may expect unfair behavior of others). However, when BPD patients had to judge the amount of a repayment received from their trustee during a trust game, no differences were detected in the experience of the partner's fairness between patients and healthy subjects (Franzen et al., 2011).

Exchange games with virtual partners allow for experimental manipulating of specific features of the co-players behaviors to directly investigate their effects on interaction behavior. When social emotional cues were available to infer the intentions of a co-player during interaction, emotional facial expressions have been shown to differentially affect interaction behavior in BPD patients and healthy controls (Franzen et al., 2011; Polgár, Fogd, Unoka, Sirály, & Csukly, 2014). These findings suggest that BPD patients differ in the manner in which they integrate emotional recognition with other social-cognitive processes, and this seems to result in altered use of social emotional signals to guide their interaction behavior. It should be noted that BPD patients are not incapable of using information regarding others' emotional states—inferred from facial expressions—to guide their behavior. Rather, findings suggest that emotional cues have less impact on social decision-making in BPD patients compared to healthy individuals.

Empathy

Studies that used self-report questionnaires and experimental approaches found impaired cognitive empathy but intact or superior affective empathy in BPD (Guttman & Laporte, 2000; Harari et al., 2010; New et al., 2012; see also Jeung & Herpertz, 2014). In contrast, applying the MET, Dziobek et al. (2011) found both cognitive and affective empathy to be dysfunctional in BPD and linked these impairments to alteration of cerebral activation of the superior temporal sulcus and gyrus during cognitive empathy and of the insula during emotional empathy. This profile differs from that described for other personality disorders, for example narcisistic personality disorder with deficits in affective but not cognitive empathy (Ritter et al., 2011).

Social Perception and Knowledge

Maladaptive social schemas assessed by questionnaires have been observed in several studies in BPD. BPD has been linked particularly to schemas of disconnection and rejection as well as of impaired autonomy and performance (e.g., Butler, Brown, Beck, & Grisham, 2002; Jovev & Jackson, 2004; Nordahl & Nysæter, 2005). Nevertheless, some findings suggest that other dysfunctional beliefs are similarly present in BPD patients (Arntz, Dietzel, & Dreessen, 1999). This agrees with data of a recent study in adolescent BPD patients pointing to higher scores in most maladaptive schema domains and the lack of a specific pattern (Lawrence, Allen, & Chanen, 2011). The authors emphasize that both diagnostic criteria and schema profiles were unrelated to each other and both were highly heterogeneous. Early maladaptive schemas have been related to reduced emotion recognition abilities in BPD: A prevalence of schemas in the domain of "impaired autonomy and performance" and "overvigilance and inhibition" were linked with deficits in the recognition of positive emotional states in the eye region of a face (Unoka et al., 2014), pointing to a link between alterations in social emotional perception and social knowledge. An indirect hint to alterations in understanding of social norms comes from a study by Baron-Cohen et al. (2001). They applied an interview to assess social functioning in different domains of social life and found increased "domain disorganization" in BPD, that is, a lack of demarcation of behaviors and emotional expression between social domains, suggesting that the understanding of social roles may be less differentiated in BPD. Similarly, an electrophysiological study by Gutz, Renneberg, Roepke, and Niedeggen (2015) has found that cues of social inclusion during an inclusion condition of a virtual ball-tossing game evoke a large P300-deflection in BPD patients but not in healthy subjects. This may be interpreted as an alteration of social knowledge in BPD, that is, altered expectations in regard to the behavior of partners in a specific interaction context.

Attributional Style

In contrast to studies on emotion recognition and ToM, findings regarding attributional style in BPD are sparse. Moritz, Schilling, Wingenfeld, Kother, and Wittekind (2011) found a predominantly internal attribution style with the Internal, Personal and Situational Attributions Questionnaire (Kinderman & Bentall, 1997) that was observed for both positive and negative events. This effect was not modulated by depressive symptoms and may point to a generalized overemphasizing of the relevance of the self in BPD. A study by Winter et al. (2015) found a more stable and global attributional style in BPD linked with a stronger attribution of negative events to the self and positive events to external causes. This dysfunctional attributional style was linked to alterations in self-referential processing in the manner of a devaluation of the self. Further studies have to investigate how alterations of the attributional style may be related to impairments in more basal cognitive and social cognitive processes such as alterations of the self-image as one of the *Diagnostic and Statistical Manual of Mental Disorders* (5th ed. [*DSM-V*]) diagnostic criteria for BPD (Winter, Bohus, & Lis, 2017).

Finally, it has to be mentioned that alterations in social cognitive function have been linked to alterations in various neural structures (for reviews, see Krause-Utz, Elzinga, et al., 2014; Krause-Utz, Winter, Niedtfeld, & Schmahl, 2014; O'Neill & Frodl, 2012; Ruocco, Amirthavasagam, & Zakzanis, 2012; Stone, 2014). Among the most often replicated findings is a hyperactivation of the amygdala that has been linked to emotional processing particularly of negative valenced social information (Hazlett et al., 2012). Although many studies support the assumption of alterations in fronto-limbic networks and their association with emotion processing and regulatory control processes in BPD, further studies have to clarify the exact contribution of theses alterations to social functioning in BPD.

Broadly, most of the data on social cognition in BPD patients—briefly reviewed—support a complex pattern of alterations in different domains of social cognition which is opposed to a deficit model that characterizes the schizophrenia spectrum. Findings suggest that a hypersensitivity to negative emotions goes along with a hyposensitivity to positive social cues. This might explain why, on the one hand, BPD patients outperform healthy controls in some social cognition tasks, but on the other hand, BPD results in a distortion of the evaluation of social relations, a lack in belonging, and feelings of loneliness. An overattribution of meaning to interpersonal encounters as suggested by findings of hypermentalizing attributes an excessive salience to social emotional stimuli with a higher than normal recruitment of emotion processing brain networks, resulting in excessive emotional reactions and attention toward social stimuli.

Although it is very likely that social cognitive impairments are implicated in decreased social functioning in BPD, the direct connection between social cognition and psychosocial outcomes has rarely been tested. Nevertheless, it is clear that social cognitive functioning is altered in patients with BPD and constitutes a promising target for cognitive remediation and psychotherapeutical interventions.

■ SOCIAL COGNITION ABNORMALITIES IN OTHER PERSONALITY DISORDERS

Avoidant Personality Disorder

Avoidant personality disorder (AvPD) is characterized by severe deficits in interpersonal relationships that cause significant disability (Grant et al., 2004) and are associated with receiving public assistance. This may be related to their avoidance of occupational activities requiring social contact (Vaughn et al., 2010).

AvPD and social phobia/social anxiety are highly comorbid and share many overlapping features, including risk factors, neurobiology, and genetic underpinnings. This has led some to hypothesize that AvPD and social phobia may be a single entity or reflect a spectrum of social anxiety. Due to the lack of evidence for treatment outcomes in AvPD, treatment strategies developed for social anxiety/social phobia are usually extrapolated to treat AvPD. These include medications such as antidepressants or anxiolytics (Herpertz et al., 2007; Ripoll, Triebwasser, & Siever, 2011)—none of which specifically target the core social cognitive dysfunctions—and cognitive-behavioral therapy including exposure and social skills training (Emmelkamp et al., 2006).

At the neural level, the social anxiety spectrum is characterized by exaggerated amygdala reactivity to social emotional stimuli—particularly fear-related stimuli—and abnormal connectivity patterns within the neural networks subserving social threat processing and emotion regulation—including the amygdala, the medial prefrontal cortex, the insula, and the cingulate cortex, among other areas (Gorka et al., 2015; Marazziti et al., 2015).

Antisocial Personality Disorder

Individuals with antisocial personality disorder (Dolan & Fullam, 2004) appear to only show subtle social cognitive abnormalities. Key deficits are mostly related to the lack of empathic concern regarding the impact of their actions (Rice & Derish, 2014). Studies demonstrate only subtle impairment in emotion recognition and social perception, manifested for example as difficulty appreciating fearful vocal affect (Blair, Budhani, Colledge, & Scott, 2005) and posture (Munoz, 2009).

This finding is consistent with fMRI studies describing reduced amygdala reactivity to fearful facial expressions (Marsh & Blair, 2008; Jones, Laurens, Herba, Barker, & Vilding, 2009). This hypothetical "fear blindness" could interfere with socialization and contribute to the development of antisocial behaviors (van Zwieten et al., 2013), although causality cannot be established, as individuals with antisocial tendencies are also less likely to develop and employ social cognitive skills to decipher the internal states of others (Stellwagen & Kerig, 2013).

■ **PSYCHOTHERAPEUTICAL APPROACHES**

Social cognitive deficits have been recognized as influential for the overall outcome of mental disorders. Most psychotherapeutic approaches tailored to specific personality disorders comprise modules that aim at improving social cognitive functioning. Examples are dialectical behavior therapy, mentalization-based therapy, or schema-focused therapy in BPD. Results of prospective studies have revealed high remission rates (e.g., for BPD; Zanarini, Frankenburger, Reich, & Fitzmaurice, 2012). Nevertheless, findings indicate persistent serious social problems in, for example, up to 50% of treated BPD clients (see Lis & Bohus, 2013). There has been increased investment in the development of training interventions during the past few years that target specifically social cognitive functions. The available approaches have primarily been designed for individuals suffering from schizophrenia, providing the first promising data on the effectiveness of these trainings (see Kurtz & Richardson, 2012; Statucka & Walder, 2013). Nevertheless, most of the available programs, such as the social cognition and interaction training (Penn, Roberts, Combs, & Sterne, 2007), are group-based and are time- and effort-intensive in nature. Computer-assisted trainings may complement these attempts by allowing for a more cost-efficient way of practicing social cognitive functions. In contrast to software that has been designed to improve cognitive functions, only a few computer-based trainings exist for improving social cognition. These focus on cognitive processes with social emotional stimuli (e.g., www.brainhq.com, which provides modules to train perception for and memory of facial stimuli via matching tasks), or on single circumscribed functions such as affect control during emotional working memory tasks (Schweizer, Grahn, Hampshire, Mobbs, & Dalgleish, 2013). Although there is still a lack in computer-assisted trainings that more specifically target those social cognitive processes linked to personality disorders, first findings suggest that they may constitute useful tools to improve functioning in this domain.

■ **CONCLUSION AND FUTURE DIRECTIONS**

During the past few decades, empirical research on social cognition in personality disorders has dramatically advanced our understanding of the pathophysiology of the severe social dysfunction that characterizes personality disorders. Nevertheless, research in this area is still young, and many questions have to be answered to allow the widespread clinical application of social cognitive enhancement interventions.

Elucidating the neurobiological underpinnings of social cognition is particularly important since social dysfunctions have been shown to be rather persistent and not sufficiently addressed by conventional treatment approaches.

Future studies should compare refined phenotypes and intermediate phenotypes within the personality disorders. These "biomarkers" and more homogeneous subgroups of patients may more closely reflect neurobiological factors compared to the broad, heterogeneous categorical personality disorders. For example, BPD has a very high clinical heterogeneity. With nine *DSM-IV* criteria and a threshold of five positive criteria for a diagnosis of BPD, there are 151 theoretically possible ways of diagnosing this disorder. To refine the group of studied patients, it may be useful to perform studies on personality-disordered patients matched for a clinical dimension such as social cognition impairment, which represents a dimension consistent with the RDoC initiative. The development of standardized measures and batteries of social cognition is necessary to allow for comparison of data across studies. The relationship between changes in social cognitive measures and social and interpersonal functioning in the real world also needs to be established.

■ **REFERENCES**

Abbott, G. R., & Green, M. J. (2012). Facial affect recognition and schizotypal personality characteristics. *Early Interv Psychiatry, 7*(1). doi:10.1111/j.1751-7893.2012.00346.x

Adolphs, R. (2002). Recognizing emotion from facial expressions: psychological and neurological mechanisms. *Behav Cogn Neurosci Rev, 1*(1), 21–62.

Adolphs, R., Gosselin, F., Buchanan, T. W., Tranel, D., Schyns, P., & Damasio, A. R. (2005). A mechanism for impaired fear recognition after amygdala damage. *Nature, 433*(7021), 68–72. doi:10.1038/nature03086

American Psychiatric Association. (1994). *Diagnostic and statistical manual of mental disorders* (4th ed.). Washington, DC: American Psychiatric Association.

American Psychiatric Association. (2013). *Diagnostic and statistical manual of mental disorders* (5th ed.). Washington, DC: American Psychiatric Association.

Arntz, A., Bernstein, D., Oorschot, M., & Schobre, P. (2009). Theory of mind in borderline and cluster-C personality disorder. *J Nerv Ment Dis, 197*(11), 801–807. doi:10.1097/NMD.0b013e3181be78fb

Arntz, A., Dietzel, R., & Dreessen, L. (1999). Assumptions in borderline personality disorder: specificity, stability and relationship with etiological factors. *Behav Res Ther, 37*(6), 545–557. doi:10.1016/S0005-7967(98)00152-1

Averbeck, B. B., Bobin, T., Evans, S., & Shergill, S. S. (2011). Emotion recognition and oxytocin in patients with schizophrenia. *Psychol Med*, 1–8. doi:10.1017/s0033291711001413

Bakermans-Kranenburg, M. J., & van IJzendoorn, M. H. (2013). Sniffing around oxytocin: review and meta-analyses of trials in healthy and clinical groups with implications for pharmacotherapy. *Transl Psychiatry, 3*, e258. doi:10.1038/tp.2013.34

Ball, S. A., & Young, J. (2001). *Early maladaptive schemas questionnaire—research.* Unpublished test. Yale University School of Medicine, New Haven, CT.

Baron-Cohen, S., & Wheelwright, S. (2004). The empathy quotient: an investigation of adults with Asperger syndrome or high functioning autism, and normal sex differences. *J Autism Dev Disord, 34*(2), 163–175.

Baron-Cohen, S., Wheelwright, S., Hill, J., Raste, Y., & Plumb, I. (2001). The "Reading the Mind in the Eyes" Test revised version: a study with normal adults, and adults with Asperger syndrome or high-functioning autism. *J Child Psychol Psychiatry, 42*(2), 241–251.

Baumert, A., Schlösser, T., & Schmitt, M. (2014). Economic games. a performance-based assessment of fairness and altruism. *Eur J Psychol Assess, 30*(3), 178–192.

Baumgarten, M., Süß, H.-M., & Weis, S. (2014). The cue is the key: the relevance of cue and context information in social understanding tasks of the Magdeburg Test of Social Intelligence. *Eur J Psychol Assess, 31*(1), 38–44. doi:10.1027/1015-5759/a000204

Benuzzi, F., Pugnaghi, M., Meletti, S., Lui, F., Serafini, M., Baraldi, P., & Nichelli, P. (2007). Processing the socially relevant parts of faces. *Brain Res Bull, 74*(5), 344–356. doi:10.1016/j.brainresbull.2007.07.010

Bertsch, K., Gamer, M., Schmidt, B., Schmidinger, I., & Herpertz, S. (2012). *Effects of intranasal oxytocin administration on face processing in borderline personality disorder.* Paper presented at the ESSPD meeting.

Bertsch, K., Gamer, M., Schmidt, B., Schmidinger, I., Walther, S., Kastel, T., . . . Herpertz, S. C. (2013). Oxytocin and reduction of social threat hypersensitivity in women with borderline personality disorder. *Am J Psychiatry, 170*(10), 1169–1177. doi:10.1176/appi.ajp.2013.13020263

Billeke, P., & Aboitiz, F. (2013). Social cognition in schizophrenia: from social stimuli processing to social engagement. *Front Psychiatry, 4*, 4. doi:10.3389/fpsyt.2013.00004

Blair, R. J. R., Budhani, S., Colledge, E., & Scott, S. (2005). Deafness to fear in boys with psychopathic tendencies. *J Child Psychol Psychiatry, 46*(3), 327–336. doi:10.1111/j.1469-7610.2004.00356.x

Blair, R. J., & Mitchell, D. G. (2009). Psychopathy, attention and emotion. *Psychol Med, 39*(4), 543–555. doi:10.1017/s0033291708003991

Brune, M., Abdel-Hamid, M., Lehmkamper, C., & Sonntag, C. (2007). Mental state attribution, neurocognitive functioning, and psychopathology: what predicts poor social competence in schizophrenia best? *Schizophr Res, 92*(1–3), 151–159. doi:S0920-9964(07)00058-8 [pii]10.1016/j.schres.2007.01.006

Bungert, M., Liebke, L., Thome, J., Haeussler, K., Bohus, M., & Lis, S. (2015). Rejection sensitivity and symptom severity in patients with borderline personality disorder: effects of childhood maltreatment and self-esteem. *Borderline Personal Disord Emot Dysregul, 2*, 4. doi:10.1186/s40479-015-0025-x

Butler, A. C., Brown, G. K., Beck, A. T., & Grisham, J. R. (2002). Assessment of dysfunctional beliefs in borderline personality disorder. *Behav Res Ther, 40*(10), doi:10.1016/S0005-7967(02)00031-1

Corrigan, P. W., & Green, M. F. (1993). Schizophrenic patients' sensitivity to social cues: the role of abstraction. *Am J Psychiatry, 150*(4), 589–594.

Corrigan, P. W., & Nelson, D. R. (1998). Factors that affect social cue recognition in schizophrenia. *Psychiatry Res, 78*(3), 189–196.

Couture, S. M., Penn, D. L., & Roberts, D. L. (2006). The functional significance of social cognition in schizophrenia: a review. *Schizophr Bull, 32*(Suppl 1), S44–S63. doi:10.1093/schbul/sbl029

Crick, N. R., & Dodge, K. A. (1994). A review and reformulation of social information-processing mechanisms in children's social adjustment. *Psychol Bull, 115*, 74–101. doi:http://dx.doi.org/10.1037/0033-2909.115.1.74

Cusi, A. M., Nazarov, A., Macqueen, G. M., & McKinnon, M. C. (2013). Theory of mind deficits in patients with mild symptoms of major depressive disorder. *Psychiatry Res, 210*(2), 672–674. doi:10.1016/j.psychres.2013.06.018

Daros, A. R., Uliaszek, A. A., & Ruocco, A. C. P. (2014). Perceptual biases in facial emotion recognition in borderline personality disorder. *PD: TRT, 5*(1), 79-84.

Daros, A. R., Zakzanis, K. K., & Ruocco, A. C. (2013). Facial emotion recognition in borderline personality disorder. *Psychol Med, 43*(9), 1953–1963. doi:10.1017/S0033291712002607

Davis, M. C., Lee, J., Horan, W. P., Clarke, A. D., McGee, M. R., Green, M. F., & Marder, S. R. (2013). Effects of single dose intranasal oxytocin on social cognition in schizophrenia. *Schizophr Res, 147*(2–3), 393–397. doi:10.1016/j.schres.2013.04.023

Davis, M. H. (1983). Measuring individual differences in empathy: evidence for a multidimensional approach. *J Pers Soc Psychol, 44*, 113–126.

Decety, J., & Jackson, P. L. (2004). The functional architecture of human empathy. *Behav Cogn Neurosci Rev, 3*(2), 71–100. doi:10.1177/1534582304267187

Dickey, C. C., Panych, L. P., Voglmaier, M. M., Niznikiewicz, M. A., Terry, D. P., Murphy, C., . . . McCarley, R. W. (2011). Facial emotion recognition and facial affect display in schizotypal personality disorder. *Schizophr Res, 131*(1–3), 242–249. doi:10.1016/j.schres.2011.04.020

Dickey, C. C., Vu, M. A., Voglmaier, M. M., Niznikiewicz, M. A., McCarley, R. W., & Panych, L. P. (2012). Prosodic abnormalities in schizotypal personality disorder. *Schizophr Res, 142*(1–3), 20–30. doi:10.1016/j.schres.2012.09.006

Dinsdale, N., & Crespi, B. J. (2013). The borderline empathy paradox: evidence and conceptual models for empathic enhancements in borderline personality disorder. *J Pers Disord, 27*(2), 172–195. doi:10.1521/pedi.2013.27.2.172

Dolan, M., & Fullam, R. (2004). Theory of mind and mentalizing ability in antisocial personality disorders with and without psychopathy. *Psychol Med 34*(6), 1093–1102. doi:10.1017/S0033291704002028

Domes, G., Czieschnek, D., Weidler, F., Berger, C., Fast, K., & Herpertz, S. C. (2008). Recognition of facial affect in borderline personality disorder. *J Pers Disord, 22*, 135–147. doi:10.1521/pedi.2008.22.2.135

Domsalla, M., Koppe, G., Niedtfeld, I., Vollstädt-Klein, S., Schmahl, C., Bohus, M., & Lis, S. (2013). Cerebral processing of social rejection in patients with borderline personality disorder. *Soc Cogn Affect Neurosci, 9*(11), 1789–1797. doi:10.1093/scan/nst176

Doop, M. L., & Park, S. (2009). Facial expression and face orientation processing in schizophrenia. *Psychiatry Res, 170*(2–3), 103–107. doi:S0165-1781(09)00218-2 [pii]10.1016/j.psychres.2009.06.009

Downey, G., & Feldman, S. I. (1996). Implications of rejection sensitivity for intimate relationships. *J Pers Soc Psychol, 70*(6), 1327–1343.

Dziobek, I., Fleck, S., Kalbe, E., Rogers, K., Hassenstab, J., Brand, M., . . . Convit, A. (2006). Introducing MASC: a movie for the assessment of social cognition. *J Autism Dev Disord, 36*(5), 623–636. doi:10.1007/s10803-006-0107-0

Dziobek, I., Preissler, S., Grozdanovic, Z., Heuser, I., Heekeren, H. R., & Roepke, S. (2011). Neuronal correlates of altered empathy and social cognition in borderline personality disorder. *Neuroimage 57*(2), 539–548. doi:10.1016/j.neuroimage.2011.05.005

Dziobek, I., Rogers, K., Fleck, S., Bahnemann, M., Heekeren, H. R., Wolf, O. T., & Convit, A. (2008). Dissociation of cognitive and emotional empathy in adults with Asperger syndrome using the Multifaceted Empathy Test (MET). *J Autism Dev Disord, 38*(3), 464–473. doi:10.1007/s10803-007-0486-x

Eisenberg, N., & Miller, P. A. (1987). The relation of empathy to prosocial and related behaviors. *Psychol Bull, 101*(1), 91–119.

Emmelkamp, P. M., Benner, A., Kuipers, A., Feiertag, G. A., Koster, H. C., & van Apeldoorn, F. J. (2006). Comparison of brief dynamic and cognitive-behavioural therapies in avoidant personality disorder. *Br J Psychiatry, 189*, 60–64. doi:10.1192/bjp.bp.105.012153

Erwin, R. J., Gur, R. C., Gur, R. E., Skolnick, B., Mawhinney-Hee, M., & Smailis, J. (1992). Facial emotion discrimination: I. Task construction and behavioral findings in normal subjects. *Psychiatry Res, 42*(3), 231–240.

Fertuck, E. A., Jekal, A., Song, I., Wyman, B., Morris, M. C., Wilson, S. T., . . . Stanley, B. (2009). Enhanced "Reading the Mind in the Eyes" in borderline personality disorder compared to healthy controls. *Psychol Med, 39*(12), 1979–1988. doi:10.1017/S003329170900600X

Fischer-Shofty, M., Brune, M., Ebert, A., Shefet, D., Levkovitz, Y., & Shamay-Tsoory, S. G. (2013). Improving social perception in schizophrenia: the role of oxytocin. *Schizophr Res, 146*(1–3), 357–362. doi:10.1016/j.schres.2013.01.006

Fischer-Shofty, M., Shamay-Tsoory, S. G., & Levkovitz, Y. (2013). Characterization of the effects of oxytocin on fear recognition in patients with schizophrenia and in healthy controls. *Front Neurosci, 7*, 127. doi:10.3389/fnins.2013.00127

Franzen, N., Hagenhoff, M., Baer, N., Schmidt, A., Mier, D., Sammer, G., . . . Lis, S. (2011). Superior "theory of mind" in borderline personality disorder: an analysis of interaction behavior in a virtual trust game. *Psychiatry Res, 187*(1-2), 224–233. doi:10.1016/j.psychres.2010.11.012

Frick, C., Lang, S., Kotchoubey, B., Sieswerda, S., Dinu-Biringer, R., Berger, M., . . . Barnow, S. (2012). Hypersensitivity in borderline personality disorder during mindreading. *PLoS One, 7*(8), e41650. doi:10.1371/journal.pone.0041650

Frith, C. D. (2008). Social cognition. *Philos Trans R Soc Lond B Biol Sci, 363*(1499), 2033–2039. doi:10.1098/rstb.2008.0005

Fyfe, S., Williams, C., Mason, O. J., & Pickup, G. J. (2008). Apophenia, theory of mind and schizotypy: perceiving meaning and intentionality in randomness. *Cortex, 44*(10), 1316–1325. doi:10.1016/j.cortex.2007.07.009

Gamer, M., Zurowski, B., & Buchel, C. (2010). Different amygdala subregions mediate valence-related and attentional effects of oxytocin in humans. *Proc Natl Acad Sci U S A, 107*(20), 9400–9405. doi:10.1073/pnas.1000985107

Gawronski, B., & Bodenhausen, G. V. (2014). Social-cognitive theories. In B. Gawronski & G. V. Bodenhausen (Eds.), *Theory and explanation in social psychology* (pp. 65–83). New York: Guilford Press.

Ghiassi, V., Dimaggio, G., & Brune, M. (2010). Dysfunctions in understanding other minds in borderline personality disorder: a study using cartoon picture stories. *Psychother Res, 20*(6), 657–667. doi:10.1080/10503307.2010.501040

Goldberg, T. E., Goldman, R. S., Burdick, K. E., Malhotra, A. K., Lencz, T., Patel, R. C., . . . Robinson, D. G. (2007). Cognitive improvement after treatment with second-generation antipsychotic medications in first-episode schizophrenia: is it a practice effect? *Arch Gen Psychiatry, 64*(10), 1115–1122. doi:10.1001/archpsyc.64.10.1115

Goldman, M. B., Gomes, A. M., Carter, C. S., & Lee, R. (2011). Divergent effects of two different doses of intranasal oxytocin on facial affect discrimination in schizophrenic patients with and without polydipsia. *Psychopharmacology, 216*(1), 101–110. doi:10.1007/s00213-011-2193-8

Gooding, D. C., & Pflum, M. J. (2011). Theory of mind and psychometric schizotypy. *Psychiatry Res, 188*(2), 217–223. doi:10.1016/j.psychres.2011.04.029

Gorka, S. M., Fitzgerald, D. A., Labuschagne, I., Hosanagar, A., Wood, A. G., Nathan, P. J., . . . Dodhia, S. (2015). Oxytocin modulation of amygdala functional connectivity to fearful faces in generalized social anxiety disorder. *Neuropsychopharmacology 40*(2), 278–286.

Grant, B. F., Hasin, D. S., Stinson, F. S., Dawson, D. A., Chou, S. P., Ruan, W. J., & Pickering, R. P. (2004). Prevalence, correlates, and disability of personality disorders in the United States: results from the national epidemiologic survey on alcohol and related conditions. *J Clin Psychiatry, 65*(7), 948–958.

Green, M. F. (2006). Cognitive impairment and functional outcome in schizophrenia and bipolar disorder. *J Clin Psychiatry*, *67*(10), e12.

Green, M. F., Penn, D. l., Bentall, R. F., Carpenter, W. T., Gaebel, W., Gur, R. C., . . . Heinssen, R. (2008). Social cognition in schizophrenia: an NIMH workshop on definitions, assessment, and research opportunities. *Schizophr Bull*, *34*(6), 1211–1220.

Gumley, A., Braehler, C., & Macbeth, A. (2014). A meta-analysis and theoretical critique of oxytocin and psychosis: prospects for attachment and compassion in promoting recovery. *Br J Clin Psychol*, *53*(1), 42–61. doi:10.1111/bjc.12041

Guttman, H. A., & Laporte, L. (2000). Empathy in families of women with borderline personality disorder, anorexia nervosa, and a control group. *Fam Process*, *39*(3), 345–358. doi:10.1111/j.1545-5300.2000.39306.x

Gutz, L., Renneberg, B., Roepke, S., & Niedeggen, M. (2015). Neural processing of social participation in borderline personality disorder and social anxiety disorder. *J Abnorm Psychol*, *124*, 421–431. doi:10.1037/a0038614

Hagenhoff, M., Franzen, N., Gerstner, L., Koppe, G., Sammer, G., Netter, P., . . . Lis, S. (2013). Reduced sensitivity to emotional facial expressions in borderline personality disorder: effects of emotional valence and intensity. *J Pers Disord*, *27*(1), 19–35. doi:10.1521/pedi.2013.27.1.19

Hansen, C. H., & Hansen, R. D. (1988). Finding the face in the crowd: an anger superiority effect. *J Pers Soc Psychol*, *54*(6), 917–924.

Happe, F. G. E. (1994). An advanced test of theory of mind: understanding of story characters' thoughts and feelings by able autistic, mentally handicapped, and normal children and adults. *J Autism Dev Disord*, *24*(2), 129–154.

Harari, H., Shamay-Tsoory, S. G., Ravid, M., & Levkovitz, Y. (2010). Double dissociation between cognitive and affective empathy in borderline personality disorder. *Psychiatry Res*, *175*(3), 277–279. doi:10.1016/j.psychres.2009.03.002

Harvey, P. D., & Bowie, C. R. (2012). Cognitive enhancement in schizophrenia: pharmacological and cognitive remediation approaches. *Psychiatr Clin North Am*, *35*(3), 683–698. doi:10.1016/j.psc.2012.06.008

Hasler, G. (2012). Can the neuroeconomics revolution revolutionize psychiatry? *Neurosci Biobehav Rev*, *36*(1), 64–78. doi:10.1016/j.neubiorev.2011.04.011

Hazlett, E. A., Zhang, J., New, A. S., Zelmanova, Y., Goldstein, K. E., Haznedar, M. M., . . . Chu, K. W. (2012). Potentiated amygdala response to repeated emotional pictures in borderline personality disorder. *Biol Psychiatry*, *72*(6), 448–456. doi:10.1016/j.biopsych.2012.03.027

Heider, F. (1982). *The psychology of interpersonal relations*. Hillsdale, NJ: Lawrence Erlbaum Associates.

Herpertz, S. C., & Bertsch, K. (2014). The social-cognitive basis of personality disorders. *Curr Opin Psychiatry*, *27*(1), 73–77. doi:10.1097/YCO.0000000000000026

Herpertz, S. C., Zanarini, M., Schulz, C. S., Siever, L., Lieb, K., & Moller, H. J. (2007). World Federation of Societies of Biological Psychiatry (WFSBP) guidelines for biological treatment of personality disorders. *World J Biol Psychiatry*, *8*(4), 212–244. doi:10.1080/15622970701685224

Herpertz, S., Lischke, A., Berger, C., & Gamer, M. (2012). *Effects of oxytocin on emotional processing in borderline personality disorder* [Abstract]. 2nd International Congress on Borderline Personality Disorder and Allied Disorders.

Hessling, R. M., Anderson, C. A., & Russell, D. W. (2002). Attributional style. In R. Fernandez-Ballesteros (Ed.), *Encyclopedia of psychological assessment* (pp. 116–120). London: SAGE.

Hooker, C. I., Bruce, L., Fisher, M., Verosky, S. C., Miyakawa, A., & Vinogradov, S. (2012). Neural activity during emotion recognition after combined cognitive plus social cognitive training in schizophrenia. *Schizophr Res, 139*(1-3), 53–59. doi:10.1016/j.schres.2012.05.009

Hooker, C., & Park, S. (2002). Emotion processing and its relationship to social functioning in schizophrenia patients. *Psychiatry Res, 112*(1), 41–50. doi:S0165178102001774 [pii]

Huang, J., Wang, Y., Jin, Z., Di, X., Yang, T., Gur, R. C., . . . Chan, R. C. (2013). Happy facial expression processing with different social interaction cues: an fMRI study of individuals with schizotypal personality traits. *Prog Neuropsychopharmacol Biol Psychiatry, 44*, 108–117. doi:10.1016/j.pnpbp.2013.02.004

Inoue, Y., Tonooka, Y., Yamada, K., & Kanba, S. (2004). Deficiency of theory of mind in patients with remitted mood disorder. *J Affect Disord, 82*(3), 403–409. doi:10.1016/j.jad.2004.04.004

Insel, T., Cuthbert, B., Garvey, M., Heinssen, R., Pine, D. S., Quinn, K., . . . Wang, P. (2010). Research domain criteria (RDoC): toward a new classification framework for research on mental disorders. *Am J Psychiatry, 167*(7), 748–751. doi:167/7/748 [pii]10.1176/appi.ajp.2010.09091379

Itier, R. J., & Batty, M. (2009). Neural bases of eye and gaze processing: the core of social cognition. *Neurosci Biobehav Rev, 33*(6), 843–863. doi:10.1016/j.neubiorev.2009.02.004

Jeung, H., & Herpertz, S. C. (2014). Impairments of interpersonal functioning: empathy and intimacy in borderline personality disorder. *Psychopathology, 47*(4), 220–234. doi:10.1159/000357191

Jeung, H., Schwieren, C., & Herpertz, S. C. (2016). Rationality and self-interest as economic-exchange strategy in borderline personality disorder: game theory, social preferences, and interpersonal behavior. *Neurosci Biobehav Rev, 71*, 849–864. doi:10.1016/j.neubiorev.2016.10.030

Jones, A. P., Laurens, K. R., Herba, C. M., Barker, G. J., & Vilding, E. (2009). Amygdala hypoactivity to fearful faces in boys with conduct problems and callous-unemotional traits. *Am J Psychiatry 166*(1), 95–102. doi:10.1176/appi.ajp.2008.07071050

Jovev, M., & Jackson, H. J. (2004). Early maladaptive schemas in personality disordered individuals. *J Pers Disord, 18*, 467–478. doi:10.1521/pedi.18.5.467.51325

Kinderman, P., & Bentall, R. P. (1997). Causal attributions in paranoia and depression: internal, personal, and situational attributions for negative events. *J Abnorm Psychol, 106*(2), 341–345.

King-Casas, B., Sharp, C., Lomax-Bream, L., Lohrenz, T., Fonagy, P., & Montague, P. R. (2008). The rupture and repair of cooperation in borderline personality disorder. *Science, 321*(5890), 806–810. doi:10.1126/science.1156902

Kishida, K. T., King-Casas, B., & Montague, P. R. (2010). Neuroeconomic approaches to mental disorders. *Neuron, 67*(4), 543–554. doi:10.1016/j.neuron.2010.07.021

Kishida, K. T., & Montague, P. R. (2012). Imaging models of valuation during social interaction in humans. *Biol Psychiatry, 72*(2), 93–100. doi:10.1016/j.biopsych.2012.02.037

Kliemann, D., Dziobek, I., Hatri, A., Baudewig, J., & Heekeren, H. R. (2012). The role of the amygdala in atypical gaze on emotional faces in autism spectrum disorders. *J Neurosci, 32*(28), 9469–9476. doi:10.1523/jneurosci.5294-11.2012

Kohler, C. G., Walker, J. B., Martin, E. A., Healey, K. M., & Moberg, P. J. (2010). Facial emotion perception in schizophrenia: a meta-analytic review. *Schizophr Bull, 36*(5), 1009–1019. doi:10.1093/schbul/sbn192

Krause-Utz, A., Elzinga, B. M., Oei, N. Y., Spinhoven, P., Bohus, M., & Schmahl, C. (2014). Susceptibility to distraction by social cues in borderline personality disorder. *Psychopathology, 47*(3), 148–157. doi:10.1159/000351740

Krause-Utz, A., Winter, D., Niedtfeld, I., & Schmahl, C. (2014). The latest neuroimaging findings in borderline personality disorder. *Curr Psychiatry*, *16*(3). doi:10.1007/s11920-014-0438-z

Kurtz, M. M., & Richardson, C. L. (2012). Social cognitive training for schizophrenia: a meta-analytic investigation of controlled research. *Schizophr Bull 38*(5), 1092–1104. doi:10.1093/schbul/sbr036

Lawrence, K., Allen, J., & Chanen, A. (2011). A study of maladaptive schemas and borderline personality disorder in young people. *Cogn Ther Res*, *35*(1), 30–39.

Lazarus, S. A., Cheavens, J. S., Festa, F., & Zachary Rosenthal, M. (2014). Interpersonal functioning in borderline personality disorder: a systematic review of behavioral and laboratory-based assessments. *Clin Psychol Rev*, *34*(3), 193–205. doi:10.1016/j.cpr.2014.01.007

Lee, L., Harkness, K. L., Sabbagh, M. A., & Jacobson, J. A. (2005). Mental state decoding abilities in clinical depression. *J Affect Disord*, *86*(2–3), 247–258. doi:10.1016/j.jad.2005.02.007

Lemerise, E. A., & Arsenio, W. F. (2000). An integrated model of emotion processes and cognition in social information processing *Child Dev*, *71*(1), 107–118.

Li, H., Chan, R. C., McAlonan, G. M., & Gong, Q. Y. (2010). Facial emotion processing in schizophrenia: a meta-analysis of functional neuroimaging data. *Schizophr Bull*, *36*(5), 1029–1039. doi:10.1093/schbul/sbn190

Lindenmayer, J. P., McGurk, S. R., Khan, A., Kaushik, S., Thanju, A., Hoffman, L., . . . Herrmann, E. (2012). Improving social cognition in schizophrenia: a pilot intervention combining computerized social cognition training with cognitive remediation. *Schizophr Bull*, *39*(3), 507–517. doi:10.1093/schbul/sbs120

Lis, S., & Bohus, M. (2013). Social interaction in borderline personality disorder. *Curr Psychiatry Rep*, *15*(338). doi:10.1007/s11920-012-0338-z

Lis, S., & Kirsch, P. (2016). Neuroeconomic approaches in mental disorders. In M. Reuter & C. Montag (Eds.), *Neuroeconomics* (pp. 311–330). Heidelberg: Springer.

Loughland, C. M., Williams, L. M., & Gordon, E. (2002a). Schizophrenia and affective disorder show different visual scanning behavior for faces: a trait versus state-based distinction? *Biol Psychiatry*, *52*(4), 338–348.

Loughland, C. M., Williams, L. M., & Gordon, E. (2002b). Visual scanpaths to positive and negative facial emotions in an outpatient schizophrenia sample. *Schizophr Res*, *55*(1–2), 159–170.

Loughland, C. M., Williams, L. M., & Harris, A. W. (2004). Visual scanpath dysfunction in first degree relatives of schizophrenia probands: evidence for a vulnerability marker? *Schizophr Res*, *67*(1), 11–21.

Maat, A., Cahn, W., Gijsman, H. J., Hovens, J. E., Kahn, R. S., & Aleman, A. (2014). Open, randomized trial of the effects of aripiprazole versus risperidone on social cognition in schizophrenia. *Eur Neuropsychopharmacol*, *24*, 575–584.

Malaspina, D., & Coleman, E. (2003). Olfaction and social drive in schizophrenia. *Arch Gen Psychiatry*, *60*(6), 578–584. doi:10.1001/archpsyc.60.6.57860/6/578

Mancuso, F., Horan, W. P., Kern, R. S., & Green, M. F. (2011). Social cognition in psychosis: multidimensional structure, clinical correlates, and relationship with functional outcome. *Schizophr Res*, *125*, 143–151.

Marazziti, D., Abelli, M., Baroni, S., Carpita, B., Ramacciotti, C. E., Dell'osso, L., . . . Phan, K. L. (2015). Neurobiological correlates of social anxiety disorder: an update. *CNS Spect* *20*(2), 100–111.

Marsh, A. A., & Blair, R. J. (2008). Deficits in facial affect recognition among antisocial populations: a meta-analysis. *Neurosci Biobehav Rev*, *32*(3), 454–465. doi:10.1016/j.neubiorev.2007.08.003

Matzke, B., Herpertz, S. C., Berger, C., Fleischer, M., & Domes, G. (2014). Facial reactions during emotion recognition in borderline personality disorder: a facial electromyography study. *Psychopathology, 47*, 101–110. doi:10.1159/000351122

Mayer, J. D., Salovey, P., & Caruso, D. R. (2002). *Mayer-Salovey-Caruso Emotional Intelligence Test (MSCEIT).* Toronto: Multi-Health Systems.

Meyer-Lindenberg, A., Domes, G., Kirsch, P., & Heinrichs, M. (2011). Oxytocin and vasopressin in the human brain: social neuropeptides for translational medicine. *Nat Rev Neurosci, 12*(9), 524–538. doi:10.1038/nrn3044

Meyer-Lindenberg, A., & Tost, H. (2012). Neural mechanisms of social risk for psychiatric disorders. *Nat Neurosci, 15*(5), 663–668. doi:10.1038/nn.3083

Mier, D., Lis, S., Esslinger, C., Sauer, C., Hagenhoff, M., Ulferts, J., . . . Kirsch, P. (2013). Neuronal correlates of social cognition in borderline personality disorder. *Soc Cogn Affect Neurosci, 8*(5), 531–537. doi:10.1093/scan/nss028

Mikhailova, E. S., Vladimirova, T. V., Iznak, A. F., Tsusulkovskaya, E. J., & Sushko, N. V. (1996). Abnormal recognition of facial expression of emotions in depressed patients with major depression disorder and schizotypal personality disorder. *Biol Psychiatry, 40*(8), 697–705. doi:10.1016/0006-3223(96)00032-7

Millan, M. J., & Bales, K. L. (2013). Towards improved animal models for evaluating social cognition and its disruption in schizophrenia: the CNTRICS initiative. *Neurosci Biobehav Rev, 37*(9 Pt B), 2166–2180. doi:10.1016/j.neubiorev.2013.09.012

Miller, D. T., & Ross, M. (1975). Self-serving biases in the attribution of causality: fact or fiction? *Psychol Bull, 82*(2), 213–225. https://doi.org/10.1037/h0076486

Mitchell, A. E., Dickens, G. L., & Picchioni, M. M. (2014). Facial emotion processing in borderline personality disorder: a systematic review and meta-analysis. *Neuropsychol Rev, 24*(2), 166–184. doi:10.1007/s11065-014-9254-9

Montag, C., Dziobek, I., Richter, I. S., Neuhaus, K., Lehmann, A., Sylla, R., . . . Gallinat, J. (2011). Different aspects of theory of mind in paranoid schizophrenia: evidence from a video-based assessment. *Psychiatry Res, 186*(2–3), 203–209.

Montag, C., Ehrlich, A., Neuhaus, K., Dziobek, I., Heekeren, H. R., Heinz, A., & Gallinat, J. (2010). Theory of mind impairments in euthymic bipolar patients. *J Affect Disord, 123*(1–3), 264–269.

Moritz, S., Schilling, L., Wingenfeld, K., Kother, U., & Wittekind, C. (2011). Psychotic-like cognitive biases in borderline personality disorder. *J Behav Ther Exp Psychiatry, 42*(349–354).

Munoz, L. C. (2009). Callous-unemotional traits are related to combined deficits in recognizing afraid faces and body poses. *J Am Acad Child Adolesc Psychiatry, 48*(5), 554–562. doi:10.1097/CHI.0b013e31819c2419

New, A. S., aan het Rot, M., Ripoll, L. H., Perez-Rodriguez, M. M., Lazarus, S., Zipursky, E., . . . Siever, L. J. (2012). Empathy and alexithymia in borderline personality disorder: clinical and laboratory measures. *J Pers Disord, 26*(5), 660–675. doi:10.1521/pedi.2012.26.5.660

Nordahl, H. M., & Nysæter, T. E. (2005). Schema therapy for patients with borderline personality disorder: a single case series. *J Behav Ther Exp Psychiatry, 36*(3), 254–264. doi:10.1016/j.jbtep.2005.05.007

Nuechterlein, K. H., & Green, M. F. (2006). *MATRICS™ (Measurement and Treatment Research to Improve Cognition in Schizophrenia) Consensus Cognitive Battery (MCCB™)* Los Angeles, CA: MATRICS Assessment.

O'Neill, A., & Frodl, T. (2012). Brain structure and function in borderline personality disorder. *Brain Struct Funct, 217*(4), 767–782.

Ochsner, K. N. (2008). The social-emotional processing stream: five core constructs and their translational potential for schizophrenia and beyond. *Biol Psychiatry*, *64*(1), 48–61. doi:10.1016/j.biopsych.2008.04.024

Pedersen, C. A., Gibson, C. M., Rau, S. W., Salimi, K., Smedley, K. L., Casey, R. L., . . . Penn, D. L. (2011). Intranasal oxytocin reduces psychotic symptoms and improves theory of mind and social perception in schizophrenia. *Schizophr Res*, *132*(1), 50–53. doi:10.1016/j.schres.2011.07.027

Penn, D. L., Roberts, D. L., Combs, D., & Sterne, A. (2007). Best practices: the development of the Social Cognition and Interaction Training program for schizophrenia spectrum disorders. *Psychiatr Serv*, *58*(4), 449–451. doi:10.1176/appi.ps.58.4.449

Perez-Rodriguez, M. M., Derish, N., & New, A. (2014). The use of oxytocin in personality disorders: rationale and current status. *Curr Treat Opt Psychiatry*, *1*(4), 345–357. doi:10.1007/s40501-014-0026-1

Perez-Rodriguez, M. M., Mahon, K., Russo, M., Ungar, A. K., & Burdick, K. E. (2014). Oxytocin and social cognition in affective and psychotic disorders. *Eur Neuropsychopharmacol*, *25*(2), 265–282. doi:10.1016/j.euroneuro.2014.07.012

Perlick, D., Stastny, P., Mattis, S., & Teresi, J. (1992). Contribution of family, cognitive and clinical dimensions to long-term outcome in schizophrenia. *Schizophr Res*, *6*(3), 257–265.

Peterson, C., Semmel, A., von Baeyen, C., Abramson, l. Y., Metalsky, G. I., & Seligman, M. E. P. (1982). The Attributional Style Questionnaire. *Cogn Ther Res*, *6*, 287–299.

Pflum, M. J., Gooding, D. C., & White, H. J. (2013). Hint, hint: theory of mind performance in schizotypal individuals. *J Nerv Ment Dis*, *201*(5), 394–399. doi:10.1097/NMD.0b013e31828e1016

Pinkham, A. E. (2014). Social cognition in schizophrenia. *J Clin Psychiatry*, *75*(Suppl. 2), 14–19. doi:10.4088/JCP.13065su1.04

Pinkham, A. E., Loughead, J., Ruparel, K., Overton, E., Gur, R. E., & Gur, R. C. (2011). Abnormal modulation of amygdala activity in schizophrenia in response to direct- and averted-gaze threat-related facial expressions. *Am J Psychiatry*, *168*(3), 293–301. doi:10.1176/appi.ajp.2010.10060832

Polgár, P., Fogd, D., Unoka, Z. S., Sirály, E., & Csukly, G. (2014). Altered social decision making in borderline personality disorder: an Ultimatum Game study. *J Pers Disord*, *28*(6), 841–852. doi:10.1521/pedi_2014_28_142

Preissler, S., Dziobek, I., Ritter, K., Heekeren, H. R., & Roepke, S. (2010). Social cognition in borderline personality disorder: evidence for disturbed recognition of the emotions, thoughts, and intentions of others. *Front Behav Neurosci*, *4*, 182. doi:10.3389/fnbeh.2010.00182

Premack, D., & Woodruff, G. (1978). Does the chimpanzee have a theory of mind? *Behav Brain Sci*, *4*, 515–526.

Renneberg, B., Herm, K., Hahn, A., Staebler, K., Lammers, C. H., & Roepke, S. (2012). Perception of social participation in borderline personality disorder. *Clin Psychol Psychother*, *19*(6), 473–480. doi:10.1002/cpp.772

Rice, T. R., & Derish, N. E. (2014). Oxytocin and callous-unemotional traits: towards a social-cognitive approach to forensic analysis. *Int J Adolesc Med Health*, *27*(2). doi:doi.org/10.1515/ijamh-2015-5011

Ripoll, L. H., Triebwasser, J., & Siever, L. J. (2011). Evidence-based pharmacotherapy for personality disorders. *Int J Neuropsychopharmacol*, *14*(9), 1257–1288. doi:10.1017/s1461145711000071

Ripoll, L. H., Zaki, J., Perez-Rodriguez, M. M., Snyder, R., Strike, K. S., Boussi, A., . . . New, A. S. (2013). Empathic accuracy and cognition in schizotypal personality disorder. *Psychiatry Res*, *210*(1), 232–241. doi:10.1016/j.psychres.2013.05.025

Ritter, K., Dziobek, I., Preissler, S., Rüter, A., Vater, A., Fydrich, T., Lammers, C. H., . . .
Roepke, S. (2011). Lack of empathy in patients with narcissistic personality disorder.
Psychiatry Res, 187(1–2), 241–247.

Robin, M., Pham-Scottez, A., Curt, F., Dugre-Le Bigre, C., Speranza, M., Sapinho, D.,
. . . Kedia, G. (2012). Decreased sensitivity to facial emotions in adolescents with
borderline personality disorder. *Psychiatry Res, 200*(2–3), 417–421. doi:10.1016/
j.psychres.2012.03.032

Roepke, S., Vater, A., Preissler, S., Heekeren, H. R., & Dziobek, I. (2013). Social cognition
in borderline personality disorder. *Front Neurosci, 6*, 195. doi:10.3389/fnins.2012.00195

Roncone, R., Falloon, I. R., Mazza, M., De Risio, A., Pollice, R., Necozione, S., . . . Casacchia,
M. (2002). Is theory of mind in schizophrenia more strongly associated with clinical and
social functioning than with neurocognitive deficits? *Psychopathology, 35*(5), 280–288.
doi:psp35280 [pii]

Ruocco, A. C., Amirthavasagam, S., & Zakzanis, K. K. (2012). Amygdala and hippocampal
volume reductions as candidate endophenotypes for borderline personality disorder: a
meta-analysis of magnetic resonance imaging studies. *Psychiatry Res, 201*(3), 245–252.
doi:10.1016/j.pscychresns.2012.02.012

Sabatinelli, D., Fortune, E. E., Li, Q., Siddiqui, A., Krafft, C., Oliver, W. T., . . . Jeffries, J.
(2011). Emotional perception: meta-analyses of face and natural scene processing.
Neuroimage, 54(3), 2524–2533. doi:10.1016/j.neuroimage.2010.10.011

Samuel, D., & Ball, S. (2013). The factor structure and concurrent validity of the Early
Maladaptive Schema Questionnaire: Research Version. *Cogn Ther Res, 37*, 150–159.

Schilbach, L., Timmermans, B., Reddy, V., Costall, A., Bente, G., Schlicht, T., & Vogeley,
K. (2013). Toward a second-person neuroscience. *Behav Brain Sci, 36*(4), 393–414.
doi:10.1017/S0140525X12000660

Schilling, L., Wingenfeld, K., Lowe, B., Moritz, S., Terfehr, K., Kother, U., & Spitzer, C.
(2012). Normal mind-reading capacity but higher response confidence in borderline
personality disorder patients. *Psychiatry Clin Neurosci, 66*(4), 322–327. doi:10.1111/
j.1440-1819.2012.02334.x

Schlegel, K., Grandjean, D., & Scherer, K. R. (2014). Introducing the Geneva emotion recognition test: an example of Rasch-based test development. *Psychol Assess, 26*(2), 666–
672. doi:10.1037/a0035246

Schmahl, C., Herpertz, S. C., Bertsch, K., Ende, G., Flor, H., Kirsch, P., . . . Bohus, M.
(2014). Mechanisms of disturbed emotion processing and social interaction in borderline personality disorder: state of knowledge and research agenda of the German
Clinical Research Unit. *Borderline Personal Disord Emot Dysregul, 1*, 12. doi:10.1186/
2051-6673-1-12

Schonenberg, M., Christian, S., Gausser, A. K., Mayer, S. V., Hautzinger, M., & Jusyte, A.
(2014). Addressing perceptual insensitivity to facial affect in violent offenders: first evidence for the efficacy of a novel implicit training approach. *Psychol Med, 44*(5), 1043–
1052. doi:10.1017/s0033291713001517

Schweizer, S., Grahn, J., Hampshire, A., Mobbs, D., & Dalgleish, T. (2013). Training the
emotional brain: improving affective control through emotional working memory
training. *J Neurosci, 33*(12), 5301–5311. doi:10.1523/JNEUROSCI.2593-12.2013

Shamay-Tsoory, S. G., & Aharon-Peretz, J. (2007). Dissociable prefrontal networks for cognitive and affective theory of mind: a lesion study. *Neuropsychologia, 45*(13), 3054–3067.
doi:10.1016/j.neuropsychologia.2007.05.021

Sharp, C., Ha, C., Carbone, C., Kim, S., Perry, K., Williams, L., & Fonagy, P. (2013).
Hypermentalizing in adolescent inpatients: treatment effects and association with borderline traits. *J Pers Disord, 27*(1), 3–18. doi:10.1521/pedi.2013.27.1.3

Sharp, C., Monterosso, J., & Montague, P. R. (2012). Neuroeconomics: a bridge for translational research. *Biol Psychiatry, 72*(2), 87–92. doi:10.1016/j.biopsych.2012.02.029

Sharp, C., Pane, H., Ha, C., Venta, A., Patel, A. B., Sturek, J., & Fonagy, P. (2011). Theory of mind and emotion regulation difficulties in adolescents with borderline traits. *J Am Acad Child Adolesc Psychiatry, 50*(6), 563–573 e561. doi:10.1016/j.jaac.2011.01.017

Shean, G., Bell, E., & Cameron, C. D. (2007). Recognition of nonverbal affect and schizotypy. *J Psychol, 141*(3), 281–291. doi:10.3200/jrlp.141.3.281-292

Siever, L. J., & Davis, K. L. (2004). The pathophysiology of schizophrenia disorders: perspectives from the spectrum. *Am J Psychiatry, 161*(3), 398–413.

Staebler, K., Helbing, E., Rosenbach, C., & Renneberg, B. (2011). Rejection sensitivity and borderline personality disorder. *Clin Psychol Psychother, 18*(4), 275–283. doi:10.1002/cpp.705

Stanley, B., & Siever, L. J. (2010). The interpersonal dimension of borderline personality disorder: toward a neuropeptide model. *Am J Psychiatry, 167*(1), 24–39. doi:appi.ajp.2009.09050744 [pii]10.1176/appi.ajp.2009.09050744 [doi]

Statucka, M., & Walder, D. J. (2013). Efficacy of social cognition remediation programs targeting facial affect recognition deficits in schizophrenia: a review and consideration of high-risk samples and sex differences. *Psychiatry Res 206*(2–3), 125–139. doi:10.1016/j.psychres.2012.12.00

Stellwagen, K. K., & Kerig, P. K. (2013). Ringleader bullying: association with psychopathic narcissism and theory of mind among child psychiatric inpatients. *Child Psychiatry Hum Dev, 44*(5), 612–620. doi:10.1007/s10578-012-0355-5

Stoffers, J. M., Vollm, B. A., Rucker, G., Timmer, A., Huband, N., & Lieb, K. (2012). Psychological therapies for people with borderline personality disorder. *Cochrane Database Syst Rev, 8*, CD005652. doi:10.1002/14651858.CD005652.pub2

Stone, M. H. (2014). The spectrum of borderline personality disorder: a neurophysiological view. *Curr Top Behav Neurosci, 21*, 23–46. doi:10.1007/7854_2014_308

Thome, J., Liebke, L., Bungert, M., Schmahl, C., Domes, G., Bohus, M., & Lis, S. (2015). Confidence in facial emotion recognition in borderline personality disorder. *Personal Disord, 7*(2), 159–168. doi:10.1037/per0000142

Tomasello, M., Carpenter, M., Call, J., Behne, T., & Moll, H. (2005). Understanding and sharing intentions: the origins of cultural cognition. *Behav Brain Sci, 28*(5), 675–691; discussion 691-735. doi:10.1017/s0140525x05000129

Tronick, E., Als, H., Adamson, L., Wise, S., & Brazelton, T. B. (1978). The infant's response to entrapment between contradictory messages in face-to-face interaction. *J Am Acad Child Psychiatry, 17*(1), 1–13.

Unoka, Z. S., Fogd, D., Seres, I., Kéri, S., & Csukly, G. (2014). Early maladaptive schema-related impairment and co-occurring current major depressive episode-related enhancement of mental state decoding ability in borderline personality disorder. *J Pers Disord, 29*(2), 145–162. doi:10.1521/pedi_2014_28_146

van 't Wout, M., van Rijn, S., Jellema, T., Kahn, R. S., & Aleman, A. (2009). Deficits in implicit attention to social signals in schizophrenia and high risk groups: behavioural evidence from a new illusion. *PLoS One, 4*(5), e5581. doi:10.1371/journal.pone.0005581

van Zwieten, A., Meyer, J., Hermens, D. F., Hickie, I. B., Hawes, D. J., Glozier, N., . . . Guastella, A. J. (2013). Social cognition deficits and psychopathic traits in young people seeking mental health treatment. *PLoS One, 8*(7), e67753. doi:10.1371/journal.pone.0067753

Vaughn, M. G., Fu, Q., Beaver, D., DeLisi, M., Perron, B., & Howard, M. (2010). Are personality disorders associated with social welfare burden in the United States? *J Pers Disord, 24*(6), 709–720. doi:10.1521/pedi.2010.24.6.709

Vrana, S. R., & Gross, D. (2004). Reactions to facial expressions: effects of social context and speech anxiety on responses to neutral, anger, and joy expressions. *Biol Psychol, 66*(1), 63–78. doi:10.1016/j.biopsycho.2003.07.004

Waldeck, T. L., & Miller, L. S. (2000). Social skills deficits in schizotypal personality disorder. *Psychiatry Res, 93*(3), 237–246.

Weiner, B. (1986). *An attributional theory of motivation and emotion.* New York: Springer.

Weiner, B. (1992). *Human motivation: metaphors, theories and research.* Newbury Park, CA: SAGE.

Williams, K. D., & Jarvis, B. (2006). Cyberball: a program for use in research on interpersonal ostracism and acceptance. *Behav Res Methods, 38*, 174–180.

Winking, J., & Mizer, N. (2013). Natural-field dictator game shows no altruistic giving. *Evol Hum Behav, 34*, 288–293.

Winter, D., Bohus, M., & Lis, S. (2017). Understanding negative self-evaluations in borderline personality disorder-a review of self-related cognitions, emotions, and motives. *Curr Psychiatry Rep, 19*(3), 17. doi:10.1007/s11920-017-0771-0

Winter, D., C., H., Koplin, K., Schmahl, C., Bohus, M., & Lis, S. (2015). Negative evaluation bias for positive self-referential information in borderline personality disorder. *PLoS One, 10*(1). doi:10.1371/journal.pone.0117083

Wischniewski, J., & Brüne, M. (2013). How do people with borderline personality disorder respond to norm violations? Impact of personality factors on economic decision-making. *J Pers Disord, 27*(4), 531–546. doi:10.1521/pedi_2012_26_036

Wolkenstein, L., Schonenberg, M., Schirm, E., & Hautzinger, M. (2011). I can see what you feel, but I can't deal with it: impaired theory of mind in depression. *J Affect Disord, 132*(1-2), 104–111. doi:10.1016/j.jad.2011.02.010

Zanarini, M. C., Frankenburg, F. R., Hennen, J., Reich, D. B., & Silk, K. R. (2004). Axis I comorbidity in patients with borderline personality disorder: 6-year follow-up and prediction of time to remission. *Am J Psychiatry, 161*(11), 2108–2114. doi:10.1176/appi.ajp.161.11.2108

Zanarini, M. C., Frankenburg, F. R., Vujanovic, A. A., Hennen, J., Reich, D. B., & Silk, K. R. (2004). Axis II comorbidity of borderline personality disorder: description of 6-year course and prediction to time-to-remission. *Acta Psychiatr Scand, 110*(6), 416–420. doi:10.1111/j.1600-0447.2004.00362.x

Zanarini, M. C., Frankenburger, F. R., Reich, D. B., & Fitzmaurice, G. (2012). Attainment and stability of sustained symptomatic remission and recovery among patients with borderline personality disorder and axis II comparison subjects: a 16-year prospective follow-up study. *Am J Psychiatry, 169*(5), 476–483.

10 Attachment in Personality Disorders

■ M. MERCEDES PEREZ-RODRIGUEZ,
NICOLE E. DERISH, NEREA PALOMARES,
SUKHBIR KAUR, ARMANDO
CUESTA-DIAZ, AND STEFANIE LIS

■ INTRODUCTION

Definition of Attachment

Attachment theory, pioneered by the British psychoanalyst John Bowlby (1969), posits that early relationships with significant others have a significant effect on later interpersonal relationships.

While the concept of attachment was first introduced to characterize early childhood relations between mother and infant and the consequences for the social development of the infant, attachment theory was extended to include later stages of social development in children, adolescents, and adults.

Attachment theory is based on the assumption that early experiences lead to the formation of a "working model" of the real world, which plays a central role in subsequent social relationships throughout later life. This representational structure involves beliefs, expectations, and rules, which constitute mental representations of the self and others and relationships with others (Bowlby, 1982).

In early life, the function of the "attachment system" is to provide children with a sense of security, which facilitates exploration. The caregiver provides a "secure base" by being available and sensitively responsive. If the infant trusts in this secure base, he or she is then enabled to explore the environment and return to the safety of the attachment figure in case of distress (Bowlby, 1988).

Supporting the attachment theory, there is evidence that early childhood experiences influence attachments to others in later life and that attachment style predicts social functioning, interpersonal difficulties, and psychopathology (Korver-Nieberg, Berry, Meijer, & de Haan, 2014).

Attachment Styles

Attachment styles characterize differences between individuals in attachment behaviors. Attachment styles are assumed to be shaped during early childhood and be stable over time within subjects (Chopik, Edelstein, & Fraley, 2013). Ainsworth, Blehar, Waters, and Wall (1978) identified three distinct attachment styles: secure, anxious-resistant or ambivalent, and avoidant. They suggested that the responsiveness of the maternal behavior strongly impacts the infant's attachment style. Later research has supported the view that attachment styles are the result of the complex interaction between the infant's inherited vulnerabilities and environmental influences, including parenting styles (Gervai, 2009; Letourneau, Giesbrecht, Bernier, & Joschko, 2014; Gervai, 2009; see "Neurobiology of Attachment" section).

Bartholomew and Horowitz (1991) defined four adult attachment styles based on different combinations of positive versus negative self and other representations: secure (positive self/positive others), anxious-preoccupied (negative self/positive others), dismissive (positive self/negative others), and fearful-avoidant (negative self/negative others).

Secure attachment is associated with positive views of the self and others and comfort and independence in close relationships. Those who are anxiously attached tend to have less positive views of themselves and others. They are excessively preoccupied and worried and, as a result, seek high levels of intimacy and emotional reassurance. Dismissive attachment is associated with self-sufficiency, negative views of others, and a tendency to distance oneself from partners. Those with fearful-avoidant attachment have mixed feelings about close relationships. While they desire closeness, they feel uncomfortable trusting others. They have a negative view of themselves and tend to seek less intimacy (Hazan & Shaver, 1994).

Attachment, Social Functioning, and Psychopathology

Attachment styles are associated with social cognitive processing (Suslow et al., 2009; Vrtička, Bondolfi, Sander, & Vuilleumier, 2012) and play a key role in social competence (Groh et al., 2014). In fact, attachment styles have a significant impact on social functioning, quality of life, and mental health and have been linked to personality disorders as well as to many psychiatric disorders such as psychoses, eating disorders, depression, anxiety disorders, and posttraumatic stress disorder (Calkins, Propper, & Mills-Koonce, 2013; Cassidy, Jones, & Shaver, 2013).

Instruments Used to Assess Attachment Behaviors

Several methods are available to assess attachment behaviors depending on the developmental stage of the individuals under investigation. In toddlers and young children, behavioral observations are the main method to assess attachment, while self-report questionnaires and observer-based interviews are most commonly used in older subjects (Ravitz, Maunder, Hunter, Sthankiya, & Lancee, 2010).

A caveat of self-reports is that they measure not so much the actual attachment style but rather the subjective perception of attachment behaviors. These may be biased and differ from actual behavior, particularly among populations with impaired insight and self-knowledge. Observer-based methods can also be influenced by expectations and biases (Ravitz et al., 2010).

Instruments Used to Assess Attachment Behaviors in Children

The most widely used attachment instrument in toddlers aged between six months and two years, is the ***strange situation paradigm*** (Ainsworth, Blehar, 1978). In this laboratory paradigm, infants are separated from their caregiver for short durations of time. The child's behavior is scored during this separation and the subsequent reunion.

Using this paradigm, secure attachment is seen in 60% of the infants. Securely attached infants show distress during the separation but calm down quickly after seeking active proximity to the caregiver during reunion. Around 20% of the infants show an anxious-ambivalent attachment style. They react with extreme distress to separation and need much longer to calm down during reunion. During reunion, they seek proximity but also the punishment of their caregiver for the previous abandonment. An anxious-avoidant attachment style is observed in another 20% of infants. They do not seem to be distressed by the separation and avoid contact during reunion, focusing on other objects (e.g., play tools).

The Cassidy-Marvin paradigm is a similar method as the strange situation test that is used for children in kindergarten age (Main & Cassidy, 1988). Walters and Deane's Attachment Style Questionnaire is another validated method to examine attachment behaviors in children (van IJzendoorn, Vereijken, Bakermans-Kranenburg, & Riksen-Walraven, 2004).

Instruments Used to Assess Attachment Behaviors in Adults

Attachment has been investigated in adults based on the assumption that romantic and other relationships in adults also are determined by attachment behaviors (Weinstein, Perez-Rodriguez, & Siever, 2014). There are multiple measurement instruments of attachment style in adults, including interviews and self-report questionnaires, as reviewed by Ravitz et al. (2010). These authors discuss various methods for assessment of attachment styles in regard to e.g. their theoretical background, test criteria as validity and reliability and type of approach (categorical vs. dimensional). Most instruments assess insecure attachment behavior and define secure attachment as the absence of insecure attachment behaviors. The Experiences in Close Relationships Inventory (Brennan, Clark, & Shaver, 1998a), the Adult Attachment Interview (Bakermans-Kranenburg & van IJzendoorn, 2009), and the Relationship Questionnaire are among the most widely used attachment measures in psychosocial research.

The Experiences in Close Relationships Inventory (Brennan et al., 1998a) was derived from a factor analysis of previously existing attachment measures. It yields two subscales mapping to two dimensions of anxiety and avoidance. The Adult Attachment Interview (Bakermans-Kranenburg & van IJzendoorn, 2009) is a one-hour attachment-history interview, including questions about early relationships and attachment and adult personality. The Relationship Questionnaire (Bartholomew & Horowitz, 1991) is a forced-choice instrument in which the four styles of attachment proposed by the authors (secure, anxious-preoccupied, dismissive, and fearful-avoidant) are described in brief paragraphs.

■ NEUROBIOLOGY OF ATTACHMENT

Earlier attachment models were based on the assumption that the degree of maternal-sensitive responsiveness was the main factor explaining the variance in infant attachment security. However, mounting evidence from genetic studies suggests that the development of attachment behaviors can be understood as the result of complex interactions between biological (genetic) and environmental mechanisms (Gervai, 2009; Letourneau et al., 2014).

Historically, the interaction between genes and the environment has been understood under the traditional diathesis-stress framework, which posits that insecure attachment styles, and subsequent psychopathology, are the result of the combination of both biological vulnerabilities (the diathesis; e.g., difficult temperament) and negative, unresponsive, harsh parenting (the stressor). Conversely, warm, responsive parenting that avoids coercion is assumed to be protective against the risk caused by biological vulnerabilities (Kochanska, Brock, Chen, Aksan, & Anderson, 2015).

A more recent model, the differential susceptibility hypothesis, proposes that biological vulnerabilities may be better conceptualized as plasticity factors rather than risk factors. Under suboptimal parenting, children with high plasticity genetic factors (i.e., highly sensitive to environmental influences) have worse outcomes than their peers; however, they do better than their peers under optimal parenting conditions. Conversely, the environment has very little impact among those with low plasticity traits (Belsky, Hsieh, & Crnic, 1998; Gervai, 2009; Kochanska et al., 2015).

As the interaction between attachment styles, biological factors, and environmental factors in the development of psychopathology is further understood, improvements in evidence-based risk assessment and clinical management of psychiatric disorders can be expected, with interventions that may be carried out as early as the prenatal period and infancy (Steele & Siever, 2010).

What follows is a brief review of the biological systems which have been explored in relation to attachment behavior and psychopathological traits related to personality disorders (Steele & Siever, 2010).

Serotoninergic System

Although there are some unreplicated reports of direct associations between serotonergic gene polymorphisms and attachment (Lakatos et al., 2003), most of the studies suggest a more complex relationship between serotonergic genes and attachment (Spangler, Johann, Ronai, & Zimmermann, 2009). For example, several investigators have reported that serotonergic polymorphisms moderate the effect of maternal care on attachment styles (Salo, Jokela, Lehtimaki, & Keltikangas-Jarvinen, 2011). Supporting the differential susceptibility hypothesis, Salo and colleagues observed that, among serotonin receptor 2A gene T102C polymorphism T/T genotype carriers, early maternal nurturance was strongly and inversely correlated to avoidant attachment (i.e., T/T carriers were more influenced by quality of maternal care than C-carriers); conversely, among C-allele carriers, maternal nurturance was not significantly related to attachment style.

Other studies have focused on the effect of serotonergic polymorphisms as moderators of the effect of different attachment styles on psychopathological outcomes. Kochanska, Philibert, and Barry (2009) found evidence of a gene–environment interaction between the short/long polymorphism in the serotonin transporter gene promoter (5-HTTLPR) and infant attachment with regard to self-regulation in early childhood. Carriers of the 5-HTTLPR short allele who were insecurely attached showed poor regulatory capacities. Conversely, short 5-HTTLPR allele carriers with secure attachment models had regulatory capacities equal to those homozygous for the 5-HTTLPR long allele. A similar interaction between the short/long 5-HTTLPR polymorphism and attachment was observed by Zimmermann, Mohr, and Spangler (2009), who reported that adolescents who carried the 5-HTTLPR short allele but were securely attached showed more agreeable autonomy in interactions with their parents, while those who were insecurely attached showed more hostile autonomy (see also Kochanska, Philibert, & Barry, 2009). Both of these studies suggest that attachment—likely through epigenetic mechanisms—may modulate expression of genes related to behavioral dysregulation (Levy, Beeney, & Temes, 2011), which is a core feature of borderline and antisocial personality disorders. In fact, recent developments in the field of epigenetics suggest that all of the gene–environment interactions described here likely are further modulated by epigenetic processes, which influence phenotypic outcomes by regulating gene expression (van IJzendoorn, Caspers, Bakermans-Kranenburg, Beach, & Philibert, 2010).

Dopaminergic System

Several studies have reported an association between the 7-repeat allele of the 48 bp VNTR polymorphism in the D4 dopaminergic receptor and insecure, disorganized attachment (Gervai et al., 2005; Lakatos et al., 2000, 2002; Gervai, 2009), which was enhanced by the presence of the -521T allele in the promoter region of the gene (van IJzendoorn & Bakermans-Kranenburg, 2006).

Other studies have also suggested that the 7-repeat allele of the 48 bp VNTR polymorphism of the D4 receptor moderates the relationship between environmental risk factors, such as maternal unresolved loss or levels of atypical maternal behavior, and attachment disorganization (Bakermans-Kranenburg, van IJzendoorn, Pijlman, Mesman, & Juffer, 2008; Gervai et al., 2007). For example, Bakermans-Kranenburg et al. reported an 18.8-fold increase in the odds of attachment disorganization when maternal unresolved loss was present, in comparison to children with neither of those risk factors. Interestingly, the 7-repeat allele also predicted a positive response to therapeutic interventions in toddlers with aggressive behavioral problems (Bakermans-Kranenburg et al., 2008).

In line with the differential susceptibility model, it may be hypothesized that the DRD4 7-repeat allele is a potential risk factor under adversity conditions, such as maternal unresolved trauma history, but also sensitizes the individual to therapeutic disciplinary interventions, exerting a positive effect on behavioral outcomes (Steele & Siever, 2010).

Neuropeptides

There is likely a reciprocal influence between developmental and environmental experiences that promote attachment insecurity and the endogenous opioidergic and oxytocinergic systems. Neuropeptide system dysregulation may contribute to dysregulation of brain networks involved in social cognition and attachment (Ripoll, Snyder, Steele, & Siever, 2013).

Oxytocin

Mounting nonhuman research data suggests that oxytocin is an essential modulator of parental care and attachment (Rilling, 2013; Rilling & Young, 2014). A similar role of oxytocin in humans is supported by studies directly assessing attachment behaviors, as well as by data linking the oxytocinergic system with social processes and behaviors, such as the reading of social cues and the appropriate establishment of trust (Stanley & Siever, 2010; Perez-Rodriguez, Derish, & New, 2014; Hammock, 2015; Rilling & Young, 2014; Weinstein et al., 2014). Moreover, data suggests that, in humans, oxytocin also plays a role in social connectedness in the context of romantic partnerships (Stanley & Siever, 2010).

Evidence of the role of oxytocin in human parenting and attachment stems from observational and interventional studies (Rilling & Young, 2014; Swain et al., 2014). The first approach involves correlating parental behavior and peripheral oxytocin concentrations. Although these studies are limited by the lack of robust evidence of a strong correlation between peripheral and central (brain) oxytocin levels (Rilling & Young, 2014), they overall suggest a link between peripheral oxytocin levels and parental behavior. For example, plasma oxytocin concentrations during early pregnancy and the immediate postpartum period were associated with attachment thoughts; maternal bonding behaviors such as affectionate touch, vocalizations, and eye gaze; and frequent infant monitoring (Feldman, Weller, Zagoory-Sharon, & Levine, 2007). The same group found that peripheral oxytocin levels increased after parent–infant interaction among mothers who provided high levels of affectionate contact and among fathers with high levels of stimulatory contact (Feldman, Gordon, Schneiderman, Weisman, & Zagoory-Sharon, 2010). In another study, researchers observed that low plasma oxytocin levels were related to less parental touch toward the infants (Feldman et al., 2012). Oxytocin may also play a role in the lower responsiveness of depressed mothers to their children. Indeed, salivary oxytocin levels were found to be lower in mothers, fathers, and children within depressed mothers' families, compared to those in nondepressed mothers' families. Children of depressed mothers in this sample had lower empathy and level of social engagement (Apter-Levy, Feldman, Vakart, Ebstein, & Feldman, 2013).

Interventional studies involve administering intranasal oxytocin and measuring its effect on attachment-related behaviors. After administering intranasal oxytocin to fathers, there was an increase in both fathers and children in peripheral oxytocin levels and in key parenting behaviors that support parental-infant bonding (Weisman, Zagoory-Sharon, & Feldman, 2012). Furthermore, among women with postpartum depression, exogenous oxytocin also increases maternal protective behavior in the presence of a socially intrusive stranger (Mah, Bakermans-Kranenburg, van IJzendoorn, & Smith, 2015).

There is also evidence that oxytocinergic genes modulate attachment behaviors (Rilling & Young, 2014). For example, Feldman et al. (2012) found that risk alleles in the oxytocin receptor gene and in the CD38 gene (coding for an ectoenzyme that mediates the release of brain oxytocin) were both associated with low parental touch, and the interaction between high plasma oxytocin and low-risk CD38 alleles predicted longer duration of parent–infant gaze synchrony (Feldman et al., 2012).

The relationship between the oxytocinergic system and attachment is likely complex. In fact, attachment style has been shown to modulate the effects of intranasal oxytocin (Bartz, Simeon, et al., 2011; Bartz, Zaki, Bolger, & Ochsner, 2011), such that the effects of oxytocin differ across attachment styles (Weisman, Zagoory-Sharon, & Feldman, 2013), ranging from positive (i.e., prosocial) to negative. For example, oxytocin decreased trust and cooperation among those anxiously attached (Bartz, Simeon, et al., 2011), and administration of oxytocin to the parent diminished social gaze toward the unavailable father among infants experiencing low parent–infant social synchrony (Weisman et al., 2013).

Oxytocin also plays a key role in encoding social memories and associating these memories to the reward of a social stimulus. The effects of exogenous oxytocin on attachment representations are also mediated by attachment style. Less anxiously attached individuals, in response to oxytocin (vs. placebo), will remember their mother as more caring and close, but more anxiously attached individuals experience an opposite effect (Bartz et al., 2010).

Epigenetic modification of oxytocinergic genes is likely the mechanism through which developmental experiences—and, more broadly, the environment—interact with an individual's genetic vulnerability to give rise to the intra- and interindividual variability in specific social behaviors, including attachment. (Jack, Connelly, & Morris, 2012). Supporting this hypothesis, epigenetic modification of the oxytocin receptor gene has been shown to influence neural activity during the processing of anger and fear (Puglia, Lillard, Morris, & Connelly, 2015).

Opiates

It has been hypothesized that oxytocin facilitates affiliation and social attachment by modulating reward pathways (Young, Lim, Gingrich, & Insel, 2001). The endogenous opiate system has been implicated in attachment behavior (Depue & Morrone-Strupinsky, 2005; Nelson & Panksepp, 1998; Panksepp, 2005). Animal data suggests that opiate functioning is involved in the regulation of attachment behavior by mediating the soothing and comforting of infants by their mothers (Panksepp, Herman, Vilberg, Bishop, & DeEskinazi, 1980).

Social mammals seek affiliative interactions for pleasure and also to relieve negative affect. These two motivational states are modulated by μ-opioid receptor activity in the brain (Loseth, Ellingsen, & Leknes, 2014). The μ-opioid receptor may facilitate the association between affiliative behavior and reward, playing a significant role in affiliative bonds (Depue & Morrone-Strupinsky, 2005). Depue and Morrone-Strupinsky proposed that the capacity to experience affiliative reward via opiate functioning plays a key role in determining individual differences in affiliation. This is consistent with recent positron emission tomography data in humans showing an inverse correlation between the avoidance dimension of attachment and μ-opioid receptor availability in the thalamus, anterior cingulate cortex, frontal cortex, amygdala, and insula (Nummenmaa et al., 2015).

Opiates have also been found to mediate and diminish the intensity of emotions in the context of social exclusion and separation (Panksepp, Herman, Conner, Bishop, & Scott, 1978). Opiate dysregulation may thus interfere with the maintenance of attachment and interpersonal well-being in disorders such as borderline personality disorder (Stanley & Siever, 2010).

Consistent with the differential susceptibility model, the A118G polymorphism of the μ-opioid receptor gene was found to moderate the impact of early maternal care on fearful attachment in a sample of psychiatric patients (Troisi et al., 2012). Those carrying the minor 118 G allele had relatively high scores on fearful attachment regardless of the quality of maternal care. By contrast, early maternal care had a major impact for patients carrying the A/A genotype. A/A carriers with higher levels of early maternal care reported the lowest levels of fearful attachment, while those who reported lower levels of early maternal care scored highest on fearful attachment.

■ EVIDENCE OF ATTACHMENT ABNORMALITIES IN PERSONALITY DISORDERS

Abnormal interpersonal functioning is one of the core diagnostic criteria for personality disorders (American Psychiatric Association [APA], 2013). Moreover, in the dimensional model for personality disorders described in Section III of the *Diagnostic and Statistical Manual of Mental Disorders* (fifth edition [*DSM-5*]), abnormal capacity for and desire for intimacy with others (closely related to attachment) is listed as a core diagnostic criterion for personality disorders (APA, 2013). What follows is a review of attachment abnormalities in each of the personality disorders.

Cluster A Personality Disorders

Schizotypal Personality Disorder

Given that schizotypal personality disorder (SPD) is characterized by social and interpersonal deficits and acute discomfort with close relationships (APA, 2013), it is surprising that attachment abnormalities remain mostly unexplored in this population. Moreover, the quality of parental care (Giakoumaki et al., 2013; Meins, Jones, Fernyhough, Hurndall, & Koronis, 2008) and early maternal separation (Anglin, Cohen, & Chen, 2008) have been shown to predict the development of schizotypal personality traits later in life.

The few studies examining attachment in SPD patients have reported significant differences in attachment measures compared to healthy controls. Our group recently observed that SPD patients, compared to healthy controls, had significantly higher levels of attachment avoidance and attachment anxiety, measured with the Experiences in Close Relationships Inventory, as well as lower perceived social support and less diverse, smaller social networks (Ripoll et al., 2013). Riggs and colleagues (2007) found that the Adult Attachment Interview "Unresolved Trauma" and "Unresolved Loss" scales predicted SPD scores. Fossati et al. (2003) found an avoidance attachment pattern with limited social interactions in SPD patients.

Other studies have focused on the relationship between attachment styles and symptoms of dimensional schizotypy, a construct that overlaps in symptom dimensions with schizophrenia and can be divided into positive and negative schizotypy. These studies were performed in nonclinical samples (see Korver-Nieberg et al., 2014 for a review). In a young adult sample, Wilson and Constanzo (1996) reported that secure attachment was associated with low positive and negative schizotypy: Anxious attachment was associated with positive schizotypy and avoidant attachment with both positive and negative schizotypy. In university students, Berry, Wearden, Barrowclough, and Liversidge (2006) found correlations between anxious and avoidant attachment and positive psychotic symptoms and social anhedonia, respectively. The same group also found correlations between attachment anxiety and avoidance and all schizotypy subscales. The strongest correlations were between attachment anxiety and cognitive disorganization and between avoidance and introvertive anhedonia. Moreover, they reported that attachment avoidance predicted schizotypy symptoms (Berry, Band, Corcoran, Barrowclough, & Wearden, 2007).

In a convenience sample of young undergraduates, Meins et al. (2008) found associations between anxious attachment and paranoia (a symptom of positive schizotypy), and both attachment anxiety and avoidance were associated with negative schizotypy. Also in undergraduates, Sheinbaum, Bedoya, Ros-Morente, Kwapil, and Barrantes-Vidal (2013) measured dimensional schizotypy using the Wisconsin Schizotypy Scales and found associations between preoccupied attachment and positive schizotypy, dismissing attachment with negative schizotypy, and fearful attachment and both positive and negative schizotypy. Later some of the authors reported that fearful attachment mediated the relationship between childhood trauma and psychotic-like experiences (Sheinbaum, Kwapil, & Barrantes-Vidal, 2014).

Abnormal attachment may also play a role in the development of SPD. Early studies showed that individuals with SPD remembered their parenting as being underprotective, differentiating them from BPD, characterized by affectionless control and thus causing negative overinvolvement (Torgersen & Alnaes, 1992). Moreover, Rosenstein and Horowitz (1996), using the Adult Attachment Interview, found that adolescents with SPD tended to show a preoccupied attachment style, characterized by avoidance, with a high concordance between adolescent and maternal attachment styles.

Schizoid Personality Disorder

Individuals with SPD show a pervasive pattern of social detachment with limited desire for social intimacy and a restricted range of emotions; however, they may acknowledge having painful feelings related to social interactions (*DSM-5*; APA, 2013). Schizoid patients have been classically associated with a detached attachment (Brennan & Shaver, 1998b). However, it remains unclear whether this is based on a pattern of dismissing attachment or nonattachment (Meyer, Pilkonis, & Beevers, 2004). In a study by Bogarerts Vanheule, and Desmet (2006), the authors found that SPD was strongly associated with insecure attachment among child molesters. They hypothesized that schizoid individuals may be blocked from engaging in adult relationships due to prior bad experiences, while they may be more emotionally congruent to children and feel more comfortable in relating to them (Bogaerts et al., 2006; Cosyns, De Doncker, Hamelinck, Koeck, & De Ruyter, 1994).

Paranoid Personality Disorder

There is very little research exploring the relationship between paranoid personality disorder and attachment styles. There are several studies that have linked attachment styles with paranoid traits. For example, paranoid delusions have been linked to adverse childhood experiences, such as neglect and being raised in institutionalized care, causing insecure attachment that may have led to the development of paranoid thinking (Bentall & Fernyhough, 2008). Sitko, Bentall, Shevlin, O'Sullivan, and Sellwood (2014) found that the association between neglect and paranoia was fully mediated by both anxious and avoidant attachment. Others (Wickham, Sitko, & Bentall, 2015) have also found that paranoia is closely linked to negative self-esteem, which is consistent with the complex cognitive model of persecutory delusions proposed by Freeman, Garety, Kuipers, Fowler, and Bebbington (2002), according to which beliefs are hypothesized to arise from a search of meaning for experiences that are anomalous or emotionally significant. In a large cross-sectional community sample, Varghese et al. (2013) described an association between insecure adult attachment and delusional-like experiences. It has been hypothesized that the combination of low self-esteem and high levels of attachment anxiety could lead to paranoid social references (Korver-Nieberg et al., 2013). In a small study by Rankin Bentall, Hill, and Kinderman (2005), paranoid patients and paranoid patients in remission reported disturbed relationships with their parents, specifically perceived as high overprotection and low care, which is in line with the attachment representations seen in patients with positive symptoms in schizophrenia (Helgeland & Torgersen, 1997).

Cluster B Personality Disorders

Borderline Personality Disorder

Interpersonal difficulties and emotional dysregulation have been core aspects of the diagnosis of borderline personality disorder (BPD) from the earliest (Stern, 1938) to the most recent (APA, 2013) descriptions of this disorder. Moreover, many of the symptoms of BPD, such as impulsive and self-injurious behaviors or excessive anger, are most often triggered by interpersonal interactions (Levy, 2005). Even benign separations from significant others may be experienced as intense rejection (Fossati, 2012).

Individuals with BPD describe intense desire for intimacy, coupled with extreme fear of dependency and an increased sensitivity for rejection. An association between BPD and maladaptive insecure attachment styles has been consistently replicated in previous studies (Barone, 2003; Barone, Fossati, & Guiducci, 2011; Nickell, Waudby, & Trull, 2002). Preoccupied and fearful attachment styles have been found to be more specific to BPD than other insecure attachment styles and were correlated with features of interpersonal disturbance in BPD (Choi-Kain, Fitzmaurice, Zanarini, Laverdiere, & Gunderson, 2009; Scott et al., 2013). Attachment anxiety and avoidance have also been correlated with BPD symptoms such as reactive aggression, anger, and self-harm (Critchfield, Levy, Clarkin, & Kernberg, 2008). The longitudinal McLean Study of Adult Development (Gunderson et al., 2011) found that core affectively oriented interpersonal symptoms, related to intolerance of aloneness and conflicts over dependency, persisted much longer than other interpersonal behavioral symptoms among BPD patients (Choi-Kain, Zanarini, Frankenburg, Fitzmaurice, & Reich, 2010).

According to some authors, the prevalence and severity of insecure attachment styles found among BPD patients suggest a key role of abnormal attachment in the pathogenesis of BPD (Agrawal, Gunderson, Holmes, & Lyons-Ruth, 2004; Fonagy & Bateman, 2008; Fossati, 2012). In fact, it has been hypothesized that the attachment abnormalities in mothers with BPD may cause difficulties in early maternal care, including bonding, internalization, affect attunement, and attachment with the infant. This, in turn, may have a detrimental developmental impact on the offspring and may contribute to the intergenerational transmission of BPD (Chlebowski, 2013; Gratz et al., 2014; Hobson, Patrick, Crandell, Garcia-Perez, & Lee, 2005; Macfie, 2009; Macfie, Swan, Fitzpatrick, Watkins, & Rivas, 2014).

Several models have been proposed for the role of attachment in the development of interpersonal dysfunction and BPD. According to the psychoanalytic theory, aggression and negative emotions in early childhood impair the normal development of distinct representations of the self and others (Gunderson, 1996). In BPD, this impairment has been conceptualized as a protective mechanism that avoids the child having to recognize the hostility that may be present in the caregiver (Fonagy, 2000).

Other theories posit that the prominent rejection hypersensitivity found in BPD, which is expressed as overreaction to rejection cues due to anxious expectations, is a result of childhood rejection experiences (Bowlby, 1969).

More recent models have been developed, which are grounded on the emerging knowledge about the neurobiology of attachment and of BPD. For example, the neuropeptide model (Stanley & Siever, 2010) of BPD hypothesizes that attachment insecurity in BPD may be caused by endogenous opioid dysregulation (Prossin, Love, Koeppe, Zubieta, & Silk, 2010) and alterations in the oxytocinergic system (Ripoll et al., 2013). Other models suggest that attachment abnormalities in BPD are related to abnormalities in brain circuits subserving social/emotional processing and social cognition (Minzenberg, Poole, & Vinogradov, 2008).

Antisocial Personality Disorder

Antisocial personality disorder (AsPD) is characterized by a failure to conform to social norms, impulsivity, aggressiveness, and/or irresponsibility, followed by a lack of remorse for one's own actions (APA, 2013). Individuals with AsPD usually do not care about the safety of self or others. As a consequence of those symptoms, patients with AsPD struggle with difficulties in their daily interactions with others.

Indeed, attachment problems have been identified by several authors as the basis of antisocial behaviors (Allen et al., 1996; Fagot & Kavanagh, 1990; Allen et al., 2002; Fearon, Bakermans-Kranenburg, van IJzendoorn, Lapsley, & Roisman, 2010). Bowlby (1977) argued that children who had difficulties connecting with their caregivers could subsequently develop behavioral problems due to their lack of trust, empathy, and concern toward others. In a recent study, Kim, Kochanska, Boldt, Nordling, and Bleness (2014) observed the response to discomfort in toddlers during a transgression task and concluded that secure attachment was a moderating factor for the relationship between discomfort at toddler age and later antisocial behaviors at school. Insecure toddlers were seen as more oppositional, callous, and aggressive at school. This same group observed that the quality of the relationship between mother and child was a moderator between children's tense discomfort and externalizing problems at school (Kim et al., 2014). In regard to early attachment (until 18 months of life), the children's personality also seemed to impact parents' responses: those children more prone to anger and more difficult to handle provoked a more power-assertive discipline among parents one year later. In insecure relationships, the forceful discipline increased the risk of rule-violation behavior and children's resentful opposition, which then predicted antisocial conduct (Grazyna Kochanska & Kim, 2012). Low maternal care seems to be significantly associated with greater callous-unemotional traits and uncaring behavior in the offspring and future aggression and psychopathic traits (Kimonis, Cross, Howard, & Donoghue, 2013; Gao, Raine, Chan, Venables, & Mednick, 2010). Furthermore, parental stress seems to be related to antisocial behaviors, callousness, and impulsivity in children between the ages of 6 and 12 (Fite, Goodnight, Bates, Dodge, & Pettit, 2008).

A study in a psychiatric population relating attachment to clinical diagnosis and personality traits (Rosenstein & Horowitz, 1996) showed that when maternal attachment was insecure, adolescents were more likely to have a substance abuse disorder, narcissistic or antisocial personality disorder, and other antisocial traits. Those data have been confirmed in other studies where insecure attachment was a predictor of a more violent interaction in adulthood (Holtzworth-Munroe, Meehan, Herron, Rehman, & Stuart, 2000; Babcock, Jacobson, Gottman, & Yerington, 2000; Bruce & Laporte, 2015; Lawson & Bunyan, 2013). Other studies showed that a neglecting attachment was related to drug abuse disorders (Henry et al., 2008) and alcohol consumption (Patock-Peckham & Morgan-Lopez, 2010). Conversely, it appears that a good parental attachment in adolescence may predict a lower risk for antisocial behaviors (Sousa et al., 2011). Maltreatment in childhood has also been hypothesized to be a risk factor for antisocial behavior. Shi et al. (2012) showed that child maltreatment predicted antisocial symptomatology. Dutton, Saunders, Starzomski, and Bartholomew (1994) reported that violent men reported higher rates of exposure to violence, rejection by the father, and an insecure attachment to the mother during childhood.

The current knowledge of the neural basis of AsPD further supports a role of early attachment experiences in the pathophysiology of the disorder. In fact, the regions involved in the neurobiology of AsPD closely overlap with areas involved in social cognitive processes, including the amygdala. For example, AsPD patients are characterized by impaired facial emotion processing (Yoder & Decety, 2014), a reduced response of the amygdala to emotional stimuli, and weaker functional connectivity between the amygdala and the ventromedial prefrontal cortex (Herpers, Scheepers, Bons, Buitelaar, & Rommelse, 2014). An interesting paper reviewing the neuroscience of aggression and antisocial behavior in children with callous-unemotional traits proposes that impairments in eye contact and fear recognition may be associated with violence and callousness (Dadds & Rhodes, 2008). Social eye contact develops in the first months of life and is likely related to parental attachment (Dadds et al., 2006).

Although biomarkers such as low levels of cortisol and other hormonal dysfunctions have been studied in patients with AsPD (Herpers et al., 2014), to our knowledge no studies have related those impairments to attachment measures.

Narcissistic Personality Disorder

Narcissistic personality disorder is characterized by a grandiose sense of self-importance, a belief that one is unique or special, a lack of empathy toward others, envy, arrogance, and a strong sense of entitlement (APA, 2013). Those symptoms cause difficulties in interpersonal relationships since the person requires excessive attention and admiration. Both Kohut (1968) and Kernberg and Haven (1984) agreed in the view of narcissism as a personality structure preventing feelings and awareness of weakness, fragmentation, and dependence. This point of view would understand narcissism as a defensive structure underlying feelings of inferiority, anxiety, and neediness (Kealy, Hadjipavlou, & Ogrodniczuk, 2015).

Psychodynamic theories have described two forms of narcissism—grandiose narcissism (arrogance and beliefs of superiority) and vulnerable narcissism (emotional lability and vulnerability)—which commonly are presented simultaneously by the patients, although one can be more prominent than the other. Two distinct theories aim to explain how self-esteem may play a role in the development of the disorder and how this role is mediated by parental attachment. The first, defended by Millon, Ebel, Le Goffic, and Ehresmann (1981) proposed that children reporting high parental affection with a low level of monitoring and control showed grandiose narcissism as well as vulnerable narcissism. The second, defended by

Kernberg (1975), proposed that narcissism appeared in children who experienced a lack of parental affection, parental coldness, and high parental expectations and understood narcissism as a defensive form of self-regard. This theory is also supported by Horton and Tritch (2014) and Horton, Bleau, and Drwecki (2006). Otway and Vignoles (2006) suggested that both theories are possibly valid and both coldness and parental affection could be the basis of both grandiose and vulnerable narcissism.

Studies of attachment styles in narcissistic personality disorder have suggested inconsistent results: Brennan and Shaver (1998b) found both anxious attachment and avoidant attachment to be the basis of narcissism. Recently other studies have proposed that anxious attachment, but not avoidant attachment, is related to pathological narcissism (Kealy et al., 2015; Meyer et al., 2004).

Differentiating grandiose and vulnerable narcissisms, Dickinson, Coggan, and Bennett (2003) found grandiose narcissism to be related to secure attachment and vulnerable narcissism to insecure attachment. However, other studies suggested that narcissistic grandiosity was related to insecure attachment (Kealy et al., 2015). Those differences and almost opposed results may be explained by methodological problems due to reliability of responses and different instruments used.

The role of attachment in childhood has been suggested to be a mediator between pathological narcissism and self-esteem (Maxwell et al., 2014). What seems to be a consistent agreement is the idea that emotional and empathic care from parents is related to higher levels of self-esteem, and lower levels of depression and maladjusted narcissism (Trumpeter, Watson, O'Leary, & Weathington, 2008).

Studies exploring the neurobiology of narcissistic personality disorder and its relationship to attachment are lacking. Further study will contribute to advancing our understanding of the role of attachment in this disorder.

Histrionic Personality Disorder

Older studies focused on Oedipical explanations of histrionic personality disorder (HPD), where repression was viewed as a mechanism of defense (Fenichel, 1945; Reich & Knopf, 1972). Psychoanalytical perspectives proposed the discharge of repressed sexual emotions for the treatment of HPD. Marmor (1953) argued that the fixation involved in HPD was primarily oral rather than phallic, suggesting a more pervasive disorder. Millon (1996) proposed that parents of patients with HPD were self-absorbed, and Baker, Capron, and Azorlosa (1996) reported that families of patients with HPD were high in control, intellectually and culturally oriented, and low in cohesion. Beck, Froman, and Bernal (2005) proposed that patients with HPD tend to seek attention by fulfilling an extreme of their sex-role stereotype, since they were often rewarded for their cuteness and attractiveness when they were little. Those authors stated that rejection is an extreme and devastating threat to those patients since it reminds them of their tenuous position in the world (Beck et al., 2005).

Since the mentioned studies, not much attention has been paid to the relationship of attachment and HPD. This lack of attention may be explained by a high level of functionality of these patients compared to other personality disorders, so they are less help-seeking, as well as therapists' refusal to treat them due to the high countertransference they may provoke.

Cluster C Personality Disorders

Obsessive–Compulsive Personality Disorder

Obsessive–compulsive personality disorder (OCPD) is primarily characterized by a preoccupation with perfectionism, an excessive attention to detail, and a rigid or inflexible demeanor (Sadock et al., 2010). Patients often display a dysfunction in social skills and have difficulty functioning in social environments, especially when concerning issues of defiance and control (Sadock et al., 2010). Individuals can be reluctant to delegate tasks or otherwise relinquish control over a situation.

Interpersonal dysfunction is explicitly included in the following *DSM-5* criteria for OCPD: "(1) Is excessively devoted to work and productivity to the exclusion of leisure activities and friendships (not accounted for by obvious economic necessity); (2) Is reluctant to delegate tasks or to work with others unless they submit to exactly his or her way of doing things; (3) Adopts a miserly spending style toward both self and others; money is viewed as something to be hoarded for future catastrophes" (APA, 2013). Predominant themes of maintaining control over the external environment, even at the expense of interpersonal relationships, undercut many of the OCPD individual's social interactions.

Attachment dysfunction may be a key etiologic component of the etiology of OCPD, though more research is needed to establish this association. According to attachment theory, individuals with OCPD fail to form secure attachments with parental figures. One study conducted by Nordahl and Stiles (1997) measured self-reported perceptions of parental behavior in individuals with various personality disorders. The results showed that OCPD individuals reported significantly higher levels of parental overprotection and significantly lower levels of paternal care compared to healthy controls.

A similar study conducted by Wiltgen et al. (2015) measured self-reported attachment security among severely mentally ill adult inpatients. Compared to controls, individuals with OCPD showed significantly more insecure/fearful attachment styles characterized by attachment avoidance and attachment anxiety. These findings correlate with many of the behaviors central to an OCPD diagnosis. For example, high attachment avoidance is congruent with the lack of trust and the need to control, often at the expense of interpersonal functioning (Wiltgen et al., 2015).

On that same note, a comparative study by Aaronson, Bender, Skodol, and Gunderson (2006) measured and compared attachment styles among OCPD and BPD patients. The study found that, compared to OCPD, BPD patients tend to display a more insecure attachment style characterized by a high score on the dimensions of "lack of availability of the attachment figure, feared loss of the attachment figure, lack of use of the attachment figure, and separation protest" (Aaronson et al., 2006). However, little conclusive information can be gleaned about the nature of OCPD from this study, and attachment patterns in OCPD need to be compared to several other personality disorders as well as healthy controls before further conclusions can be drawn (Aaronson et al., 2006). This is, again, a testament to the need for further research on the topic of attachment and OCPD.

A number of biological models for OCPD etiology have been suggested and supported to various degrees. There is clear evidence for the heritability of this disorder, though there is dissent as to the degree of heritability (Diedrich & Voderholzer,

2015). Another hypothesis, that OCPD individuals have particularly well-branched limbic regions, has not been well supported by empirical evidence (Diedrich & Voderholzer, 2015). Another suggested biological explanation is a deficit in the OCPD brains' "empathizing system" or the "evolutionary system that enables comprehension of intentional motivated behavior characteristics of humans" and increased activity in the so-called systemizing mechanism or the "system that enables comprehension for lawful and non-intentional events"(Diedrich & Voderholzer, 2015). Again, more research is needed before a compelling case can be made for one particular model of OCPD etiology.

Avoidant Personality Disorder

Avoidant personality disorder (AvPD) is primarily characterized by a simultaneous wish for but fear of social engagement (Sadock et al., 2010). Individuals with AvPD are often very shy, timid, and reluctant to engage or participate in social activity (Sadock et al., 2010). Individuals may also be highly sensitive to criticism and rejection and may withdraw or avoid activities where there is real or perceived threat of such (Sadock et al., 2010). In this sense, the AvPD individual can be highly risk-aversive and show restraint in social behavior.

Given the reluctance or avoidance of social engagement, individuals understand-ably often have difficulties maintaining interpersonal relationships. Underlying fears of shame and ridicule often motivate many of the defensive behaviors in AvPD individuals (APA, 2013). Additionally, individuals may have low self-esteem and view themselves as inferior to others (APA, 2013).

Potential widely recognized psychosocial etiologic factors of AvPD include parental deprecation, parental overprotection, or phobic tendencies in parents or role models (Sadock et al., 2010). A compelling case, thus, can be made for the role of attachment dysfunction in the development of AvPD psychopathology.

Bartholomew and Horowitz (1991) propose that the paradigm for understanding attachment in the context of AvPD involves a disordered understanding of the self and the other. Adult avoidance is seen as the result of a childhood history of unavailable attachment figures, which leads to a theory of the self as inherently unworthy and a theory of the other as inherently cold (Bartholomew & Horowitz, 1991). The result is a desire for social intimacy that cannot be fulfilled as long as the other is viewed in a distrustful light.

This paradigm is supported by a study done by Sheldon and West (1990) which measured "desire for an attachment relationship, fear of an attachment relation-ship, and level of social skills" in individuals with AvPD. The study found that, ulti-mately, desire coupled with fear of an attachment relationship was more indicative and clinically relevant to an AvPD diagnosis than a measure of social skills (Sheldon & West, 1990). On that same note, a recent study conducted in an outpatient sample by MacDonald, Berlow, and Thomas (2013) found a relationship between attachment anxiety and AvPD.

It should be noted that AvPD and social phobia/social anxiety are highly co-morbid and share many common features, including risk factors and neurobiological underpinnings. It has been hypothesized that AvPD and social phobia may be a single condition or reflect a spectrum of social anxiety.

The social anxiety spectrum is characterized by exaggerated amygdala reactivity to social emotional stimuli—particularly those related to fear—and abnormal connectivity patterns between brain regions involved in social threat processing and emotion regulation (e.g., the amygdala, the medial prefrontal cortex, the insula, and the cingulate cortex; Gorka et al., 2014; Marazziti et al., 2015).

Dependent Personality Disorder

Dependent personality disorder (DPD) is primarily characterized by excessive clinging behavior and excessive dependence on interpersonal relations for basic care, survival, and decision-making (Sadock et al., 2010). Individuals with DPD often depend on others to take responsibility for decisions in their life. Fear of the loss of this support can result in the individual behaving in a submissive or excessively compliant manner (Sadock et al., 2010).

Many of the *DSM-5* diagnostic criteria for DPD involve dysfunction in the context of interpersonal relationships. For example, the following criteria all suggest overdependence on close relations: "(1) Has difficulty making everyday decisions without an excessive amount of advice and reassurance from others, (2) Needs others to assume responsibility for most major areas of his or her life, (3) Goes to excessive lengths to obtain nurturance and support from others, (4) Has difficulty initiating projects or doing things on his or her own" (APA, 2013). Fear of abandonment and lack of confidence in one's own ability motivate many of these diagnostic behaviors (APA, 2013). For example, individuals may never voice disagreement against a relation or acquiesce to completing unpleasant or undesired tasks out of fear that said relation would abandon them, leaving them to face their problems alone. When such a dependent relationship does end, the DPD individual urgently seeks another such relationship (APA, 2013).

Problems with attachment can play a crucial role in the etiology of DPD. As noted by Livesley, Schroeder, and Jackson (1990), attachment theory makes a crucial distinction between the concepts of "attachment" and "dependence." While attachment behavior is "any form of behavior that results in a person attaining or retaining proximity to some other differentiated and preferred individual, who is usually conceived as stronger and/or wiser" (Bowlby, 1977), dependency behaviors "are not directed towards a specific individual nor are they concerned with promoting the feelings of security that arise from proximity to attachment figures; Instead, they are more generalized behaviors designed to elicit assistance, guidance, and approval" (Livesley et al., 1990).

Livesley et al. (1990) further noted that DPD individuals scored high compared to healthy controls on scales congruent with insecure or anxious attachment styles (e.g., separation protest, secure base, and proximity seeking). A similar study by West, Rose, and Sheldon-Keller (1994) aimed to study attachment paradigms such as "compulsive care seeking, compulsive care giving, compulsive self-reliance and generalized anger toward attachment figure" among adult outpatients with dependent personality disorder and schizoid personality disorder. The study found that individuals with DPD had significantly higher scores on scales of compulsive care-seeking behavior (West et al., 1994). This theme was further supported in a more recent 2013 study by MacDonald et al. which found correlations between DPD and attachment anxiety.

■ ATTACHMENT AND PSYCHOTHERAPY

Attachment styles may be modifiable through psychotherapy. Based on a review of the literature, Taylor, Rietzschel, Danquah, and Berry (2015) argued that psychotherapeutic interventions increase attachment security and decrease attachment anxiety in different populations, such as patients with major depression or posttraumatic stress disorder.

Attachment styles also have been linked to psychotherapeutic outcomes (Levy, Ellison, Scott, & Bernecker, 2011), and there are several therapeutic modalities specifically based on attachment theory. What follows is a review of attachment-based psychotherapies used in the treatment of personality disorders.

Transference-focused psychotherapy is one of the most studied therapies based on attachment and object relations theory. This is a psychoanalytically oriented therapy which has been shown to improve symptoms and functioning and to shift attachment styles toward security (Clarkin, 2007; Doering et al., 2010; Levy et al., 2006). There is some evidence of the efficacy of transference-focused psychotherapy in the treatment of BPD and other severe personality disorders (Fischer-Kern et al., 2015; Stoffers et al., 2012; Yeomans, Levy, & Caligor, 2013). Mentalization-based therapy (Daubney & Bateman, 2015) is focused on mentalizing, defined as the "capacity to relate to others (especially significant attachment figures) by grasping their behaviors as the product of mental states, while bearing in mind the necessarily inferential nature of this process" (Peter Fonagy, Gergely, & Target, 2007). Mentalization-based therapy is concretely focused on attachment, may prevent violent and aggressive behaviors (Taubner, White, Zimmermann, Fonagy, & Nolte, 2013), and has shown some efficacy in the treatment of BPD (Stoffers et al., 2012).

The Connect Program, based on parental attachment, has also been shown to be useful in the treatment of antisocial behaviors and aggression (Moretti & Obsuth, 2009; Moretti, Obsuth, Craig, & Bartolo, 2015).

Other therapies termed "attachment-based treatments," focus on maintaining a secure attachment. A very recent review on interventions aimed at improving attachment security between mothers and children from one to three years old found that direct intervention focusing on maternal sensitivity was useful. Video feedback of the sensitive responsiveness was especially helpful (Letourneau et al., 2015).

Although several studies found no differences in treatment outcomes between insecurely and securely attached patients (Cyranowski et al., 2002; Fonagy et al., 1996), more recent studies have contradicted those results. Berant and Wald (2009) proposed that securely attached clients benefitted more from psychotherapy than insecurely attached patients. Dozier (1990) observed the same results: securely attached clients were more compliant with the treatment. Secure attachment seems to be related to the therapeutic alliance, which is a key predictor of treatment outcome. However, the strength of this relationship between treatment outcomes and attachment is still unclear (Levy et al., 2011).

■ CONCLUSION AND FUTURE DIRECTIONS

Impaired interpersonal functioning and abnormal attachment patterns are increasingly being identified as core features of personality disorders. For many years, the study of attachment was approached only from the viewpoint of psychotherapy and psychoanalysis. Despite dramatic advances in empirical research during the past decades, which have began to uncover the neurobiological basis of attachment behaviors, the exploration of the neurobiology of attachment and its relationship to treatment interventions and outcomes in personality disorders is still in its infancy.

Elucidating the neurobiological underpinnings of attachment and interpersonal dysfunction is particularly important because social/interpersonal dysfunction appears to be quite treatment-resistant and persists for many years despite conventional treatments.

Research into the neurobiology of psychiatric disorder increasingly focuses on dimensions or domains of psychopathology across diagnoses (as exemplified by the Research Domain Criteria initiative [RDoC]; Insel et al., 2010) and their underlying neurobiological substrates. Attachment is included in the RDoC framework as the dimensional construct "attachment formation and maintenance" within the social processes domain. Although attachment impairments are found across all the personality disorders, studies are lacking that analyze attachment as a dimension cutting across psychiatric disorders.

Since attachment style is strongly associated with treatment response and treatment outcomes, future studies should compare refined phenotypes and intermediate phenotypes within the personality disorders defined by attachment. These "biomarkers" and more homogeneous subgroups of patients may more closely reflect neurobiological factors compared to the broad, heterogeneous categorical personality disorders. For example, a study may recruit personality-disordered patients selected to represent two extremes along a dimension such as attachment anxiety and then test for correlations between the effect of an intervention (e.g., intranasal oxytocin) and the level of attachment anxiety. Another important area that warrants further research is the investigation of the relationship between changes in attachment and social and interpersonal functioning in the real world.

■ REFERENCES

Aaronson, C. J., Bender, D. S., Skodol, A. E., & Gunderson, J. G. (2006). Comparison of attachment styles in borderline personality disorder and obsessive-compulsive personality disorder. *Psychiatr Q, 77*(1), 69–80. doi:10.1007/s11126-006-7962-x [doi]

Agrawal, H. R., Gunderson, J., Holmes, B. M., & Lyons-Ruth, K. (2004). Attachment studies with borderline patients: a review. *Harvard Rev Psychiatry, 12*(2), 94–104. doi:10.1080/10673220490447218

Ainsworth, Blehar, Waters, & Wall, S. (1978). Scoring System for Interactive Behaviors In The Strange Situation. In Patterns of attachment.

Ainsworth, M. S., Blehar, M. C., Waters, E., & Wall, S. (1978). *Patterns of attachment: A psychological study of the strange situation.* Oxford: Lawrence Erlbaum.

Allen, G. C., Hall, G., Michalowski, S., Newman, W., Spiker, S., Weissinger, A. K., & Thompson, W. F. (1996). High-level transgene expression in plant cells: effects of a strong scaffold attachment region from tobacco. *Plant Cell, 8*(5), 899–913.

Allen, J. P., Marsh, P., McFarland, C., McElhaney, K. B., Land, D. J., Jodl, K. M., & Peck, S. (2002). Attachment and autonomy as predictors of the development of social skills and delinquency during midadolescence. *J Consult Clin Psychol, 70*(1), 56–66.

Anglin, D. M., Cohen, P. R., & Chen, H. (2008). Duration of early maternal separation and prediction of schizotypal symptoms from early adolescence to midlife. *Schizophr Res*, 103(1–3), 143–150. doi:10.1016/j.schres.2008.02.016

American Psychiatric Association. (2013). *Diagnostic and statistical manual of mental disorders* (5th ed.). Washington, DC: American Psychiatric Association.

Apter-Levy, Y., Feldman, M., Vakart, A., Ebstein, R. P., & Feldman, R. (2013). Impact of maternal depression across the first 6 years of life on the child's mental health, social engagement, and empathy: the moderating role of oxytocin. *Am J Psychiatry*, 170(10), 1161–1168. doi:10.1176/appi.ajp.2013.12121597

Babcock, J. C., Jacobson, N. S., Gottman, J. M., & Yerington, T. P. (2000). Attachment, emotional regulation, and the function of marital violence: differences between secure, preoccupied, and dismissing violent and nonviolent husbands. *J Fam Violence*, 15, 391–409.

Baker, J. D., Capron, E. W., & Azorlosa, J. (1996). Family environment characteristics of persons with histrionic and dependent personality disorders. *J Pers Disord*, 10, 82–87.

Bakermans-Kranenburg, M. J., & van IJzendoorn, M. H. (2009). The first 10,000 Adult Attachment Interviews: distributions of adult attachment representations in clinical and non-clinical groups. *Attach Hum Dev*, 11(3), 223–263. doi:10.1080/14616730902814762

Bakermans-Kranenburg, M. J., van IJzendoorn, M. H., Pijlman, F. T. A., Mesman, J., & Juffer, F. (2008). Experimental evidence for differential susceptibility: dopamine D4 receptor polymorphism (DRD4 VNTR) moderates intervention effects on toddlers' externalizing behavior in a randomized controlled trial. *Dev Psychol*, 44, 293–300. doi:10.1037/0012-1649.44.1.293

Barone, L. (2003). Developmental protective and risk factors in borderline personality disorder: a study using the Adult Attachment Interview. *Attach Hum Dev*, 5(1), 64–77. doi:10.1080/1461673031000078634

Barone, L., Fossati, A., & Guiducci, V. (2011). Attachment mental states and inferred pathways of development in borderline personality disorder: a study using the Adult Attachment Interview. *Attach Hum Dev*, 13(5), 451–469. doi:10.1080/14616734.2011.602245

Bartholomew, K., & Horowitz, L. M. (1991). Attachment styles among young adults: a test of a four-category model. *J Pers Soc Psychol*, 61(2), 226–244.

Bartz, J. A., Zaki, J., Bolger, N., & Ochsner, K. N. (2011). Social effects of oxytocin in humans: context and person matter. *Trends Cogn Sci*, 15(7), 301–309. doi:10.1016/j.tics.2011.05.002

Bartz, J. A., Zaki, J., Ochsner, K. N., Bolger, N., Kolevzon, A., Ludwig, N., & Lydon, J. E. (2010). Effects of oxytocin on recollections of maternal care and closeness. *Proc Natl Acad Sci U S A*, 107(50), 21371–5. doi:10.1073/pnas.1012669107

Bartz, J., Simeon, D., Hamilton, H., Kim, S., Crystal, S., Braun, A., . . . Hollander, E. (2011). Oxytocin can hinder trust and cooperation in borderline personality disorder. *Soc Cogn Affect Neurosci*, 6(5), 556–563. doi:10.1093/scan/nsq085

Beck, C. T., Froman, R. D., & Bernal, H. (2005). Acculturation level and postpartum depression in Hispanic mothers. *MCN Am J Matern Child Nurs*, 30(5), 299–304. doi:00005721-200509000-00006 [pii]

Belsky, J., Hsieh, K. H., & Crnic, K. (1998). Mothering, fathering, and infant negativity as antecedents of boys' externalizing problems and inhibition at age 3 years: differential susceptibility to rearing experience? *Dev Psychopathol*, 10(2), 301–319.

Bentall, R. P., & Fernyhough, C. (2008). Social predictors of psychotic experiences: specificity and psychological mechanisms. *Schizophr Bull*, 34(6), 1012–1020. doi:10.1093/schbul/sbn103

Berant, E., & Wald, Y. (2009). Self-reported attachment patterns and Rorschach-related scores of ego boundary, defensive processes, and thinking disorders. *J Pers Assess, 91*(4), 365–372.

Berry, K., Band, R., Corcoran, R., Barrowclough, C., & Wearden, A. (2007). Attachment styles, earlier interpersonal relationships and schizotypy in a non-clinical sample. *Psychol Psychother, 80*(Pt 4), 563–576. doi:10.1348/147608307x188368

Berry, K., Wearden, A., Barrowclough, C., & Liversidge, T. (2006). Attachment styles, interpersonal relationships and psychotic phenomena in a non-clinical student sample. *Pers Individ Diff, 41*, 707–718.

Bogaerts, S., Vanheule, S., & Desmet, M. (2006). Personality disorders and romantic adult attachment: a comparison of secure and insecure attached child molesters. *Int J Offender Ther Comp Criminol, 50*(2), 139–147. doi:10.1177/0306624x05278515

Bowlby, J. (1969). *Attachment and loss. Vol 1: Attachment.* New York: Basic Books.

Bowlby, J. (1977). The making and breaking of affectional bonds. I. Aetiology and psychopathology in the light of attachment theory. An expanded version of the Fiftieth Maudsley Lecture, delivered before the Royal College of Psychiatrists, 19 November 1976. *Br J Psychiatry, 130*, 201–210.

Bowlby, J. (1982). Attachment and loss: retrospect and prospect. *Am J Orthopsychiatry, 52*, 664–678. doi:10.1111/j.1939–0025.1982.tb01456.x

Bowlby, J. (1988). Developmental psychiatry comes of age. *Am J Psychiatry, 145*(1), 1–10.

Brennan, K. A., Clark, C. L., & Shaver, P. R. (1998a). Self-report measurement of adult attachment: an integrative overview. In J. A. Simpson & W. S. Rholes (Eds.), *Attachment theory and close relationships* (pp. 46–76). New York: Guilford Press.

Brennan, K. A., & Shaver, P. R. (1998b). Attachment styles and personality disorders: their connections to each other and to parental divorce, parental death, and perceptions of parental caregiving. *J Pers, 66*(5), 835–878.

Bruce, M., & Laporte, D. (2015). Childhood trauma, antisocial personality typologies and recent violent acts among inpatient males with severe mental illness: exploring an explanatory pathway. *Schizophr Res, 162*(1–3), 285–290.

Calkins, S. D., Propper, C., & Mills-Koonce, W. R. (2013). A biopsychosocial perspective on parenting and developmental psychopathology. *Dev Psychopathol, 25*(4 Pt 2), 1399–1414. doi:10.1017/s0954579413000680

Cassidy, J., Jones, J. D., & Shaver, P. R. (2013). Contributions of attachment theory and research: a framework for future research, translation, and policy. *Dev Psychopathol, 25*(4 Pt 2), 1415–1434. doi:10.1017/s0954579413000692

Chlebowski, S. M. (2013). The borderline mother and her child: a couple at risk. *Am J Psychother, 67*(2), 153–164.

Choi-Kain, L. W., Fitzmaurice, G. M., Zanarini, M. C., Laverdiere, O., & Gunderson, J. G. (2009). The relationship between self-reported attachment styles, interpersonal dysfunction, and borderline personality disorder. *J Nerv Ment Dis, 197*(11), 816–821. doi:10.1097/NMD.0b013e3181bea56e

Choi-Kain, L. W., Zanarini, M. C., Frankenburg, F. R., Fitzmaurice, G. M., & Reich, D. B. (2010). A longitudinal study of the 10-year course of interpersonal features in borderline personality disorder. *J Pers Disord, 24*(3), 365.

Chopik, W. J., Edelstein, R. S., & Fraley, R. C. (2013). From the cradle to the grave: age differences in attachment from early adulthood to old age. *J Pers, 81*(2), 171–183. doi:10.1111/j.1467–6494.2012.00793.x

Clarkin, J. F. (2007). [The empirical development of transference-focused psychotherapy]. *Sante mentale Quebec, 32*(1), 35–56.

Cosyns, P., De Doncker, D., Hamelinck, L., Koeck, S., & De Ruyter, B. (1994). *Interpenitentiaire begeleiding van daders van seksueel geweld. UFC jaarverslag* [Treatment of sex offenders in detention]. Antwerp, Belgium: Universitaire Instelling Antwerpen.

Critchfield, K. L., Levy, K. N., Clarkin, J. F., & Kernberg, O. F. (2008). The relational context of aggression in borderline personality disorder: using adult attachment style to predict forms of hostility. *J Clin Psychol, 64*(1), 67–82. doi:10.1002/jclp.20434

Cyranowski, J. M., Bookwalla, J., Feske, U., Houck, P., Pilkonis, P., Kostelnik, B., & Frank, E. (2002). Adult attachment profiles, interpersonal difficulties, and response to interpersonal psychotherapy in women with recurrent major depression. *J Soc Clin Psychol, 21*, 191–217.

Dadds, M. R., Perry, Y., Hawes, D. J., Merz, S., Riddell, A. C., Haines, D. J., . . . Abeygunawardane, A. I. (2006). Attention to the eyes and fear-recognition deficits in child psychopathy. *Br J Psychiatry, 189*, 280–281.

Dadds, M. R., & Rhodes, T. (2008). Aggression in young children with concurrent callous-unemotional traits: can the neurosciences inform progress and innovation in treatment approaches? *Phil Trans Royal Soc London B Biol Sci, 363*(1503), 2567–2576.

Daubney, M., & Bateman, A. (2015). Mentalization-based therapy (MBT): an overview. *Aust Psychiatry, 23*(2), 132–135. doi:10.1177/1039856214566830

Depue, R. A., & Morrone-Strupinsky, J. V. (2005). A neurobehavioral model of affiliative bonding: implications for conceptualizing a human trait of affiliation. *Behav Brain Sci, 28*(3), 313–350; discussion 350–395. doi:10.1017/s0140525x05000063

Dickinson, P., Coggan, C., & Bennett, S. (2003). TRAVELLERS: a school-based early intervention programme helping young people manage and process change, loss and transition. Pilot phase findings. *Aust N Z J Psychiatry, 37*(3), 299–306.

Diedrich, A., & Voderholzer, U. (2015). Obsessive-compulsive personality disorder: a current review. *Curr Psychiatry Rep, 17*(2), 2–014–0547–0548. doi:10.1007/s11920-014-0547-8

Doering, S., Hörz, S., Rentrop, M., Fischer-Kern, M., Schuster, P., Benecke, C., . . . Buchheim, P. (2010). Transference-focused psychotherapy v. treatment by community psychotherapists for borderline personality disorder: randomised controlled trial. *Br J Psychiatry, 196*(5), 389–395.

Dozier, M. (1990). Attachment organization and treatment use for adults with serious psychopathological disorders. *Dev Psychopathol, 2*(1), 47–60.

Dutton, D. G., Saunders, K., Starzomski, A., & Bartholomew, K. (1994). Intimacy anger and insecure attachment as precursors of abuse in intimate relationships. *J Appl Soc Psychol, 24*(15 SRC—GoogleScholar), 1367–1386.

Fagot, B. I., & Kavanagh, K. (1990). The prediction of antisocial behavior from avoidant attachment classifications. *Child Devel, 61*(3), 864–873.

Fearon, R. P., Bakermans-Kranenburg, M. J., van IJzendoorn, M. H., Lapsley, A.-M., & Roisman, G. I. (2010). The significance of insecure attachment and disorganization in the development of children's externalizing behavior: a meta-analytic study. *Child Devel, 81*(2), 435–456.

Feldman, R., Gordon, I., Schneiderman, I., Weisman, O., & Zagoory-Sharon, O. (2010). Natural variations in maternal and paternal care are associated with systematic changes in oxytocin following parent-infant contact. *Psychoneuroendocrinology, 35*(8), 1133–1141. doi:10.1016/j.psyneuen.2010.01.013

Feldman, R., Weller, A., Zagoory-Sharon, O., & Levine, A. (2007). Evidence for a neuroendocrinological foundation of human affiliation: Plasma oxytocin levels across pregnancy and the postpartum period predict mother-infant bonding. *Psychol Sci, 18*, 965–970. doi:10.1111/j.1467-9280.2007.02010.x

Feldman, R., Zagoory-Sharon, O., Weisman, O., Schneiderman, I., Gordon, I., Maoz, R., . . . Ebstein, R. P. (2012). Sensitive parenting is associated with plasma oxytocin and polymorphisms in the OXTR and CD38 genes. *Biol Psychiatry, 72*(3), 175–181. doi:10.1016/j.biopsych.2011.12.025

Fenichel, O. (1945). *The psychoanalytic theory of neuroses.* New York: Norton.

Fischer-Kern, M., Doering, S., Taubner, S., Horz, S., Zimmermann, J., Rentrop, M., . . . Buchheim, A. (2015). Transference-focused psychotherapy for borderline personality disorder: change in reflective function. *Br J Psychiatry, 207*(2), 173–174.

Fite, J. E., Goodnight, J. A., Bates, J. E., Dodge, K. A., & Pettit, G. S. (2008). Adolescent aggression and social cognition in the context of personality: impulsivity as a moderator of predictions from social information processing. *Aggress Behav, 34*(5), 511–520.

Fonagy, P. (2000). Attachment and borderline personality disorder. *J Am Psychoanal Assoc, 48*(4), 1129–1146; discussion 1175–1187.

Fonagy, P., & Bateman, A. (2008). The development of borderline personality disorder—a mentalizing model. *J Pers Disord, 22*(1), 4–21. doi:10.1521/pedi.2008.22.1.4

Fonagy, P., Gergely, G., & Target, M. (2007). The parent-infant dyad and the construction of the subjective self. *J Child Psychol Psychiatry, 48*(3–4), 288–328.

Fonagy, P., Leigh, T., Steele, M., Steele, H., Kennedy, R., Mattoon, G., . . . Gerber, A. (1996). The relation of attachment status, psychiatric classification, and response to psychotherapy. *J Consult Clin Psychol, 64*(1), 22–31.

Fossati, A. (2012). Adult attachment in the clinical management of borderline personality disorder. *J Psychiatr Pract, 18*(3), 159–71. doi:10.1097/01.pra.0000415073.36121.64

Fossati, A., Feeney, J. A., Donati, D., Donini, M., Novella, L., Bagnato, M., . . . Maffei, C. (2003). Personality disorders and adult attachment dimensions in a mixed psychiatric sample: a multivariate study. *J Nerv Ment Dis, 191*(1), 30–37. doi:10.1097/01.nmd.0000044443.94975.3a

Freeman, D., Garety, P. A., Kuipers, E., Fowler, D., & Bebbington, P. E. (2002). A cognitive model of persecutory delusions. *Br J Clin Psychol, 41*(Pt 4), 331–347.

Gao, Y., Raine, A., Chan, F., Venables, P. H., & Mednick, S. A. (2010). Early maternal and paternal bonding, childhood physical abuse and adult psychopathic personality. *Psychol Med, 40*(6), 1007–1016.

Gervai, J. (2009). Environmental and genetic influences on early attachment. *Child Adolesc Psychiatry Ment Health, 3*(1), 25. doi:10.1186/1753-2000-3-25

Gervai, J., Nemoda, Z., Lakatos, K., Ronai, Z., Toth, I., Ney, K., & Sasvari-Szekely, M. (2005). Transmission disequilibrium tests confirm the link between DRD4 gene polymorphism and infant attachment. *Am J Med Genet Neuropsychiatr Genet, 132 B*, 126–130. doi:10.1002/ajmg.b.30102

Gervai, J., Novak, A., Lakatos, K., Toth, I., Danis, I., Ronai, Z., & Lyons-Ruth, K. (2007). Infant genotype may moderate sensitivity to maternal affective communications: attachment disorganization, quality of care, and the DRD4 polymorphism. *Soc Neurosci, 2*(3–4), 307–319. doi:10.1080/17470910701391893

Giakoumaki, S. G., Roussos, P., Zouraraki, C., Spanoudakis, E., Mavrikaki, M., Tsapakis, E. M., & Bitsios, P. (2013). Sub-optimal parenting is associated with schizotypic and anxiety personality traits in adulthood. *Eur Psychiatry, 28*(4), 254–260. doi:10.1016/j.eurpsy.2012.07.002

Gorka, S. M., Fitzgerald, D. a, Labuschagne, I., Hosanagar, A., Wood, A. G., Nathan, P. J., & Phan, K. L. (2014). Oxytocin modulation of amygdala functional connectivity to fearful faces in generalized social anxiety disorder. *Neuropsychopharmacology, 40*(2), 278–286. doi:10.1038/npp.2014.168

Gratz, K. L., Kiel, E. J., Latzman, R. D., Elkin, T. D., Moore, S. A., & Tull, M. T. (2014). Emotion: empirical contribution. Maternal borderline personality pathology and infant emotion regulation: examining the influence of maternal emotion-related difficulties and infant attachment. *J Pers Disord, 28*(1), 52–69. doi:10.1521/pedi.2014.28.1.52

Groh, A. M., Fearon, R. P., Bakermans-Kranenburg, M. J., van IJzendoorn, M. H., Steele, R. D., & Roisman, G. I. (2014). The significance of attachment security for children's social competence with peers: a meta-analytic study. *Attach Hum Dev, 16*(2), 103–36. doi:10.1080/14616734.2014.883636

Gunderson, J. G. (1996). The borderline patients's intolerance of aloneness: Insecure attachments and therapist availability. *Am J Psychiatry, 153*, 752–758.

Gunderson, J. G., Stout, R. L., McGlashan, T. H., Shea, M. T., Morey, L. C., Grilo, C. M., . . . Skodol, A. E. (2011). Ten-year course of borderline personality disorder: psychopathology and function from the Collaborative Longitudinal Personality Disorders study. *Arch Gen Psychiatry, 68*, 827–837. doi:10.1001/archgenpsychiatry.2011.37

Hammock, E. A. (2015). Developmental perspectives on oxytocin and vasopressin. *Neuropsychopharmacology, 40*(1), 24–42. doi:10.1038/npp.2014.120

Hazan, C., & Shaver, P. R. (1994). Deeper into attachment theory. *Psychol Inq, 5*(1), 68–79. doi:10.1207/s15327965pli0501_15

Helgeland, M. I., & Torgersen, S. (1997). Maternal representations of patients with schizophrenia as measured by the Parental Bonding Instrument. *Scand J Psychol, 38*(1), 39–43.

Henry, S. D., van der Wegen, P., Metselaar, H. J., Scholte, B. J., Tilanus, H. W., & van der Laan, L. J. W. (2008). Hydroxyethyl starch-based preservation solutions enhance gene therapy vector delivery under hypothermic conditions. *Liver Transplant, 14*(12), 1708–1717.

Herpers, P. C. M., Scheepers, F. E., Bons, D. M. A., Buitelaar, J. K., & Rommelse, N. N. J. (2014). The cognitive and neural correlates of psychopathy and especially callous-unemotional traits in youths: a systematic review of the evidence. *Dev Psychopathol, 26*(1), 245–273.

Hobson, R. P., Patrick, M., Crandell, L., Garcia-Perez, R., & Lee, A. (2005). Personal relatedness and attachment in infants of mothers with borderline personality disorder. *Dev Psychopathol, 17*(2), 329–347.

Holtzworth-Munroe, A., Meehan, J. C., Herron, K., Rehman, U., & Stuart, G. L. (2000). Testing the Holtzworth-Munroe and Stuart (1994) batterer typology. *J Consult Clin Psychol, 68*(6), 1000–1019.

Horton, R. S., Bleau, G., & Drwecki, B. (2006). Parenting narcissus: what are the links between parenting and narcissism? *J Pers, 74*(2), 345–376. doi:JOPY378 [pii]

Horton, R. S., & Tritch, T. (2014). Clarifying the links between grandiose narcissism and parenting. *J Psychol, 148*(2), 133–143.

Insel, T., Cuthbert, B., Garvey, M., Heinssen, R., Pine, D. S., Quinn, K., . . . Wang, P. (2010). Research domain criteria (RDoC): toward a new classification framework for research on mental disorders. *Am J Psychiatry, 167*(7), 748–751. doi:167/7/748 [pii]

Jack, A., Connelly, J. J., & Morris, J. P. (2012). DNA methylation of the oxytocin receptor gene predicts neural response to ambiguous social stimuli. *Front Hum Neurosci, 6*. doi:10.3389/fnhum.2012.00280

Kealy, D., Hadjipavlou, G. A., & Ogrodniczuk, J. S. (2015). On overvaluing parental overvaluation as the origins of narcissism. *Proc Natl Acad Sci U S A, 112*(23), E2986.

Kernberg, O. F. (1975). [Treatment of narcissistic personality disorders]. *Psyche, 29*(10), 890–905.

Kernberg, O. F., & Haven, C. T. (1984). *Severe personality disorders: psychotherapeutic strategies*. New Haven, CT: Yale University Press.

Kim, S., Kochanska, G., Boldt, L. J., Nordling, J. K., & Bleness, J. J. (2014). Developmental trajectory from early responses to transgressions to future antisocial behavior: evidence for the role of the parent-child relationship from two longitudinal studies. *Dev Psychopathol, 26*(1), 93–109.

Kimonis, E. R., Cross, B., Howard, A., & Donoghue, K. (2013). Maternal care, maltreatment and callous-unemotional traits among urban male juvenile offenders. *J Youth Adolesc, 42*(2), 165–177.

Kochanska, G., Brock, R. L., Chen, K. H., Aksan, N., & Anderson, S. W. (2015). Paths from mother-child and father-child relationships to externalizing behavior problems in children differing in electrodermal reactivity: a longitudinal study from infancy to age 10. *J Abnorm Child Psychol, 43*(4), 721–734. doi:10.1007/s10802–014–9938-x

Kochanska, G., & Kim, S. (2012). Toward a new understanding of legacy of early attachments for future antisocial trajectories: evidence from two longitudinal studies. *Dev Psychopathol, 24*(3), 783–806.

Kochanska, G., Philibert, R. A., & Barry, R. A. (2009). Interplay of genes and early mother-child relationship in the development of self-regulation from toddler to preschool age. *J Child Psychol Psychiatry, 50*(11), 1331–1338. doi:10.1111/j.1469–7610.2008.02050.x

Kohut, H. (1968). The psychoanalytic treatment of narcissisticppersonality disorders. Outline of a systematic approach. *Psychoanal Study Child, 23*, 86–113.

Korver-Nieberg, N., Berry, K., Meijer, C. J., & de Haan, L. (2014). Adult attachment and psychotic phenomenology in clinical and non-clinical samples: a systematic review. *Psychol Psychother, 87*(2), 127–154. doi:10.1111/papt.12010

Korver-Nieberg, N., Fett, A. K., Meijer, C. J., Koeter, M. W., Shergill, S. S., de Haan, L., & Krabbendam, L. (2013). Theory of mind, insecure attachment and paranoia in adolescents with early psychosis and healthy controls. *Aust N Z J Psychiatry, 47*(8), 737–745. doi:10.1177/0004867413484370

Lakatos, K., Nemoda, Z., Birkas, E., Ronai, Z., Kovacs, E., Ney, K., . . . Gervai, J. (2003). Association of D4 dopamine receptor gene and serotonin transporter promoter polymorphisms with infants' response to novelty. *Mol Psychiatry, 8*(1), 90–97. doi:10.1038/sj.mp.4001212

Lakatos, K., Nemoda, Z., Toth, I., Ronai, Z., Ney, K., Sasvari- Szekely, M., & Gervai, J. (2002). Further evidence for the role of the dopamine D4 receptor (DRD4) gene in attachment disorganization: interaction of the exon III 48-bp repeat and the -521 C/T promoter polymorphisms. *Mol Psychiatry, 7*, 27–31. doi:10.1038/sj/mp/4000986

Lakatos, K., Toth, I., Nemoda, Z., Ney, K., Sasvari-Szekely, M., & Gervai, J. (2000). Dopamine D4 receptor (DRD4) gene polymorphism is associated with attachment disorganization in infants. *Mol Psychiatry, 5*, 633–637. doi:10.1038/sj.mp.4000773

Lawson, L., & Bunyan, C. (2013). Midwives: the next generation. *Midwives, 16*(4), 46–47.

Letourneau, N., Giesbrecht, G. F., Bernier, F. P., & Joschko, J. (2014). How do interactions between early caregiving environment and genes influence health and behavior? *Biol Res Nurs, 16*(1), 83–94. doi:10.1177/1099800412463602

Letourneau, N., Tryphonopoulos, P., Giesbrecht, G., Dennis, C.-L., Bhogal, S., & Watson, B. (2015). Narrative and meta-analytic review of interventions aiming to improve maternal-child attachment security. *Infant Mental Health J, 36*(4), 366–387.

Levy, K. N. (2005). The implications of attachment theory and research for understanding borderline personality disorder. *Dev Psychopathol, 17*(4), 959–986.

Levy, K. N., Beeney, J. E., & Temes, C. M. (2011). Attachment and its vicissitudes in borderline personality disorder. *Curr Psychiatry Rep*, *13*(1), 50–59. doi:10.1007/s11920-010-0169-8

Levy, K. N., Ellison, W. D., Scott, L. N., & Bernecker, S. L. (2011). Attachment style. *J Clin Psychol*, *67*, 193–203. doi:10.1002/jclp.20756

Levy, K. N., Meehan, K. B., Kelly, K. M., Reynoso, J. S., Weber, M., Clarkin, J. F., & Kernberg, O. F. (2006). Change in attachment patterns and reflective function in a randomized control trial of transference-focused psychotherapy for borderline personality disorder. *J Consult Clin Psychol*, *74*(6), 1027–1040.

Livesley, W. J., Schroeder, M. L., & Jackson, D. N. (1990). Dependent personality disorder and attachment problems. *J Pers Disord*, *4*(2), 131–140. doi:10.1521/pedi.1990.4.2.131; M3: doi:10.1521/pedi.1990.4.2.131

Loseth, G. E., Ellingsen, D.-M., & Leknes, S. (2014). State-dependent μ-opioid modulation of social motivation. *Front Behav Neurosci*, *8*, 430. doi:10.3389/fnbeh.2014.00430

MacDonald, K., Berlow, R., & Thomas, M. L. (2013). Attachment, affective temperament, and personality disorders: a study of their relationships in psychiatric outpatients. *J Affect Disord*, *151*(3), 932–941. doi:10.1016/j.jad.2013.07.040 [doi]

Macfie, J. (2009). Development in children and adolescents whose mothers have borderline personality dis v24 n3 (1988): 415-426order. *Child Dev Perspect*, *3*(1), 66. doi:10.1111/j.1750-8606.2008.00079.x

Macfie, J., Swan, S. A., Fitzpatrick, K. L., Watkins, C. D., & Rivas, E. M. (2014). Mothers with borderline personality and their young children: Adult Attachment Interviews, mother-child interactions, and children's narrative representations. *Dev Psychopathol*, *26*(2), 539–551. doi:10.1017/s095457941400011x

Mah, B. L., Bakermans-Kranenburg, M. J., Van, I. M. H., & Smith, R. (2015). Oxytocin promotes protective behavior in depressed mothers: a pilot study with the enthusiastic stranger paradigm. *Depress Anxiety*, *32*(2), 76–81. doi:10.1002/da.22245

Main, M., & Cassidy, J. (1988). Categories of response to reunion with the parent at age 6: Predictable from infant attachment classifications and stable over a 1-month period. *Dev Psychol*, *24*(3), 415–426. doi:10.1037/0012-1649.24.3.415

Marazziti, D., Abelli, M., Baroni, S., Carpita, B., Ramacciotti, C. E., & Dell'Osso, L. (2015). Neurobiological correlates of social anxiety disorder: an update. *CNS Spectr*, *20*(2), 100–111. doi:10.1017/s109285291400008x

Marmor, J. (1953). Orality in the hysterical personality. *J Am Psychoanal Assoc*, *1*(4), 657–671.

Maxwell, J. E., Sherman, S. K., Stashek, K. M., O'Dorisio, T. M., Bellizzi, A. M., & Howe, J. R. (2014). A practical method to determine the site of unknown primary in metastatic neuroendocrine tumors. *Surgery*, *156*(6), 1359–1365; discussion 1365.

Meins, E., Jones, S. R., Fernyhough, C., Hurndall, S., & Koronis, P. (2008). Attachment dimensions and schizotypy in a non-clinical sample. *Pers Individ Diff*, *44*(4), 1000–1011. doi:http://dx.doi.org/10.1016/j.paid.2007.10.026

Meyer, B., Pilkonis, P. A., & Beevers, C. G. (2004). What's in a (neutral) face? Personality disorders, attachment styles, and the appraisal of ambiguous social cues. *J Pers Disord*, *18*(4), 320–336. doi:10.1521/pedi.18.4.320.40344

Millon, T. (1996). *Disorders of personality: DSM-IV and beyond* (2nd ed.). New York: Wiley.

Millon, R., Ebel, J. P., Le Goffic, F., & Ehresmann, B. (1981). Ribonucleic acid-protein crosslinking in Escherichia coli ribosomal 30S subunits by the use of two new heterobifunctional reagents: 4-azido-2,3,5,6-tetrafluoropyridine and 4-azido-3,5-dichloro-2,6-difluoropyridine. *Biochem Biophys Res Comm*, *101*(3), 784–791.

Minzenberg, M. J., Poole, J. H., & Vinogradov, S. (2008). A neurocognitive model of borderline personality disorder: effects of childhood sexual abuse and relationship to adult social attachment disturbance. *Dev Psychopathol, 20*(1), 341–368. doi:10.1017/s0954579408000163

Moretti, M. M., & Obsuth, I. (2009). Effectiveness of an attachment-focused manualized intervention for parents of teens at risk for aggressive behaviour: The Connect Program. *J Adolesc, 32*(6), 1347–1357.

Moretti, M. M., Obsuth, I., Craig, S. G., & Bartolo, T. (2015). An attachment-based intervention for parents of adolescents at risk: mechanisms of change. *Attach Hum Dev, 17*(2), 119–135.

Nelson, E. E., & Panksepp, J. (1998). Brain substrates of infant-mother attachment: contributions of opioids, oxytocin, and norepinephrine. *Neurosci Biobehav Rev, 22*(3), 437–452. doi:S0149-7634(97)00052-3 [pii]

Nickell, A. D., Waudby, C. J., & Trull, T. J. (2002). Attachment, parental bonding and borderline personality disorder features in young adults. *J Pers Disord, 16*(2), 148–159.

Nordahl, H. M., & Stiles, T. C. (1997). Perceptions of parental bonding in patients with various personality disorders, lifetime depressive disorders, and healthy controls. *J Pers Disord, 11*(4), 391–402.

Nummenmaa, L., Manninen, S., Tuominen, L., Hirvonen, J., Kalliokoski, K. K., Nuutila, P., . . . Sams, M. (2015). Adult attachment style is associated with cerebral mu-opioid receptor availability in humans. *Hum Brain Mapp, 36*(9), 3621–3628. doi:10.1002/hbm.22866

Otway, L. J., & Vignoles, V. L. (2006). Narcissism and childhood recollections: a quantitative test of psychoanalytic predictions. *Person Social Psychol Bull, 32*(1), 104–116.

Panksepp, J. (2005). Why does separation distress hurt? Comment on MacDonald and Leary (2005). *Psychol Bull, 131*(2), 237–240. doi:2005-01973-005 [pii]

Panksepp, J., Herman, B., Conner, R., Bishop, P., & Scott, J. P. (1978). The biology of social attachments: opiates alleviate separation distress. *Biol Psychiatry, 13*, 607–618.

Panksepp, J., Herman, B. H., Vilberg, T., Bishop, P., & DeEskinazi, F. G. (1980). Endogenous opioids and social behavior. *Neurosci Biobehav Rev, 4*(4), 473–487. doi:0149-7634(80)90036-6 [pii]

Patock-Peckham, J. A., & Morgan-Lopez, A. A. (2010). Direct and mediational links between parental bonds and neglect, antisocial personality, reasons for drinking, alcohol use, and alcohol problems. *J Stud Alcohol Drugs, 71*(1), 95–104.

Perez-Rodriguez, M. M., Derish, N., & New, A. (2014). The Use of Oxytocin in Personality Disorders: Rationale and Current Status. *Curr Treat Options Psychiatry, 1*(4), 345–357. doi:10.1007/s40501-014-0026-1

Prossin, A. R., Love, T. M., Koeppe, R. A., Zubieta, J. K., & Silk, K. R. (2010). Dysregulation of regional endogenous opioid function in borderline personality disorder. *Am J Psychiatry, 167*, 925–933. doi:10.1176/appi.ajp.2010.09091348

Puglia, M. H., Lillard, T. S., Morris, J. P., & Connelly, J. J. (2015). Epigenetic modification of the oxytocin receptor gene influences the perception of anger and fear in the human brain. *Proc Natl Acad Sci U S A, 112*(11), 3308–3313. doi:10.1073/pnas.1422096112

Rankin, P., Bentall, R., Hill, J., & Kinderman, P. (2005). Perceived relationships with parents and paranoid delusions: comparisons of currently ill, remitted and normal participants. *Psychopathology, 38*(1), 16–25. doi:10.1159/000083966

Ravitz, P., Maunder, R., Hunter, J., Sthankiya, B., & Lancee, W. (2010). Adult attachment measures: a 25-year review. *J Psychosom Res, 69*(4), 419–432. doi:10.1016/j.jpsychores.2009.08.006

Reich, P., & Knopf, B. (1972). [Specific tonsillar angina in a homosexual young man with gonorrheal urethritis]. *Das Deutsche Gesundheitswesen, 27*(25), 1191–1194.

Riggs, S. A., Paulson, A., Tunnell, E., Sahl, G., Atkison, H., & Ross, C. A. (2007). Attachment, personality, and psychopathology among adult inpatients: self-reported romantic attachment style versus Adult Attachment Interview states of mind. *Dev Psychopathol, 19*(1), 263–291. doi:10.1017/s0954579407070149

Rilling, J. K. (2013). The neural and hormonal bases of human parental care. *Neuropsychologia, 51*(4), 731–747. doi:10.1016/j.neuropsychologia.2012.12.017

Rilling, J. K., & Young, L. J. (2014). The biology of mammalian parenting and its effect on offspring social development. *Science, 345*(6198), 771–776. doi:10.1126/science.1252723

Ripoll, L. H., Snyder, R., Steele, H., & Siever, L. J. (2013). The neurobiology of empathy in borderline personality disorder. *Curr Psychiatry Rep, 15*(3), 344. doi:10.1007/s11920-012-0344-1

Ripoll, L. H., Zaki, J., Perez-Rodriguez, M. M., Snyder, R., Strike, K. S., Boussi, A., . . . New, A. S. (2013). Empathic accuracy and cognition in schizotypal personality disorder. *Psychiatry Res, 210*(1), 232–241. doi:10.1016/j.psychres.2013.05.025

Rosenstein, D. S., & Horowitz, H. A. (1996). Adolescent attachment and psychopathology. *J Consult Clin Psychol, 64*(2), 244–253.

Sadock, B. J., Sadock, V. A., Belkin, G. S., Sussman, N., Perry, R., & Ahmad, S. (2010). Personality disorders. In *Kaplan & Sadock's pocket handbook of clinical psychiatry* (pp. 325–329). Philadelphia: Wolters Kluwer.

Salo, J., Jokela, M., Lehtimaki, T., & Keltikangas-Jarvinen, L. (2011). Serotonin receptor 2A gene moderates the effect of childhood maternal nurturance on adulthood social attachment. *Genes Brain Behav, 10*(7), 702–709. doi:10.1111/j.1601-183X.2011.00708.x

Scott, L. N., Kim, Y., Nolf, K. A., Hallquist, M. N., Wright, A. G., Stepp, S. D., . . . Pilkonis, P. A. (2013). Preoccupied attachment and emotional dysregulation: specific aspects of borderline personality disorder or general dimensions of personality pathology? *J Pers Disord, 27*(4), 473–495. doi:10.1521/pedi_2013_27_099

Sheinbaum, T., Bedoya, E., Ros-Morente, A., Kwapil, T. R., & Barrantes-Vidal, N. (2013). Association between attachment prototypes and schizotypy dimensions in two independent non-clinical samples of Spanish and American young adults. *Psychiatry Res, 210*(2), 408–413. doi:10.1016/j.psychres.2013.07.020

Sheinbaum, T., Kwapil, T. R., & Barrantes-Vidal, N. (2014). Fearful attachment mediates the association of childhood trauma with schizotypy and psychotic-like experiences. *Psychiatry Res, 220*(1–2), 691–693. doi:10.1016/j.psychres.2014.07.030

Sheldon, A. E., & West, M. (1990). Attachment pathology and low social skills in avoidant personality disorder: an exploratory study. *Can J Psychiatry, 35*(7), 596–599.

Shi, X., Yasumoto, S., Kurahashi, H., Nakagawa, E., Fukasawa, T., Uchiya, S., & Hirose, S. (2012). Clinical spectrum of SCN2A mutations. *Brain Dev, 34*(7), 541–545.

Sitko, K., Bentall, R. P., Shevlin, M., O'Sullivan, N., & Sellwood, W. (2014). Associations between specific psychotic symptoms and specific childhood adversities are mediated by attachment styles: an analysis of the National Comorbidity Survey. *Psychiatry Res, 217*(3), 202–209. doi:10.1016/j.psychres.2014.03.019

Sousa, C., Herrenkohl, T. I., Moylan, C. A., Tajima, E. A., Klika, J. B., Herrenkohl, R. C., & Russo, M. J. (2011). Longitudinal study on the effects of child abuse and children's exposure to domestic violence, parent-child attachments, and antisocial behavior in adolescence. *J Interpers Violence, 26*(1), 111–136. doi:10.1177/0886260510362883 [doi]

Spangler, G., Johann, M., Ronai, Z., & Zimmermann, P. (2009). Genetic and environmental influence on attachment disorganization. *J Child Psychol Psychiatry, 50*(8), 952–961.

Stanley, B., & Siever, L. J. (2010). The interpersonal dimension of borderline personality disorder: toward a neuropeptide model. *Am J Psychiatry, 167,* 24–39. doi:10.1176/appi. ajp.2009.09050744

Steele, H., & Siever, L. (2010). An attachment perspective on borderline personality disorder: advances in gene-environment considerations. *Curr Psychiatry Rep, 12*(1), 61–67. doi:10.1007/s11920–009–0091–0

Stern, A. (1938). Psychoanalytic investigation of and therapy in the border line group of neuroses. *Psychoanal Q, 7,* 467–489. Retrieved from http://www.pep-web.org/document.php?id=paq.007.0467a

Stoffers, J. M., Vollm, B. A., Rucker, G., Timmer, A., Huband, N., & Lieb, K. (2012). Psychological therapies for people with borderline personality disorder. *Cochrane Database Syst Rev, 8,* CD005652. doi:10.1002/14651858.CD005652.pub2

Suslow, T., Kugel, H., Rauch, A. V., Dannlowski, U., Bauer, J., Konrad, C., . . . Ohrmann, P. (2009). Attachment avoidance modulates neural response to masked facial emotion. *Hum Brain Mapp, 30,* 3553–3562. doi:10.1002/hbm.20778

Swain, J. E., Kim, P., Spicer, J., Ho, S. S., Dayton, C. J., Elmadih, A., & Abel, K. M. (2014). Approaching the biology of human parental attachment: brain imaging, oxytocin and coordinated assessments of mothers and fathers. *Brain Res, 1580,* 78–101. doi:10.1016/j.brainres.2014.03.007

Taubner, S., White, L. O., Zimmermann, J., Fonagy, P., & Nolte, T. (2013). Attachment-related mentalization moderates the relationship between psychopathic traits and proactive aggression in adolescence. *J Abnorm Child Psychol, 41*(6), 929–938.

Taylor, P., Rietzschel, J., Danquah, A., & Berry, K. (2015). Changes in attachment representations during psychological therapy. *Psychother Res, 25*(2), 222–238. doi:10.1080/10503307.2014.886791

Torgersen, S., & Alnaes, R. (1992). Differential perception of parental bonding in schizotypal and borderline personality disorder patients. *Compr Psychiatry, 33*(1), 34–38.

Troisi, A., Frazzetto, G., Carola, V., Di Lorenzo, G., Coviello, M., Siracusano, A., & Gross, C. (2012). Variation in the mu-opioid receptor gene (OPRM1) moderates the influence of early maternal care on fearful attachment. *Soc Cogn Affect Neurosci, 7*(5), 542–547. doi:10.1093/scan/nsr037

Trumpeter, N. N., Watson, P. J., O'Leary, B. J., & Weathington, B. L. (2008). Self-functioning and perceived parenting: relations of parental empathy and love inconsistency with narcissism, depression, and self-esteem. *J Genet Psychol, 169*(1), 51–71. doi:10.3200/GNTP.169.1.51–71 [doi]

van IJzendoorn, M. H., & Bakermans-Kranenburg, M. J. (2006). DRD4 7-repeat polymorphism moderates the association between maternal unresolved loss or trauma and infant disorganization. *Attach Hum Dev, 8,* 291–307. doi:10.1080/14616730601048159

van IJzendoorn, M. H., Caspers, K., Bakermans-Kranenburg, M. J., Beach, S. R. H., & Philibert, R. (2010). Methylation matters: Interaction between methylation density and serotonin transporter genotype predicts unresolved loss or trauma. *Biol Psychiatry, 68,* 405–407. doi:10.1016/j.biopsych.2010.05.008

van IJzendoorn, M. H., Vereijken, C. M. J. L., Bakermans-Kranenburg, M. J., & Riksen-Walraven, J. M. (2004). Assessing attachment security with the attachment Q sort: Meta-analytic evidence for the validity of the observer AQS. *Child Dev, 75*(4), 1188–1213. doi:10.1111/j.1467–8624.2004.00733.x

Varghese, D., Scott, J. G., Bor, W., Williams, G. M., Najman, J. M., & McGrath, J. J. (2013). The association between adult attachment style and delusional-like experiences in a community sample of women. *J Nerv Ment Dis, 201*(6), 525–529. doi:10.1097/NMD.0b013e318294a257

Vrtička, P., Bondolfi, G., Sander, D., & Vuilleumier, P. (2012). The neural substrates of social emotion perception and regulation are modulated by adult attachment style. *Social Neurosci, 7*(5), 473–493. doi:10.1080/17470919.2011.647410

Weinstein, L., Perez-Rodriguez, M. M., & Siever, L. (2014). Personality disorders, attachment and psychodynamic psychotherapy. *Psychopathology, 47*(6), 425–436. doi:10.1159/000366135

Weisman, O., Zagoory-Sharon, O., & Feldman, R. (2012). Oxytocin administration to parent enhances infant physiological and behavioral readiness for social engagement. *Biol Psychiatry, 72*(12), 982–989. doi:10.1016/j.biopsych.2012.06.011

Weisman, O., Zagoory-Sharon, O., & Feldman, R. (2013). Oxytocin administration alters HPA reactivity in the context of parent-infant interaction. *Eur Neuropsychopharmacol, 23*(12), 1724–1731. doi:10.1016/j.euroneuro.2013.06.006

West, M., Rose, M. S., & Sheldon-Keller, A. (1994). Assessment of patterns of insecure attachment in adults and application to dependent and schizoid personality disorders. *J Pers Disord, 8*(3), 249–256. doi:10.1521/pedi.1994.8.3.249; M3: doi:10.1521/pedi.1994.8.3.249

Wickham, S., Sitko, K., & Bentall, R. P. (2015). Insecure attachment is associated with paranoia but not hallucinations in psychotic patients: the mediating role of negative self-esteem. *Psychol Med, 45*(7), 1495–1507. doi:10.1017/s0033291714002633

Wilson, J. S., & Costanzo, P. R. (1996). A Preliminary Study of Attachment, Attention, and Schizotypy in Early Adulthood. *J Social Clin Psychol, 15*(2), 231–260.

Wiltgen, A., Adler, H., Smith, R., Rufino, K., Frazier, C., Shepard, C., . . . Fowler, J. C. (2015). Attachment insecurity and obsessive-compulsive personality disorder among inpatients with serious mental illness. *J Affect Disord, 174*, 411–415. doi:10.1016/j.jad.2014.12.011 [doi]

Yeomans, F. E., Levy, K. N., & Caligor, E. (2013). Transference-focused psychotherapy. *Psychotherapy, 50*(3), 449–453. doi:10.1037/a0033417

Yoder, K. J., & Decety, J. (2014). Spatiotemporal neural dynamics of moral judgment: a high-density ERP study. *Neuropsychologia, 60*, 39–45.

Young, L. J., Lim, M. M., Gingrich, B., & Insel, T. R. (2001). Cellular mechanisms of social attachment. *Horm Behav, 40*(2), 133–138. doi:10.1006/hbeh.2001.1691

Zimmermann, P., Mohr, C., & Spangler, G. (2009). Genetic and attachment influences on adolescents' regulation of autonomy and aggressiveness. *J Child Psychol Psychiatry, 50*(11), 1339–1347. doi:10.1111/j.1469-7610.2009.02158.x

11 Suicide and Nonsuicidal Self-Injury

Prevalence in Patients with Personality Disorders

■ PAUL SOLOFF AND CHRISTIAN SCHMAHL

■ SUICIDAL BEHAVIOR

Suicidal behavior is a complex, multidimensional behavior, with clinical, psychosocial, and biologic etiologies. A current stress-diathesis model of suicidal behavior holds that the likelihood of suicidal behavior increases when acute stressors (such as depression, substance use, or interpersonal rejection) are experienced by patients with pre-existing and chronic vulnerabilities, including maladaptive personality traits (Mann, 2003; Mann & Stoff, 1997). Traits such as impulsivity, aggressiveness, and affective instability are risk factors for suicidal behavior across diagnoses. At times of emotional crisis, they impair executive cognitive functioning and adaptive responding, predispose individuals to disinhibited behavior, and increase the likelihood of suicidal outcomes.

Maladaptive personality traits are the defining characteristics of personality disorders (PDs). Suicide studies report that a PD diagnosis increases the likelihood of suicide seven-fold in men and six-fold in women, independent of comorbid Axis I disorders (see Schneider et al., 2006, for review). Prevalence rates of PD diagnoses among suicides varies considerably with setting, age, gender, and method of study. Large sample psychological autopsy studies, using structured diagnostic interviews with informants, report a comorbid PD diagnosis in 29.3% to 72.3% of suicides, with some gender differences. Among male suicides, 72.3% have at least one PD; among female suicides, the rate is 66.7% (Isomesta et al., 1996; Schneider et al., 2006, for review). A PD diagnosis is reported in 28% to 41% of adolescent and young adult suicides (Black et al., 2004; Rich & Runeson, 1992).

Cluster B PDs are the most frequently diagnosed PDs among suicides, found in 9% to 33% of cases, followed by Cluster C (10%) and Cluster A disorders (0.4%) (Isomesta et al., 1996; Schneider et al., 2006, for review). Co-occurrence of more than one PD cluster increases the risk of suicide 16-fold in men and 20-fold in women, adjusted for comorbid Axis I disorders. Cluster B diagnoses are more predictive of suicide in women, Cluster C in men (Schneider et al., 2006). In a large psychological autopsy study in Finland, suicides associated with a Cluster B disorder were comorbid with a depressive syndrome or substance use disorder in 95% of cases (Isomesta et al., 1996).

Borderline personality disorder (BPD) is the most frequent Cluster B diagnosis found in suicides, occurring in 28.1% of suicides in men and 25.6% in women (Black et al., 2004; Schneider et al., 2006, for review). Among Cluster C suicides, Isomesta et al. (1996) found small numbers of dependent (7%) and avoidant subjects (6%), though 12% were termed Cluster C not otherwise specified. Cluster A disorders are infrequently diagnosed in large samples of suicides; however, in a small psychological autopsy study of Israeli military recruits (aged 18–21), schizoid PD was found in 16 of 43 suicides (37.2%; Apter et al., 1993).

Attempters Are Not Completers

Suicide attempters and completers represent distinct but overlapping clinical populations; however, a history of prior attempt is a strong predictor of repeat attempts and completion. Although only 10% to 15% of suicide attempters become completers, 30% to 40% of completers have a history of prior suicide attempts (Maris, Berman, & Silverman, 2000). The number of attempts far exceeds the number of suicides. The Centers for Disease Control and Prevention (2012) estimates 150.61 "self-harm nonfatal injuries" per 100,000 population compared to 12.1 suicides (or 12.4 "nonfatal self-harm injuries" for every suicide death).

Among psychiatric inpatients, the presence of a comorbid Cluster B PD is a robust predictor of past suicide attempts across diagnoses (Mann & Stoff, 1997). BPD, the most prevalent Cluster B diagnosis among attempters, is defined, in part, by "recurrent suicidal behavior, gestures or threats, or self-mutilating behavior" (American Psychiatric Association [APA], 2013). BPD is the only *Diagnostic and Statistical Manual of Mental Disorders* (fifth edition [*DSM-5*]) diagnosis to include this criterion. (Suicidal behavior has been termed "the borderline patient's behavioral specialty"; Gunderson & Ridolfi, 2001). BPD patients with histories of self-mutilation (nonsuicidal self-injury [NSSI]) are at higher risk for suicide attempts (Soloff et al., 1994). Among patients with BPD, lifetime number of suicide attempts predicts the occurrence of high lethality attempts. For some BPD patients, medical lethality of attempts increases with recurrent episodes (Soloff et al., 2012).

Because of the high prevalence of suicidal behavior in BPD (partly attributable to the *DSM* definition), research on suicide attempts and NSSI in PD patients has focused largely on BPD. A history of suicide attempts is reported in 46% to 92% of BPD inpatients and outpatients at time of initial assessment. (In contrast, among subjects with antisocial personality disorder (AsPD), suicide attempts have been reported in approximately 7.7%–11%; Black et al., 2004; Soloff et al., 1994; Zanarini et al., 2007; Zisook et al., 1994). Results of these studies vary widely due to differences in sample characteristics and methods of diagnosis (Frances, Fyer, & Clarkin, 1986; Verona, Patrick, & Joiner, 2001). Comorbidity with AsPD increases the risk of high lethality suicide attempts in BPD. AsPD is highly comorbid among BPD suicide completers. In this context, the interaction of the personality traits of impulsivity and aggressiveness increases the risk of a fatal outcome (McGirr et al., 2007; Soloff et al., 2007).

BPD patients are often recurrent attempters. with an average of three or more lifetime attempts at time of initial assessment (Black et al., 2004; Soloff et al., 1994; Zisook et al., 1994). In a naturalistic longitudinal study, 25% of BPD subjects admitted to the study (from inpatient, outpatient, and community recruitment) attempted suicide within the first two years of follow-up (Soloff & Fabio, 2008). Recurrent suicidal behaviors of low lethality are the most frequent pattern among BPD attempters. Rates of suicidal behavior and NSSI in BPD diminish with time. Longitudinal studies report near-total remission of these behaviors by 10 years of follow-up (Zanarini et al., 2007). Recurrent low-lethality attempts are found among younger BPD patients early in the clinical course, while suicide completion tends to occur later in life after many years of symptomatic behavior, poor psychosocial function, progressive isolation, and failed treatment. A 27-year naturalistic follow-up study of BPD inpatients in Montreal found the average age at time of suicide was 37 years (Heikkinen et al., 1997; Paris & Zweig-Frank, 2001). Despite remission of suicidal behaviors and NSSI for the majority of BPD subjects, 3% to 10% of BPD patients do complete suicide (Paris & Zweig-Frank, 2001). In contrast, completed suicide is reported in approximately 5% of individuals with AsPD (Verona, Patrick, & Joiner, 2001).

Epidemiology of NSSI in BPD

NSSI is a very common dysfunctional behavior, closely linked to emotion dysregulation in BPD (Welch et al., 2008). In a dysfunctional attempt to regulate aversive emotional states, a high percentage of BPD patients (69%–90%; Zanarini et al., 2008) show NSSI, mainly in the form of skin-cutting (Chapman, Gratz, & Brown, 2006; Kleindienst et al., 2008; Klonsky, 2007; Nock & Prinstein, 2004). NSSI can be differentiated from suicide attempts by the fact that, while NSSI tends to be repetitive, suicide attempts in general are single events (Herpertz, 1995). There are also differences regarding the motives— that is, tension/dissociation reduction for NSSI (Favazza, 1998; Kleindienst et al., 2008) versus the wish to die for suicide—and the methods, with cutting, burning, and head-banging being the three most frequent methods used for NSSI (Herpertz, 1995; Kleindienst et al., 2008). On the other hand, there is also a close epidemiological link between NSSI and suicide: in a German study approximately half of the adolescents with repetitive NSSI also had a history of suicide attempts (Brunner et al., 2007). NSSI doubles the risk for suicide attempts (Stone et al., 1987).

In general, NSSI is a very frequent phenomenon in adolescence. Approximately 18% of adolescents (age 14-18) show this type of behavior, with astonishing similarity of prevalence around the globe (Muehlenkamp et al., 2012). In a study in German-speaking countries, 10.7% of adolescents reported NSSI one to five times within the last six months; 3.4% reported injuring themselves more often (Plener et al., 2013). The highest frequencies of NSSI appear to be present at age 15/16, with a clear drop in prevalence between 17 and 29 (Moran, 2012). The *DSM-5* has included NSSI as condition for further study in its recent edition (APA, 2013), pointing out that NSSI can exist in several psychiatric conditions and is not limited to BPD.

■ EXPLANATORY MODELS FOR SUICIDE AND NSSI

Trait vulnerabilities associated with suicidal behavior and NSSI may be heritable (e.g., as endophenotypes), or acquired (e.g., as a result of childhood sexual abuse or head trauma). These are temperamental dispositions toward behaviors that constitute clinical risk factors for suicidal behavior. In PD patients, trait vulnerabilities may include impulsivity, aggressiveness, emotion dysregulation, and impaired executive cognitive function. These vulnerabilities are highly prevalent in patients with Cluster B PDs and are manifested clinically in suicide risk factors such as impulsive aggression, disinhibited high-risk behaviors (e.g., with sex, spending, drugs), inappropriate anger and hostility, and mood lability. Among subjects with BPD, deficits in executive cognitive functions have been reported in planning, attention, cognitive flexibility, processing speed, learning and memory, and visuospatial ability (Ruocco, 2005). Deficits in memory function among suicide attempters, independent of diagnosis, include overgeneralized and delayed recall of autobiographic memory (a subset of episodic memory). The inability to quickly recall memories of past outcomes of behavior, especially during emotional crises, contributes to impaired problem-solving and adaptive responding (Pollock & Williams, 2001). Impulsive aggression, emotion dysregulation, and executive cognitive impairment in PD subjects increases the risk of suicidal behavior at times of stress.

Trait vulnerabilities may be mediated by structural and functional abnormalities in brain networks that regulate mood, impulse, cognition, and behavior. At times of stress, especially in the face of strong negative emotion, these dysfunctional networks contribute a vulnerability to loss of cognitive control over impulse, affect, and behavior. Neuroimaging studies in PD patients have advanced our understanding of these abnormalities and their role in suicidal and self-injurious behavior. This chapter highlights these advances.

The most prominent motives for NSSI in these patients are a reduction of aversive inner tension and dissociation (Chapman, Gratz, & Brown, 2006; Kleindienst et al., 2008). Nock and Prinstein (2004) in their model of NSSI distinguish between automatic (subjective) and social reinforcement of NSSI, with subdifferentiation of positive and negative reinforcement. Reduction of unpleasant feelings or tension by NSSI constitutes an example of automatic negative reinforcement. In an extension of this model, Chapman and co-authors (2006) suggest that NSSI primarily serves to help the individual avoid unpleasant experiences and feelings, leading to temporary relief.

■ NEUROBIOLOGICAL MECHANISMS

Structural and Functional Neuroimaging in PD

Neuroimaging studies have reported structural and functional abnormalities of "the suicidal brain" across multiple diagnostic categories using magnetic resonance imaging (MRI), diffusion tensor imaging, positron-emission tomography, single photon emission computed tomography (SPECT), and functional MRI (fMRI) techniques. Due to the wide divergence of diagnoses and methods, there is little consensus on results (Desmyter, Van Heeringen, & Audenaert, 2011, for review). Suicidal behavior is a complex higher order behavioral variable which cannot be attributed to a specific neural abnormality independent of diagnostic context. Relevant studies among subjects with PDs deal primarily with "impulsive PDs," that is, BPD and/or AsPD, and focus attention on the diathesis to suicidal behavior reflected in personality traits such as impulsivity, aggression, affective instability, and executive cognitive impairment. Structural abnormalities are widely reported in fronto-temporo-limbic networks in these studies, despite important differences in methods, including comorbid Axis I disorders and use of psychoactive medications. A review of this literature supports the hypothesis that trait vulnerabilities for suicidal behavior in BPD (such as impulsive aggression and emotion dysregulation) are mediated by structural or functional aberrations in fronto-temporo-limbic networks.

In a small sample of BPD subjects with no comorbid major depressive disorder or substance use disorders ($n = 8$), Tebartz van Elst et al. (2003) reported decreased volumes in orbitofrontal cortex (OFC; right., diminished 24%), anterior cingulate cortex (ACC; right, diminished 26%), bilateral hippocampus (HIP; diminished

20%–21%), and amygdala (AMY; diminished 23%–25%) using manually drawn regions of interest (ROIs). An expanded BPD sample (*n* = 20) from the same group, analyzed by computer-driven voxel-based morphometry, found volume loss only in basolateral AMY (left), but not in OFC or ACC (Rüsch et al., 2003). Among BPD subjects compared to age- and sex-matched controls, diminished grey matter volume in the OFC (left, Brodmann's area [BA] 10) is related to increased impulsivity (Hazlett et al., 2005). Increased white matter volume in OFC (left, BA 47) is associated with increased impulsivity, irritability, and assaultiveness (Hazlett et al., 2005). OFC is involved in regulation of affect, impulse, and behavior through response inhibition, providing "top-down" cortical control over limbic ("bottom-up") hyperarousal (Davidson, Putnam, & Larson, 2000; Gross & Thompson, 2006; Ochsner & Gross, 2006; Phillips, Ladouceur, & Drevets, 2008). In concert with the ACC, the OFC assesses the relevance of external stimuli for response, focuses attention, directs expression of affect and impulse, and motivates adaptive responding. Through extensive connections to AMY and the extended limbic system, OFC helps regulate emotional responses to provocative environmental stimuli (e.g., angry faces.). Response inhibition is a critical function of the OFC, directly involved in the diathesis to suicidal behavior.

Dorsolateral prefrontal cortex (DLPFC) is diminished bilaterally in BPD compared to control subjects (Sala et al., 2011). Volume of grey matter in DLPFC is also inversely related to impulsivity (Sala et al., 2011). In BPD subjects, compared to age- and sex-matched controls, increased volumes in DLPFC (BA 44, bilaterally) are correlated with increased hostility and irritability/assaultiveness (on the Buss-Durkee Hostility Inventory; Hazlett et al., 2005). DLPFC is involved in processing working memory and in the process of voluntary emotion regulation, including the cognitive processes of suppression and reappraisal (Phillips, Ladouceur, & Drevets, 2008; Phillips et al., 2008, for review).

ACC is also diminished in BPD (Soloff et al., 2008; Tebartz van Elst et al., 2003). Volume of grey matter in ACC (left, BA 24) is inversely related to impulsivity (Hazlett et al., 2005). ACC is activated by tasks which involve competing choices, error detection, conflict resolution, and decision-making. It also plays a major role in emotion regulation.

Loss of volume in HIP is the most replicated finding in MRI studies of BPD (Brambilla et al., 2004; Driessen et al., 2000; Irle, Lange, & Sachsse, 2005; Rüsch et al., 2003; Sala et al., 2011; Schmahl et al., 2003; Soloff et al., 2008; Soloff et al., 2012; Tebartz van Elst et al., 2003; Zetzsche et al., 2007). Importantly, HIP volume has been found to be inversely correlated with history, severity, and duration of childhood abuse, a significant risk factor for suicide attempts in BPD, and with posttraumatic stress disorder symptoms and aggression (Driessen et al., 2000; Irle, Lange, & Sachsse, 2005; Sala et al., 2011; Schmahl et al., 2003; Zetzsche et al., 2007). HIP provides declarative, episodic, and working memory functions to the OFC, processes emotional input from the AMY and associated limbic structures, and forwards representations of emotion to the higher cortical centers for processing. HIP is involved (with right posterior inferior frontal gyrus and left posterior AMY) in the recall of autobiographical memory, which is needed for future planning and adaptive coping during stressful situations (Pollock & Williams, 2001; Williams & Broadbent, 1986, for review). The behavioral consequences of abnormalities in these critical fronto-temporo-limbic structures in PD patients would increase the risk of disinhibited impulsive-aggressive behavior, emotion dysregulation, and impaired memory function.

Few structural MRI studies have ascertained PD subjects for histories of suicidal behavior or compared attempters to non-attempters, controlling for diagnosis. In a first imaging study of BPD subjects ascertained specifically for suicidal behavior, Soloff et al. (2012) found that BPD attempters had decreased grey volumes in left insula compared to BPD non-attempters. The insula is a limbic integration area, forwarding limbic input to higher cortical centers. Among its many psychological functions, it processes subjective awareness of emotion in self (e.g., the somatic sensations of "feelings") and appraises emotional states in others (e.g., empathy; Augustine, 1996, for review). In fMRI studies, the insula is activated by tasks involving trust, co-operation, and sensitivity to social exclusion (King-Casas et al., 2008). High-lethality BPD attempters, compared to low-lethality attempters, had diminished volumes in a broad fronto-temporo-limbic network that included right middle-superior temporal cortex, right middle-inferior OFC, right insula, left fusiform gyrus, left lingual gyrus, and right parahippocampal gyrus. This study suggested that lethality of attempt is related to grey matter concentrations in specific brain networks (Soloff, White, & Diwadkar, 2014).

Structural abnormalities *do not prove* functional impairment. Impulsive PD subjects have also been studied with functional neuroimaging techniques such as PET, SPECT, and fMRI. These functional techniques have been widely applied in PD patients to the study of trait vulnerabilities relevant to suicidal behavior such as impulsive aggression and emotion dysregulation.

Impulsive Aggression

PET studies of violent and aggressive subjects demonstrate areas of decreased glucose metabolism (decreased rCMRglu) or hypo-perfusion (rCBF) in areas of prefrontal, frontal, and temporal cortex independent of diagnosis. Early PET studies among PD patients reported an inverse relationship between aggression and glucose uptake in a fronto-temporal network including anterior medial frontal and (left) anterior frontal cortex (orbital frontal cortex) and (right) temporal cortex (Goyer et al., 1994). A SPECT study of "impulsivity-related PDs" (all BPD and AsPD), found decreased perfusion (rCBF) in prefrontal cortex, lateral temporal cortex, and ventrolateral PFC in impulsive PDs compared to healthy control subjects (Goethals et al., 2005). Subjects in this study were inpatients, selected for impulsive behaviors, with no Axis I comorbidity and free of psychoactive medication for six weeks. De la Fuente et al. (1997) also conducted a PET study of BPD subjects with no comorbid Axis I disorders. They reported decreased glucose uptake in multiple ROIs in frontal cortex, medial and anterior PFC, and ACC (but also in bilateral caudate, thalamus, and basal ganglia). Soloff et al. (2003) reported diminished glucose uptake in OFC bilaterally in nondepressed female subjects with BPD. The hypo-metabolic pattern was related to measures of impulsivity (Barratt Impulsiveness Scale) and aggression (Lifetime History of Aggression Soloff et al., 2003). As in structural studies, results in functional studies differ depending on sample characteristics and method of imaging. However, the areas of aberrant structure and function overlap in many studies, suggesting a specific neural basis for impulsive aggression in these subjects.

Defects in connectivity between critical regions may also play a role in mediating trait vulnerabilities. New et al. (2007) reported decreased connectivity between OFC and AMY in impulsive-aggressive subjects with BPD. These investigators suggested that the normal balance between inhibitory behavioral control, mediated through the OFC, and emotional arousal, generated by AMY, may be disrupted in subjects with impulsive PDs; that is, the vulnerability to impulsive-aggressive behavior in these subjects may be related to a failure of connectivity.

An extensive body of older research has established a relationship between indices of diminished central serotonergic function, suicidal behavior, and impulsive aggression (independent of suicidal behavior) in depressed patients and impulsive PD subjects (Audenaert et al., 2006; Mann, 2003, for review). Suicidal behavior and impulsive aggression in PD patients is associated with diminished levels of cerebrospinal fluid (CSF) 5-HIAA and blunted neuroendocrine responses to serotonergic agonists (e.g., d, or d,l fenfluramine [FEN] and meta-chlorophenylpiperazine [m-CPP]). These studies have been extended by use of neuroimaging techniques to identify specific networks involved in impulsive-aggressive and suicidal behavior in PD subjects.

In PET studies, augmentation with the serotonergic agents d,l FEN or m-CPP has been used to assess metabolic responses to serotonergic challenge. Among PD subjects meeting criteria for intermittent explosive disorder (IED; defined by impulsive aggression but including BPD), FEN-PET studies demonstrate a blunted metabolic response (decreased glucose uptake) in orbitofrontal, ventromedial, and cingulate cortex (Siever et al., 1999). Among female subjects ascertained specifically for BPD, FEN activation resulted in decreased glucose uptake in OFC (right medial and orbital prefrontal cortex), left middle and superior temporal cortex, left parietal cortex, and left caudate (Soloff et al., 2000). Responses to m-CPP among impulsive-aggressive subjects with IED included diminished metabolism relative to control subjects in OFC (left medial posterior OFC) and ACC but increased metabolism in posterior cingulate. Aggression was inversely related to metabolic response in lateral frontal cortex among IED subjects (New et al., 2002).

Using alpha [C-11] m-Tryptophan, Leyton et al. (2001) assessed serotonin synthesis through radioligand "trapping" in a small mixed-gender sample of subjects with BPD. Lower alpha [C-11] m-Tryptophan trapping suggests decreased serotonin synthesis. Gender differences were prominent; however, the combined-gender BPD sample had decreased trapping in OFC, medial frontal cortex (left), ACC, and fusiform gyrus (right) There was an inverse relationship between impulsivity and radioligand trapping in medial frontal gyrus, ACC, temporal gyrus, and striatum. This study suggested that impulsivity was related to diminished synthesis of serotonin in specific brain regions in BPD subjects compared to controls.

In a PET study of impulsive female BPD subjects, Soloff et al. (2007) used [18 F] altanserin, a 5-HT2a receptor antagonist, to assess receptor binding capacity. Increased receptor binding implies diminished central serotonergic neurotransmission and postsynaptic upregulation. Binding was increased in BPD compared to control subjects in HIP, independent of depressed mood, degree of impulsivity, aggression, suicidality, or history of childhood abuse. (Because HIP volume is diminished in some MRI studies of BPD, results were also corrected for volume.) When the analysis was restricted to suicide attempters ($n = 12$), altanserin binding was significantly increased in HIP, medial temporal cortex, and occipital cortex (with a trend in lateral OFC) compared to control subjects.

Overlapping results of structural and metabolic studies in impulsive PD subjects suggest that impulsive aggression is mediated through specific fronto-temporo-limbic brain networks and related to diminished metabolic and serotonergic function in these networks. Dysfunction in these networks could contribute to emotion dysregulation and self-destructive behavior at times of stress.

Emotion Dysregulation

Emotion dysregulation is a risk factor for suicidal behavior and NSSI in BPD and other impulsive PDs and has been studied extensively using fMRI techniques. fMRI protocols demonstrate activation in neural networks involved in cognitive processing during task performance, such as tests of response inhibition, conflict resolution, or recall of episodic memory. When emotional stimuli are paired with the cognitive tasks, fMRI paradigms demonstrate the effects of affective arousal and affective interference with cognitive processing during task performance. Tests of emotion regulation may also involve voluntary suppression of an emotional response to aversive stimuli or cognitive reappraisal (Koenigsberg et al., 2009). These paradigms can be used to model the effects of negative emotion on cognitive function, which is clinically the most relevant stressor for the risk of suicidal behavior.

The simplest fMRI paradigms involve passive exposure of subjects to affectively valenced faces or pictures during scanning to generate affective arousal. Using pictures from the International Affective Pictures System, Herpertz et al. (2001) first reported that aversive pictures increased activation in AMY in BPD compared to control subjects. Donegan et al. (2003) reported similar results using the Ekman faces (neutral, happy, sad, fearful faces). However, BPD subjects activated AMY more strongly than controls for all four faces, including the neutral face, which they subjectively interpreted as hostile. (This latter finding is of special interest to psychotherapists.)

To study the effects of negative emotion on cognitive processing and behavior in subjects with BPD, Silbersweig et al. (2007) used an affective linguistic Go No-Go task, which involved discriminating words written in italics from those in plain type, incorporating words with strong negative affective valence (i.e. "meaningful to subjects with BPD"). Go No-Go tasks require response inhibition and are known to activate the OFC. In the negative emotional context, BPD subjects responded with *decreased* activation compared to controls in medial and OFC, suggesting *diminished response inhibition*; decreased activation in DLPFC and HIP, suggesting less working and episodic memory function; and diminished activation in subgenual ACC, suggesting less error recognition, conflict resolution, and emotion regulation. However, there was *increased* activation in AMY, indicating hyperarousal. BPD subjects did more poorly than controls on actual behavioral performance of the Go No-Go task, making more errors in the negative context. This paradigm demonstrated affective interference with cognitive function in the face of negative emotion in both brain networks and behavioral performance. Emotion dysregulation occurs when cognitive control ("top-down" regulation), fails in face of strong limbic ("bottom-up") hyperarousal (Silbersweig et al., 2007). It is important to note that areas of functional impairment in emotion dysregulation paradigms (i.e., OFC, ACC, DLPFC) closely parallel brain regions found to be structurally or metabolically abnormal in impulsive PD subjects.

Executive Cognitive Deficits, Affective Interference, and Cognitive Function

BPD subjects have deficits of executive cognitive functions in formal neuropsychological testing (Ruocco, 2005). These complex cognitive functions require the integrity and connectivity of OFC, ACC, DLPFC, superior parietal cortex, HIP, and many other areas (depending, in part, on the task modality). Adaptive behavior depends on healthy connectivity between cortical "control" regions and the diverse areas of the limbic system for regulation of emotion, impulses, and behavior. However, in BPD subjects, these areas may have structural, functional, and connectivity abnormalities compared to healthy control subjects. In addition, negative emotions interfere with neural processing in BPD compared to control subjects, resulting in impaired task performance (Soloff et al., 2015b).

Personality traits such as impulsivity and aggressiveness are also associated with structural, functional, and connectivity abnormalities in BPD; however, it is unclear whether, or how, these personality traits actually modulate neural processing during cognitive task performance. A recent fMRI study of female BPD subjects correlated personality traits of impulsivity and aggression with activation metrics during performance of a Go No-Go task, a measure of motor impulsiveness and response inhibition, modified to include positive, negative, and neutral Ekman faces as targets. In the negative (vs. positive) affective condition, impulsivity and aggression had significant but differing effects on neural processing during response inhibition. Effects were in opposite directions, and in different anatomical regions, suggesting that impulsivity and aggression are mediated by separate neural networks in BPD. In addition, the effects of impulsivity in BPD subjects differed markedly from impulsivity in healthy controls, suggesting a disorder-specific interaction of this personality trait with brain responses. Negative affect and impulsivity (but not aggression) had adverse and independent effects on task performance (Soloff et al., 2015a). The disruptive effects of negative affect on impulsive and aggressive PD subjects may be attributable to an interaction of the affective stimulus with the pre-existing neurobiology of personality traits, resulting in affective interference with neural processing and cognitive functions. That is, the diathesis to suicidal behavior in BPD may be "hard-wired" as aberrations in specific neural networks related to personality trait vulnerabilities and "triggered" by negative affective experiences.

The Endogenous Opioid System

The endogenous opioid system (EOS) has been suggested to be closely related to NSSI (Bandelow et al., 2010; Stanley & Siever, 2009). Two hypotheses have been formulated in this domain (cf. Tiefenbacher et al., 2005). According to the pain hypothesis, an increased EOS activity leads to hypoalgesia, and self-injurers use this behavior to reach a normal level of pain sensitivity (Barron & Sandman, 1983, 1985). The addiction hypothesis posits that self-injurers use their behavior to repetitively stimulate the EOS and develop a dependent behavioral pattern (Sandman & Hetrick, 1995; Thompson et al., 1995). However, data on the EOS in the context of NSSI in BPD is conflicting: Plasma β-endorphin immunoreactivity was low in patients with nonmajor depression, many of whom met criteria for BPD (Cohen et al., 1984). Coid, Allolio, and Rees (1983) reported raised plasma met-enkephalin levels. Pickar et al. (1982) reported low levels of opioid activity in CSF. In the Coid, Allolio, and Rees (1983) study, all subjects showed self-injurious behavior which was in most cases carried out in the absence of pain and was followed by relief of tension and/or dysphoria. In a more recent study in patients with Cluster B PDs, those with NSSI had significantly lower levels of CSF β-endorphin and met-enkephalin when compared with a non-NSSI group (Stanley et al., 2010). BPD patients' hypoalgesia could not be reversed by the opioid antagonist naloxone (Russ et al., 1994), but the longer-acting antagonist naltrexone was able to reduce dissociative symptoms as well as NSSI (Bohus et al., 1999; Roth, Ostroff, & Hoffman, 1996; Simeon & Knutelska, 2005; Sonne et al., 1996). A randomized, placebo-controlled trial of naltrexone in patients with BPD revealed small to medium effects on dissociation but no effect on NSSI frequencies (Schmahl et al., 2012).

Pain Processing and NSSI

Interestingly, many BPD patients report analgesic phenomena during self-injury (Shearer, 1994). Since pain appears to have an important emotion-regulating effect in BPD (Klonsky, 2007), it is crucial to explore the effects of pain on emotions at the neurobiological level. A large body of experimental research investigating pain perception in individuals with BPD points to reduced sensitivity in BPD patients (Bohus et al., 2000; Cardenas-Morales et al., 2011; Ludäscher et al., 2007; McCown et al., 1993; Russ et al., 1992; Schmahl et al., 2006; Schmahl et al., 2004; Schmahl et al., 2010). To further disentangle analgesic states in BPD, Schmahl et al. (2004) applied laser-evoked pain and a spatial discrimination task to test both pain perception and thresholds. In this study, subjective ratings and electroencephalography were measured. In accordance with previous findings, Schmahl and his colleagues were able to show that subjective pain ratings were lower in BPD patients and that pain thresholds were altered. Interestingly, no differences where observed in discrimination task performance of laser-evoked brain potentials. Accordingly, the analgesic state in BPD cannot be explained by an impairment of the sensory-discriminative component of pain. Aiming to explore neural correlates of reduced pain sensitivity in BPD, several studies used fMRI to assess brain activation in response to painful stimulation. In a first study by Schmahl et al. (2006), patients with BPD and NSSI underwent an fMRI scan while heat stimuli were applied to their hands. While BPD patients showed increased pain thresholds and smaller overall activation in response to standardized temperature stimuli (compared to healthy controls [HC]), the overall activation was similar in response to individually adjusted heat stimuli. However, BPD patients showed increased DLPFC activation along with decreased activations of the posterior parietal cortex. Moreover, painful heat stimulation evoked neural deactivation in the AMY and the perigenual ACC in participants with BPD. The observed interaction between increased pain-induced response in the DLPFC coupled with deactivations in the ACC and the AMY could be interpreted as an antinociceptive mechanism in BPD. While sensory discrimination processes remain intact, this mechanism may modulate pain circuits primarily by an increased top-down-regulation of emotional components of pain or an altered affective appraisal of pain.

To further explore neural processing of NSSI behavior in patients with BPD, Kraus et al. (2010) used script-driven imagery of self-injury. The authors compared different experimental sections of the script (situation-triggering SIB, emotional and cognitive reactions to the triggering situation, the act of SIB, relaxation after SIB) with a neutral baseline section. During the reactions to the trigger situation, patients compared to HCs showed significantly reduced activation in the orbitofrontal cortex. Most importantly, only BPD patients showed an increase of activation in the DLPFC during this section. When asked to imagine the self-injurious act itself, a significant decline in activation in the mid-cingulate gyrus was evoked in BPD patients. OFC deactivation in the BPD group might be related to a failure to inhibit or modulate their emotional reactivity.

Examining the neural mechanisms underlying the role of self-inflicted pain as a means of affect regulation in BPD more directly, Niedtfeld et al. (2010) conducted a fMRI study using picture stimuli to elicit negative affect and thermal stimuli to induce heat pain. Although the authors found an attenuation of activation in limbic areas (AMY, insula) in response to sensory stimulation, it was neither specific to patients with BPD nor to painful stimulation. The authors argue that possible mechanisms causing AMY deactivation over time could include an attentional shift caused by sensory stimuli per se (Pessoa et al., 2002), the automatic use of cognitive regulation strategies or (re-) appraisal (Ochsner et al., 2004), or habituation processes (Breiter et al., 1996). In order to identify brain mechanisms potentially underlying the limbic deactivation observed in their initial data analysis (Niedtfeld et al., 2010), the authors reanalyzed their findings of pain-mediated emotion regulation in BPD by measuring functional connectivity using psychophysiological interaction analyses. Guided by the intention to reveal potential neural mechanisms responsible for the potential role of pain in affect regulation in BPD, their analyses focused on connectivity between those regions that had previously been identified to be involved in emotional processing, namely the AMY, insula, and ACC (Niedtfeld et al., 2012). Results of their analyses indicated that there is a modulating effect of pain on the processing of negative pictures in BPD patients. More precisely, they observed that painful sensory stimuli, as opposed to warmth perception, resulted in enhanced negative coupling between (para-) limbic and prefrontal structures in BPD, thus indicating inhibition of limbic arousal (Niedtfeld et al., 2012). Moreover, the authors stated that in healthy participants this pattern was only noticeable when negative pictures were paired with warm stimuli and interpreted this finding as the result of automatic emotion regulation processes in response to a negative state of arousal (Ochsner et al., 2004). It is important to note that the statistically significant clusters in the prefrontal cortex, related to enhanced inhibitory coupling in BPD under pain, were located in close spatial proximity in the right medial frontal gyrus (BA 8 and BA 9)—that is, in regions previously associated with emotion regulation processes. For instance, a study by McRae and colleagues (2010) found that BA 8 was activated in the course of attentional shift processes, while activation in the DLPFC (BA 9) was observed when participants were asked to reappraise presented stimuli (Boettiger & D'Esposito, 2005; Ochsner et al., 2002). It is also interesting to note Niedtfeld et al.'s (2012) observation that the DLPFC showed enhanced coupling to the posterior insula. As already mentioned, the insular cortex is known to play a critical role in pain processing (Rainville, 2002) as well as in the affective appraisal of pain perception (Treede et al., 2000). Hence, one could speculate that the connectivity between DLPFC and posterior insula in BPD may imply an altered, possibly positive, appraisal of pain, whereas connectivity between BA 8 and AMY and ACC may reflect a neuronal correlate of attentional shift. Niedtfeld and colleagues (2017) recently demonstrated that the observed pattern of AMY deactivation with painful stimuli is tends to normalize after successful dialectical behavior therapy treatment.

Additional evidence for an altered appraisal mechanism of pain in patients with BPD stems from an fMRI study by Kluetsch and colleagues (2012). Analyses of functional connectivity in brain activation during pain processing in BPD showed that patients with BPD exhibited less connectivity between the posterior cingulate cortex and DLPFC when exposed to painful heat rather than neutral temperature stimulation. Moreover, Kluetsch and colleagues (2012) reported that participants with BPD showed reduced integration of the left retrosplenial cortex, the right inferior temporal gyrus, and the left superior frontal gyrus in the default mode network. Thus the authors discuss their findings as a possible indicator for a cognitive and affective appraisal of pain in patients with BPD that is less self-relevant and aversive. In sum, the overall reported results on pain processing in BPD suggest that NSSI may be interpreted as an attempt to compensate for a deficient emotion regulation mechanism in BPD patients. More specifically, the reported findings implicate that the soothing effect of pain in BPD seems to be mediated by different emotion regulation processes (attentional shift and altered appraisal of pain).

Using incision-induced pain, which takes into account tissue damage and thus provides a more valid model for NSSI, a stress-reducing effect of an incision into the forearm in terms of reduced subjective arousal and increased heart rate could be demonstrated (Reitz et al., 2012). These findings were recently replicated in an fMRI study, where a decrease of AMY activity after incision and an additional restitution of poststress AMY-mPFC coupling following incision in BPD patients was demonstrated (Reitz et al., 2015). The additional tension-reducing effect of seeing blood could recently be experimentally demonstrated in a study where painful stimuli were combined with artificial blood (Naoum et al., 2016).

■ REFERENCES

American Psychiatric Association. (2013). Borderline personality disorder. In *Diagnostic and statistical manual of mental disorders* (5th ed., pp. 663–666). Washington, DC: American Psychiatric Publishing.

Apter, A., Bleich, A., King, R. A., Kron, S., Fluch, A., Kotler, M., & Cohen, D. J. (1993). Death without warning? A clinical postmortem study of suicide in 43 Israeli adolescent males. *Arch Gen Psychiatry, 50*(2), 138–142.

Audenaert, K., Peremans, K., Goethals, I., & Van Heeringen, C. (2006). Functional imaging, serotonin and the suicidal brain. *Acta Neurol Belg, 106*(3), 125–131.

Augustine, J. R. (1996). Circuitry and functional aspects of the insular lobe in primates including humans. *Brain Res Rev, 22*(3), 229–244.

Bandelow, B., Schmahl, C., Falkai, P., & Wedekind, D. (2010). Borderline personality disorder: a dysregulation of the endogenous opioid system? *Psychol Rev, 117*(2), 623–636.

Barron, J., & Sandman, C. A. (1983). Relationship of sedative-hypnotic response to self-injurious behavior and stereotypy by mentally retarded clients. *Am J Ment Defic, 88*(2), 177–186.

Barron, J., & Sandman, C. A. (1985). Paradoxical excitement to sedative-hypnotics in mentally retarded clients. *Am J Ment Defic, 90*(2), 124–129.

Black, D. W., Blum, N., Pfohl, B., & Hale, N. (2004). Suicidal behavior in borderline personality disorder: prevalence, risk factors, prediction, and prevention. *J Pers Disord, 18*(3), 226–239.

Boettiger, C. A., & D'Esposito, M. (2005). Frontal networks for learning and executing arbitrary stimulus-response associations. *J Neurosci, 25*(10), 2723–2732. doi:10.1523/JNEUROSCI.3697-04.2005

Bohus, M., Landwehrmeyer, G. B., Stiglmayr, C. E., Limberger, M. F., & d Christian, G. S. (1999). An open-label trial. *Clin Psychiatry, 60*, 598–603.

Bohus, M., Limberger, M., Ebner, U., Glocker, F. X., Schwarz, B., Wernz, M., & Lieb, K. (2000). Pain perception during self-reported distress and calmness in patients with borderline personality disorder and self-mutilating behavior. *Psychiatry Res, 95*(3), 251–260.

Brambilla, P., Soloff, P. H., Sala, M., Nicoletti, M. A., Keshavan, M. S., & Soares, J. C. (2004). Anatomical MRI study of borderline personality disorder patients. *Psychiatry Res Neuroimag, 131*(2), 125–133. doi:10.1016/j.pscychresns.2004.04.003

Breiter, H. C., Etcoff, N. L., Whalen, P. J., Kennedy, W. A., Rauch, S. L., Buckner, R. L., . . . Rosen, B. R. (1996). Response and habituation of the human amygdala during visual processing of facial expression. *Neuron, 17*(5), 875–887.

Brunner, R., Parzer, P., Haffner, J., Steen, R., Roos, J., Klett, M., & Resch, F. (2007). Prevalence and psychological correlates of occasional and repetitive deliberate self-harm in adolescents. *Arch Pediatr Adolesc Med, 161*(7), 641–649.

Cardenas-Morales, L., Fladung, A. K., Kammer, T., Schmahl, C., Plener, P. L., Connemann, B. J., & Schonfeldt-Lecuona, C. (2011). Exploring the affective component of pain perception during aversive stimulation in borderline personality disorder. *Psychiatry Res, 186*(2–3), 458–460. doi:10.1016/j.psychres.2010.07.050

Centers for Disease Control and Prevention. (2012). Table 35. Death rates for suicide, by sex, race, Hispanic origin, and age: United States, selected years 1950–2010 [Data file]. Retrieved March 31, 2014, from http://www.cdc.gov/nchs/data/hus/2012/035.pdf.

Chapman, A. L., Gratz, K. L., & Brown, M. Z. (2006). Solving the puzzle of deliberate self-harm: The experiential avoidance model. *Behav Res Ther, 44*(3), 371–394.

Cohen, M. R., Pickar, D., Extein, I., Gold, M. S., & Sweeney, D. R. (1984). Plasma cortisol and B-endorphin immunoreactivity in nonmajor and major depression. *Am J Psychiatry, 141*(625632), 1949.

Coid, J., Allolio, B., & Rees, L. (1983). Raised plasma metenkephalin in patients who habitually mutilate themselves. *Lancet, 322*(8349), 545–546.

Davidson, R. J., Putnam, K. M., & Larson, C. L. (2000). Dysfunction in the neural circuitry of emotion regulation—a possible prelude to violence. *Science, 289*(5479), 591–594.

De la Fuente, J., Goldman, S., Stanus, E., Vizuete, C., Morlán, I., Bobes, J., & Mendlewicz, J. (1997). Brain glucose metabolism in borderline personality disorder. *J Psychiatr Res, 31*(5), 531–541.

Desmyter, S., Van Heeringen, C., & Audenaert, K. (2011). Structural and functional neuroimaging studies of the suicidal brain. *Progr Neuropsychopharmacol Biol Psychiatry, 35*(4), 796–808.

Donegan, N. H., Sanislow, C. A., Blumberg, H. P., Fulbright, R. K., Lacadie, C., Skudlarski, P., . . . Wexler, B. E. (2003). Amygdala hyperreactivity in borderline personality disorder: implications for emotional dysregulation. *Biol Psychiatry, 54*(11), 1284–1293.

Driessen, M., Herrmann, J., Stahl, K., Zwaan, M., Meier, S., Hill, A., . . . Petersen, D. (2000). Magnetic resonance imaging volumes of the hippocampus and the amygdala in women with borderline personality disorder and early traumatization. *Arch Gen Psychiatry, 57*(12), 1115–1122.

Favazza, A. R. (1998). The coming of age of self-mutilation. *J Nerv Ment Dis*, *186*(5), 259–268.

Frances, A., Fyer, M., & Clarkin, J. (1986). Personality and suicide. *Ann N Y Acad Sci*, *487*(1), 281–295.

Goethals, I., Audenaert, K., Jacobs, F., Van den Eynde, F., Bernagie, K., Kolindou, A., . . . Van Heeringen, C. (2005). Brain perfusion SPECT in impulsivity-related personality disorders. *Behav Brain Res*, *157*(1), 187–192.

Goyer, P. F., Andreason, P. J., Semple, W. E., Clayton, A. H., King, A. C., Compton-Toth, B. A., . . . Cohen, R. M. (1994). Positron-emission tomography and personality disorders. *Neuropsychopharmacology*, *10*(1), 21–28.

Gross, J. J., & Thompson, R. A. (2006). Conceptual foundations. In G. J. J. (Ed.), *Handbook of emotion regulation* (pp. 5–18). New York: Guilford Press.

Gunderson, J. G., & Ridolfi, M. E. (2001). Borderline personality disorder: suicidality and self-mutilation. *Ann N Y Acad Sci*, *932*, 61–73.

Hazlett, E. A., New, A. S., Newmark, R., Haznedar, M. M., Lo, J. N., Speiser, L. J., . . . Buchsbaum, M. S. (2005). Reduced anterior and posterior cingulate gray matter in borderline personality disorder. *Biol Psychiatry*, *58*(8), 614–623.

Heikkinen, M., Isometsa, E. T., Henriksson, M. M., Marttunen, M. J., Aro, H. M., & Lonnqvist, J. K. (1997). Psychosocial factors and completed suicide in personality disorders. *Acta Psychiatr Scand*, *95*(1), 49–57.

Herpertz, S. (1995). Self-injurious behaviour Psychopathological and nosological characteristics in subtypes of self-injurers. *Acta Psychiatr Scand*, *91*(1), 57–68.

Herpertz, S., Dietrich, T. M., Wenning, B., Krings, T., Erberich, S. C., Willmes, K., . . . Sass, H. (2001). Evidence of abnormal amygdala functioning in borderline personality disorder: a functional MRI study. *Biol Psychiatry*, *50*(4), 292–298.

Irle, E., Lange, C., & Sachsse, U. (2005). Reduced size and abnormal asymmetry of parietal cortex in women with borderline personality disorder. *Biol Psychiatry*, *57*(2), 173–182.

Isometsa, E. T., Henriksson, M. M., Heikkinen, M. E., Aro, H. M., Marttunen, M. J., Kuoppasalmi, K. I., & Lönnqvist, J. K. (1996). Suicide among subjects with personality disorders. *Am J Psychiatry*, *153*, 667–673.

King-Casas, B., Sharp, C., Lomax-Bream, L., Lohrenz, T., Fonagy, P., & Montague, P. R. (2008). The rupture and repair of cooperation in borderline personality disorder. *Science*, *321*(5890), 806–810.

Kleindienst, N., Bohus, M., Ludäscher, P., Limberger, M. F., Kuenkele, K., Ebner-Priemer, U. W., . . . Schmahl, C. (2008). Motives for nonsuicidal self-injury among women with borderline personality disorder. *J Nerv Ment Dis*, *196*(3), 230–236.

Klonsky, E. D. (2007). The functions of deliberate self-injury: a review of the evidence. *Clin Psychol Rev*, *27*(2), 226–239. doi:10.1016/j.cpr.2006.08.002

Kluetsch, R. C., Schmahl, C., Niedtfeld, I., Densmore, M., Calhoun, V. D., Daniels, J., . . . Lanius, R. A. (2012). Alterations in default mode network connectivity during pain processing in borderline personality disorder default mode network, pain processing, and BPD. *Arch Gen Psychiatry*, *69*(10), 993–1002. doi:10.1001/archgenpsychiatry.2012.476

Koenigsberg, H. W., Fan, J., Ochsner, K. N., Liu, X., Guise, K. G., Pizzarello, S., . . . Goodman, M. (2009). Neural correlates of the use of psychological distancing to regulate responses to negative social cues: a study of patients with borderline personality disorder. *Biol Psychiatry*, *66*(9), 854–863.

Kraus, A., Valerius, G., Seifritz, E., Ruf, M., Bremner, J., Bohus, M., & Schmahl, C. (2010). Script-driven imagery of self-injurious behavior in patients with borderline personality disorder: a pilot FMRI study. *Acta Psychiatr Scand*, *121*(1), 41–51.

Leyton, M., Okazawa, H., Diksic, M., Paris, J., Rosa, P., Mzengeza, S., . . . Benkelfat, C. (2001). Brain regional α-[11C] methyl-L-tryptophan trapping in impulsive subjects with borderline personality disorder. *Am J Psychiatry, 158*(5), 775–782.

Ludäscher, P., Bohus, M., Lieb, K., Philipsen, A., & Schmahl, C. (2007). Elevated pain thresholds correlate with dissociation and aversive arousal in patients with borderline personality disorder. *Psychiatry Res, 149*(1–3), 291–296.

Mann, J. J. (2003). Neurobiology of suicidal behaviour. *Nature Rev Neurosci, 4*(10), 819–828.

Mann, J. J., & Stoff, D. M. (1997). A synthesis of current findings regarding neurobiological correlates and treatment of suicidal behavior. *Ann N Y Acad Sci, 836,* 352–363.

Maris, R. W., Berman, A. L., & Silverman, M. M. (2000). *Comprehensive textbook of suicidology.* New York: Guilford Press.

McCown, W., Galina, H., Johnson, J., de Simone, P. A., & Posa, J. (1993). Borderline personality disorder and laboratory-induced cold pressor pain: evidence of stress-induced analgesia. *J Psychopathol Behav Assess, 15*(2), 87–95.

McGirr, A., Paris, J., Lesage, A., Renaud, J., & Turecki, G. (2007). Risk factors for suicide completion in borderline personality disorder: a case-control study of cluster B comorbidity and impulsive aggression. *J Clin Psychiatry, 68*(5), 721–729.

McRae, K., Hughes, B., Chopra, S., Gabrieli, J. D., Gross, J. J., & Ochsner, K. N. (2010). The neural bases of distraction and reappraisal. *J Cogn Neurosci, 22*(2), 248–262. doi:10.1162/jocn.2009.21243

Moran, P., Coffey, C., Romaniuk, H., Olsson, C., Borschmann, R., Carlin, J. B., & Patton, G. C. (2012). The natural history of self-harm from adolescence to young adulthood: a population-based cohort study. *Lancet, 379*(9812), 236–243.

Muehlenkamp, J. J., Claes, L., Havertape, L., & Plener, P. L. (2012). International prevalence of adolescent non-suicidal self-injury and deliberate self-harm. *Child Adolesc Psychiatry Ment Health, 6*(10), 1–9.

Naoum, J., Reitz, S., Krause-Utz, A., Kleindienst, N., Willis, F., Kuniss, S., . . . Schmahl, C. (2016). The role of seeing blood in non-suicidal self-injury in female patients with borderline personality disorder. *Psychiatry Res, 246,* 676–682.

New, A. S., Hazlett, E. A., Buchsbaum, M. S., Goodman, M., Mitelman, S. A., Newmark, R., . . . Siever, L. J. (2007). Amygdala-prefrontal disconnection in borderline personality disorder. *Neuropsychopharmacology, 32*(7), 1629–1640.

New, A. S., Hazlett, E. A., Buchsbaum, M. S., Goodman, M., Reynolds, D., Mitropoulou, V., . . . Platholi, J. (2002). Blunted prefrontal cortical 18fluorodeoxyglucose positron emission tomography response to meta-chlorophenylpiperazine in impulsive aggression. *Archives of General Psychiatry, 59*(7), 621–629.

Niedtfeld, I., Kirsch, P., Schulze, L., Herpertz, S. C., Bohus, M., & Schmahl, C. (2012). Functional connectivity of pain-mediated affect regulation in borderline personality disorder. *PLoS One, 7*(3), e33293. doi:10.1371/journal.pone.0033293

Niedtfeld, I., Schulze, L., Kirsch, P., Herpertz, S. C., Bohus, M., & Schmahl, C. (2010). Affect regulation and pain in borderline personality disorder: a possible link to the understanding of self-injury. *Biol Psychiatry, 68*(4), 383–391. doi:10.1016/j.biopsych.2010.04.015

Niedtfeld, I., Winter, D., Schmitt, R., Bohus, M., Schmahl, C., & Herpertz, C. S. (2017). Pain-mediated affect regulation is reduced after dialectical behavior therapy in borderline personality disorder. *Soc Cogn Affect Neurosci, 12*(5), 739–747.

Nock, M. K., & Prinstein, M. J. (2004). A functional approach to the assessment of self-mutilative behavior. *J Consult Clin Psychol, 72*(5), 885–890.

Ochsner, K. N., Bunge, S. A., Gross, J. J., & Gabrieli, J. D. (2002). Rethinking feelings: an FMRI study of the cognitive regulation of emotion. *J Cogn Neurosci, 14*(8), 1215–1229. doi:10.1162/089892902760807212

Ochsner, K. N., & Gross, J. J. (2006). The neural architecture of emotion regulation. In J. J. Gross (Ed.), *Handbook of emotion regulation* (pp. 87–89). New York: Guilford Press.

Ochsner, K. N., Ray, R. D., Cooper, J. C., Robertson, E. R., Chopra, S., Gabrieli, J. D., & Gross, J. J. (2004). For better or for worse: neural systems supporting the cognitive down- and up-regulation of negative emotion. *NeuroImage, 23*(2), 483–499. doi:10.1016/j.neuroimage.2004.06.030

Paris, J., & Zweig-Frank, H. (2001). A 27-year follow-up of patients with borderline personality disorder. *Compr Psychiatry, 42*(6), 482–487.

Pessoa, L., McKenna, M., Gutierrez, E., & Ungerleider, L. G. (2002). Neural processing of emotional faces requires attention. *Proc Natl Acad Sci U S A, 99*(17), 11458–11463. doi:10.1073/pnas.172403899

Phillips, M. L., Ladouceur, C. D., & Drevets, W. C. (2008). A neural model of voluntary and automatic emotion regulation: implications for understanding the pathophysiology and neurodevelopment of bipolar disorder. *Mol Psychiatry, 13*(9), 829, 833–857. doi:10.1038/mp.2008.65

Phillips, M. L., Travis, M. J., Fagiolini, A., & Kupfer, D. J. (2008). Medication effects in neuroimaging studies of bipolar disorder. *Am J Psychiatry, 165*(3), 313–320.

Pickar, D., Cohen, M. R., Naber, D., & Cohen, R. M. (1982). Clinical studies of the endogenous opioid system. *Biol Psychiatry, 17*(11), 1243–1276.

Plener, P. L., Fischer, C. J., In-Albon, T., Rollett, B., Nixon, M. K., Groschwitz, R. C., & Schmid, M. (2013). Adolescent non-suicidal self-injury (NSSI) in German-speaking countries: comparing prevalence rates from three community samples. *Soc Psychiatry Psychiatr Epidemiol, 48*(9), 1439–1445.

Pollock, L. R., & Williams, J. M. G. (2001). Effective problem solving in suicide attempters depends on specific autobiographical recall. *Suicide Life Threat Behav, 31*(4), 386–396.

Rainville, P. (2002). Brain mechanisms of pain affect and pain modulation. *Curr Opin Neurobiol, 12*(2), 195–204.

Reitz, S., Kluetsch, R., Niedtfeld, I., Knorz, T., Lis, S., Paret, C., . . . Baumgärtner, U. (2015). Incision and stress regulation in borderline personality disorder: neurobiological mechanisms of self-injurious behaviour. *Br J Psychiatry, 207*(2), 165–172 .

Reitz, S., Krause-Utz, A., Pogatzki-Zahn, E. M., Ebner-Priemer, U., Bohus, M., & Schmahl, C. (2012). Stress regulation and incision in borderline personality disorder--a pilot study modeling cutting behavior. *J Pers Disord, 26*(4), 605–615. doi:10.1521/pedi.2012.26.4.605

Rich, C., & Runeson, B. S. (1992). Similarities in diagnostic comorbidity between suicide among young people in Sweden and the United States. *Acta Psychiatr Scand, 86*(5), 335–339.

Roth, A. S., Ostroff, R. B., & Hoffman, R. E. (1996). Naltrexone as a treatment for repetitive self-injurious behavior: an open-label trial. *J Clin Psychiatry, 57*(6), 233–237.

Ruocco, A. C. (2005). The neuropsychology of borderline personality disorder: a meta-analysis and review. *Psychiatry Res, 137*(3), 191–202.

Rüsch, N., van Elst, L. T., Ludaescher, P., Wilke, M., Huppertz, H. J., Thiel, T., . . . Ebert, D. (2003). A voxel-based morphometric MRI study in female patients with borderline personality disorder. *NeuroImage, 20*(1), 385–392.

Russ, M. J., Roth, S. D., Lerman, A., Kakuma, T., Harrison, K., Shindledecker, R. D., . . . Mattis, S. (1992). Pain perception in self-injurious patients with borderline personality disorder. *Biol Psychiatry, 32*(6), 501–511.

Russ, M. J., Roth, S. D., Kakuma, T., Harrison, K., & Hull, J. W. (1994). Pain perception in self-injurious borderline patients: naloxone effects. *Biological Psychiatry, 35*(3), 207–209.

Sala, M., Caverzasi, E., Lazzaretti, M., Morandotti, N., De Vidovich, G., Marraffini, E., . . . Brambilla, P. (2011). Dorsolateral prefrontal cortex and hippocampus sustain impulsivity and aggressiveness in borderline personality disorder. *J Affect Disord, 131*(1–3), 417–421.

Sandman, C. A., & Hetrick, W. P. (1995). Opiate mechanisms in self-injury. *Ment Retard Dev Disabil Res Rev, 1*(2), 130–136.

Schmahl, C., Bohus, M., Esposito, F., Treede, R. D., Di Salle, F., Greffrath, W., . . . Seifritz, E. (2006). Neural correlates of antinociception in borderline personality disorder. *Arch Gen Psychiatry, 63*(6), 659–667. doi:10.1001/archpsyc.63.6.659

Schmahl, C., Greffrath, W., Baumgartner, U., Schlereth, T., Magerl, W., Philipsen, A., . . . Treede, R. D. (2004). Differential nociceptive deficits in patients with borderline personality disorder and self-injurious behavior: laser-evoked potentials, spatial discrimination of noxious stimuli, and pain ratings. *Pain, 110*(1–2), 470–479. doi:10.1016/j.pain.2004.04.035

Schmahl, C., Kleindienst, N., Limberger, M., Ludäscher, P., Mauchnik, J., Deibler, P., . . . Herpertz, S. (2012). Evaluation of naltrexone for dissociative symptoms in borderline personality disorder. *Internat Clin Psychopharmacol, 27*(1), 61–68.

Schmahl, C., Meinzer, M., Zeuch, A., Fichter, M., Cebulla, M., Kleindienst, N., . . . Bohus, M. (2010). Pain sensitivity is reduced in borderline personality disorder, but not in posttraumatic stress disorder and bulimia nervosa. *World J Biol Psychiatry, 11*(2 Pt 2), 364–371. doi:10.3109/15622970701849952

Schmahl, C., Vermetten, E., Elzinga, B. M., & Bremner, J. D. (2003). Magnetic resonance imaging of hippocampal and amygdala volume in women with childhood abuse and borderline personality disorder. *Psychiatry Res: Neuroimag, 122*(3), 193–198.

Schneider, B., Wetterling, T., Sargk, D., Schneider, F., Schnabel, A., Maurer, K., & Fritze, J. (2006). Axis I disorders and personality disorders as risk factors for suicide. *Eur Arch Psychiatry Clin Neurosci, 256*(1), 17–27.

Shearer, S. L. (1994). Phenomenology of self-injury among inpatient women with borderline personality disorder. *J Nerv Ment Dis, 182*(9), 524–526.

Siever, L. J., Buchsbaum, M. S., New, A. S., Spiegel-Cohen, J., Wei, T., Hazlett, E. A., . . . Mitropoulou, V. (1999). d,l-fenfluramine response in impulsive personality disorder assessed with [18F]fluorodeoxyglucose positron emission tomography. *Neuropsychopharmacology, 20*(5), 413–423.

Silbersweig, D., Clarkin, J. F., Goldstein, M., Kernberg, O. F., Tuescher, O., Levy, K. N., . . . Stern, E. (2007). Failure of frontolimbic inhibitory function in the context of negative emotion in borderline personality disorder. *Am J Psychiatry, 164*(12), 1832–1841.

Simeon, D., & Knutelska, M. (2005). An open trial of naltrexone in the treatment of depersonalization disorder. *J Clin Psychopharmacol, 25*(3), 267–270.

Soloff, P. H., & Fabio, A. (2008). Prospective predictors of suicide attempts in borderline personality disorder at one, two, and two-to-five year follow-up. *J Pers Disord, 22*(2), 123–134. doi:10.1521/pedi.2008.22.2.123

Soloff, P. H., Lis, J. A., Kelly, T., Cornelius, J., & Ulrich, R. (1994). Self-mutilation and suicidal behavior in borderline personality disorder. *J Pers Disord, 8*(4), 257–267.

Soloff, P. H., Meltzer, C. C., Becker, C., Greer, P. J., Kelly, T. M., & Constantine, D. (2003). Impulsivity and prefrontal hypometabolism in borderline personality disorder. *Psychiatry Res Neuroimag, 123*(3), 153–163.

Soloff, P. H., Meltzer, C. C., Greer, P. J., Constantine, D., & Kelly, T. M. (2000). A fenfluramine-activated FDG-PET study of borderline personality disorder. *Biol Psychiatry, 47*(6), 540–547.

Soloff, P. H., Nutche, J., Goradia, D., & Diwadkar, V. (2008). Structural brain abnormalities in borderline personality disorder: a voxel-based morphometry study. *Psychiatry Res: Neuroimag, 164*(3), 223–236.

Soloff, P. H., Price, J. C., Meltzer, C. C., Fabio, A., Frank, G. K., & Kaye, W. H. (2007). 5HT 2A receptor binding is increased in borderline personality disorder. *Biol Psychiatry, 62*(6), 580–587.

Soloff, P. H., Pruitt, P., Sharma, M., Radwan, J., White, R., & Diwadkar, V. A. (2012). Structural brain abnormalities and suicidal behavior in borderline personality disorder. *J Psychiatr Res, 46*(4), 516–525. doi:10.1016/j.jpsychires.2012.01.003

Soloff, P. H., Ramaseshan, K., Abraham, K., Burgess A., Chowdury, A., & Diwadkar, V. A. (2015a). Impulsivity and aggression mediate regional brain responses in borderline personality disorder: an fMRI study. Paper presented at the ISSPD XIV meeting, Montreal, Canada, October 13–16.

Soloff, P. H., White, R., & Diwadkar, V. A. (2014). Impulsivity, aggression and brain structure in high and low lethality suicide attempters with borderline personality disorder. *Psychiatry Res Neuroimag, 222*(3), 131–139.

Soloff, P. H., White, R., Omari, A., Ramaseshan, K., & Diwadkar, V. A. (2015b). Affective context interferes with brain responses during cognitive processing in borderline personality disorder: fMRI evidence. *Psychiatry Res Neuroimag, 233*(1), 23–35.

Sonne, S., Rubey, R., Brady, K., Malcolm, R., & Morris, T. (1996). Naltrexone treatment of self-injurious thoughts and behaviors. *J Nerv Ment Dis, 184*(3), 192–194.

Stanley, B., Sher, L., Wilson, S., Ekman, R., Huang, Y.-Y., & Mann, J. J. (2010). Non-suicidal self-injurious behavior, endogenous opioids and monoamine neurotransmitters. *J Affect Disord, 124*(1), 134–140.

Stanley, B., & Siever, L. J. (2009). The interpersonal dimension of borderline personality disorder: toward a neuropeptide model. *Am J Psychiatry, 167*(1), 24–39.

Tebartz van Elst, L., Hesslinger, B., Thiel, T., Geiger, E., Haegele, K., Lemieux, L., . . . Ebert, D. (2003). Frontolimbic brain abnormalities in patients with borderline personality disorder: a volumetric magnetic resonance imaging study. *Biol Psychiatry, 54*(2), 163–171.

Thompson, T., Symons, F., Delaney, D., & England, C. (1995). Self-injurious behavior as endogenous neurochemical self-administration. *Ment Retard Dev Disabil Res Rev, 1*(2), 137–148.

Tiefenbacher, S., Novak, M. A., Lutz, C. K., & Meyer, J. S. (2005). The physiology and neurochemistry of self-injurious behavior: a nonhuman primate model. *Front Biosci, 10*(1), 1–11.

Treede, R.-D., Apkarian, A. V., Bromm, B., Greenspan, J. D., & Lenz, F. A. (2000). Cortical representation of pain: functional characterization of nociceptive areas near the lateral sulcus. [Review]. *Pain, 87*(2), 113–119.

Verona, E., Patrick, C. J., & Joiner, T. E. (2001). Psychopathy, antisocial personality, and suicide risk. *J Abnorm Psychol, 110*(3), 462.

Welch, S. S., Linehan, M. M., Sylvers, P., Chittams, J., & Rizvi, S. L. (2008). Emotional responses to self-injury imagery among adults with borderline personality disorder. *J Consult Clin Psychol, 76*(1), 45–51. doi:10.1037/0022-006X.76.1.45

Williams, J. M., & Broadbent, K. (1986). Autobiographical memory in suicide attempters. *J Abnorm Psychol, 95*(2), 144–149.

Zanarini, M. C., Frankenburg, F. R., Reich, D. B., Fitzmaurice, G., Weinberg, I., & Gunderson, J. G. (2008). The 10-year course of physically self-destructive acts reported by borderline patients and axis II comparison subjects. *Acta Psychiatr Scand, 117*(3), 177–184.

Zanarini, M. C., Frankenburg, F. R., Reich, D. B., Silk, K. R., Hudson, J. I., & McSweeney, L. B. (2007). The subsyndromal phenomenology of borderline personality disorder: a 10-year follow-up study. *Am J Psychiatry, 164*(6), 929–935.

Zetzsche, T., Preuss, U. W., Frodl, T., Schmitt, G., Seifert, D., Munchhausen, E., . . . Meisenzahl, E. M. (2007). Hippocampal volume reduction and history of aggressive behaviour in patients with borderline personality disorder. *Psychiatry Res, 154*(2), 157–170.

Zisook, S., Goff, A., Sledge, P., & Shuchter, S. R. (1994). Reported suicidal behavior and current suicidal ideation in a psychiatric outpatient clinic. *Ann Clin Psychiatry, 6*(1), 27–31.

Neurobiology of Categorical Diagnoses of Personality Disorder

12 The Neurobiology and Genetics of Schizotypal Personality Disorder

■ DANIEL R. ROSELL AND LARRY J. SIEVER

■ INTRODUCTION

This chapter focuses on the neurobiology of schizotypal personality disorder (SPD) as well as *schizotypy* or attenuated schizophrenia-spectrum traits present among the general population, as opposed to clinical cohorts. A greater understanding of the neurobiology of SPD will hopefully lead to (a) enhancements of the diagnosis and treatment of this complex, impairing, yet understudied, condition and (b) an improved understanding of the etiopathogenesis of schizophrenia, as well as the assessment of novel therapeutics without important confounds such as the effects of antipsychotic treatment and bouts of acute psychosis.

We first focus on the characterization of the SPD construct, as the quality of neurobiological correlates depends on psychometric validity. We then turn our attention to the genetics and development of SPD, followed by a review of studies employing nonimaging, laboratory measures. Then we discuss anatomical, functional, and neurochemical imaging findings. Finally we provide some general conclusions, address controversies in the field, and make suggestions for future directions.

■ ORIGINS AND CHARACTERIZATION OF THE SPD CONSTRUCT

SPD was formally introduced in the third edition of the *Diagnostic and Statistical Manual of Mental Disorders* (*DSM-III*) in 1980. Prior to this, schizoid and paranoid personality disorder diagnoses had been in use in *DSM-I* and *-II*. The term *schizoid personality* was originally used by Bleuler to refer to a constellation of enduring attenuated schizophrenia-spectrum traits which he believed reflected a diathesis to developing schizophrenia proper (Bleuler, 2010). Schizoid personality soon became applied relatively broadly, however, to patients who were shy and avoided intimacy and close relationships; and the significance of schizoid personality as a schizophrenia-spectrum condition ultimately dissipated (Siever & Gunderson, 1983).

The term "schizotype" or "schizotypal disorder" was coined by Rado in 1953, as a condensation of "schizophrenia genotype," which he used to describe a population of patients manifesting anhedonia, avoidance of emotional expression and thought, excessive dependency, and a vulnerability to disordered thinking (Rado, 1953). Although

Rado conjectured these patients carried a genetic liability for schizophrenia, his focus was in fact on psychodynamic mechanisms of psychopathology.

At the time of development of *DSM-III* and criteria for SPD, use of the term "borderline," which appeared to be applied to both a pathological personality syndrome (note: borderline personality disorder [BPD] proper had yet to be introduced prior to *DSM-III*) and a constellation of stable psychopathological traits believed to reflect a genetic diathesis to schizophrenia (i.e., borderline schizophrenia) (Spitzer et al., 1979). To complicate matters further, descriptions of both the borderline personality and borderline schizophrenia constructs consisted of paranoid ideation and transient periods of impaired reality testing, providing further confusion as to whether these two conditions were divergent or unitary.

Thus introduction of SPD in *DSM-III* was significant in that (a) it was specifically differentiated from the co-introduced BPD diagnosis (note: transient or quasi-psychotic symptoms were not included in the BPD criteria) and (b) for the first time it formally operationalized the personality syndrome believed to carry a genetic vulnerability for schizophrenia, which had long been envisaged. Following the introduction of SPD and BPD, numerous studies sought to (a) examine the validity of distinguishing between these two personality disorders and (b) verify the relationship between SPD and schizophrenia. We do not focus on the former issue in this review but rather refer the reader to a number of useful references (Baron et al., 1985; George & Soloff, 1986; Kavoussi & Siever, 1992; McGlashan, 1987; Plakun et al., 1987; Rosenberger & Miller, 1989; Serban et al., 1987; Silk et al., 1990; Spitzer & Endicott, 1979; Torgersen, 1984; Widiger et al., 1986). We discuss in greater detail throughout this chapter, however, studies that have examined the relationship between SPD and schizophrenia.

Following studies that addressed the validity of SPD as a diagnostic entity, investigators began to focus on the structure of schizotypal symptoms in personality-disordered patients (Bergman et al., 1996) (as well as the unaffected family members of schizophrenia patients [Bergman et al., 2000]) and schizotypy in nonclinical populations (Cohen et al., 2010; Compton et al., 2009; Raine et al., 1994). Both SPD (Battaglia et al., 1997; Hummelen et al., 2012) and schizotypy (Cohen et al., 2010; Raine et al., 1994) have consistently been shown to manifest a three-factor solution: The *cognitive–perceptual* factor subsumes odd beliefs/magical thinking, perceptual disturbances, referential thinking, and paranoia/suspiciousness. The *oddness* or *disorganized* factor consists of odd speech/thought processes and odd appearance/behavior. The *interpersonal* factor comprises no close friends and excessive social anxiety. Constricted/inappropriate affect belongs to the oddness factor when personality-disordered populations are assessed with a structured clinical interview and when nonclinical participants are assessed with self-report questionnaires; however, constricted/inappropriate affect is part of the interpersonal domain. Although this may owe to differences in the structure of SPD versus schizotypy in nonclinical populations, we suspect, as others have suggested (Hummelen et al., 2012), that observed affect deviations may be a separate dimension from subjective abnormalities. Finally, some models indicate that no close friends and social anxiety represent separate factors, thus leading to a four-factor model (Cohen et al., 2010), which has similarly been described in nonpsychotic family members of schizophrenia patients (Lien et al., 2010).

When SPD diagnostic criteria were examined along with the criteria of the nine other personality disorders in a treatment-seeking population with at least one personality disorder listed in the fourth edition, text revision of the *DSM* (*DSM-IV-R*), the cognitive-perceptual and oddness factors were replicated; however, the interpersonal factor was not: The "no close friends" criterion coalesced only with the identical criterion of schizoid personality disorder (SzPD), and, remarkably, the "social anxiety" criterion was not associated with any coherent factor. Additionally, the "paranoid/suspiciousness" criterion loaded onto a factor that consisted of a number of paranoid personality disorder (PPD) criteria, rather than the cognitive-perceptual factor (Hummelen et al., 2012). Oddness criteria were highly specific to SPD, whereas those of the cognitive-perceptual factor were also correlated with a diagnosis of BPD. Remarkably, however, BPD was not shown to be more common in patients with SPD relative to the total sample of personality-disordered patients. Antisocial personality disorder (AsPD) and PPD were found to be more common in SPD patients (Hummelen et al., 2012).

Therefore, neurobiological studies of SPD and schizotypy could address a number of important issues raised by these psychometric studies, such as the nature of interpersonal symptoms, the differences between observed affective abnormalities compared to subjective ones, how cognitive-perceptual symptoms in SPD differed from those in BPD, whether the paranoia/suspiciousness of SPD was different from that of PPD, and what the convergent and divergent properties of SPD and highly comorbid conditions such as AsPD and obsessive-compulsive disorder are.

■ HERITABILITY, DEVELOPMENT, AND MOLECULAR GENETICS

SPD and psychometric schizotypy have repeatedly been shown to be heritable; however, heritability estimates for SPD have ranged from 20% to 70% (Coolidge et al., 2001; Kendler et al., 2006, 2007; Torgersen et al., 2000). There is conflicting evidence as to whether the genetic liability of SPD also contributes to the heritability of PPD and SzPD (Kendler et al., 2006, 2015). In one twin study, however, in which all *DSM-IV* personality disorders were examined, there was support for a shared environmental factor contributing to all three Cluster A personality disorders but not a shared genetic component (Kendler et al., 2008).

With respect to the multidimensional nature of schizotypy, there is emerging evidence that there are both genetic and environmental factors that influence the broad construct of schizotypy, as well as ones that underlie individual schizotypy dimensions more specifically (Lin et al., 2007; Linney et al., 2003). One study also found evidence for three phenomenologically distinct latent classes of SPD—one with predominantly positive symptoms, one with predominantly negative symptoms, and the other characterized by interpersonal anxiety/sensitivity (Battaglia et al., 1999). The former two were found to be influenced by both genetic and environmental influences, whereas the latter class appeared to be determined by environmental but not genetic factors.

A handful of studies have addressed the role of genetic and environmental factors on the development and temporal stability of schizotypy during childhood and adolescence, as well as adulthood. Similar to what has been observed in adult populations, schizotypy in adolescence has also been shown to exhibit a three-factor structure (cognitive-perceptual, interpersonal, and disorganization). Moreover, it has also been shown that there are genetic and environmental influences that contribute to the broad schizotypy construct, as well as specific dimensions, in adolescence. One study demonstrated that the heritability of schizotypy was found to occur at two separate time points in adolescence: age 11 to 13 and age 14 to 16 (Ericson et al., 2011). Each of these heritable factors was influenced by both additive genetic factors as well as unique environmental influences (i.e., those not shared by siblings) (Ericson et al., 2011). While these heritability factors at these two developmental time points promoted development of all three schizotypy factors, there were additional genetic and environmental effects specific to the interpersonal-affective and disorganization dimensions at each developmental time point (Ericson et al., 2011).

One study has described that the genetic influences of SPD and PPD appeared to be, temporally, highly stable during adulthood (Kendler et al., 2015). Further, it was described that the temporal stability of SPD and Cluster A symptomatology appears to derive predominantly from genetic as opposed to environmental influences.

It is reasonable to speculate that environmental contributions to the development of schizotypy and SPD consist of psychological trauma. Multiple forms of childhood adversity—including physical abuse by anyone including parent or caretaker, witnessing fighting in the home, parental/caretaker neglect, and sexual abuse—were strongly associated with SPD (Lentz et al., 2010). In a study of schoolchildren 8 to 16 years of age, multiple forms of peer victimization were associated with SPD in both males and females (Fung & Raine, 2012). Schizotypy scores were found to be more than doubled in participants with significant levels of victimization (Fung & Raine, 2012). A recent twin study, however, has questioned the significance of childhood trauma as a significant contributor to Cluster A personality disorders, after taking into account family history and genetic factors (Berenz et al., 2013).

A number of genes have been identified that contribute to the development of SPD and schizotypal traits. Savitz et al. recently examined the interaction between a number of dopaminergic genes and childhood trauma on the development of schizotypal traits in a cohort of participants with a family history of bipolar disorder (Savitz et al., 2010). They found increasing levels of childhood trauma were related to greater schizotypal symptoms, specifically in participants with the Val allele of the Val158Met COMT gene polymorphism (Savitz et al., 2010), which is associated with greater dopamine degradation than the Met allele (Chen et al., 2004). A number of other genes have been identified that are associated with specific schizotypy dimensions. In an unselected population, variants of the Disrupted In Schizophrenia 1 (DISC1) gene, which is involved in regulating neuronal proliferation and differentiation, were shown to be associated with lower levels of social anhedonia but not with other schizotypy dimensions (e.g., perceptual aberrations, physical anhedonia) (Tomppo et al., 2009). Common variants of ZNF804A, a zinc finger protein associated with schizophrenia, were shown to be associated with suspiciousness/referential thinking but not a variety of other schizotypal dimensions and related features, such as cognitive function (Stefanis et al., 2013). Variants of the p250GAP gene, which encodes for a protein involved in N-methyl-D-aspartate receptor function, have been shown to be associated with increased total schizotypy scores in unaffected participants, with specific involvement of the interpersonal/affective schizotypy domain (Ohi et al., 2012).

QUANTITATIVE ENDOPHENOTYPES: OCULOMOTOR FUNCTION, EVENT-RELATED POTENTIALS, AND NEUROCOGNITION

Oculomotor Function

Oculomotor function represents a well characterized and noninvasive means to examine central nervous system integrity. In particular, smooth pursuit eye movements (SPEM) and anti-saccades (AS) have been used to assess executive and inhibitory processes that depend on fronto-temporal and fronto-striatal neural circuitry. Given the well-described SPEM (Ivleva et al., 2014) and AS abnormalities (Radant et al., 2015) in schizophrenia, these oculomotor functions have also been examined in SPD and psychometric schizotypy in order to determine their role in psychosis vulnerability more broadly.

A number of studies have examined SPEM and AS abnormalities in nonclinical participants psychometrically assessed with standard self-report measures of schizotypy. Aberrant SPEM performance has been observed consistently in participants with elevated levels of schizotypy, irrespective of whether these elevations were due to the positive or negative facets (Gooding et al., 2000; O'Driscoll et al., 1998; Smyrnis et al., 2007). On the other hand, deviant AS performance has been shown to occur in participants with elevated levels of cognitive-perceptual or positive schizotypal traits, whereas an association with negative or deficit dimensions of schizotypy is less consistent (O'Driscoll et al., 1998; Gooding, 1999; Gooding et al., 2005; Holahan & O'Driscoll, 2005; Smyrnis et al., 2003). As we describe further later, SPEM abnormalities have been more consistently described in clinical populations with SPD or schizotypal traits than have AS deficits.

An additional issue is whether the relationship between oculomotor abnormalities and schizotypy occurs as a continuous variable among all participants or only within the subgroup with divergent levels of schizotypal traits. This has important implications for a key issue in personality disorder research, that is, whether personality disorder phenomenologies exist on a continuum with "normality" or are taxonic/categorical. Most studies, such as the ones described, are consistent with the taxonic model. The few that have been suggestive of a continuous relationship have either involved individuals with a broader age range (Lenzenweger & O'Driscoll, 2006), or have employed oculomotor measures that isolate predictive or executive processes, as well as examined schizotypy in a factor-specific manner (Kattoulas et al., 2011). Therefore, whether schizotypy is a continuous or taxonic construct may depend on the population, component of schizotypy, and type of oculomotor task.

Oculomotor abnormalities have also been examined in personality-disordered patients with SPD or SPD traits. An early study demonstrated that in a cohort of male college students, a diagnosis of SPD or significant SPD traits occurred with significantly greater frequency in those with poor eye tracking compared to those with high-accuracy tracking (Siever et al., 1984). Subsequently, it was observed that undergraduate students meeting criteria for SPD manifested poorer quality eye tracking than healthy comparison participants (Lencz et al., 1993). Patients meeting full criteria for SPD as well as personality-disordered patients with two or more SPD traits both exhibited poorer qualitative SPEM compared to healthy comparison participants; however, personality-disordered patients with fewer than two SPD traits did not differ from controls on SPEM qualitative ratings (Siever et al., 1994). Further, the "deficit" symptoms of SPD (poor social rapport, oddness, social anxiety/isolation) were positively associated with SPEM impairments, whereas the positive or psychotic-like symptoms were either unrelated or positively associated depending on how these traits were measured. Two studies have examined SPD participants in comparison to a healthy group as well as a group with schizophrenia. Both of these studies found that it was easier to observe a significant difference between schizophrenia patients and controls than SPD and controls (Brenner et al., 2001; Mitropoulou et al., 2011). Finally, abnormalities of AS performance in SPD has been less well described than smooth pursuit deficits (Brenner et al., 2001; Cadenhead et al., 2002). We suspect that SPEM impairments may be a more global marker of SPD/schizotypy, whereas AS deficits may have a more restricted involvement. On the other hand, AS performance may also be influenced by other personality trait variables (Nguyen et al., 2008) that could act as confounds.

Event-Related Potentials

Event related potentials (ERPs) are voltage changes, as measured by electroencephalogram, that occur in response to specific stimuli and are used as neural correlates of specific sensory, motor, or cognitive processes. The advantages of employing ERPs are high temporal resolution and noninvasiveness. An ERP is designated according to whether it results in positive (P) or negative (N) voltage deflections and the latency or amount of time after test stimulus (typically measured in milliseconds) the voltage deflection occurs. The three best characterized ERPs in schizotypy are the P50, P300, and N400.

The P50 ERP has been used to assess the early, automatic process of "sensory gating." Typically, a P50 wave that occurs after a repeated auditory stimulus will be reduced in amplitude relative to the one associated with initial stimulus exposure: This phenomenon has been termed *P50 suppression*. Reduced P50 suppression is a widely replicated finding in both patients with SPD (Cadenhead et al., 2000; Hazlett et al., 2015) and as a function of schizotypy in nonclinical participants (Croft et al., 2001; Wang et al., 2004). The magnitude of effect of reduced P50 suppression in SPD is less than that of schizophrenia (Hazlett et al., 2015).

There is accumulating evidence that smoking is an important moderating variable between schizotypy and P50 suppression. In heavy smokers, there appears to be a positive association between P50 suppression and schizotypy, as opposed to the characteristic inverse correlation, which is most robust in those who are either light smokers or nonsmokers (Croft et al., 2004; Wan et al., 2006). Deficits of P50, particularly reductions in the amplitude of the initial or conditioning stimulus, may be related to greater number and intensity of SPD traits (an index of global severity) in patients with SPD (Hazlett et al., 2015). While only a few studies have examined whether specific schizotypy dimensions are related to P50 suppression deficits, it appears that the "positive" symptomatology (cognitive-perceptual, as well as mood/anxiety and attention/concentration difficulties) are primarily involved (Croft et al., 2001, 2004; Evans et al., 2007), as opposed to social or introvertive anhedonia, which is a core "negative" symptom.

The P300 ERP (also referred to as P3 or P3b) is believed to reflect a relatively late, active, cognitive process associated with decision-making regarding perceptual information. Classically, the P300 has been assessed with "oddball tasks" in which participants are asked to identify outlier stimuli such as a deviant auditory tone. Numerous studies have demonstrated P300 abnormalities in SPD/schizotypy, consisting of both reduced amplitudes and greater latency (Kimble et al., 2000; Klein et al., 1999; Mannan et al., 2001; Niznikiewicz et al., 2000; Salisbury et al., 1996). Furthermore, P300 abnormalities in SPD may also be intermediate to that of schizophrenia (Shin et al., 2010). Preliminary evidence suggests altered P300 may be associated with the cognitive-perceptual domain of schizotypy, including paranoia/suspiciousness (Li et al., 2011).

The N400 ERP has been used to examine processes related to language, semantic memory, or, more fundamentally, how meaningful stimuli and concepts are related to each other. Thus the N400 has been considered functionally salient to SPD and schizotypy due to impairments in language use, thought process, and meaning attribution. The N400 is commonly examined by comparing the amplitude elicited by a *target stimulus* that is congruous with a preceding *priming stimulus*, compared to an incongruous target stimulus. For example, the word *mouse* (congruous target) will normally elicit a less negative N400 amplitude than the word *monkey* (incongruous target) following the sentence fragment (priming stimulus): *The cat chased the* . . . . The difference in amplitude in response to congruous relative to incongruous target stimuli has been termed the *N400 effect* and is generally considered an index of how context is used to generate meaning.

Numerous studies have described N400 abnormalities in both patients with SPD as well as healthy participants psychometrically assessed for schizotypy (Kiang et al., 2010; Niznikiewicz et al., 1999, 2004). A matter of ongoing debate, however, is the extent to which relatively early and automatic, *predictive* mechanisms underlie N400 abnormalities in SPD/schizotypy as opposed to later, controlled, *integrative* ones (which may also rely on working memory) (de Loye et al., 2013; Kiang & Kutas, 2005; Kostova et al., 2014; Niznikiewicz et al., 2002). Moreover, the domain(s) that schizotypy N400 abnormalities may contribute to remain(s) unclear, as different studies have separately implicated the cognitive-perceptual (Kiang et al., 2010), interpersonal (Kiang & Kutas, 2005), and disorganized (Prevost et al., 2010) schizotypy dimensions.

Neurocognition

As the critical role of cognitive impairment in determining functional outcomes in schizophrenia has been widely examined (Green, 2006), characterizing the neuropsychological profile of patients with SPD has also become an area of growing interest. Generally speaking, the cognitive impairments observed in SPD are more circumscribed, less severe (McClure et al., 2008; Mitropoulou et al., 2005, 2011), and possibly more pharmacologically responsive relative to the cognitive deficits of schizophrenia (McClure et al., 2007, 2010; Rosell et al., 2015; Siegel et al., 1996). Most consistently, deficits of various forms of executive function (Diforio et al., 2000; Trestman et al., 1995; Voglmaier et al., 1997), verbal learning and memory (Bergman et al., 1998), context processing (McClure et al., 2008), and working memory (Kopp, 2007; McClure et al., 2007; Mitropoulou et al., 2005; Roitman et al., 2000) have been observed in patients with SPD. Finally, cognitive function in SPD has been shown to be impaired not only in relation to healthy participants but in comparison to other (non-Cluster A) personality disorders, including avoidant personality disorder, further supporting the specificity of this finding (McClure et al., 2013; Mitropoulou et al., 2002).

The central role of working memory to the cognitive deficits of SPD has been emerging. Similar to schizophrenia, attenuated working memory function appears to be an important determinant of functional impairment in SPD (McClure et al., 2013). Various forms of working memory deficits have been demonstrated in SPD patients including auditory (Mitropoulou et al., 2005), visual-verbal (McClure et al., 2008), and nonverbal or visuospatial (McClure et al, 2007; Roitman et al., 2000). There is evidence that aberrant verbal working memory underlies impairments in other cognitive areas (McClure et al., 2007; Mitropoulou et al., 2005). The deficit or negative symptoms of SPD and schizotypy have primarily been associated with cognitive impairment in SPD and schizotypy, as opposed to the positive symptoms or cognitive-perceptual dimension (Daly et al., 2012; McClure et al., 2008; Mitropoulou et al., 2002; Suhr and Spitznagel, 2001; Szoke et al., 2009). A putative pathophysiological mechanism of working memory impairment in SPD that has received support is understimulation of prefrontal dopamine 1 receptors, which may owe to corticolimbic hypodopaminergia and a compensatory, albeit insufficient, upregulation of prefrontal dopamine 1 receptors (Thompson et al., 2014). Preliminary evidence from our group supports a role for dopamine 1 receptor agonists, such as dihydrexidine, to enhance working memory in patients with SPD (Rosell et al., 2015).

■ STRUCTURAL BRAIN IMAGING

Numerous studies have examined structural/morphological neuroanatomical differences in SPD compared to healthy participants, as well as those with schizophrenia and other personality disorders. The primary focus has been on neocortical regions, particularly the frontal and temporal cortices. Although less well examined, the parietal lobe has also been implicated, as well as medial temporal lobe regions and the striatum.

One of the earliest and most consistent structural findings in SPD has been reduced temporal lobe volume (Dickey et al., 1999). The temporal lobe was originally of interest due to its involvement in schizophrenia (Sun et al., 2009). The structural abnormalities of the temporal lobe in SPD have been shown to be more restricted than those of schizophrenia in terms of the regions and subregions involved; the involvement of white matter integrity; and temporal progression (Hazlett et al., 2008; Kawasaki et al., 2004; Takahashi et al., 2010). While the superior temporal gyrus (STG) has been consistently observed in SPD, there is also some, albeit conflicting, evidence for the middle temporal gyrus and the fusiform gyrus; however, the inferior temporal gyrus has more often than not been shown to not be involved in SPD (Takahashi et al., 2006, 2011). Nevertheless, reduced STG (total and subregion) volumes have been associated with greater severity of SPD symptoms, logical memory, and odd speech/thought process (Dickey et al., 1999). Finally, reductions in STG volume provides a fair to good capacity to diagnostically discriminate between controls and SPD patients (Hazlett et al., 2014).

The frontal lobe, particularly the prefrontal cortex, has also been of particular interest in SPD given (a) the presence of prefrontal cortical pathology in schizophrenia, as well as (b) the characteristic cognitive deficits of the schizophrenia spectrum which implicate prefrontal impairments. Both early and more recent studies have provided evidence for reduced prefrontal gray matter volumes; however, unlike temporal lobe findings, consistent involvement of specific prefrontal subregions has not been identified. Further, there has been evidence for increased prefrontal cortical thickness in SPD and schizotypy (Hazlett et al., 2008, 2014; Kuhn et al., 2012). Our group has demonstrated *increased* volume of Brodmann's area (BA) 10, which, in contrast, is decreased in schizophrenia (Hazlett et al., 2008). Interestingly, greater BA 10 volumes in SPD is associated with *lower* SPD symptom severity, which may suggest BA 10 volume increases play a compensatory/protective role (Hazlett et al., 2014).

Although there has been relatively greater focus on frontal and temporal cortical regions, structural neuroanatomical differences of the striatum have also been identified. Two early studies by the same group demonstrated smaller caudate volumes in male and female medication-naïve patients with SPD; furthermore, greater caudate volume reduction was associated with poorer cognitive performance (Koo et al., 2006; Levitt et al., 2002). Additionally, shape abnormalities of the caudate have been examined, first on a more global level (Levitt et al., 2004) and, more recently, using methods that allow for a local or subregion approach (Levitt et al., 2009). These studies have demonstrated aberrant morphology of the right caudate, particularly the caudate head; furthermore, these morphological differences were correlated with verbal learning memory performance. In two studies by our group, caudate volumes were not found to differ from healthy controls or patients with schizophrenia (Chemerinski et al., 2013; Shihabuddin et al., 2001); nevertheless, we found a positive correlation between schizotypal psychotic-like symptoms and caudate volumes (Shihabuddin et al., 2001). Collectively, these findings suggest reduced caudate volumes in SPD may mitigate the development of overt psychosis at the expense of cognitive function.

Similar to findings in the caudate, differential putamen size in SPD has also been conflicting (Chemerinski et al., 2013; Shihabuddin et al., 2001). In a recent report by our group, we observed larger putamen size in patients with SPD compared to healthy controls, and an inverse correlation was observed between putamen size and symptoms of paranoia/suspiciousness (Chemerinski et al., 2013). In schizophrenia, greater loss of putamen volume over time is associated with poorer outcomes (Mitelman et al., 2009). Therefore, protection from the development of overt psychosis in patients with SPD may be associated with putamen size.

▪ FUNCTIONAL BRAIN IMAGING

Differences in neural activity with functional magnetic resonance imaging was examined in neuroleptic-naïve men with SPD compared to healthy controls in a paradigm using auditory stimuli of deviant pitch and duration. They found the SPD group exhibited increased activity of the STG (which manifests anatomical differences in SPD, as described) relative to control participants. Moreover, STG activity in response to deviant auditory stimuli was significantly associated with greater levels of the "odd speech/thought process" SPD symptom and poorer verbal learning memory performance (Dickey et al., 2008).

Functional imaging studies have examined neural correlates of cognitive and executive function impairments. Performance of a working memory task in patients with SPD was associated with differential neural activity compared to healthy participants, despite similar levels of task performance (Vu et al., 2013). Specifically, SPD was associated with decreased working memory task–induced activation of the posterior cingulate gyrus, STG, and middle frontal gyrus. These activation differences in SPD were not related to working memory task performance. We also previously found decreased activity of brain regions involved in working memory tasks (viz., the left ventral prefrontal cortex, superior frontal gyrus, intraparietal cortex, and posterior inferior gyrus) in SPD patients relative to control participants despite similarities in working memory performance (Koenigsberg et al., 2005). Future research is needed to expand our knowledge of working memory performance in schizotypy/SPD.

Interpersonal and affective impairments also play an important role in SPD and schizotypy, and functional imaging studies have begun to identify their neural correlates. One study compared neural activity in a high- versus low-stress task in a control group and a group with high levels of positive and negative schizotypy. Only the group with high levels of negative schizotypy (specifically, physical anhedonia) exhibited less deactivation of limbic and striatal regions during the high-stress task. Additionally, among all three groups combined, physical anhedonia scores were negatively correlated with the degree of striatal and limbic deactivation during the high-stress task (Soliman et al., 2011).

We examined whole amygdala activity while viewing affectively valenced pictures in patients with SPD compared to controls and a BPD group. The SPD group demonstrated greater amygdala activity to emotional pictures during the first presentation but significantly attenuated activity upon repeat exposures, compared to both the control and BPD groups. Attenuated amygdala activity in response to repeated negative emotional stimuli was associated with greater dissociative symptoms (Hazlett et al., 2012).

Finally, functional neurobiological differences in facial expressions and other affectively salient social cues have been described in schizotypy. Less deactivation of the right anterior cingulate cortex was observed in a group with SPD compared to controls in response to a dynamic facial affect processing stimulus. Moreover, social cues associated with "blame" resulted in different patterns of neural activity in the posterior cingulate gyrus and STG in SPD patients compared to controls (Huang et al., 2013).

Hooker and coworkers examined regional brain activity and schizotypal symptoms to positive facial expressions in adults with high and low levels of social anhedonia—a core dimension of schizotypy. Participants with high levels of social anhedonia exhibited less activity of the ventrolateral prefrontal cortex (VLPFC) in response to positive versus neutral facial expressions compared to participants with low levels of social anhedonia. Furthermore, low VLPFC activity in response to positive facial expressions was associated with greater state levels of schizotypal symptomatology (cognition, paranoia, positive affect, productivity) most notably in those with high levels of social anhedonia (Hooker et al., 2014).

A further study examined changes in neural activity in response to images of social rejection in participants with high compared to low levels of a measure of *unusual experiences* (an index of positive schizotypy). They found that while viewing images depicting rejection relative to neutral scenes, the high schizotypy group exhibited deactivation of the dorsal anterior cingulate cortex (dACC)—a region involved in cognitive control—whereas dACC activity was increased in the low schizotypy group (Premkumar et al., 2012).

■ **NEUROCHEMICAL BRAIN IMAGING**

The importance of the dopaminergic system in the schizophrenia spectrum has been well documented (Toda & Abi-Dargham, 2007), and a handful of studies to date have examined dopamine neurochemistry in patients with SPD and psychometric schizotypy with methods such as single photon emission computed tomography (SPECT) and positron emission tomography (PET). One of the earliest studies, by our group, used SPECT to assess striatal presynaptic dopamine in patients with SPD compared to healthy controls (Abi-Dargham et al., 2004). This technique consists of comparing striatal binding of the D2 receptor radioligand, [(123)I]Iodobenzamide (IBZM) before and after amphetamine infusion: greater amphetamine-induced decreases in [(123)I]IBZM binding signifies greater presynaptic dopamine. We found no differences in baseline [(123)I]IBZM striatal binding (i.e., no differences in striatal D2 receptor levels between SPD patients and healthy controls), however, there was greater amphetamine-induced decrease in striatal [(123)I]IBZM binding in patients with SPD compared to controls. Levels of presynaptic dopamine release were similar to those of patients with remitted schizophrenia, but less than acutely ill or psychotic schizophrenic patients.

The majority of related studies have examined dopaminergic neurochemistry in psychometric schizotypy, or schizotypal traits in healthy, non-clinical participants as assessed by well validated questionnaires such as the Schizotypal Personality Questionnaire (SPQ) or the Chapman scales. Soliman and coworkers used PET to examine changes in striatal binding of [(11)C]raclopride (a D2 receptor radioligand) before and after a psychological stress task involving mental arithmetic in three groups: healthy controls, non-clinical participants scoring high on the Chapman's Physical Anhedonia scale (a measure of negative schizotypy) and Perceptual Aberrations (a measure of positive schizotypy) (Soliman et al., 2008). Only participants scoring high on Physical Anhedonia exhibited relatively higher presynaptic dopamine levels in response to psychological stress (Soliman et al., 2008).

In a study of healthy participants characterized with the SPQ, amphetamine-induced changes in [(18)C]fallypride binding was used to identify relationships between presynaptic dopamine release in the striatum with schizotypal traits (Woodward et al., 2011). The primary finding was the positive correlation between dopamine release in the whole striatum with the total SPQ score. Further analyses revealed that this relationship was primarily related to the disorganized factor of the SPQ (consisting primarily of eccentric behavior and odd speech/disorganized thought process) and the associative striatum (involved in higher-order cognitive processes). Exploratory, voxel-wise analyses demonstrated positive correlations with total SPQ scores and the left medial prefrontal gyrus (roughly corresponding to BA 9/10) and the left supramarginal gyrus. Further exploratory analyses identified a more extensive set of cortical and subcortical brain regions in which presynaptic dopamine release was positively correlated with the disorganized SPQ factor (Woodward et al., 2011).

In a recent study, Chen and coworkers examined the relation between schizotypy and D2 receptor availability using [(123)I]IBZM SPECT in a large group of nonclinical adults characterized with the SPQ. Striatal D2 receptor availability was not found to be correlated with total SPQ scores; however, the disorganized SPQ factor was positively correlated with D2 receptor availability in the right striatum (Chen et al., 2012). Thus, increased dopaminergic activity has been associated with the psychotic-like symptoms and decreased activity with the deficit-like symptoms of SPD.

■ **SUMMARY AND CONCLUSIONS**

SPD illustrates many of the limitations of phenomenology-based classification and, therefore, the importance of genetic and neurobiological characterization of psychiatric diagnostic constructs. To name a few, SPD sits at the intersection of syndromes and personality (or what had, until the fifth edition of the *DSM*, been referred to as Axis I and Axis II disorders). The debate over whether psychiatric conditions are taxonic/categorical or lie on a continuum with normality is also exemplified given the existence of schizotypy, SPD, and schizophrenia. Finally, there are a number of examples of apparent symptom overlap between SPD and other personality disorders, most notably, paranoia/suspiciousness, the cognitive-perceptual criteria domain (specifically with BPD), and social anxiety. It is not clear if such symptom overlap represents true convergence or, rather, the difficulty in differentiating between two separate phenomenological dimensions which have similar symptomatic outcomes.

SPD is heritable and associated with an increased risk for schizophrenia. There is conflicting evidence as to whether SPD and other Cluster A personality disorders are genetically linked. There is even some evidence that they are not but rather share a common environmental pathogenic factor. There appear to be genetic factors that contribute to the development of schizotypy in general and others that promote specific dimensions. Many of the genes involved in schizophrenia have also been shown to promote schizotypy, and, as predicted by heritability studies, certain genetic polymorphisms are associated with specific schizotypy dimensions. There appear to be heritability time periods during adolescence and adulthood, including both genetic and environmental factors for SPD.

Based on certain neurobiological findings, SPD appears to simply be a milder or intermediate form of schizophrenia. Other findings, however, reveal important distinctions between SPD and schizophrenia, which may represent either (a) the absence of critical pathogenic factors (be they genetic and/or environmental) that otherwise would promote the development of schizophrenia proper or (b) the presence of compensatory mechanisms that may mitigate frank psychosis, albeit at the expense of other processes, such as cognition.

Future directions include refined characterization of the interpersonal domain of SPD. We suspect that the pathological personality dimensions that lead to lack of close friends and social anxiety in SPD likely differ from those associated with other personality disorders such as AsPD and AvPD or social phobia. Understanding, for example, the neurochemical basis of the interpersonal symptoms of SPD has critical clinical implications given, in our experience, these criteria are the ones patients find most symptomatic. Therefore, to dismiss the interpersonal symptoms as "nonspecific" as opposed to "difficult to differentiate phenomenologically yet neurobiologically distinct" would be a mistake in terms of developing novel therapeutics.

Identifying the etiopathogenetic mechanisms that differentiate SPD from schizophrenia is essential as it may lead to interventions which may allow for early interventions designed to thwart the development of schizophrenia in high-risk prodromal patients. Finally, given the significance of working memory deficits in determining functional impairment in schizophrenia and SPD, further assessment of the neurochemistry and novel therapeutics in both conditions remains essential.

■ REFERENCES

Abi-Dargham, A., Kegeles, L. S., Zea-Ponce, Y. et al. (2004). Striatal amphetamine-induced dopamine release in patients with schizotypal personality disorder studied with single photon emission computed tomography and [123I]iodobenzamide. *Biol Psychiatry*, *55*(10), 1001–1006.

Baron, M., Gruen, R., Asnis, L., & Lord, S. (1985). Familial transmission of schizotypal and borderline personality disorders. *Am J Psychiatry*, *142*(8), 927–934.

Battaglia, M., Cavallini, M. C., Macciardi, F., & Bellodi, L. (1997). The structure of DSM-III-R schizotypal personality disorder diagnosed by direct interviews. *Schizophr Bull*, *23*(1), 83–92.

Battaglia, M., Fossati, A., Torgersen, S. et al. (1999). A psychometric-genetic study of schizotypal disorder. *Schizophr Res*, *37*(1), 53–64.

Berenz, E. C., Amstadter, A. B., Aggen, S, H. et al. (2013). Childhood trauma and personality disorder criterion counts: a co-twin control analysis. *J Abnorm Psychol*, *122*(4), 1070–1076.

Bergman, A. J., Harvey, P. D., Mitropoulou, V. et al. (1996). The factor structure of schizotypal symptoms in a clinical population. *Schizophr Bull*, *22*(3), 501–509.

Bergman, A. J., Harvey, P. D., Roitman, S. L. et al. (1998). Verbal learning and memory in schizotypal personality disorder. *Schizophr Bull*, *24*(4), 635–641.

Bergman, A. J., Silverman, J. M., Harvey, P. D., Smith, C. J., & Siever, L. J. (2000). Schizotypal symptoms in the relatives of schizophrenia patients: an empirical analysis of the factor structure. *Schizophr Bull*, *26*(3), 577–586.

Bleuler, E. (2010). Dementia praecox or the group of schizophrenias. *Vertex*, *21*(93), 394–400.

Brenner, C. A., McDowell, J. E., Cadenhead, K. S., & Clementz, B. A. (2001). Saccadic inhibition among schizotypal personality disorder subjects. *Psychophysiology*, *38*(3), 399–403.

Cadenhead, K. S., Light, G. A., Geyer, M. A., & Braff, D. L. (2000). Sensory gating deficits assessed by the P50 event-related potential in subjects with schizotypal personality disorder. *Am J Psychiatry*, *157*(1), 55–59.

Cadenhead, K. S., Light, G. A., Geyer, M. A., McDowell, J. E., & Braff, D. L. (2002). Neurobiological measures of schizotypal personality disorder: defining an inhibitory endophenotype? *Am J Psychiatry*, *159*(5), 869–871.

Chemerinski, F., Byne, W., Kolaitis, J, C, et al. (2013). Larger putamen size in antipsychotic-naive individuals with schizotypal personality disorder. *Schizophr Res*, *143*(1), 158–164.

Chen, J., Lipska, B. K., Halim, N. et al. (2004). Functional analysis of genetic variation in catechol-O-methyltransferase (COMT): effects on mRNA, protein, and enzyme activity in postmortem human brain. *Am J Hum Genet*, *75*(5), 807–821.

Chen, K. C., Lee, I. H., Yeh, T. L. et al. (2012). Schizotypy trait and striatal dopamine receptors in healthy volunteers. *Psychiatry Res*, *201*(3), 218–221.

Cohen, A. S., Matthews, R. A., Najolia, G. M., & Brown, L. A. (2010). Toward a more psychometrically sound brief measure of schizotypal traits: introducing the SPQ-Brief Revised. *J Pers Disord*, *24*(4), 516–537.

Compton, M. T., Goulding, S. M., Bakeman, R., & McClure-Tone, E. B. (2009). Confirmation of a four-factor structure of the Schizotypal Personality Questionnaire among undergraduate students. *Schizophr Res*, *111*(1–3), 46–52.

Coolidge, F. L., Thede, L. L., & Jang, K. L. (2001). Heritability of personality disorders in childhood: a preliminary investigation. *J Pers Disord*, *15*(1), 33–40.

Croft, R. J., Dimoska, A., Gonsalvez, C. J., & Clarke, A. R. (2004). Suppression of P50 evoked potential component, schizotypal beliefs and smoking. *Psychiatry Res*, *128*(1), 53–62.

Croft, R. J., Lee, A., Bertolot, J., & Gruzelier, J. H. (2001). Associations of P50 suppression and desensitization with perceptual and cognitive features of "unreality" in schizotypy. *Biol Psychiatry, 50*(6), 441–446.

Daly, M. P., Afroz, S., & Walder, D. J. (2012). Schizotypal traits and neurocognitive functioning among nonclinical young adults. *Psychiatry Res, 200*(2–3), 635–640.

de Loye, C., Beaucousin, V., Bohec, A. L., Blanchet, A., & Kostova, M. (2013). An event-related potential study of predictive and integrative semantic context processing in subjects with schizotypal traits. *Psychophysiology, 50*(11), 1109–1119.

Dickey, C. C., McCarley, R. W., Voglmaier, M. M. et al. (1999). Schizotypal personality disorder and MRI abnormalities of temporal lobe gray matter. *Biol Psychiatry, 45*(11), 1393–1402.

Dickey, C. C., Morocz, I. A., Niznikiewicz, M. A. et al. (2008). Auditory processing abnormalities in schizotypal personality disorder: an fMRI experiment using tones of deviant pitch and duration. *Schizophr Res, 103*(1–3), 26–39.

Diforio, D., Walker, E. F., & Kestler, L. P. (2000). Executive functions in adolescents with schizotypal personality disorder. *Schizophr Res, 42*(2), 125–134.

Ericson, M., Tuvblad, C., Raine, A., Young-Wolff, K., & Baker, L. A. (2011). Heritability and longitudinal stability of schizotypal traits during adolescence. *Behav Genet, 41*(4), 499–511.

Evans, L. H., Gray, N. S., & Snowden, R. J. (2007). Reduced P50 suppression is associated with the cognitive disorganisation dimension of schizotypy. *Schizophr Res, 97*(1–3), 152–162.

Fung, A. L., & Raine A. (2012). Peer victimization as a risk factor for schizotypal personality in childhood and adolescence. *J Pers Disord, 26*(3), 428–434.

George, A., & Soloff, P. H. (1986). Schizotypal symptoms in patients with borderline personality disorders. *Am J Psychiatry, 143*(2), 212–215.

Gooding, D. C. (1999). Antisaccade task performance in questionnaire-identified schizotypes. *Schizophr Res, 35*(2), 157–166.

Gooding, D. C., Miller, M. D., & Kwapil, T. R. (2000). Smooth pursuit eye tracking and visual fixation in psychosis-prone individuals. *Psychiatry Res, 93*(1), 41–54.

Gooding, D. C., Shea, H. B., & Matts, C. W. (2005). Saccadic performance in questionnaire-identified schizotypes over time. *Psychiatry Res, 133*(2–3), 173–186.

Green, M. F. (2006). Cognitive impairment and functional outcome in schizophrenia and bipolar disorder. *J Clin Psychiatry, 67*(10), e12.

Hazlett, E. A., Buchsbaum, M. S., Haznedar, M. M. et al. (2008). Cortical gray and white matter volume in unmedicated schizotypal and schizophrenia patients. *Schizophr Res, 101*(1–3), 111–123.

Hazlett, E. A., Lamade, R. V., Graff, F. S. et al. (2014). Visual-spatial working memory performance and temporal gray matter volume predict schizotypal personality disorder group membership. *Schizophr Res, 152*(2–3), 350–357.

Hazlett, E. A., Rothstein, E. G., Ferreira, R., Silverman, J. M., Siever, L. J., & Olincy, A. (2015). Sensory gating disturbances in the spectrum: similarities and differences in schizotypal personality disorder and schizophrenia. *Schizophr Res, 161*(2–3), 283–290.

Hazlett, E. A., Zhang, J., New, A. S. et al. (2012). Potentiated amygdala response to repeated emotional pictures in borderline personality disorder. *Biol Psychiatry, 72*(6), 448–456.

Holahan, A. L., & O'Driscoll, G. A. (2005). Antisaccade and smooth pursuit performance in positive- and negative-symptom schizotypy. *Schizophr Res, 76*(1), 43–54.

Hooker, C. I., Benson, T. L., Gyurak, A., Yin, H., Tully, L. M., & Lincoln, S. H. (2014). Neural activity to positive expressions predicts daily experience of schizophrenia-spectrum symptoms in adults with high social anhedonia. *J Abnorm Psychol, 123*(1), 190–204.

Huang, J., Wang, Y., Jin, Z. et al. (2013). Happy facial expression processing with different social interaction cues: an fMRI study of individuals with schizotypal personality traits. *Prog Neuropsychopharmacol Biol Psychiatry, 44,* 108–117.

Hummelen, B., Pedersen, G., & Karterud, S. (2012). Some suggestions for the DSM-5 schizotypal personality disorder construct. *Compr Psychiatry, 53*(4), 341–349.

Ivleva, E. I., Moates, A. F., Hamm, J. P. et al. (2014). Smooth pursuit eye movement, prepulse inhibition, and auditory paired stimuli processing endophenotypes across the schizophrenia-bipolar disorder psychosis dimension. *Schizophr Bull, 40*(3), 642–652.

Kattoulas, E., Evdokimidis, I., Stefanis, N. C., Avramopoulos, D., Stefanis, C. N., & Smyrnis, N. (2011). Predictive smooth eye pursuit in a population of young men: II. Effects of schizotypy, anxiety and depression. *Exp Brain Res, 215*(3–4), 219–226.

Kavoussi, R. J., & Siever, L. J. (1992). Overlap between borderline and schizotypal personality disorders. *Compr Psychiatry, 33*(1), 7–12.

Kawasaki, Y., Suzuki, M., Nohara, S. et al. (2004). Structural brain differences in patients with schizophrenia and schizotypal disorder demonstrated by voxel-based morphometry. *Eur Arch Psychiatry Clin Neurosci, 254*(6), 406–414.

Kendler, K. S., Aggen, S. H., Czajkowski, N. et al. (2008). The structure of genetic and environmental risk factors for DSM-IV personality disorders: a multivariate twin study. *Arch Gen Psychiatry, 65*(12), 1438–1446.

Kendler, K. S., Aggen, S. H., Neale, M. C. et al. (2015). A longitudinal twin study of cluster A personality disorders. *Psychol Med, 45*(7), 1531–1538.

Kendler, K. S., Czajkowski, N., Tambs, K. et al. (2006). Dimensional representations of DSM-IV cluster A personality disorders in a population-based sample of Norwegian twins: a multivariate study. *Psychol Med, 36*(11), 1583–1591.

Kendler, K. S., Myers, J., Torgersen, S., Neale, M. C., & Reichborn-Kjennerud, T. (2007). The heritability of cluster A personality disorders assessed by both personal interview and questionnaire. *Psychol Med, 37*(5), 655–665.

Kiang, M., & Kutas, M. (2005). Association of schizotypy with semantic processing differences: an event-related brain potential study. *Schizophr Res, 77*(2–3), 329–342.

Kiang, M., Prugh, J., & Kutas, M. (2010). An event-related brain potential study of schizotypal personality and associative semantic processing. *Int J Psychophysiol, 75*(2), 119–126.

Kimble, M., Lyons, M., O'Donnell, B., Nestor, P., Niznikiewicz, M., & Toomey, R. (2000). The effect of family status and schizotypy on electrophysiologic measures of attention and semantic processing. *Biol Psychiatry, 47*(5), 402–412.

Klein, C., Berg, P., Rockstroh, B., & Andresen, B. (1999). Topography of the auditory P300 in schizotypal personality. *Biol Psychiatry, 45*(12), 1612–1621.

Koenigsberg, H. W., Buchsbaum, M. S., Buchsbaum, B. R. et al. (2005). Functional MRI of visuospatial working memory in schizotypal personality disorder: a region-of-interest analysis. *Psychol Med, 35*(7), 1019–1030.

Koo, M. S., Levitt, J. J., McCarley, R. W. et al. (2006). Reduction of caudate nucleus volumes in neuroleptic-naive female subjects with schizotypal personality disorder. *Biol Psychiatry, 60*(1), 40–48.

Kopp, B. (2007). Mnemonic intrusions into working memory in psychometrically identified schizotypal individuals. *J Behav Ther Exp Psychiatry, 38*(1), 56–74.

Kostova, M., Bohec, A. L., & Blanchet, A. (2014). Event-related brain potential study of expectancy and semantic matching in schizotypy. *Int J Psychophysiol, 92*(2), 67–73.

Kuhn, S., Schubert, F., & Gallinat, J. (2012). Higher prefrontal cortical thickness in high schizotypal personality trait. *J Psychiatr Res, 46*(7), 960–965.

Lencz, T., Raine, A., Scerbo, A. et al. (1993). Impaired eye tracking in undergraduates with schizotypal personality disorder. *Am J Psychiatry, 150*(1), 152–154.

Lentz, V., Robinson, J., & Bolton, J. M. (2010). Childhood adversity, mental disorder comorbidity, and suicidal behavior in schizotypal personality disorder. *J Nerv Ment Dis, 198*(11), 795–801.

Lenzenweger, M. F., & O'Driscoll, G. A. (2006). Smooth pursuit eye movement and schizotypy in the community. *J Abnorm Psychol, 115*(4), 779–786.

Levitt, J. J., McCarley, R. W., Dickey, C. C. et al. (2002). MRI study of caudate nucleus volume and its cognitive correlates in neuroleptic-naive patients with schizotypal personality disorder. *Am J Psychiatry, 159*(7), 1190–1197.

Levitt, J. J., Styner, M., Niethammer, M. et al. (2009). Shape abnormalities of caudate nucleus in schizotypal personality disorder. *Schizophr Res, 110*(1–3), 127–139.

Levitt, J. J., Westin, C. F., Nestor, P. G. et al. (2004). Shape of caudate nucleus and its cognitive correlates in neuroleptic-naive schizotypal personality disorder. *Biol Psychiatry, 55*(2), 177–184.

Li, X. B., Huang, J., Cheung, E. F., Gong, Q. Y., & Chan, R. C. (2011). Event-related potential correlates of suspicious thoughts in individuals with schizotypal personality features. *Soc Neurosci, 6*(5–6), 559–568.

Lien, Y. J., Tsuang, H. C., Chiang, A. et al. (2010). The multidimensionality of schizotypy in nonpsychotic relatives of patients with schizophrenia and its applications in ordered subsets linkage analysis of schizophrenia. *Am J Med Genet B Neuropsychiatr Genet, 153B*(1), 1–9.

Lin, C. C., Su, C. H., Kuo, P. H., Hsiao, C. K., Soong, W. T., & Chen, W. J. (2007). Genetic and environmental influences on schizotypy among adolescents in Taiwan: a multivariate twin/sibling analysis. *Behav Genet, 37*(2), 334–344.

Linney, Y. M., Murray, R. M., Peters, E. R., MacDonald, A. M., Rijsdijk, F., & Sham, P. C. (2003). A quantitative genetic analysis of schizotypal personality traits. *Psychol Med, 33*(5), 803–816.

Mannan, M. R., Hiramatsu, K. I., Hokama, H., & Ohta, H. (2001). Abnormalities of auditory event-related potentials in students with schizotypal personality disorder. *Psychiatry Clin Neurosci, 55*(5), 451–457.

McClure, M. M., Barch, D. M., Flory, J. D., Harvey, P. D., & Siever, L. J. (2008). Context processing in schizotypal personality disorder: evidence of specificity of impairment to the schizophrenia spectrum. *J Abnorm Psychol, 117*(2), 342–354.

McClure, M. M., Barch, D. M., Romero, M. J. et al. (2007). The effects of guanfacine on context processing abnormalities in schizotypal personality disorder. *Biol Psychiatry, 61*(10), 1157–1160.

McClure, M. M., Harvey, P. D., Bowie, C. R., Iacoviello, B., & Siever, L. J. (2013). Functional outcomes, functional capacity, and cognitive impairment in schizotypal personality disorder. *Schizophr Res, 144*(1–3), 146–150.

McClure, M. M., Harvey, P. D., Goodman, M. et al. (2010). Pergolide treatment of cognitive deficits associated with schizotypal personality disorder: continued evidence of the importance of the dopamine system in the schizophrenia spectrum. *Neuropsychopharmacology, 35*(6), 1356–1362.

McClure, M. M., Romero, M. J., Bowie, C. R., Reichenberg, A., Harvey, P. D., & Siever, L. J. (2007). Visual-spatial learning and memory in schizotypal personality disorder: continued evidence for the importance of working memory in the schizophrenia spectrum. *Arch Clin Neuropsychol, 22*(1), 109–116.

McGlashan, T. H. (1987). Testing DSM-III symptom criteria for schizotypal and borderline personality disorders. *Arch Gen Psychiatry, 44*(2), 143–148.

Mitelman, S. A., Canfield, E. L., Chu, K. W. et al. (2009). Poor outcome in chronic schizophrenia is associated with progressive loss of volume of the putamen. *Schizophr Res,* *113*(2–3), 241–245.

Mitropoulou, V., Friedman, L., Zegarelli, G. et al. (2011). Eye tracking performance and the boundaries of the schizophrenia spectrum. *Psychiatry Res, 186*(1), 18–22.

Mitropoulou, V., Harvey, P. D., Maldari, L. A. et al. (2002). Neuropsychological performance in schizotypal personality disorder: evidence regarding diagnostic specificity. *Biol Psychiatry, 52*(12), 1175–1182.

Mitropoulou, V., Harvey, P. D., Zegarelli, G., New, A. S., Silverman, J. M., & Siever, L. J. (2005). Neuropsychological performance in schizotypal personality disorder: importance of working memory. *Am J Psychiatry, 162*(10), 1896–1903.

Nguyen, H. N., Mattingley, J. B., & Abel, L. A. (2008). Extraversion degrades performance on the antisaccade task. *Brain Res, 1231*, 81–85.

Niznikiewicz, M. A., Friedman, M., Shenton, M. E. et al. (2004). Processing sentence context in women with schizotypal personality disorder: an ERP study. *Psychophysiology, 41*(3), 367–371.

Niznikiewicz, M. A., Shenton, M. E., Voglmaier, M. et al. (2002). Semantic dysfunction in women with schizotypal personality disorder. *Am J Psychiatry, 159*(10), 1767–1774.

Niznikiewicz, M. A., Voglmaier, M., Shenton, M. E. et al. (1999). Electrophysiological correlates of language processing in schizotypal personality disorder. *Am J Psychiatry, 156*(7), 1052–1058.

Niznikiewicz, M. A., Voglmaier, M. M., Shenton, M. E. et al. (2000). Lateralized P3 deficit in schizotypal personality disorder. *Biol Psychiatry, 48*(7), 702–705.

O'Driscoll, G. A., Lenzenweger, M. F., & Holzman, P. S. (1998). Antisaccades and smooth pursuit eye tracking and schizotypy. *Arch Gen Psychiatry, 55*(9), 837–843.

Ohi, K., Hashimoto, R., Nakazawa, T. et al. (2012). The p250GAP gene is associated with risk for schizophrenia and schizotypal personality traits. *PLoS One, 7*(4), e35696.

Plakun, E. M., Muller, J. P., & Burkhardt, P. E. (1987). The significance of borderline and schizotypal overlap. *Hillside J Clin Psychiatry, 9*(1), 47–54.

Premkumar, P., Ettinger, U., Inchley-Mort, S. et al. (2012). Neural processing of social rejection: the role of schizotypal personality traits. *Hum Brain Mapp, 33*(3), 695–706.

Prevost, M., Rodier, M., Renoult, L. et al. (2010). Schizotypal traits and N400 in healthy subjects. *Psychophysiology, 47*(6), 1047–1056.

Radant, A. D., Millard, S. P., Braff, D. L. et al. (2015). Robust differences in antisaccade performance exist between COGS schizophrenia cases and controls regardless of recruitment strategies. *Schizophr Res, 163*(1–3), 47–52.

Rado, S. (1953). Dynamics and classification of disordered behavior. *Am J Psychiatry, 110*(6), 406–416.

Raine, A., Reynolds, C., Lencz, T., Scerbo, A., Triphon, N., & Kim, D. (1994). Cognitive-perceptual, interpersonal, and disorganized features of schizotypal personality. *Schizophr Bull, 20*(1), 191–201.

Roitman, S. E., Mitropoulou, V., Keefe, R. S. et al. (2000). Visuospatial working memory in schizotypal personality disorder patients. *Schizophr Res, 41*(3), 447–455.

Rosell, D. R., Zaluda, L. C., McClure, M. M. et al. (2015). Effects of the D1 dopamine receptor agonist dihydrexidine (DAR-0100A) on working memory in schizotypal personality disorder. *Neuropsychopharmacology, 40*(2), 446–453.

Rosenberger, P. H., & Miller, G. A. (1989). Comparing borderline definitions: DSM-III borderline and schizotypal personality disorders. *J Abnorm Psychol, 98*(2), 161–169.

Salisbury, D. F., Voglmaier, M. M., Seidman, L. J., & McCarley, R. W. (1996). Topographic abnormalities of P3 in schizotypal personality disorder. *Biol Psychiatry, 40*(3), 165–172.

Savitz, J., van der Merwe, L., Newman, T. K., Stein, D. J., & Ramesar, R. (2010). Catechol-o-methyltransferase genotype and childhood trauma may interact to impact schizotypal personality traits. *Behav Genet, 40*(3), 415–423.

Serban, G., Conte, H. R., & Plutchik, R. (1987). Borderline and schizotypal personality disorders: mutually exclusive or overlapping? *J Pers Assess, 51*(1), 15–22.

Shihabuddin, L., Buchsbaum, M. S., Hazlett, E. A. et al. (2001). Striatal size and relative glucose metabolic rate in schizotypal personality disorder and schizophrenia. *Arch Gen Psychiatry, 58*(9), 877–884.

Shin, Y. W., Krishnan, G., Hetrick, W. P. et al. (2010). Increased temporal variability of auditory event-related potentials in schizophrenia and schizotypal personality disorder. *Schizophr Res, 124*(1–3), 110–118.

Siegel, B. V., Jr., Trestman, R. L., O'Flaithbheartaigh, S. et al. (1996). D-amphetamine challenge effects on Wisconsin Card Sort Test. Performance in schizotypal personality disorder. *Schizophr Res, 20*(1–2), 29–32.

Siever, L. J., Coursey, R. D., Alterman, I. S., Buchsbaum, M. S., & Murphy, D. L. (1984). Impaired smooth pursuit eye movement: vulnerability marker for schizotypal personality disorder in a normal volunteer population. *Am J Psychiatry, 141*(12), 1560–1566.

Siever, L. J., Friedman, L., Moskowitz, J. et al. (1994). Eye movement impairment and schizotypal psychopathology. *Am J Psychiatry, 151*(8), 1209–1215.

Siever, L. J., & Gunderson, J. G. (1983). The search for a schizotypal personality: historical origins and current status. *Compr Psychiatry, 24*(3), 199–212.

Silk, K. R., Westen, D., Lohr, N. E., Benjamin, J., & Gold, L. (1990). DSM-III and DSM-III-R schizotypal symptoms in borderline personality disorder. *Compr Psychiatry, 31*(2), 103–110.

Smyrnis, N., Evdokimidis, I., Mantas, A. et al. (2007). Smooth pursuit eye movements in 1,087 men: effects of schizotypy, anxiety, and depression. *Exp Brain Res, 179*(3), 397–408.

Smyrnis, N., Evdokimidis, I., Stefanis, N. C. et al. (2003). Antisaccade performance of 1,273 men: effects of schizotypy, anxiety, and depression. *J Abnorm Psychol, 112*(3), 403–414.

Soliman, A., O'Driscoll, G. A., Pruessner, J. et al. (2011). Limbic response to psychosocial stress in schizotypy: a functional magnetic resonance imaging study. *Schizophr Res, 131*(1–3), 184–191.

Soliman, A., O'Driscoll, G. A., Pruessner, J. et al. (2008). Stress-induced dopamine release in humans at risk of psychosis: a [11C]raclopride PET study. *Neuropsychopharmacology, 33*(8), 2033–2041.

Spitzer, R. L., & Endicott, J. (1979). Justification for separating schizotypal and borderline personality disorders. *Schizophr Bull, 5*(1), 95–104.

Spitzer, R. L., Endicott, J., & Gibbon, M. (1979). Crossing the border into borderline personality and borderline schizophrenia: the development of criteria. *Arch Gen Psychiatry, 36*(1), 17–24.

Stefanis, N. C., Hatzimanolis, A., Avramopoulos, D. et al. (2013). Variation in psychosis gene ZNF804A is associated with a refined schizotypy phenotype but not neurocognitive performance in a large young male population. *Schizophr Bull, 39*(6), 1252–1260.

Suhr, J. A., & Spitznagel, M. B. (2001). Factor versus cluster models of schizotypal traits. II: relation to neuropsychological impairment. *Schizophr Res, 52*(3), 241–250.

Sun, J., Maller, J. J., Guo, L., & Fitzgerald, P. B. (2009). Superior temporal gyrus volume change in schizophrenia: a review on region of interest volumetric studies. *Brain Res Rev, 61*(1), 14–32.

Szoke, A., Meary, A., Ferchiou, A., Trandafir, A., Leboyer, M., & Schurhoff, F. (2009). Correlations between cognitive performances and psychotic or schizotypal dimensions. *Eur Psychiatry, 24*(4), 244–250.

Takahashi, T., Suzuki, M., Zhou, S. Y. et al. (2010). A follow-up MRI study of the superior temporal subregions in schizotypal disorder and first-episode schizophrenia. *Schizophr Res*, *119*(1–3), 65–74.

Takahashi, T., Suzuki, M., Zhou, S. Y. et al. (2006). Temporal lobe gray matter in schizophrenia spectrum: a volumetric MRI study of the fusiform gyrus, parahippocampal gyrus, and middle and inferior temporal gyri. *Schizophr Res*, *87*(1–3), 116–126.

Takahashi, T., Zhou, S. Y., Nakamura, K. et al. (2011). A follow-up MRI study of the fusiform gyrus and middle and inferior temporal gyri in schizophrenia spectrum. *Prog Neuropsychopharmacol Biol Psychiatry*, *35*(8), 1957–1964.

Thompson, J. L., Rosell, D. R., Slifstein, M. et al. (2014). Prefrontal dopamine D1 receptors and working memory in schizotypal personality disorder: a PET study with [(1)(1)C] NNC112. *Psychopharmacology*, *231*(21), 4231–4240.

Toda, M., & Abi-Dargham, A. (2007). Dopamine hypothesis of schizophrenia: making sense of it all. *Curr Psychiatry Rep*, *9*(4), 329–336.

Tomppo, L., Hennah, W., Miettunen, J. et al. (2009). Association of variants in DISC1 with psychosis-related traits in a large population cohort. *Arch Gen Psychiatry*, *66*(2), 134–141.

Torgersen, S. (1984). Genetic and nosological aspects of schizotypal and borderline personality disorders: a twin study. *Arch Gen Psychiatry*, *41*(6), 546–554.

Torgersen, S., Lygren, S., Oien, P. A. et al. (2000). A twin study of personality disorders. *Compr Psychiatry*, *41*(6), 416–425.

Trestman, R. L., Keefe, R. S., Mitropoulou, V. et al. (1995). Cognitive function and biological correlates of cognitive performance in schizotypal personality disorder. *Psychiatry Res*, *59*(1–2), 127–136.

Voglmaier, M. M., Seidman, L. J., Salisbury, D., & McCarley, R. W. (1997). Neuropsychological dysfunction in schizotypal personality disorder: a profile analysis. *Biol Psychiatry*, *41*(5), 530–540.

Vu, M. A., Thermenos, H. W., Terry, D. P. et al. (2013). Working memory in schizotypal personality disorder: fMRI activation and deactivation differences. *Schizophr Res*.

Wan, L., Crawford, H. J., & Boutros, N. (2006). P50 sensory gating: impact of high vs. low schizotypal personality and smoking status. *Int J Psychophysiol*, *60*(1), 1–9.

Wang, J., Miyazato, H., Hokama, H., Hiramatsu, K., & Kondo, T. (2004). Correlation between P50 suppression and psychometric schizotypy among non-clinical Japanese subjects. *Int J Psychophysiol*, *52*(2), 147–157.

Widiger, T. A., Frances, A., Warner, L., & Bluhm, C. (1986). Diagnostic criteria for the borderline and schizotypal personality disorders. *J Abnorm Psychol*, *95*(1), 43–51.

Woodward, N. D., Cowan, R. L., Park, S. et al. (2011). Correlation of individual differences in schizotypal personality traits with amphetamine-induced dopamine release in striatal and extrastriatal brain regions. *Am J Psychiatry*, *168*(4), 418–426.

13 The Neurobiological Basis of Borderline Personality Disorder

■ ROBERT O. FRIEDEL, CHRISTIAN SCHMAHL, AND MARIJN DISTEL

■ INTRODUCTION

It is the intent of this chapter to provide an overview of the biological underpinnings of borderline personality disorder (BPD). In the categorical diagnostic approach used in the *Diagnostic and Statistical Manual of Mental Disorders* (fifth edition [*DSM-5*]; American Psychiatric Association, [APA], 2013), BPD is defined as multiple subsets of at least five of nine multisymptomatic criteria that may range from mild to severe. Because there are no requirements on the order or maximal number of criteria up to nine, BPD may present in as many as 126 heterogenous combinations of these criteria as calculated from the following equation applicable under these conditions: $C = n!/(n - r)! (r!)$. Factor analysis of the nine criteria of BPD has resulted in four groupings or domains consistent with those described in *DSM-5* for personality disorders in general: affectivity, impulse control, cognitive, and interpersonal functioning. Because of the marked heterogeneity of symptoms that may be present in patients with BPD and the likelihood that each symptom is grounded in specific distributed processing neural networks, in this chapter we pursue a minimalist approach and describe the main neurobiological findings associated with the *individual symptoms* of the disorder. Given this approach and the limitations of space, this review is selective rather than comprehensive.

A number of the authors who initially described the symptoms, nature, and treatment of BPD proposed that it resulted, in part, from inherent risk factors (e.g., Stern, 1938; Knight, 1953; Kernberg, 1967; Grinker et al., 1968). This proposal has been verified by quantitative genetic neuroimaging (Mauchnik & Schmahl, 2010) and other biological studies (Skodol et al., 2002; Goodman et al., 2004). To place this issue in perspective, as noted, recent studies estimate the heritability of BPD at 42% to 67% (Distel et al., 2008, 2009; Kendler et al., 2011; Torgersen et al., 2012), ranking it as one of the most heritable of all psychiatric disorders (Flint et al., 2010). There is evidence that psychosocial risk factors, such as early abandonment, deficient nurturing, and early, sustained physical and sexual abuse are also important, but not essential, risk factors for the disorder (Gunderson, 2009).

BPD typically has its onset and may be readily diagnosed from the early teenage to early adult years. The disorder, therefore, begins to significantly affect most of those who suffer from it during a critical period of their biopsychosocial development. It appears to be ubiquitous, and the lifetime prevalence varies from 1.2% to 5.9% depending on the sampling and statistical methods used, making it one of the most prevalent of personality disorders (Sansone & Sansone, 2011). BPD also has a high co-occurrence with other mental disorders including mood disorders (75.0%), anxiety disorders (74.2%), other personality disorders (73.9%), and substance use disorders (72.9% ;Grant et al., 2008). The high prevalence of co-occurring disorders may be accounted for, in part, by overlapping genetic diathesis as suggested by the recent findings on the comorbidity of attention deficit hyperactivity disorder (ADHD) symptoms and borderline personality traits (Distel et al., 2011a).

Treatment of BPD with psychotherapy and medications was consistently unsuccessful until relatively low to moderate doses of first-generation antipsychotic agents (FGAs) appeared to be effective in significantly reducing some of the core symptoms of the disorder (Brinkley et al., 1979; Goldberg et al., 1986; Soloff et al., 1986). Further studies supported these initial findings and extended them to second-generation antipsychotic agents (SGAs) and to mood stabilizers (Saunders & Silk, 2009; Stoffers et al., 2010). A number of BPD-specific psychotherapies were then developed and also found to be effective in ameliorating some symptoms of BPD in subjects with the disorder, most of whom were treated simultaneously with medications (Linehan, 1993; Stoffers et al., 2012). Finally, a recent review of the neurobiological underpinnings of BPD in childhood and adolescence suggests that the biological abnormalities demonstrated consistently in adults are also observed in childhood, further supporting a neurobiological diathesis to the disorder (Winsper et al., 2016).

Thus the total body of evidence indicates that BPD has a strong neurobiological basis and that it is important to understand the biological underpinnings of the disorder to interpret properly the results of existing and new information added to its rapidly expanding data base (Ruocco & Carcone, 2016; Visintin et al., 2016). The material in this chapter is presented in five sections: one describing the structure of genetic and environmental risk factors for BPD and four describing our current knowledge about the anatomy and pathophysiology of symptom in each of the four domains of the disorder. The chapter concludes with a discussion of the clinical, research, and educational implications of this information.

■ THE QUANTITATIVE AND MOLECULAR GENETICS OF BPD

It has long been recognized that mental disorders run in families. This also holds for BPD. First degree relatives of an individual with BPD have a three- to four-fold increase in risk of the disorder compared to first-degree relatives without a family member with BPD. Also, the four main domains of BPD symptoms—affective, behavioral, cognitive, and interpersonal—aggregate in families (Gunderson et al., 2011b). Resemblance within families can arise from shared genetic factors, shared environmental factors, or both. Using correlations between family members of different genetic relatedness, twin family studies can estimate the relative influence of each of them. If genetic factors are important for a trait or disorder, family members who are genetically more similar (e.g., monozygotic twins) will resemble each other more than family members who are genetically less similar (e.g., dizygotic twins or non-twin siblings). These studies showed that 42% to 67% of the variance in BPD, or borderline personality features, can be explained by genetic factors (Distel et al., 2008, 2009; Torgersen et al., 2008,

2012). Environmental factors that are shared within families do not explain familial resemblance in BPD, which is a common finding for personality traits and disorders in general.

BPD often co-occurs with other mental disorders. About 80% of the individuals with BPD also have a lifetime anxiety disorder, mood disorder, or substance use disorder (Tomko et al., 2013). Twin family studies can be used to study shared etiology between traits and disorders. Using this methodology, substantial genetic correlations were found between BPD and bipolar disorder, major depression, schizophrenia, ADHD, anger, alcohol use, cannabis use, and smoking behavior (Reichborn-Kjennerud et al., 2010; Distel et al., 2011a, 2012; Long et al., 2017). Regarding personality disorder comorbidity, BPD is genetically most closely related to antisocial personality disorder, which may reflect genetic risk for impulsive aggression (Torgersen et al., 2008; Kendler et al., 2008).

Heritability estimates for the main features of BPD have also been established with estimates ranging from 26% to 35% for affective instability, identity problems, negative relationships, and self-harm/impulsivity (Distel et al., 2010). The association between main features of BPD can be accounted for by a latent BPD construct (Distel et al., 2010; Kendler et al., 2011; Gunderson et al., 2011a). Genes and environmental factors thus influence the association between the main features in similar ways through the latent BPD construct. In addition, there are genetic and environmental factors specific to each main feature, with a specific genetic loading for affective instability that suggests it is a core component in the etiology of BPD as it is derived mainly from the latent BPD factor (Distel et al., 2010; Kendler et al., 2011). Reichborn-Kjennerud et al. (2013) conducted multivariate genetic analyses for the nine BPD criteria in the fourth edition of the *DSM* (*DSM-IV*) and found similar results. The highest heritability estimates were found for the criteria "suicidal behavior" (48.6%), "impulsive self-harm" (44.6%), "feelings of emptiness" (38.4%), and "affective instability" (33.5%). For the other criteria heritability estimates range from 21.2% to 27.8%. Again, one highly heritable BPD factor influenced all nine BPD criteria. In addition to this single, heritable BPD factor, the criteria "affective instability," "feelings of emptiness," and "intense anger" were influenced by what the authors called the *affective factor*, which was influenced by genetic factors for 29.3% and by environmental factors for 70.7%. Another factor called *interpersonal* influenced the criteria "unstable relationships" and "avoidance of abandonment" and was also mainly influenced by environmental factors (97.8%). As opposed to the highly heritable BPD factor, criteria-specific influences were mainly unique and environmental in origin. In this group of factors, only for the criteria "impulsivity/self-harm" (27%), "suicidal behavior" (14.4%), "feelings of emptiness" (17.6%), and "intense anger" (9%), were significant criterion-specific genetic influences found. Summarizing, there is strong evidence that there are genetic factors that make an individual vulnerable to all symptoms/components of BPD, but there may also be additional neurobiological systems that influence only part of the symptoms, for example impulsivity/self-harm.

Molecular Genetic Studies

The specific genetic variants and their associated neurobiological systems have not yet been identified convincingly in BPD. Molecular genetic research has mainly focused on the association between BPD and genetic polymorphisms involved in the serotonergic and dopaminergic neurotransmitter systems. For reviews see Calati et al. (2013) and Amad et al. (2014). Both the serotonergic and the dopaminergic systems are involved in emotional processing and the regulation of impulsive behavior (Joyce et al., 2014). The dopamine system has also been implicated in cognitive-perceptual behaviors. Dysfunction in these processes are core symptoms of BPD. Although several associations between serotonergic candidate genes and BPD have been found, they explained only very small proportions of the variance, and results could often not be replicated. A meta-analyses for three serotonergic polymorphisms showed no association (Calati et al., 2013). Associations between BPD and dopaminergic candidate genes have also been inconsistent. The disappointing results so far suggest that many genes with small effects are probably involved in the development of BPD. In addition, gene by gene interactions may play an important role. Evidence for gene by gene interaction has been found between several genes involved in the serotonergic system (Ni et al., 2009) and between the COMT gene (involved in breaking down dopamine) and 5-HTTLPR (the serotonin transporter gene) (Tadic et al., 2009). Recently, the first genome-wide association study has been conducted in two Dutch samples ($N = 7,125$) which showed a promising signal in a region on chromosome 5. This result was replicated in an independent third sample ($N = 1,301$; Lubke et al., 2013). Overall, molecular genetic studies of BPD are confronted with significant methodological challenges, as noted, to achieve valid results (Flint et al., 2010).

Genetic–Environmental Correlations and Interactions

There is a strong correlation between having experienced traumatic life events and the development of BPD. Genetic factors and environmental influences are often interrelated (e.g., Perroud et al., 2016). This also seems to be the case for BPD (for a review of gene by environment interaction studies that are relevant to BPD, see Carpenter & Trull, 2013), although many studies suffer from methodological limitations such as small sample sizes, lack of replication samples, and imprecise measurements of environmental influences. Genotype–environment correlation refers to the role of genetic factors in exposure to environments. Parents with (symptoms of) BPD may create an unstable family environment for their children. In addition, they pass on the genes that make them more vulnerable to develop BPD. Individuals who have difficulties regulating their emotions will have more conflicts with others than individuals who are able to regulate their emotions adequately. Individuals who have an inherited desire for excitement will create environments that give them exciting experiences. These examples illustrate passive, evocative, and active genotype–environment correlation, respectively.

Genes and environment may also interact with each other. Someone's sensitivity to environmental influences then depends on his or her genetic vulnerability (Kendler & Eaves, 1986). Gene–environment interaction can be studied with latent genetic effects or with measured genes. Distel et al. (2011b) used the first approach and found evidence for correlated genetic factors for BPD features and certain life events. Evidence for gene–environment interaction was also found, but results must be interpreted with caution because spurious gene–environment correlation was also found. Wilson et al. (2012) found that a measured gene tryptophan hydroxylase I significantly strengthened the association between childhood abuse and the development of BPD in later life.

Epigenetics in BPD

In addition to genetic variations, epigenetic modifications may also contribute to mental disorders. Epigenetic modifications are changes in gene activity that are not caused by changes in the nucleotide sequence. Epigenetic modification can arise, for example, from DNA methylation, whereby a methyl group is added to the DNA nucleotides making transcription impossible, or from histone modification whereby an added methyl group can result in a repressed or activated gene expression depending on the location of the added methyl group. Evidence suggests that environmental factors can induce epigenetic changes which can influence the onset and course of psychiatric disorders. For BPD it is hypothesized that early adverse life events may influence the development of BPD through epigenetic modifications of developmental or stress-related genes (Perroud et al., 2011, 2016). Dammann et al. (2011) measured methylation levels of 14 neuropsychiatric genes that were previously linked to BPD, schizophrenia, or depressive disorders in 26 BPD patients and 11 controls. The average methylation level of five of them was significantly higher in the blood from BPD patients compared to controls. Using a genome-wide approach, several CpG sites were identified that exhibited significantly increased methylation in the blood of BPD patients (Teschler et al., 2013). Using a whole-genome methylation scan of BPD subjects, a highly relevant biological result was observed for cg04927004 close to miR124-3 that was significantly associated with BPD and severity of childhood maltreatment (Prados et al., 2015).

Not surprisingly, early data is beginning to emerge that suggests treatment may affect altered epigenetic processes in BPD patients. In one study, there was a positive correlation of the methylation status of brain-derived neurotrophic factor (BDNF) exons CpG I and IV with levels of childhood trauma experienced in BPD subjects compared to controls (Perroud et al., 2013). After a four-week intensive dialectical behavioral therapy (DBT) treatment program, BPD patients who responded well to the treatment showed a decrease in BDNF methylation status whereas nonresponders showed an increase in methylation during treatment. Further research needs to be conducted in medication-free subjects, or samples where this variable is controlled with respect to drug class and dosage, to determine whether BDNF methylation levels may have relevance in predicting the success of psychotherapy in BPD.

■ AFFECTIVE DYSREGULATION IN BPD

Affective dysregulation, characterized by a hypersensitivity to emotional stimuli, intense emotional reactivity, a delayed return to emotional baseline, and deficits in emotional control, is a core feature of BPD (Carpenter & Trull, 2013). Affective instability is considered by many experts to be the most common and stable diagnostic criterion of BPD (Stern, 1938; Lieb et al., 2004; Glenn & Klonsky, 2009; Gunderson et al., 2011b). It also represents one of the most detrimental characteristics of the disorder because it is closely linked to suicidal and parasuicidal behavior, extreme anger, and pervasive feelings of emptiness (Stiglmayr et al., 2005).

Several neuroimaging studies have used functional MRI (fMRI) during emotional challenge (e.g., presentation of emotionally arousing pictures or facial expressions) to investigate the neural correlates of emotional responding in individuals with BPD compared to healthy individuals: The majority of fMRI studies have observed a hyperreactivity of the amygdala in response to negative emotional stimuli in BPD patients as compared to healthy controls (HCs; Herpertz et al., 2001; Donegan et al., 2003; Minzenberg et al., 2007; Koenigsberg et al., 2009; Niedtfeld et al., 2010; Schulze et al., 2011; Krause-Utz et al., 2012). A recent study also demonstrated a slower return of amygdala activation to baseline in BPD (Kamphausen et al., 2013). The amygdala plays an important role in the detection of emotionally salient events, processing of emotions, and initiating stress and fear responses (Ochsner & Gross, 2007). Therefore, increased and prolonged limbic activation during emotional challenge may reflect the clinically well-observed features of emotional hypersensitivity and intense, long-lasting emotional reactions in individuals with BPD (Kamphausen et al., 2013). A recent meta-analysis points confirmed amygdala hyperactivity during processing of negative emotions relative to neutral conditions in patients with BPD compared to HCs (Schulze et al., 2016). Besides amygdala hyperreactivity, increased activation in the insula has been observed in emotional challenge studies in BPD patients, emphasizing the role of this brain area in disturbed emotion processing in BPD (Beblo et al., 2006; Niedtfeld et al., 2010; Schulze et al., 2011; Krause-Utz et al., 2012; Ruocco et al., 2013). The insula has been associated with the encoding of unpleasant feelings, interoceptive awareness, perceived social exclusion, and pain perception (Damasio et al., 2000; Menon & Uddin, 2010).

Furthermore, BPD patients were shown to exhibit limbic hyperreactivity in response to neutral pictures of facial expressions or interpersonal scenes (Donegan et al. 2003; Koenigsberg et al. 2009; Niedtfeld et al., 2010; Krause-Utz et al., 2012). This was related to higher arousal ratings of these pictures (Donegan et al., 2003; Krause-Utz et al., 2012). Resembling findings of behavioral emotion recognition studies, amygdala hyperreacitvity to neutral social pictures suggest a negativity bias, that is, a tendency to interpret normative neutral stimuli as emotionally arousing in individuals with BPD (Lis & Bohus, 2013). Inconsistencies of emotional challenging studies in BPD may further be attributable to a moderating effect of situational variables such as dissociation; this is discussed in more detail in the section on cognitive-perceptual disturbances.

In addition to limbic hyperreactivity, numerous functional neuroimaging studies revealed a hypoactivation of frontal brain regions in response to emotionally arousing or trauma-related stimuli. For example, Minzenberg and colleagues (2007) demonstrated amygdala hyperreactivity to fearful faces in BPD patients but also decreased activation in the anterior cingulate cortex (ACC). In a positron emission tomography (PET) study, Prossin et al. (2010) measured the selective radiotracer [(11)C] carfentanil, a potent synthetic opioid, during induced sadness states in BPD patients and HCs. Sadness induction was associated with greater reductions in endogenous opioid system activation in BPD patients than in the comparison group in the pregenual anterior cingulate, left orbitofrontal cortex (OFC), left ventral pallidum, left amygdala, and left inferior temporal cortex. Two fMRI studies applied functional connectivity to investigate the coupling between limbic and frontal brain areas during emotional challenge (Cullen et al., 2011; Kamphausen et al., 2013). Cullen and colleagues reported a stronger coupling between the amygdala and perigenual ACC during the processing of fearful stimuli. In the study by Kamphausen and colleagues, BPD patients not only showed prolonged amygdala activation but also stronger coupling between this area and the ventromedial PFC during experimentally induced fear conditions in BPD patients compared to healthy participants.

Recently, Scherpiet and colleagues (2013) investigated whether individuals with BPD have abnormal activation patterns in the anticipation of emotional stimuli. They presented either visual cues steadily preceding negative pictures or visual cues that ambiguously announced the valence of the upcoming picture. Compared to HCs, patients with BPD exhibited diminished activation in the left middle cingulate cortex, and dorsal ACC as well as increased activation in the left posterior cingulate cortex, perigenual ACC, and lingual gyrus during the anticipation of negative pictures. When processing visual cues that ambiguously announced upcoming pictures, BPD patients showed diminished activation in the left middle cingulate cortex and in parts of the dorsolateral prefrontal cortex (DLPFC). Results of this study suggest a hypervigilance to emotionally relevant cues and unbalanced fronto-limbic brain activation during the anticipation phase, highlighting effects related to expectancy in emotion processing in BPD.

Neuroimaging studies have also been aimed at investigating neuroanatomical alterations of brain regions involved in emotion processing on a structural level in patients with BPD. In several studies, reduced volume was observed in limbic(-related) brain regions, most prominently in the amygdala, hippocampus, ACC, and insula in patients with BPD (Driessen et al., 2000; Rüsch et al., 2003; Schmahl et al., 2003; van Elst et al., 2003; Brambilla et al., 2004; Hazlett et al., 2005; Irle et al., 2005; Leinsinger et al., 2006; Zetzsche et al., 2006; Minzenberg et al. 2008; Soloff et al., 2008; Schmahl et al. 2009; Goodman et al., 2011; Soloff et al., 2012). Reduced hippocampal and amygdala volumes could be confirmed in meta-analyses (Nunes et al., 2009; Ruocco et al., 2012).

Additional factors possibly underlying disturbed emotion processing in BPD may be related to alterations in neurotransmitter levels. Proton magnetic resonance spectroscopy was used to study the concentration of neurometabolites. Results from an initial study showed increased concentrations of creatine in the left amygdala in BPD patients, which can be interpreted as a marker for increased energy metabolism (van Elst et al., 2003). A later study reported reduced levels of N-acetylaspartate and creatine in the amygdala (Hoerst et al., 2010b). Lower levels of N-acetylaspartate concentration have been detected in the DLPFC of BPD patients, indicating that the quantity of neurons in this cerebral control region might be reduced (van Elst et al., 2001).

Current conceptualizations of BPD and previous neuroimaging research suggest that emotion dysregulation stems from deficient "top-down" frontal control mechanisms involved in regulating hyperactive "bottom-up" emotion-generating limbic structures (Ochsner & Gross, 2014). To investigate neural correlates of explicit or cognitive processes of emotion regulation, experimental research investigated the process of reappraisal (Ochsner et al., 2002). During explicit emotion regulation tasks, subjects were instructed to change their affective response to emotional pictures by predetermined cognitive reappraisal strategies. Three studies revealed abnormalities in the explicit regulation of negative emotions through reappraisal in BPD, which were presumably mediated by a reduced recruitment of prefrontal networks (Koenigsberg et al., 2009; Schulze et al., 2011; Lang et al., 2012). More specifically, the study by Koenigsberg and colleagues found diminished activity in the DLPFC and ventrolateral prefrontal cortex when patients with BPD tried to cognitively distance themselves from negative stimuli. Similarly, cognitive reappraisal yielded decreased recruitment of the left OFC and increased activation of the insula in patients with BPD relative to healthy participants (Schulze et al., 2011). In an attempt to clarify the role of trauma history on top-down regulation of emotional responses in BPD patients, Lang et al.

(2012) compared trauma-exposed BPD patients to trauma-exposed healthy subjects without posttraumatic stress disorder (PTSD) and nontraumatized healthy subjects. In this study, BPD patients as well as healthy individuals with trauma history recruited brain regions associated with up- and downregulation of negative emotions (e.g., ACC) to a lesser extent, which might reflect compensatory changes associated with trauma exposure (Lang et al., 2012).

Findings of these studies are in line with the assumption that diminished emotion regulation abilities in BPD are associated with a decreased capacity to activate prefrontal regions involved in emotion control. However, it is interesting to note that individuals with BPD did not differ from HCs on behavioral measures of reappraisal success (Koenigsberg et al., 2009; Schulze et al., 2011; Lang et al., 2012). This suggests that individuals with BPD are less apt than HCs in self-monitoring and making online assessments of their regulatory abilities and perhaps of their own emotional states.

Schnell and Herpertz investigated the influence of DBT, which involves teaching of emotion regulation skills, on neural correlates of emotion dysregulation using a longitudinal study design (Schnell & Herpertz, 2007). Although, due to limited sample size, these findings have to be regarded with caution, successful psychotherapy was indeed associated with significant neural changes (i.e., decreases in amygdala and insula activity in response to negative pictures). Findings from a larger controlled study on the effects of DBT on neural emotion processing confirmed these initial findings and revealed a decrease of amygdala hyperactivity in DBT responders compared to nonresponders (Schmitt et al., 2016).

To investigate the role of pain in the context of emotion regulation, Niedtfeld and colleagues (2010) applied thermal stimuli to BPD patients while they viewed emotionally arousing pictures. A decrease of limbic activation was observed in both BPD patients and HCs that was not specific to painful stimulation as opposed to nonpainful warmth perception. In a data reanalysis, Niedtfeld and colleagues (2012) focused on patterns of functional connectivity between the amygdala, insula, and ACC. They found a stronger negative coupling between paralimbic and prefrontal structures— especially in parts of the medial frontal gyrus and DLPFC (Brodmann's areas 8 and 9)—in BPD patients who received pain stimuli in addition to emotionally arousing pictures. These results are in line with the assumption of a modulating effect of pain on affective processing in BPD. Using incision-induced pain, which takes into account tissue damage and thus provides a more valid model for nonsuicidal self-injury, a stress-reducing effect of an incision into the forearm in terms of reduced subjective arousal and increased heart rate could be demonstrated (Reitz et al., 2012). These findings were recently replicated in an fMRI study, where an additional reduction of amygdala hyperactivity and restitution of poststress amygdala-medial prefrontal cortex coupling following incision was shown (Reitz et al., 2015). A shift from amygdala deactivation to normal activation in response to pain stimulation could also be demonstrated after DBT treatment (Niedtfeld et al., 2017).

■ IMPULSIVE AGGRESSION IN BPD

Impulsive aggression in BPD is defined by two criteria in *DSM-5*. Criterion 4 requires "at least two areas that are potentially self damaging (e.g., spending, sex, substance-abuse, reckless driving, binge eating)." Criterion 5 requires "recurrent suicidal behavior, gestures, or threats, or self mutilating behavior." These actions are often precipitated by threats or expectations of separation or rejection. Self-mutilation may also occur during dissociative experiences in an attempt to relieve emotional pain, to enhance the ability to feel, or to relieve the person's sense of guilt and of being evil. Evidence suggests that impulsive-like behaviors may consist of four distinct facets: urgency, lack of premeditation, lack of perseverance, and sensation-seeking (Whiteside & Lyman, 2001). Of these, urgency, the emotionally driven failure to consider the consequences of behaviors, appears to be most commonly associated with mental disorders (Cyders & Smith, 2008). Impulsivity and aggression are related but separate constructs. Urgency, or "rash impulsivity," is associated most strongly with the impulsive, harmful, and aggressive behaviors observed in BPD (Boy et al., 2011). Impulsive aggression as defined in BPD appears to be closely related to states of stress, in contrast to other psychiatric disorders such as ADHD (Krause-Utz et al., 2013; Cackowski et al., 2014).

Structural and Functional Neuroanatomical Findings

The biological underpinnings of impulsivity and affective dysregulation are the most studied of the four dimensions of BPD. As noted in the section on genetics, the highest heritability rates for specific symptoms of the disorder are for suicidal behavior (48.6%) and impulsive self-harm (44.6%).

Technological advances in neuroimaging over the past two decades have provided new methodological approaches to the investigation of brain structures, pathways, and function related to impulsivity in subjects with and without BPD (e.g., New et al., 2007, 2013; Rusch et al., 2010; Wingenfeld et al., 2010; Coccaro et al., 2011; Carrasco et al., 2012; O'Neill & Frodl, 2012; Krause-Utz et al., 2014; Maier-Hein et al., 2014). Taken together, the evidence is consistent with dysfunction in BPD of the negative affective states generated by the amygdala especially, and other structures in the limbic system, and of their modulation and the behaviors resulting from them primarily by control networks in the prefrontal cortical regions. The cognitive control regions most frequently disrupted are the anterior orbital, medial prefrontal (e.g., ACC) and DLPFC regions of the brain as noted in the previous section of this chapter.

Effective conflict resolution, therefore, is impaired in BPD. In a comprehensive review, Coccaro et al. (2011) focused on three neural systems they consider critical to understanding the biological underpinnings of impulsive aggression: (a) those that generate aggressive impulses and the expression of emotion including the hypothalamus, amygdala, and insula; (b) those that evaluate the consequences of aggressive behaviors in response to interpersonal cues and societal norms and values such as decision-making and social-emotional information processing circuits, especially the dorsal ACC and the orbitomedial prefrontal cortex; and (c) those that subserve subsequent behavioral regulation including frontoparietal regions. They concluded that in BPD there is substantial evidence indicating functional abnormalities and volumetric reduction of medial temporal structures such as the amygdala and hippocampus and their connectivity, evidence supported by meta-analyses of these studies (Nunes et al., 2009). These changes are associated with functional hyperreactivity in limbic structures to emotionally evocative stimuli and consistent evidence of reduced baseline prefrontal metabolism and activation in BPD during emotional information processing, particularly in the medial prefrontal regions (see Krause-Utz et al., 2014).

In the first study of the relationship between structure and function of prefrontal regions and the amygdala in BPD, New et al. (2007) compared BPD subjects with aggressive intermittent explosive disorder (IED)-BPD to controls. The relative brain glucose metabolic rate of the subjects were measured at rest and after administration of meta-chlorophenylpiperazine (mCPP), a global agonist of serotonin (5-HT) receptors, with PET. Controls demonstrated a significant correlation between right orbitofrontal and ventral cortices and the ventral but not dorsal amygdala. BPD-IED subjects showed only weak coupling with no distinction between amygdala location. Citing evidence of the important roles of the ventral nucleus of the amygdala and OFC serotonin activity in the processing of aggressive behavior, the authors concluded that the prefrontal-thalamo-amygdala pathway and serotonergic activity is reduced in BPD-IED subjects, which accounts, in part, for the aggressive behavior of these individuals. In a small sample of subjects, inferior orbitofrontal white matter integrity as measured by fractional anisotropy (FA) was decreased in women with BPD and high levels of self-injurious behaviors compared to controls (Grant et al., 2007), a finding consistent with the proposal of New and her colleagues. A recent study using FA (New et al., 2013) demonstrated significant differences in the inferior longitudinal fasciculus of adolescents with BPD and controls, suggesting a neural substrate for the OFC-amygdala disconnect in adults with the disorder. Consistent with and extending these findings, a reduction in the thickness of left orbitofrontal, cingulate, and temporal cortices increased susceptibility of externalizing behavior across a continuum of healthy and clinical populations of children, and positive OFC-amygdala associations decreased susceptibility (Ameis et al., 2014).

ADHD demonstrates high comorbidity and genetic overlap with BPD (Distel et al., 2011a). McCarthy et al. (2013) reported that the resting state functional connectivity of adults with ADHD was significantly decreased within the attention networks and increased within the affective and default mode and the right cognitive control network compared with HCs and was significantly correlated with symptom severity (Cole & Schneider, 2007). Microstructural white matter damage in orbitofrontal areas has also been reported in affective disorders and PTSD (Domes et al., 2009; Nielen et al., 2009), which supports the concept that BPD shares psychobiological features with these disorders as well as with ADHD (Distel et al., 2011c).

Abnormal function in the ventral striatum, another structure often involved in limbic system activity and structurally and functionally related to the medial frontal cortices, has also been demonstrated in subjects with BPD (Perez-Rodriguez, 2012). BPD patients with BPD-IED were exposed to aggression-provoking and nonprovoking versions of the Point Subtraction Aggression Paradigm while monitored by fluorodeoxyglucose PET. Male patients demonstrated decreased striatal metabolism during both conditions while female patients did not differ from HCs. The authors suggest that these gender-related differences in frontal-striatal circuits in BPD-IED reflect sex differences in disorders of aggression and are consistent with gender differences in the modulation of the reward system by striatal dopamine and gonadal steroid hormones. Data from animal studies provide partial support and complementary information on the involvement of the ventral striatum in BPD. A reduction in gray matter density in the left nucleus accumbens region of the ventral striatum of rats with high versus low motor impulsivity has been demonstrated and is associated with reductions of glutamate decarboxylase and dendritic spine markers in this region (Caprioli et al., 2014). It is important to recall that impulsivity and aggression are related but separate constructs. As noted, "rash impulsivity," the tendency to react to emotionally provocative stimuli without serious consideration of the consequences, is associated most strongly with the harmful and aggressive behaviors observed in BPD (Boy et al., 2011).

Electrophysiological evidence supports functional neuroimaging findings of the relationship of specific brain regions to impulsivity. Evoked-response potential (ERP) results showed that the amplitudes of a component of the ERP generated in the ACC, referred to as error-related negativity (ERN), was reduced in patients with BPD, as were the P300 amplitudes after late feedback (de Bruijn et al., 2006). The results in the BPD group were associated with larger differences between correct and incorrect responses and in increased errors to the easy congruent stimuli. Control subjects corrected their errors better than patients with BPD. The reduced ERNs in BPD indicate reduced action monitoring, suggesting dysfunction in the ACC in patients with BPD.

These proposals and findings on the structural and functional underpinnings of impulsivity in BPD have been supported and further clarified in recent studies. Evaluation of the association of ACC GABA levels with functional activation and the connectivity in the frontostriatal network during interference inhibition have demonstrated impairments in patients with BPD (Wang et al., 2016). Results suggested a disconnection of the frontostriatal network correlated with ACC GABA levels, especially in subjects with high impulsivity and impulsive sensation-seeking in BPD. In another study, Herbort et al. (2016) demonstrated a negative relationship between ventral striatal loss anticipation response and impulsivity in female patients with BPD.

Neurochemical Findings

The most consistent neurochemical finding associated with aggressive impulsivity is impaired serotonergic function (see Coccaro et al., 2011). These data include increased levels of cerebrospinal fluid 5-hydroxyindoleacetic acid and homovanillic acid in only those subjects with BPD and an impulse action pattern (Chotai et al., 1998); a blunted stimulation to a serotonin stimulus, particularly in the orbital and medial prefrontal cortex, of individuals with impulsive aggression (New et al., 2002); and decreased negative emotional control in unfair game situations subsequent to ventromedial prefrontal damage (Koenigs & Tranel, 2007) or ingestion of a tryptophan-deficient beverage (Crockett et al., 2009). As noted, the prefrontal-thalamo-amygdala pathway and serotonergic activity is reduced in BPD-IED subjects (New et al., 2007). However, the comorbid diagnosis of IED in the subjects in this study is a confounding variable. A number of studies have suggested aberrations in molecular genetic mechanisms in subjects with BPD, as noted. However, association studies for BPD are sparse, and meta-analyses found no significant associations for the serotonin transporter, tryptophan hydroxylase 1, or serotonin 1-B receptor genes (Amad et al., 2014). With other evidence suggesting that impulsive aggression in BPD is highly heritable and associated with decreased serotonergic activity, the authors suggested a paradigm shift in which "plasticity/vulnerability" rather than "susceptibility" genes should be examined. Also, it is surprising that selective serotonin reuptake inhibitors (SSRIs), the medications used most commonly to enhance brain serotonergic activity, have not been shown to be as consistently effective in the pharmacological treatment of BPD as some SGAs and mood stabilizers (Lieb et al., 2010). It is possible that a small number of underpowered studies and other methodological flaws have resulted in type II errors in the meta-analyses of both the serotonin molecular genetic and the SSRI studies in subjects with BPD.

Dopamine dysfunction has also been proposed to be involved in three of the symptom domains of BPD: affective dysregulation, aggressive impulsivity, and cognitive-perceptual disturbances (Friedel, 2004b). Several lines of evidence lend support to this hypothesis and include the significant therapeutic effects of SGAs on impulsivity and other core symptoms of the disorder (Lieb et al., 2010) and genetic studies of subjects with BPD that have implicated the dopamine transporter (Joyce et al., 2009) and the DRD4 dopamine receptor (Nemoda et al, 2010). Meta-analyses did not confirm these findings (Amad et al., 2014) but support the pharmacological data on the efficacy of SGAs in decreasing impulsivity in BPD (Lieb et al., 2010). Also, dopamine 2 and 3 (D2/D3) receptor availability and dopamine levels in dopamine networks have been associated with human impulsivity (Buckholtz et al., 2010). D2/D3 autoreceptor availability (binding potential) in the substantia nigra/ventral tegmental area was inversely correlated with trait impulsivity and positively correlated with the levels of amphetamine-induced dopamine released in the striatum.

In addition to dysregulation of the serotonin and dopamine neuromodulator systems in BPD, there is early evidence of impaired function of the primary central nervous system (CNS) stimulatory and inhibitory neurotransmitter systems in BPD, glutamate and gamma-aminobutyric acid (GABA). Using magnetic resonance spectroscopy, Hoerst et al. (2010a) studied multiple neurometabolite concentrations in the ACC of BPD subjects and compared them to the results of a number of psychometric measures. They found significantly higher glutamate concentrations in subjects with BPD compared with HCs. In addition, there were positive correlations between glutamate levels and self-reported measures of impulsivity and subscores of the Borderline Symptom Checklist. Glutamate metabolism, in particular N-methyl-D-aspartate (NMDA) receptor neurotransmission, has been linked to several aspects of BPD symptomatology (Grosjean & Tsai, 2007.). A recent study revealed evidence for increased ACC glutamate being related to impulsivity, while reduced GABA was related to reduced GABA levels (Ende et al. 2016).

The inhibitory neurotransmitter GABA has also been implicated in aggressive impulsivity in BPD. Boy et al. (2011) developed measures of the four-facet model of impulsivity (Whiteside & Lynam, 2001) and evaluated concentrations of GABA in the DLPFC with MRI spectroscopy in two cohorts of men ages 19 to 35 years without a neurological or psychiatric history. There was a significant, inverse correlation between GABA levels in the DLPFC and scores on the urgency and perseverance scales when both cohorts were included in the statistical analysis of the data. Lending support to both the Hoerst and Boy studies, recently, glutamate decarboxylase gene expression, structural markers (dendritic spines and microtubules) in the nucleus accumbens core, a structure considered an integral part of the limbic system, were inversely related to trait impulsivity (premature responding) in rats (Caprioli et al., 2014).

■ DISTURBANCES OF PERCEPTION AND COGNITION IN BPD

There are two cognitive and perceptual criteria of BPD defined in *DSM-5* (APA, 2013). First, an identity disturbance that is characterized by a markedly and persistently unstable self-image or sense of self and, second, transient, paranoid ideation or severe dissociative symptoms that are stress related. Genetic risk factors for identity disturbance, criterion 3, and paranoid ideation/dissociative symptoms, criterion 9, are derived almost exclusively from the general BPD factor (Reichborn-Kjennerud et al., 2013) noted in the section on genetics in this chapter. They and the interpersonal dimension (criteria 1 and 2) show the lowest level of heritability of all BPD criteria.

Identity Disturbance in BPD

Along with the description of identity disturbance defined in criterion 3 of BPD in *DSM-5*, the manual also describes rapid shifts in self-image, goals, life plans, sexual identity, and self-values, and those of friends. Sudden role changes occur. Self-image is usually that of being bad, evil, or nonexistent. These experiences vary with the history of lack of a nurturing, supportive relationship. Performance in work or school situations depends on the degree of structure provided.

Identity disturbance in BPD has not been well-studied because it is subjective, difficult to evaluate validly and reliably, and lacks an accepted definition (Jorgensen, 2010). These problems have impeded examination of the biological underpinnings of this critical feature of BPD. Therefore, we focus on the relationship of disturbances of identity similar to BPD due to biological impairments caused by brain trauma and other disease processes. Epigenetic factors associated with trauma are addressed elsewhere in the book.

The Neurobiological Bases of Identity Disturbances Similar to Those in BPD

The first comprehensive description of the relationship between discrete, anatomical dysfunction and behaviors that we now classify as identity disturbances in BPD are contained in the reports of a railroad worker named Phineas P. Gage. (For a detailed account of this classic medical case see Antonio Damasio, 1994a.)

In 1848, Gage was a 25-year-old construction crew foreman who was skilled, highly dependable, committed, socially mature beyond his years, and liked and respected by his superiors and his men. An accidental explosion drove Gage's tamping rod upward through the front of his skull landing more than a hundred feet away. He quickly regained consciousness, mobility, and speech and promptly received medical care of his wounds by Dr. John Harlow, a professor of surgery at Harvard.

Gage's recovery progressed well but not completely. While there were no impairments of his speech functions, memory, new learning, intellectual, and physical abilities, he began to demonstrate behavior markedly different from before the accident. "he had become irreverent and capricious. His respect for the social conventions by which he had once abided had vanished. His abundant profanity offended those around him. Perhaps most troubling, he had taken leave of his sense of responsibility. He could not be trusted to honor his commitments. His employers had deemed him 'the most efficient and capable man in their employ' but now had to dismiss him." His friends stated, "Gage was no longer Gage" (Damasio et al., 1994a). He spent the final 12 years of his life in a dissolute existence, moving from job to job but never achieving his former level of performance. How are we to account for these dramatic changes in certain attitudes and behaviors, many similar to the identity and other disturbances frequently observed in patients with BPD, while other behaviors were left essentially intact?

Fortunately, Gage's skull and the iron bar were preserved at the Medical Museum at Harvard. Hannah Damasio and her colleagues reconstructed the extent of the damage done to Gage's brain by three-dimensional computer manipulation of the data obtained from these artifacts and descriptions of the wound (Damasio et al., 2004). The rod entered the left cheek under the zygomatic arch, continued in an upward, slightly posterior and medial direction, destroyed the left eye, then entered the roof of the orbit, damaging the anterior midline structures of both frontal lobes before exiting at the midline of the frontal bone. The damage was in the ventromedial prefrontal cortices of both hemispheres, the left suffering more damage than the right. There was no damage to the dorsal and lateral prefrontal cortices, including Broca's, Wernicke's, and the motor areas. The spared areas are associated with language and motor functions, the control of attention, working memory, the performance of calculations, and reasoning *not involved in the personal-social realm*. Studies of patients with lesions similar to Gage's due to midline frontal tumors and other diseases have confirmed these findings (Damasio, 1994b, 1994c).

Damage to other brain areas also leads to behavioral changes that overlap with those described, some of which resemble the impairments in identity observed in patients with BPD (Damasio, 1994c). Damage in specific areas of the right somatosensory cortices that results from strokes or other lesions affecting specific regions of the right hemisphere result in anosognosia. The patient is unaware of the severe loss of sensory and motor function of the left side of the body and has no emotional response to this life-changing disorder. Patients who suffer similar damage to the left side of the brain with equivalent impairments on the right side of the body are aware of and appropriately disturbed by their severe disabilities. In anosognosic patients, their self-image is so seriously compromised that it has little basis in reality and drastically impairs their ability to make rational, personal decisions and to plan effectively for the required changes in their future. The specific areas affected in these patients include the insula located on the internal face of the lateral sulcus, the primary somatosensory cortex at the dorsal and lateral region of the anterior parietal lobe, the secondary somatosensory cortex in the roof of the lateral sulcus and contiguous with the insula, and the connections of these areas to the anterior cingulate and prefrontal cortices, amygdala, thalamus, basal ganglia, and hippocampus.

Taken together, these findings and others suggest that specific regions of the ventromedial prefrontal lobes and of the right anterior parietal lobe are involved in a number of the identity disturbances observed in BPD. The distributed processing of information involved in complex brain functions and the lateralization of many of these functions may account for the widespread anatomical sites involved in the core features of identity.

Although there are no data that provide information on the pathophysiological bases of identity disturbances in BPD, it is noteworthy that in the human brain only the anterior cingulate and the frontal insular cortices have been shown to contain large, bipolar projection neurons referred to as Von Economo neurons (VENs; Allman et al., 2011). These authors conclude that the destruction of VENs in early frontotemporal dementia suggest they are involved in empathy, social awareness, and self-control, consistent with findings in functional neuroimaging. Other authors have suggested that VENs are involved in neuropsychiatric disorders associated with deficits in social skills and emotional function (Butti et al., 2013) and report that VENs display the highest percentage of immunostaining of any cells studied (Stimson et al., 2011).

This is a provocative finding in light of the proposal by Menon and Uddin (2010) that the anterior portion of the insula and the ACC form a "salience network" that guides behavior by selecting the most relevant internal and external stimuli and then switching attention and behavioral control to the most relevant brain networks. It is not difficult to imagine how dysregulation of this mechanism could interfere with one's self-perception.

Transient Paranoid Ideation

Transient, stress-related paranoid ideation and severe dissociative symptoms (criterion 9 of BPD) were included in *DSM-IV* in 1980 and have been retained in *DSM-5*. Their heritability falls in the midrange of the nine criteria of BPD (Reichborn-Kjennerud et al., 2013).

The Neurobiological Basis of Paranoid Ideation in BPD

Few reviews and studies of the biological underpinnings of BPD have included information or hypotheses related to paranoid ideation and other psychotic symptoms in the disorder (Friedel, 2004; Grosjean & Tsai, 2007; Barnow et al., 2010; Krause-Utz et al., 2014), primarily because of the scarcity of data available in this area. However, studies directed at this issue are beginning to appear.

For example, patients with BPD and psychotic symptoms have more deficits in cognitive inhibition as determined by an anti-saccade eye task than BPD subjects without them but fewer than schizophrenic subjects (Grootens et al., 2008). Again, we turn to information obtained from the pathophysiology of psychosis in other mental disorders to provide us with a framework for understanding these symptoms in BPD (see Fornito et al., 2013 for a review of this issue).

The striatum (Fornito et al., 2013) and thalamus (Ettinger et al., 2013) play prominent roles in psychotic disorders. Their function is modulated strongly by dopamine, and they contain a large number of D2 receptors that are elevated in drug-naive psychotic patients and that are a major target of antipsychotic agents which are strong D2 receptor antagonists (Seeman, 2002, 2013). It has been suggested that dopamine dysfunction is involved in at least three of the dimensions of BPD, especially in psychotic manifestations (Friedel, 2004), and there is growing evidence supporting this hypothesis. In addition, the striatum is strongly connected by projection neurons to multiple, functionally distinct, distributed processing systems throughout the brain.

A ventral striatal circuit is the primary pathway for mesolimbic dopamine connections and links the inferior limbic division of the striatum with key structures integrated with the extended amygdala system such as the OFC and ventromedial prefrontal cortex. Disturbances in the structures and functions of the components of this ventral pathway have been demonstrated in patients with psychotic disorders. Also, patients in at-risk mental states for psychosis have been shown to have elevated levels of dopamine in the dorsal striatum, the DLPFC, and other multimodal association areas. Fornito et al. (2013) helped clarify the relationship of the dorsal and ventral corticostriatal circuitry by demonstrating that first-episode psychosis is characterized by a dorsal to ventral gradient of hypoconnectivity to hyperconnectivity between striatal and prefrontal regions. The degree of these aberrations correlates with the severity of symptoms, which are present in first-degree relatives. Therefore, they may represent a phenotypic risk factor for psychotic states. (OK as edited. ROF)

To our knowledge, there is no study that evaluates the relationship of psychotic-like symptoms in subjects with BPD with the areas associated with psychosis in other disorders. However, comparisons of the volume of the superior temporal gyrus (BA22) demonstrate reduced volumes in schizophrenia and schizotypal personality disorder but not in BPD (Goldstein et al., 2009). These findings suggest that biological markers may help to differentiate subtle differences in the biological substrates of paranoid ideation and other symptoms in patients with BPD from those with other mental disorders.

Transient Dissociative Symptoms in BPD

Pathological dissociation comprises a complex group of symptoms that include de-personalization (detachment from one's mind, body, or self), derealization (a sense of unreality or detachment from one's surroundings), distortions of time, and am-nestic episodes (APA, 2013). Dissociative symptoms have been studied more ex-tensively than the other symptoms of the cognitive-perceptual domain of BPD (see reviews by Korzekwa et al., 2009a, 2009b; Vermetten & Spiegel, 2014) and appear to affect a significant and more severely disturbed subpopulation of patients with the dis-order (Dell, 1998). Compared to normal controls, subjects with BPD and dissociative symptoms demonstrate a more severe history of psychological and physical trauma and co-occurring PTSD than BPD subjects without dissociative symptoms (Vermetten & Spiegel, 2014). These BPD patients also appear to have a poor response to DBT (Kleindienst et al., 2011) and short-term inpatient psychotherapy (Spitzer et al., 2007)

The Neurobiological Basis of Dissociation in BPD

In contrast to most other symptoms of BPD, we know of no information on the her-itability of dissociative experiences in the disorder. The most recent report of the her-itability of dissociation in general is estimated at 45% (Pieper et al., 2011). There is a strong relationship between trauma and dissociative experiences in BPD, although only a small number of traumatized individuals have persistent, dissociative episodes (see Kozekwa et al., 2009b), suggesting that heritable risk factors are also involved in the etiology of this symptom complex. A recent study focused on genes linked to de-pressive symptoms suggests a correlation of severity of dissociation with gene expres-sion in immune system regulation and cellular signaling/second messenger systems in subjects with BPD (Schmahl et al., 2013). These findings are consistent with gene variations observed in suicidal patients with depression and patients with PTSD who demonstrate dissociative episodes.

There is little direct information on the neurobiological correlates of dissoci-ation in BPD. As noted in this chapter, serotonergic dysfunction is strongly associ-ated with BPD, and there is evidence that it may be involved in dissociative responses in a subpopulation of patients with the disorder. Impulsive patients with BPD who are challenged with mCPP, a partial serotonin agonist, have a "spacy/high," a deper-sonalization/derealization response associated with increased prolactin and cortisol levels (Stein et al., 1996). Abnormalities in the hypothalamic–pituitary–adrenal (HPA) axis in dissociation are present but may be related primarily to a history of trauma as they also occur in PTSD. In a review suggesting that NMDA is a critical mediator of BPD, Grosjean and Tsai (2007) provide a synthesis of the neuroanatomical and neurochemical correlates of BPD. They suggest that critical neuroanatomical regions involved in dissociation are the cingulate cortex, thalamus, and temporal parietal cortices. Vermetten and Spiegel (2014) extended the bases of the neurobiological underpinnings of trauma and dissociation in PTSD to those experienced in BPD. They conclude that dissociative experiences in both disorders are the result of "protective," enhanced inhibitory activity of the ventromedial prefrontal cortex that overrides the inherent/learned, stress-related increased activation of the bilateral amygdala, insula, and left thalamus. The degree of this imbalance of the top-down regulation of emotional reactivity may account for the variation of dissociative experiences reported by patients with both disorders. Recent studies demonstrated reduced amygdala activity related to acute dissociation during a working memory task (Krause-Utz et al., 2017).

Complementing and supporting these findings and theses, compared to controls, female subjects with BPD demonstrated decreased right-sided precuneus volumes while those with stronger depersonalization had a significant increase in this parietal region (Irle et al., 2005). Also, young women with BPD who had a history of severe childhood sexual and other physical abuse and pronounced dissociative symptoms demonstrated a decreased resting metabolic rate in the right temporal pole/anterior fusiform gyrus and in the left precuneus and posterior cingulate cortex compared to HCs (Lange et al., 2005). There is evidence that these areas of the brain continuously gather internal and external information and contribute to a unified view of the individual relative to the environment (Gusnard & Raichle, 2001).

■ INTERPERSONAL IMPAIRMENTS IN BPD

Interpersonal dysfunction and disorders of attachment are central features of BPD. The importance of interpersonal difficulties within borderline pathology is highlighted by the observation that this symptom domain is the slowest to improve with treatment and improves more gradually in BPD than in several other personality disorders (Choi-Kain et al., 2010; Skodal et al., 2005). In fact, certain interpersonal symptoms such as negative affect when alone, fear of abandonment, discomfort with care, and dependency are extremely slow to remit, with 15% to 25% of individuals with BPD who exhibited these symptoms at baseline failing to show improvement at 10-year follow-up (Choi-Kain et al., 2010). Another observation highlighting the importance of interpersonal symptoms in BPD is that remission from the disorder is often related to positive interpersonal events, such as entering a stable relationship (Links & Heslegrave, 2000). The nature of the interpersonal dysfunction has been characterized as an interpersonal hypersensitivity model (Gunderson & Lyons-Ruth, 2008). While there have been numerous clinical descriptions of interpersonal difficulties in BPD, only recently have there been empirical investigations of the nature of these difficulties. For example, a recent study used an event-contingent recording methodology, a method of documenting interpersonal interactions longitudinally in real time. This study identified that individuals with BPD perceived others as cold and quarrelsome, which led to an increase in their own quarrelsome behavior, resulting in further quarrelsome interactions (Sadikaj et al., 2013).

Further support for the notion that interpersonal dysfunction is a core feature of BPD is that interpersonal triggers bring about intense emotional states that interfere with proper interpretation of others' intentions (Brown et al, 2014). In this case, an electronically activated recorder (EAR) was used to measure signals in individuals with BPD compared to individuals with major depressive disorder. The EAR records approximately 47- to 50-second sound clips per day for three consecutive days. Recordings were coded for expressed positive affect and negative affect, and coder ratings were compared to participants' reports about their positive and negative affects during interpersonal events. Significant discrepancies between recalled and observed levels of negative affect and positive affect were found for BPD compared to controls for all types of interpersonal events. A recent study (Krause-Utz et al., 2014) specifically examined the hypothesis that patients with BPD, when activated by interpersonal triggers, are impaired in their cognitive ability. In an item recognition task with social distracters, compared to HCs, BPD individuals showed significantly impaired accuracy after distraction by negatively arousing stimuli (both scenes and faces) and neutral faces (but not neutral scenes). Significant negative correlations between overall accuracy and self-reported aversive inner tension were observed in BPD patients. This study supports the idea that BPD patients have an increased susceptibility to distracting (negatively arousing) social cues, which might interfere with cognitive functioning.

The specific social cognitive deficits that might underlie this interpersonal hyperreactivity have not been completely delineated. Nonetheless, there is fairly uniform evidence that individuals with BPD have disturbed "mentalizing." Most studies have found that individuals with BPD do not differ from HCs in "theory of mind" skills and are able to understand and respond to social cues. However, evidence suggests that patients with BPD are less skilled at inferring the mental states of others and may struggle to apply and utilize these abilities across contexts (Lazarus et al., 2014). Harari et al. (2010) suggest one possibility for synthesizing these findings: namely that affective empathy is intact and cognitive empathy is impaired. That is, individuals with BPD may accurately sense the emotions others are feeling but have difficulty understanding or conceptualizing the emotions and thoughts of others. Thus individuals with BPD appear to share the emotions of others but do not understand their cognitive bases. This process has been described as emotional "contagion" because of exaggerated resonance with others' emotional states. Neuroimaging data tend to support this model of excessive reactivity in the amygdala to social emotional stimuli, with a relative deficit in activation of prefrontal cortical regions thought to underlie cognitive strategies (reviewed by Jeung & Herpertz, 2014).

Exactly how a deficit in mentalizing interferes with attachment is not yet clear. It has been posited that a failure to develop the ability to perceive and interpret behavior based on underlying mental states (mentalization) may lead to difficulty interpreting and understanding interpersonal experiences, especially in contexts in which the attachment system is activated negatively (i.e., under conditions of perceived threat; Fonagy, 2003). Accordingly, this theory predicts that deficits in mentalization associated with maladaptive attachment account for the interpersonal dysfunction among individuals with BPD, as reviewed by Lazarus et al. (2014).

The Neurobiology of Attachment

Neurobiological studies of social interactions of all mammals is still in a nascent stage of development. The area with the greatest depth of understanding is the role of neuropeptides in social behavior. Since social neuroscience is a relatively new area of investigation, it is not surprising that studies in BPD are also in an early stage. Here we focus on what is known about the influence of oxytocin (OXT), arginine vasopressin (AVP), and opioids on interpersonal behavior in BPD. (See the subsection in this chapter on identity disturbances for more information on the neuroanatomical basis of impaired emotional-interpersonal reasoning and behavior.)

In healthy individuals, social stress (such as an adverse life event), stimulates the amygdala–cingulate circuit and the HPA axis. At the same time, social stress (a) encourages social approach behavior and physical contact (coping) and (b) stimulates OXT release. This promotes social approach behavior in a feedback loop; that is, positive social interactions produce OXT release, which in turn further promotes social approach behavior (Perez-Rodriguez et al., in preparation). The net effect of OXT release is the reduction of reactivity to social stressors (mediated by frontolimbic circuits and HPA axis) and the mediation of the anxiolytic and stress-protective effects of positive social interaction (e.g., "social buffering," Meyer-Lindenberg et al., 2011; "resilience," Ungar et al., 2013). Most of what is known about the effect of OXT on BPD comes from studies of the behavioral effect of intranasal OXT administration. With the exception of economic exchange games, studies have generally shown improvement of social cognition with OXT administration. Specifically, patients with BPD exhibited more and faster initial eye gaze fixation to the eyes of angry faces and heightened amygdala activation in response to angry faces compared with the health controls. These abnormal behavioral and neural patterns were normalized after OXT administration (Bertsch et al., 2013). Women with BPD had significantly reduced plasma OXT concentrations than HCs, and plasma OXT correlated negatively with experiences of childhood trauma, especially emotional neglect and abuse (Bertsch et al., 2013). During the Trier Social Stress Test, BPD patients demonstrated greater attenuation of stress-induced dysphoria compared to controls after OXT administration (Simeon et al., 2011). However, in two studies of an economic exchange game, OXT decreased cooperative behavior in BPD, especially in those with anxious attachment (Bartz et al., 2011; Ebert et al., 2013). This suggests that the context of the social interaction influences the impact of OXT administration.

AVP's primary action is to maintain fluid balance. However, many preclinical studies link AVP, and especially activation of the 1a receptor, to social behavior and specifically to aggression (Albers, 2012). However, the effects are complex. The behavioral effect of AVP administration has been primarily studied in men; these data indicate that AVP, like OXT, promotes social recognition and social cooperation (Guastella et al., 2011) in some contexts. However, it may have an opposite effect to OXT in the setting of social stress; AVP increases responsiveness to social stressors (Ebstein et al., 2009) and promotes an aggressive response to social stimuli (Thompson & Walton, 2004). One study specifically in BPD showed that micro-satellite repeats in the AVP gene associated with impulsive aggression in BPD in a small sample (Vogel et al., 2012). Overall, a model proposed by Meyer-Lindenberg et al. (2011) suggests that OXT may decrease social anxiety and enhance social cognition, while AVP increases social reward seeking and decreases social cognition. The authors note that these findings are very preliminary, but they do raise the possibility of modulation of OXT and AVP in the treatment of this core symptom of BPD. For related information on the genetically-modulated behavioral effects of OXT and AVP on the mating and maternal behavior of certain mammals, see Flint et al. (2010).

There has been a great deal of interest in the opiate system in BPD, which until recently was largely theoretical with little empirical support. For decades, researchers have theorized that at least one behavior common in BPD—self-cutting—relates to abnormalities in opiate activity. It has long been noted that BPD patients engage in self-cutting not as a suicidal act but rather because they report that it relieves psychic pain. One way of viewing cutting behavior in BPD is to consider that patients with BPD may have a pre-existing deficit in endogenous opiates. According to this view, BPD patients are self-medicating by cutting themselves, attempting to attenuate severe intrapsychic distress that healthy individuals—without such a deficit—would not be experiencing. This is consistent with the observation that opiate antagonists might decrease cutting behavior by rendering ineffective the patient's attempts to treat his or her pain (thereby decreasing the frequency of cutting) but would not relieve the underlying intrapsychic distress.

An opiate-deficit theory of BPD might explain far more than the self-injurious behavior of individuals with BPD, particularly the salient interpersonal difficulties. The endogenous opiate system not only regulates pain but also has an important role in social behavior. This system, through μ-opiate receptors, has been implicated in regulation of emotional and stress responses. Reductions in its function is associated with deficits in attachment behavior in animal models. In many species, the soothing and comforting that infants receive from maternal grooming and touching is opiate-mediated (Panksepp, 1980). In human beings, opiates are involved in normal and pathological emotion regulation (Kennedy et al., 2006) in addition to their more traditional role in modulating pain (Zubieta et al., 2001). In short, there is reason to think that endogenous opiates facilitate normal social function in healthy individuals. If the proposed model is accurate, then a deficit in endogenous opiates might help to explain not only cutting behavior and substance abuse in BPD but also the salient interpersonal dysfunction.

This view could provide a heuristic model to help patients and clinicians understand the social disruption in BPD. The satisfaction that normally accompanies closeness to other people both in early attachment and throughout life may be more difficult to achieve for patients with BPD. If individuals with BPD do not have sufficient endogenous opiate activity, then the continual craving for relationships and heightened reaction to their loss is understandable. This model could provide a better understanding of disappointment in relationships for patients and provides support for targeting the μ-opiate receptor as a novel molecular target for pharmacotherapy in BPD.

■ **CONCLUSIONS**

The heuristic value of the rapidly expanding body of knowledge on the neurobiological bases of BPD may be grouped under four headings: research, acceptance of BPD as an important brain disease, clinical treatment (medications and psychotherapy), and education.

Research

The material in this chapter suggest a number of challenges and opportunities for further research on BPD. In the area of genetics, current evidence supports the presence of one highly heritable BPD factor that influences all nine BPD criteria and that, opposed to this general factor, other, criteria-specific influences are mainly unique and more environmental in origin. (See Chapter 3.) The ubiquity of the general BPD factor suggests it may be oligogenetic and that less potent polygenetic factors operate in the specific factors. Regardless, it is important to understand the biological nature of each of these factors, that is, how are they represented in the brain anatomically, biochemically, and pathophysiologically. Also, the elucidation of epigenetic mechanisms raises exciting opportunities to integrate inherent and learned influences on the development and treatment of BPD at the brain level.

For example, dopamine (DA)- and cAMP-regulated phosphoprotein (DARRP-32) is known to be a central regulator of signaling in striatal neurons (Greengard, 2001a & b). Also, cAMP-dependent protein kinase activity regulates the phosphorylation and thus the activity level of DARPP-32 (Greengard et al., 1999). Both DA and 5-HT dysfunction are risk factors of impulsivity (Harrison et al, 1997; Van Erp & Miczek, 2000; Dalley et al., 2002). Serotonin also regulates DARPP-32 phosphorylation (Svenningsson et al., 2002a), an effect modified by fluoxetine (Svenningsson et al., 2002b). Some of the effects of diverse psychotomimetics on DA, 5-HT, and glutamate activity in humans and animals appear to be mediated by the DARPP-32 signal transduction pathway (Greengard et al., 1999). Further work by Greengard and his colleagues (Bateup et al., 2008) have demonstrated that the stimulant cocaine and the sedation-producing antipsychotic haloperidol exert differential effects on DARPP-32 phosphorylation in two striatonigral and striatopallidal cell populations, a phenomenon that can explain their opposing behavioral effects. They found that a variety of drugs that target the striatum have cell type–specific effects that were previously indiscernible. This suggests that DARPP-32 phosphorylation may mediate a portion of the reciprocal interactions of DA, 5-HT, and other neurotransmitters and psychotropic drug effects on specific symptoms of BPD and is possibly involved in the molecular mechanisms of the general genetic BPD factor.

Other research opportunities in BPD are the elucidation of central mechanisms of affect regulation, impulsive aggression, cognition and perception, and social interaction at subjective, behavioral, and neurobiological levels. As a first step, these mechanisms should be investigated with respect to BPD symptom specificity, age and gender dependence, and long-term stability following the remission of acute symptoms (Grilo et al., 2014). A different and promising area of research would seek validation of identified key neurobiological mechanisms as potential endophenotypes and to use these to tailor specific therapeutic interventions. It is proposed that endophenotypes are closer to the site of the primary causes (whether genetic or environmental) than to diagnostic categories (Almasy & Blangero, 2001), and, to be primarily state-independent, they should manifest themselves whether or not the illness is active. In addition, endophenotypes should be related to the development of the disorder and not mimic long-term consequences or secondary manifestations of the core symptoms of co-occurring mental disorders (Gottesman & Gould, 2003). This could be addressed by including remitted and adolescent patients in research projects. A major problem in neurobiological research on BPD has been that most studies have been carried out by relatively small groups or researchers, which necessarily results in mono-methodological approaches. Therefore, multidisciplinary collaboration is needed to improve the integration of structural and functional neuroimaging, neurochemistry, and neuropsychological paradigms and measurement methods.

Acceptance of BPD as an Important Brain Disease

Before existing and future research findings can be translated to the clinical setting, the acceptance of the disorder as a disease of the brain must be advanced (Friedel, 2006). It has been difficult for mental disorders, especially BPD, to gain acceptance as *bona fide* medical diseases. As Damasio (1994c) points out, the persistence of the Cartesian mind-brain dualistic model has been a serious impediment to the advance of the medical fields of both neurology and psychiatry. In addition, locked in its strong enclosure of bone, until recently, the inaccessibility of the brain provided a formidable obstacle to establishing clear evidence that mental disorders are diseases of the brain. The emergence of modern psychopharmacology in the 1950s was not sufficient to deter those who adamantly held that environmental etiologies caused even the most severe mental disorders and who continued to attribute the symptoms of the disorders to learned behaviors, especially those of parents and families. For example, during one period in the mid-20th century, many mental health professionals and researchers espoused that "shizophrenogenic mothers" played a prominent role in the etiology of the disease (Harrington, 2012), an historical episode that should serve as a reminder that lessons not learned result in behaviors repeated. As pointed out (Friedel, 2006; Harrington, 2012), schizophrenia did not become broadly accepted as a medical disorder until the 1980s when research evidence demonstrated the high heritability of the disorder and the anatomical and functional disturbances in the brains of patients with this disease. The acceptance of BPD as a valid diagnosis and a medical illness remains low (Gunderson & Links, 2014). It is our opinion that a greater effort should be made to procure and dedicate resources to didactic, clinical, and research efforts to BPD to make them proportional to the impact of this disease on individuals with the disorder, their families and society. To accomplish this task, the collaborative efforts of academic and lay advocacy communities need to be increased as they have proven successful in the areas of schizophrenia and bipolar disorder (Friedel, 2006). It can be argued that that the most promising first step would be to have the National Institute of Mental Health (NIMH) reclassify BPD as a "serious mental illness," as this would immediately increase the pool of NIMH competitive research funds available to researchers in BPD from the current $5 million annually to $400 million annually.

Clinical Treatment

Medications in BPD

Since initial reports suggesting the efficacy of FGAs in the treatment of some symptoms of BPD were published (Brinkley et al., 1979; Goldberg et al, 1986; Soloff et al., 1986), there has been a rapid increase in the use of medications in the treatment of the disorder. Also, recent evidence indicates a significant shift in the data supporting the use of medications in BPD from SSRIs and FGAs as recommended in the APA (2001) Guideline to SGAs and mood stabilizers (Abraham & Calabrese, 2008; Saunders & Silk, 2009; Lieb et al. 2010). (Also, see Chapter 2.) However, until the publication of the studies cited in this and prior reviews, there has been little information available to consider possible mechanisms of action of medications in BPD and the rationale for their proper use.

For example, a preponderance of data suggests that the therapeutic mechanism of action of antipsychotic agents in multiple mental disorders results from their inhibitory effect on D2 receptors (Seeman, 2013) and possibly serotonin 2 (5-HT2A) receptors (Meltzer, 1989). Pre- and postsynaptic DA autoreceptors are prevalent throughout the brain, especially in the ventral striatum, and are critical to the proper function of DA, a neuromodulator that affects the activity of CNS distributed processing systems related to a number of the symptoms of BPD. This information has advanced our understanding of the circuitry and molecular mechanisms of action of these agents in BPD (Friedel, 2004).

Another example involves the role of 5-HT in the etiology of BPD. The data supporting disturbances of serotonin activity in BPD are so compelling that they raise serious questions about the findings to date that medications known to enhance CNS serotonergic activity have not been demonstrated to significantly and consistently produce therapeutic effects on the symptoms of the disorder, especially aggressive impulsivity (Lieb et al., 2010). One explanation is that the studies conducted may have been underpowered or contained other methodological flaws that led to type II errors. Another possibility is that the molecular disturbances contributed by 5-HT to the symptoms of BPD occur at chemical nodal points in the 5-HT signal transduction cascade that are minimally responsive to current medications (see DARPP-32 above). In the latter event, additional basic knowledge about the neurobiological role of 5-HT in BPD may enable the development of medications that are more effective in the treatment of the disorder than those now available.

Also, existing pharmacological studies on FGAs, SGAs, and mood stabilizers indicate that they affect different synaptic transduction cascades. In the experience of one author (ROF), in some patients with moderate to severe BPD, the use of a second class of drug simultaneously may be helpful to effectively reduce the same symptom or domain of BPD if one is only partially effective (Bellino et al., 2008). This therapeutic technique is often referred to in the literature as an example of the harmful prevalence of "polypharmacy" in BPD. However, the evidence noted in this chapter suggests a complex pathophysiology and polygenetic etiology (Reichborn-Kjennerud et al., 2013; Chapter 3) of the symptoms of the disorder. Taken together, these findings provide a rationale for the multimedicinal therapeutic approach as is frequently used in other areas of medicine. The term "polypharmacy" is also used by some clinicians pejoratively even if additional medications are required to treat frequently co-occuring disorders such as ADHD and major depressive episodes, which are beginning to demonstrate a partially shared genetic etiology with BPD (Distel et al., 2011c; Chapter 3). Such statements may dissuade physicians from using multiple medications for the treatment of the symptoms of BPD and comorbid disorders and thus may limit the benefit derived from such treatment. The greater our understanding of the neurobiological processes leading to the symptoms of BPD, the more help patients suffering from the disorder will receive.

Finally, readers of the therapeutic literature on BPD are familiar with the seemingly obligatory statement in most articles and books on the topic that medications, at best, are of minimal use in treatment, and that, if used, they are merely *adjunctive* to psychotherapy. The most perplexing of these statements is contained in a guideline for medication use in BPD published by the National Collaborating Centre for Mental Health (NICE; 2009). It contends that "Drug treatment should not be used specifically for borderline personality disorder or for the individual symptoms or behavior associated with the disorder (for example, repeated self-harm, marked emotional instability, risk-taking behaviour and transient psychotic symptoms)." Ironically, the NICE guideline also recommends "nonempirically" (Schulz & Nelson, 2014) using a "sedative anti-histamine" in an immediate crisis. In a review article (Lieb et al., 2010) of a recent Cochrane report of randomized controlled trials (RCTs) of pharmacological studies on BPD (Stoffers et al, 2010), the authors disagree with the conclusions of the NICE guideline, stating "we suggest considering a reassessment of these recommendations, as there actually is encouraging evidence of the effectiveness of drug treatment for individual symptoms of borderline personality disorder." In this context, it is important to note that in the 27 RCTs included in the Cochrane meta-analyses of psychotherapy of BPD (Stoffers et al., 2012), only one were medications *not used* in some manner in the experimental group. Because of this important confounding variable in the RCTs that provide the scientific basis for the efficacy of psychotherapy of BPD, and evidence presented in this chapter indicating the strong and coherent neurobiological underpinnings of BPD, *the therapeutic interactions of pharmacotherapy and psychotherapy in the treatment of BPD require serious reconsideration and further research. (Italics added because this is an issue of major but neglected importance in the treatment of BPD!)*

Psychotherapy in BPD

In spite of the uncontrolled variable in the BPD-specific psychotherapy studies noted, these studies do suggest a significant degree of efficacy of psychotherapy in the treatment of the disorder. The data on medications suggest they are useful in reducing some of the core symptoms of affective dysregulation, aggressive impulsivity, and cognitive-perceptual disturbances of BPD (Lieb et al., 2010), which in turn suggests they enable patients to understand better the specific nature of their disorder and to learn and *apply* alternative behaviors that will enhance their resilience to the inherent and environmental risk factors associated with the disorder. These are the major roles of psychotherapy.

Also, determining further the neurobiological basis of BPD does not diminish the importance of BPD-specific psychotherapies. On the contrary, clarifying the anatomical pathways and the genetic, biochemical, and pathophysiological processes involved in the etiology and effective treatment of BPD should facilitate the task of how best to proceed with the integration of existing pharmacological and psychotherapeutic approaches that more specifically focus on the individual needs of each patient (Gunderson & Links, 2008; Oldham et al., 2014; Gunderson; with Links, 2014; Silk & Friedel, 2016). For example, as noted, an intensive course of DBT has been reported to decrease the epigenetically induced increase in methylation of BDNF exons correlated with childhood trauma in BPD subjects who responded compared to nonresponders (Perroud et al., 2013). If replicated, such epigenetic and other neurobiological findings associated with psychotherapy will provide biological mechanisms of action of psychotherapy that should improve efficacy and help withstand efforts to seriously reduce the costs of treatment of BPD by limiting it mainly to medication-based and brief psychotherapeutic approaches as medical costs come under increasing public scrutiny.

New insights into brain mechanisms associated with BPD can also be used to improve specific psychotherapeutic approaches to its treatment. An example is affective dysregulation. Functional neuroimaging has been helpful in understanding better those brain mechanisms behind affective dysregulation such as disturbed pain processing or self-injurious behaviors. It can also be used to improve other manifestations of affective dysregulation, for example, by giving feedback about brain activity while performing affective regulation strategies in the scanner (real-time fMRI). A second possibility is to define fine-grained predictors or moderators for psychotherapy response, for example, by investigating the role of brain mechanisms behind dissociation to more accurately define responders and nonresponders. Finally, there is a rapidly growing number of psychotherapy trials which use structural and/or functional imaging to assess treatment success in addition to classical treatment outcome measurements by self-reports and structured interviews. Taken together, a better understanding of the interactions between the neurobiological mechanisms and psychotherapy of BPD will help to improve treatment options for patients with the disorder.

Neurofeedback

Evidence that specific symptoms characteristic of personality disorders, especially BPD, supports the possibility that other nonpharmacological and traditional psychotherapeutic interventions may be useful in treatment. For example, Paret et al. (2016) utilized real-time fMRI to evaluate the effects of four sessions of neurofeedback training to patients with BPD. Such training resulted in alteration of resting-state amygdala-lateral prefrontal cortex connectivity, dissociation, and scores on impaired emotional awareness. Although it is not clear whether the initial disturbances were the result of inherent or epigenetic variables, such findings open up new avenues or treatment.

■ EDUCATIONAL OPPORTUNITIES

Our knowledge of the neurobiological basis of BPD has produced a significant problem but also an opportunity. In spite of the prevalence, morbidity, mortality, and increasing recognition of BPD as a brain disease by mental health clinicians and the public, there exists a significant disconnect between the effects of the disorder on society and the educational efforts and commitment of clinical and research resources devoted to it in academic training programs in the United States and much of the world. This has resulted in a growing gap between those who want and need competent and experienced care and those available to provide it.

Patients with BPD present a number of special challenges to clinicians, many of whom have seen them in their training without the benefit of a skilled faculty member to guide the trainee in evaluation and treatment. On the contrary, some are taught that it is important to learn to make the diagnosis of BPD only so that they may avoid these difficult patients in their practice (personal communication to ROF from a faculty member in the psychiatric outpatient clinic of a prestigious academic medical center in the United States). The myths about the disorder, in spite of our progress, are numerous, still believed, and passed on. Not surprisingly, they increase the discouragement of patients, their families, and clinicians from seeking and providing treatment.

To underscore this problem, the most common question one of the authors receives in response to a book and website on BPD (Friedel, 2018; www.BPDdemystified.com) is, "How can I find a clinician in my area who is skilled in the diagnosis and treatment of BPD?" The BPD Resource Center is of great assistance in identifying such clinicians when one is available, but they are not able to produce them. Although the entire number of scientific articles on BPD has more than doubled in the past decade, too few are reaching practicing clinicians and trainees. As was experienced in schizophrenia and bipolar disorder, once a mental illness has been identified as having a biological basis and is treatable, patients and their families are much more prone to seek help (Friedel, 2006). This challenge to the mental health professional community needs to be addressed vigorously.

■ REFERENCES

Abraham, P. F., & Calabrese, J. R. (2008). Evidenced-based pharmacologic treatment of borderline personality disorder: a shift from SSRIs to anticonvulsants and atypical antipsychotics? *J Affect Dis, 111*, 21–30.

Albers, H. E. (2012). The regulation of social recognition, social communication and aggression: vasopressin in the social behavior neural network. *Horm Behav, 61*, 283–292.

Allman, J. M., Tetreault, N. A., Hakeem, A. Y., Manaye, K. F., Semendeferi, K., Erwin, J. M., Park, S., Goubert, V., & Hof, P. R. (2011). The von Economo neurons in the frontoinsular and anterior cingulate cortex. *Ann N Y Acad Sciences, 1225*:59–71.

Almasy, L., & Blangero, J. (2001). Endophenotypes as quantitative risk factors for psychiatric disease: rationale and study design. *Am J Medical Genetics, 105*, 42–44.

Amad, A., Ramoz, N., Thomas, P., Jardri, R., & Gorwood, P. (2014). Genetics of borderline personality disorder: systematic review and proposal of an integrative model. *Neurosci Biobehav Revs, 40*, 6–19.

Ameis, S. H., Ducharme, S., Albaugh, M. D., Hudziak, J. J., Botteron, K. N., Lepage, C., Zhao, L., Khundrakpam, B., Collins, D. L., Lerch, J. P., Wheeler, A., Schachar, R., Evans, A. C., & Karama, S. (2014). Cortical thickness, cortico-amygdalar networks, and externalizing behaviors and healthy children. *Biol Psychiatry, 75*, 65–72.

American Psychiatric Association. (2001). Practice guideline for the treatment of patients with borderline personality disorder. *Am J Psychiatry, 158*(suppl), 1–52.

American Psychiatric Association. (2013). *Diagnostic and statistical manual of mental disorders* (5th ed.). Washington, DC: American Psychiatric Publishing.

Bateup, H. S., Svenningsson, P., Kuroiwa, M., Gong, S., Nishi, A., Heintz, N., & Greengard, P. (2008). Cell type–specific regulation of DARPP-32 phosphorylation by psychostimulant and antipsychotic drugs. *Nature Neurosci, 11*, 932–939.

Barnow, S., Limberg, A., Stopsack, M., Spitzer, C., Grabe, H. J., Freyberger, H. J., & Hamm, A. (2010). Dissociation and emotion regulation in borderline personality disorder. *Psycholog Medicine, 42*, 783–794.

Bartz, J., Simeon, D., Hamilton, H., Kim, S., Crystal, S., Braun, A., Vicens, V., & Hollander, E. (2011). Oxytocin can hinder trust and cooperation in borderline personality disorder. *Soc Cogn Affect Neurosci, 6*, 556–563.

Beblo, T., Driessen, M., Mertens, M., Wingenfeld, K., Piefke, M., Rullkoetter, N., Silva-Saavedra, A., Mensebach, C., Reddemann, L., Rau, H., Markowitsch, H. J., Wulff, H., Lange, W., Berea, C., Ollech, I., & Woermann, F. G. (2006). Functional MRI correlates of the recall of unresolved life events in borderline personality disorder. *Psycholog Medicine, 36*, 845–856.

Bellino, S., Paradiso, E., & Bogetto, F. (2008). Efficacy and tolerability of aripiprazole augmentation in sertraline-resistant patients with borderline personality disorder. *Psychiatry Res, 161*, 206–212.

Bertsch, K., Gamer, M., Schmidt, B., et al. (2013). Oxytocin and reduction of social threat hypersensitivity in women with borderline personality disorder. *Am J Psychiatry, 170*, 1169–1177.

Bertsch, K., Schmidinger, I., Neumann, I. D., & Herpertz, S. C. (2013). Reduced plasma oxytocin levels in female patients with borderline personality disorder. *Horm Behav, 63*, 424–429.

Boy, F., Evans, C. J., Edden, R. A., Lawrence, A. D., Singh, K. D., Husain, M., & Sumner, P. (2011). Dorsolateral prefrontal gamma-aminobutyric acid in men predicts individual differences in rash impulsivity. *Biol Psychiatry, 70*, 866–872.

Brambilla, P., Soloff, P. H., Sala, M., Nicoletti, M. A., Keshavan, M. S., & Soares, J. C. (2004). Anatomical MRI study of borderline personality disorder patients. *Psychiatry Res, 131*, 125–133.

Brinkley, J. R., Beitman, B. S., & Friedel, R. O. (1979). Low-dose neuroleptic regimens in the treatment of borderline patients. *Arch Gen Psychiatry, 36*, 319–326.

Brown, W. C., Tragesser, S. L., Tomko, R. L., Mehl, M. R., & Trull, T. J. (2014). Recall of expressed affect during naturalistically observed interpersonal events in those with borderline personality disorder or depressive disorder. *Assessment, 21*, 73–81.

Buckholtz, J. W., Treadway, M. T., Cowan, R. L., Woodward, N. D., Li, R., Ansari, M. S. Baldwin, R. N. Schwartzman, A. N., Shelby, E. S., Smith, C. E., Kessler, R. M., & Zald, D. H. (2010). Dopaminergic network differences in human impulsivity. *Science, 329*, 532.

Butti, C., Santos, M., Uppal, N., & Hof, P. R. (2013). Von Economo neurons: clinical and evolutionary perspectives. *Cortex, 49*, 312–326.

Cackowski, S., Reitz, A. C., Ende, G., Kleindienst, N., Bohus, M., Schmahl. C., & Krause-Utz, A. (2014). Impact of stress and attention deficit hyperactivity disorder symptoms on different components of impulsivity in borderline personality disorder. *Psychol Medicine*, 1–12.

Calati, R., Gressier, F., Balestri, M., & Serretti, A. (2013). Genetic modulation of borderline personality disorder: systematic review and meta-analysis. *J Psychiatr Res, 47*, 1275–1287.

Caprioli, D., Sawiak S. J., Merlo, E., Theobald, D. E. H., Spoelder, M., Jupp, B., Voon, V., Carpenter, T. A., Everitt, B. J., Robbins, T. W., & Dalley, J. W. (2014). Gamma aminobutyric acid and neuronal structural markers in the nucleus accumbens core underlie trait-like impulsive behavior. *Biol Psychiatry, 75*, 115–123.

Carpenter, R. W., & Trull, T. J. (2013). Components of emotion dysregulation in borderline personality disorder: a review. *Curr Psychiatry Reps, 15*, 335.

Carrasco, J. L., Tajima-Pozo, K., Díaz-Marsá, M., Casado, A., López-Ibor, J. J., Arrazola, J., & Yus, M. (2012). Microstructural white matter damage at orbitofrontal areas in borderline personality disorder. *J Affect Dis, 139*, 149–153.

Choi-Kain, L. W., Zanarini, M. C. Frances R., Frankenburg, G. M., Fitzmaurice, D. & Bradford, R. (2010). A longitudinal study of the 10-year course of interpersonal features in borderline personality disorder. *J Pers Disord, 24*, 365–376.

Chotai, J., Kullgren, G., & Asberg, M. (1998). CSF monoamine metabolites in relation to the diagnostic interview for borderline patients (DIB). *Neuropsychobiology, 38*, 207–212.

Coccaro, E. F., Sripada, C. S., Yanowitch, R. N., & Phan, K. L. (2011). Corticolimbic function in impulsive aggressive behavior. *Biol Psychiatry, 69*, 1153–1159.

Cole, M. W., & Schneider, W. (2007). The cognitive control network: integrated cortical regions with dissociable functions. *NeuroImage, 37*, 343–360.

Crockett, M. J., Clark, L., & Robbins, T. W. (2009). Reconciling the role of serotonin in behavioral inhibition and aversion: acute tryptophan depletion abolishes punishment-induced inhibition in humans. *J Neurosci, 29*, 11993–11999.

Cullen, K. R., Vizueta, N., Thomas, K. M., Han, G. J., Lim, K. O., Camchong, J., Mueller, B. A., Bell, C. H., Heller, M. D., & Schulz, S. C. (2011). Amygdala functional connectivity in young women with borderline personality disorder. *Brain Connectivity, 1*, 61–71.

Cyders, M. A., & Smith, G. A. (2008). Emotion-based dispositions to rash action: positive and negative urgency. *Psycholog Bull, 134*, 807–828.

Dalley, J. W., Theobald, D. E., Eagle, D. M., Passetti, F., & Robbins, T. W. (2002). Deficits in impulse control associated with tonically-elevated serotonergic function in rat prefrontal cortex. *Neuropsychopharmacology, 26*, 716–728.

Dalley, J. W., Mar, A. C., Economidou, D., & Robbins, T. W. (2008). Neurobehavioral mechanisms of impulsivity: Fronto-striatal systems and functional neurochemistry. *Pharmacology, Biology, and Behavior, 90*(2), 250–260.

Damasio, A. R. (1994a). *Descartes' error: emotion, reason, and the human brain* (pp. 3–33). New York, NY: Putnam Berkley.

Damasio, A. R. (1994b). *Descartes' error: emotion, reason, and the human brain* (pp. 54–70). New York: Putnam Berkley Group.

Damasio, A. R. (1994c). *Descartes' error: emotion, reason, and the human brain* (pp. 256–258). New York: Putnam Berkley Group.

Damasio, A. R., Grabowski, T. J., Bechara, A., Damasio, H., Ponto, L. L., Parvizi, J., & Hichwa, R. D. (2000). Subcortical and cortical brain activity during the feeling of self-generated emotions. *Nature Neurosci, 3*, 1049–1056.

Damasio, H., Grabowski, T., Frank, R., Galaburda, A. M., & Damasio, A. M. (2004). The return of Phineas Gage: clues about the brain from the skull of a famous patient. *Science, 264*, 1102–1105.

Dammann, G., Teschler, S., Haag, T., Altmuller, F., Tuczek, F., & Dammann, R. H. (2011). Increased DNA methylation of neuropsychiatric genes occurs in borderline personality disorder. *Epigenetics, 6*, 1454–1462.

De Bruijn, E. R., Grootens, K. P., Verkes, R. J., Buchholz, V., Hummelen, J. W., & Hulstijn, W. (2006). Neural correlates of impulsive responding in borderline personality disorder: ERP evidence for reduced action monitoring. *J Psychiatr Res, 40*, 428–437.

Dell, P. F. (1998). Axis II pathology in outpatients with dissociative identity disorder. *J Nerv Mental Dis, 186*, 352–356.

Distel, M. A., Carlier, A., Middeldorp, C. M., Derom, C. A., Lubke, G. H., & Boomsma, D. I. (2011a). Borderline personality traits and adult attention-deficit hyperactivity disorder symptoms: a genetic analysis of comorbidity. *Am J Med Gen, B, Neuropsychiatr Genet, 156B*, 817–825.

Distel, M. A., Middeldorp, C. M., Willemsen, G., Trull, T. J., Derom, C. A., & Boomsma, D. I. (2011b). Life events and borderline personality: gene-environment correlation or gene-environment interaction? *Psychol Med, 41*, 849–860.

Distel, M. A., Rebollo-Mesa, I., Willemsen, G., et al. (2009). Familial resemblance of borderline personality disorder features: genetic or cultural transmission? *PLoS ONE, 4*(4), e5334.

Distel, M. A., Roeling, M. P., Tielbeek, J. J., van Toor, D., Derom, C. A., Trull, T. J., & Boomsma, D. I. (2011c). The covariation of trait anger and borderline personality: a bivariate twin-siblings study. *J Abnorm Psychol, 12*, 458–466.

Distel, M A., Trull, T. J., de Moor, M. M., Vink, J. M., Geels, L. M., van Beek, J. H., Bartels, M., Willemsen, G., Thiery, E., Derom, C. A., Neale, M. C., & Boomsma, D. I. (2012). Borderline personality traits and substance use: genetic factors underlie the association with smoking and ever use of cannabis, but not with high alcohol consumption. *J Pers Disord, 26*, 867–879.

Distel, M. A., Trull, T. J., Derom, C. A., Thiery, E. W., Grimmer, M. A., Martin, N. G., Willemsen, G., & Boomsma, D. I. (2008). Heritability of borderline personality disorder features is similar across three countries. *Psychol Med, 38*, 1219–1229.

Distel, M. A., Willemsen, G., Ligthart, L., Derom, C. A., Martin, N. G., Neale, M. C., Trull, T. J., & Boomsma, D. I. (2010). Genetic covariance structure of the four main features of borderline personality disorder. *J Pers Disord, 24*, 427–444.

Domes, G., Schulze, L., Bottger, M., Grossmann, A., Hauenstein, K., Wirtz, P. H., Heinrichs, M., & Herpertz, S. C. (2009). The neural correlates of sex differences in emotional reactivity and emotion regulation. *Hum Brain Mapp, 31*, 758–769.

Donegan, N. H., Sanislow, C. A., Blumberg, H. P., Fulbright, R. K., Lacadie, C., Skudlarski, P., Gore, J. C., Olson, I. R., McGlashan, T. H., & Wexler, B. E. (2003). Amygdala hyperreactivity in borderline personality disorder: implications for emotional dysregulation. *Biol Psychiatry, 54*, 1284–1293.

Driessen, M., Herrmann, J., Stahl, K., Zwaan, M., Meier, S., Hill, A., Osterheider, M., & Petersen, D. (2000). Magnetic resonance imaging volumes of the hippocampus and the amygdala in women with borderline personality disorder and early traumatization. *Arch Gen Psychiatry, 57*, 1115–1122.

Ebert, A., Kolb. M., Heller, J., Edel, M. A., Roser, P., & Brüne, M. (2013). Modulation of interpersonal trust in borderline personality disorder by intranasal oxytocin and childhood trauma. *Soc Neurosci, 8*, 305–313.

Ebstein, R. P., Israel, S., Lerer, E., Uzefovsky, F., Shalev, I., Gritsenko, I., Riebold, M., Salomon, S., & Yirmiya, N. (2009). Arginine vasopressin and oxytocin modulate human social behavior. *Ann N Y Acad Sci, 1167*, 87–102.

Ende, G., Cackowski, S., van Eijk, J., Sack, M., Demirakca, T., Kleindienst, N., Bohus, M., Sobanski, E., Krause-Utz, A., & Schmahl, C. (2016). Impulsivity and aggression in female BPD and ADHD patients: association with ACC glutamate and GABA concentrations. *Neuropsychopharmacology, 41*, 410–418.

Ettinger, U., Corr, P. J., Mofidi, A., Williams, S. C. R., & Kumari, V. (2013). Dopaminergic basis of the psychosis-prone personality investigated with functional magnetic resonance imaging of procedural learning. *Front Hum Neurosci, 7*, 1–11.

Flint, J., Greenspan, R. J., & Kendler, K. S. (2010). *How genes influence behavior.* New York: Oxford University Press.

Fonagy, P. (2003). Clinical implications of attachment and mentalization: efforts to preserve the mind in contemporary treatment. Epilogue. *Bull Menninger Clin, 67*, 271–80.

Fornito, A., Harrison, B. J., Goodby, E., Dean, A., Ooi, C., Nathan, P. J., Lennox, B. R., Jones, P. B., Suckling, J., & Bullmore, E. T. (2013). Functional disconnectivity of corticostriatal circuitry as a risk phenotype for psychosis. *JAMA Psychiatry, 70*, 1143–1151.

Friedel, R. O. (2004). Dopamine dysfunction in borderline personality disorder: a hypothesis. *Neuropsychopharmacology, 29*, 1029–1039.

Friedel, R. O. (2018). *Borderline personality disorder demystified.* New York: Marlowe and Company.

Friedel, R. O. (2006). Early sea changes in borderline personality disorder. *Curr Psychiatry Rep, 8*, 1–4. Erratum in: *Curr Psychiatry Rep, 8*(3), iii.

Glenn, C. R., & Klonsky, E. D. (2009). Emotion dysregulation as a core feature of borderline personality disorder. *J Pers Disord, 23*, 20–28.

Goldberg, S. C., Schulz, S. C., Schulz, P. M., Resnick, R. J., Hamer, R. M., & Friedel, R. O. (1986). Borderline and schizotypal personality disorders treated with low-dose thiothixene vs. placebo. *Arch Gen Psychiatry, 43*, 680–686.

Goldstein, K. E., Hazlett, E. A., New A. S., Haznedar, M. M., Newmark, R. E., Zelmanova, Y., Passarelli, V., Weinstein, S. R., Canfield, E. L., Meyerson, D. A., Tang, C. Y., Buchsbaum, M. S., & Siever, L. J. (2009). Smaller superior temporal gyrus volume specificity in schizotypal personality disorder. *Schizophr Res, 112*, 14–23.

Goodman, M., Hazlett, E. A., Avedon, J. B., Siever, D. R., Chu, K. W., & New, A. S. (2011). Anterior cingulate volume reduction in adolescents with borderline personality disorder and co-morbid major depression. *J Psychiatr Res, 45*, 803–807.

Gottesman, I. I., & Gould, T. D. (2003). The endophenotype concept in psychiatry: etymology and strategic intentions. *Am J Psychiatry, 160*, 636–645.

Grant, B. F., Chou, S. P., Goldstein, R. B., Huang, B., Stinson, F. S., Saha, T. D., Smith, S. M., Dawson, D. A., Pulay, A. J., Pickering, R. P., & Ruan, W. J. (2008). Prevalence, correlates, disability, and comorbidity of DSM-IV borderline personality disorder: results from the wave 2 national epidemiologic survey on alcohol and related conditions. *J Clin Psychiatry, 69*, 533–545.

Grant, J. E., Correia, S., Brennan-Krohn, B. A., Malloy, P. F., Laidlaw, D. H., & Schulz, S. C. (2007). Frontal white matter integrity in borderline personality disorder with self injurious behavior. *J Neuropsychiatry Clin Neurosci, 19*, 383–390.

Greengard, P., Allen, P. B., & Naim, A. C. (1999). Beyond the dopamine receptor: the DARPP-32/ protein phosphatase-1 cascade. *Neuron, 23*, 435–447.

Greengard, P. (2001a) The neurobiology of dopamine signaling. *Biosci Rep, 21*, 247–269.

Greengard, P. (2001b). The neurobiology of slow synaptic transmission. *Science, 294*, 1024–1030.

Grilo, C. M., McGlashan, T. H., & Skodol, A. E. (2014). Course and outcome. In J. M. Oldham, A. E. Skodol, & D. S. Bender, (Eds.), *Textbook of personality disorders* (2nd ed., pp. 165–186). Washington, DC: American Psychiatric Publishing.

Grinker, R., Werble, B., & Drye, R. (1968). *The borderline syndrome: a behavioral study of ego functions.* New York: Basic Books.

Grootens, K. P., van Luijtelaar, G., Buitelaar, J. K., van der Laan, A., Jacobus W. Hummelen, J. W., & Verkes, R. J. (2008). Inhibition errors in borderline personality disorder with psychotic-like symptoms. *Prog Neuropsychopharmacol Biol Psychiatry, 31*, 267–273.

Grosjean, B., & Tsai, B. E. (2007). NMDA neurotransmission as a critical mediator of borderline personality disorder. *J Psychiatry Neurosci, 32*, 103–115.

Guastella, A. J., Kenyon, A. R., Unkelbach, C., Alvares, G. A., & Hickie, I. B. (2011). Arginine vasopressin selectively enhances recognition of sexual cues in male humans. *Psychoneuroendocrinology, 36*, 294–297.

Gunderson, J. G. (2009). Borderline personality disorder: ontogeny of a diagnosis. *Am J Psychiatr, 166*(5), 530–539.

Gunderson, J. G., & Links, P. S. (2008). *Borderline personality disorder: a clinical guide* (2nd ed., pp. 225–307). Arlington, VA: American Psychiatric Publishing.

Gunderson, J. G.; with Links, P. S. (2014). *Good psychiatric management for borderline personality disorder.* Washington, DC: American Psychiatric Publishing.

Gunderson, J. G., & Lyons-Ruth, K. (2008). BPD's interpersonal hypersensitivity phenotype: a gene-environment-developmental model. *J Pers Disord, 22*, 22–41.

Gunderson, J. G., Stout, R. L., McGlashan, T. H., Shea, M. T., Morey, L. C., Grilo, C. M., Zanarini, M. C., Yen, S., Markowitz, J. C., Sanislow, C., Ansell, E., Pinto, A., & Skodol, A. E. (2011a). Ten-year course of borderline personality disorder: psychopathology and function from the collaborative longitudinal personality disorders study. *Arch Gen Psychiatry, 68*, 827–837.

Gunderson, J. G., Zanarini, M. C., Choi-Kain, L. W., Mitchell, K. S., Jang, K. L., & Hudson, J. I. (2011b). Family study of borderline personality disorder and its sectors of psychopathology. *Arch Gen Psychiatry, 68,* 753–762.

Gusnard, D. A., & Raichle, M. E. (2001). Searching for a baseline: functional imaging and the resting human brain. *Nat Rev Neurosci, 2,* 685–694.

Harari, H., Shamay-Tsoory, S. G., Ravid, M., & Levkovitz, Y. (2010). Double dissociation between cognitive and affective empathy in borderline personality disorder. *Psychiatry Res, 175,* 277–279.

Harrington, A. (2012). The fall of the schizophrenogenic mother. *Lancet, 379,* 1292–1293.

Harrison, A. A., Everitt, B. J., & Robbins, T. W. (1997). Central 5-HT depletion enhances impulsive responding without affecting the accuracy of attentional performance: interactions with dopaminergic mechanisms. *Psychopharmacology (Berl), 133,* 329–342.

Hazlett, E. A., New, A. S., Newmark, R., Haznedar, M. M., Lo, J. N., Speiser, L. J., Chen, A. D., Mitropoulou, V., Minzenberg, M., Siever, L. J., & Buchsbaum, M. S. (2005). Reduced anterior and posterior cingulate gray matter in borderline personality disorder. *Biol Psychiatry, 58,* 614–623.

Herbort, M. C., Soch, J., Wüstenberg, T., Krauel, K., Pujara, M., Koenigs, M., Gallinat, J., Walter, H., Roepke, S., & Schott, B. H. (2016). A negative relationship between ventral striatal loss anticipation response and impulsivity in borderline personality disorder. *Neuroimage Clin. 12,* 724–736.

Herpertz, S. C., Dietrich, T. M., Wenning, B., Krings, T., Erberich, S. G., Willmes, K., Thron, A., & Sass, H. (2001). Evidence of abnormal amygdala functioning in borderline personality disorder: a functional MRI study. *Biol Psychiatry, 50,* 292–298.

Hoerst, M., Weber-Fahr, W., Tunc-Sharka, N., Ruf, M., Bohus, M., Schmahl, C., & Ende, G. (2010a). Correlation of glutamate levels in the anterior cingulate cortex with self-reported impulsivity in patients with borderline personality disorder. *Arch Gen Psychiatry, 67,* 946–954.

Hoerst, M., Weber-Fahr, W., Tunc-Skarka, N., Ruf, M., Bohus, M., Schmahl, C., & Ende, G. (2010b). Metabolic alterations in the amygdala in borderline personality disorder: A proton magnetic resonance spectroscopy study. *Biol Psychiatry, 67,* 399–405.

Irle, E., Lange, C., & Sachsse, U. (2005). Reduced size and abnormal asymmetry of parietal cortex in women with borderline personality disorder. *Biol Psychiatry, 57,* 173–182.

Jeung, H., & Herpertz, S. C. (2014). Impairments of interpersonal functioning: empathy and intimacy in borderline personality disorder. *Psychopathology, 47,* 220–234.

Jorgensen, C. R. (2010). Invited essay: identity and borderline personality disorder. *J Pers Disord, 24,* 344–364.

Joyce, P. R., McHugh, P. C., Light, K. J., Rowe, S., Miller, A. L., & Kennedy, M. A. (2009). Relationships between angry-impulsive personality traits and genetic polymorphisms of the dopamine transporter. *Biol Psychiatry, 66,* 717–721.

Joyce, P. R., Stephenson, J., Kennedy, M., Mulder, R. T., & McHugh, P. C. (2014). The presence of both serotonin 1A receptor (*HTR1A*) and dopamine transporter (*DAT1*) gene variants increase the risk of borderline personality disorder. *Front Genet, 4,* 313.

Kamphausen, S., Schroder, P., Maier, S., Bader, K., Feige, B., Kaller, C. P., Glauche, V., Ohlendorf, S., Tebartz van Elst, L., Kloppel, S., Jacob, G. A., Silbersweig, D., Lieb, K., & Tuscher, O. (2013). Medial prefrontal dysfunction and prolonged amygdala response during instructed fear processing in borderline personality disorder. *World J Biol Psychiatry, 14,* 307–318.

Kendler, K. S., Aggen, S. H., Czajkowski, N., Roysamb, E., Tambs, K., Torgersen, S., Neale, M. C., & Reichborn-Kjennerud, T. (2008). The structure of genetic and environmental risk factors for DSM-IV personality disorders: a multivariate twin study. *Arch Gen Psychiatry, 65,* 1438–1446.

Kendler, K. S., & Eaves, L. J. (1986). Models for the joint effect of genotype and environment on liability to psychiatric illness. *Am J Psychiatry, 143,* 279–289.

Kendler, K. S., Myers, J., & Reichborn-Kjennerud, T. (2011). Borderline personality disorder traits and their relationship with dimensions of normative personality: a web-based cohort and twin study. *Acta Psychiatr Scand, 123,* 349–359.

Kennedy, S. E., Koeppe, R. A., Young, E. A., & Zubieta, J. K. (2006). Dysregulation of endogenous opioid emotion regulation circuitry in major depression in women. *Arch Gen Psychiatry, 63,* 1199–1208.

Kernberg, O. F. (1967). Borderline personality organization. *J Am Psychoanal Assoc, 15*(3), 641–685.

Kleindienst, N., Limberger, M. F., Ebner-Priemer, U. W., Keibel-Mauchnik, J., Dyer, A., Berger, M., Schmahl, C., & Bohus, M. (2011). Dissociation predicts poor response to dialectical behavior therapy in female patients with borderline personality disorder. *J Pers Disord, 25,* 432–447.

Knight, R. P. (1953). Borderline states. *Bull Menninger Clin, 17*(1), 1–12.

Koenigs, M., & Tranel, D. (2007). Irrational economic decision-making after ventromedial prefrontal damage: evidence from the ultimatum game. *J Neurosci, 27,* 951–956.

Koenigsberg, H. W., Fan, J., Ochsner, K. N., Liu, X., Guise, K. G., Pizzarello, S., Dorantes, C., Guerreri, S., Tecuta, L., Goodman, M., New, A., & Siever, L. J. (2009). Neural correlates of the use of psychological distancing to regulate responses to negative social cues: a study of patients with borderline personality disorder. *Biol Psychiatry, 66,* 854–863.

Korzekwa, M. I., Dell, P. F., Links, P. F., Thabane, L., & Fougere, P. (2009a). Dissociation in borderline personality disorder: a detailed look. *J Trauma Dissociation, 10,* 346–367.

Korzekwa, M. I., Dell, P. F., & Pain, C. (2009b). Dissociation and borderline personality disorder: an update for clinicians. *Curr Psychiatry Rep, 11,* 82–88.

Krause-Utz, A., Bohus, M., Schmahl, C., Elzinga, B. M., Spinhoven, P., Elzinga, B. M., Oei, N. Y. L., Oei, N. Y. L., & Spinhoven, P. (2014). Susceptibility to distraction by social cues in borderline personality disorder. *Psychopathology, 47,* 148–157.

Krause-Utz, A., Oei, N. Y., Niedtfeld, I., Bohus, M., Spinhoven, P., Schmahl, C., & Elzinga, B. M. (2012). Influence of emotional distraction on working memory performance in borderline personality disorder. *Psychol Med, 42,* 2181–2192.

Krause-Utz, A., Sobanski, E., Alm, B., Valerius, G., Kleindienst, N., & Schmahl, C. (2013). Impulsivity in relation to stress in patients with borderline personality disorder with and without co-occurring attention deficit hyperactivity disorder: an exploratory study. *J Nerv Mental Dis, 201,* 116–123.

Krause-Utz, A., Winter, D., Niedtfeld, I., & Schmahl, C. (2014). The latest neuroimaging findings in borderline personality disorder. *Curr Psychiatry Rep, 16,* 438.

Krause-Utz, A., Winter, D., Schriner, F., Chiu, C. D., Lis, S., Spinhoven, P., Bohus, M., Schmahl, C., & Elzinga, B. M. (2018). Reduced amygdala reactivity and impaired working memory during dissociation in borderline personality disorder. *Eur Arch Psychiatry Clin Neurosci, 268,* 401–415.

Lang, S., Kotchoubey, B., Frick, C., Spitzer, C., Grabe, H. J., & Barnow, S. (2012). Cognitive reappraisal in trauma-exposed women with borderline personality disorder. *Neuroimage, 59,* 1727–1734.

Lange, C., Kracht, L., & Herholz, K. (2005). Reduced glucose metabolism in temporo-parietal cortices of women with borderline personality disorder. *Psychiatry Res, 139,* 115–126.

Lazarus, S. A., Cheavens, J. S., Festa, F., & Zachary Rosenthal, M. (2014). Interpersonal functioning in borderline personality disorder: a systematic review of behavioral and laboratory-based assessments. *Clin Psychol Rev, 34,* 193–205.

Leinsinger, G., Born, C., Reiser, M., Moller, H. J., & Meisenzahl, E. M. (2006). Amygdala volume and depressive symptoms in patients with borderline personality disorder. *Biol Psychiatry, 60,* 302–310.

Lieb, K., Völlm, B., Rücker, G., Timmer, A., & Stoffers, J. M. (2010). Pharmacotherapy for borderline personality disorder: Cochrane systematic review of randomised trials. *Br J Psychiatry, 196,* 4–12.

Lieb, K., Zanarini, M. C., Schmahl, C., Linehan, M. M., & Bohus, M. (2004). Borderline personality disorder. *Lancet, 364,* 453–461.

Links, P., & Heslegrave, R. (2000). Prospective studies of outcome: understanding mechanisms of change in patients with borderline personality disorder. *Psychiatr Clin North Am, 23,* 137–150.

Linehan, M. M. (1993). *Cognitive behavioral treatment of borderline personality disorder.* New York, NY: Guilford Press.

Lis, S., & Bohus, M. (2013). Social interaction in borderline personality disorder. *Curr Psychiatry Rep, 15,* 338.

Livesley, W. J., Dimaggio, G.,& Clarkin, J. F. (Eds.) (2016). *Integrated treatment for personality disorder: a modular approach.* New York: Guilford Press

Livesley, W. J. (2016). *The integrated treatment of personality disorders.* New York: Guilford Press.

Long, E. C., Aggen, S. H., Neale, M. C., Knudsen, G. P., Krueger. R. F., South, S. C., Czajkowski, N., Nesvåg, R., Ystrom, E., Torvik, F. A., Kendler, K. S., Gillespie, N. A., & Reichborn-Kjennerud, T. (2017). The association between personality disorders with alcohol use and misuse: a population-based twin study. *Drug Alcohol Depend, 174,* 171–180.

Lubke, G. H., Laurin, C., Amin, N., Hottenga, J. J., Willemsen, G., van Grootheest, G., Abdellaoui, A., Karssen, L. C., Oostra, B. A., van Duijn, C. M., Penninx, B. W., & Boomsma, D. I. (2013). Genome-wide analyses of borderline personality features. *Mol Psychiatry, 19,* 1–7.

Maier-Hein, K. H., Brunner, R., Lutz, K., Henze, R., Parzer, P., Feigl, N., Kramer, J., Meinzer, H., Resch, F., & Stieltjes, B. (2014). Disorder-specific white matter alterations in adolescent borderline personality disorder. *Biol Psychiatry, 75,* 81–88.

Mauchnik, J., & Schmahl, C. (2010). The latest neuroimaging findings in borderline personality disorder. *Curr Psychiatry Rep, 16*(3), 46–55.

McCarthy, H., Skokauskas, N., Mulligan, A., Donohoe, G., Mullins, D., Kelly, J., Johnson, K., Fagan, A., Gill, M., Meaney, J., & Frodl, T. (2013). Attention network hypoconnectivity with default and affective network hyperconnectivity in adults diagnosed with attention-deficit/hyperactivity disorder in childhood. *JAMA Psychiatry, 70,* 1329–1337.

Meltzer, H. Y. (1989). Clinical studies in the mechanism of action of clozapine: the dopamine serotonin hypothesis of schizophrenia. *Psychopharmacology Suppl, 99,* 518–527.

Menon, V., & Uddin, L. Q. (2010). Saliency, switching, attention and control: a network model of insula function. *Brain Struct Funct, 214,* 655–667.

Meyer-Lindenberg, A., Domes, G., Kirsch, P., & Heinrichs, M. (2011). Oxytocin and vasopressin in the human brain: social neuropeptides for translational medicine. *Nat Rev Neurosci, 12,* 524–538.

Minzenberg, M. J., Fan, J., New, A. S., Tang, C. Y., & Siever, L. J. (2007). Fronto-limbic dysfunction in response to facial emotion in borderline personality disorder: an event-related fMRI study. *Psychiatry Res, 155*, 231–243.

Minzenberg, M. J., Fan, J., New, A. S., Tang, C. Y., & Siever, L. J. (2008). Frontolimbic structural changes in borderline personality disorder. *J Psychiatr Res, 42*, 727–733.

National Collaborating Centre for Mental Health. (2009). *Borderline personality disorder: the NICE guideline on treatment and management.* National Clinical Practice Guideline No. 78. National Institute for Health & Clinical Excellence. Leicester, UK: British Psychological Society & Royal College of Psychiatrists.

Nemoda, Z., Lyons-Ruth, K., Szekely, A., Bertha, E., Faludi, G., & Sasvari-Szekely, M. (2010). Association between dopaminergic polymorphisms and borderline traits among at-risk young adults and psychiatric inpatients. *Behav Brain Funct, 6*, 4. doi: 10.1186/1744-9081-6-4.

New, A. S., Carpenter, D. M., Perez-Rodriguez, M. M., Ripoll, L. H., Avedon, J., Patil, U., Hazlett, E. A., & Goodman, M. (2013). Developmental differences in diffusion tensor imaging parameters in borderline personality disorder. *J Psychiatr Res, 47*, 1101–1109.

New, A. S., Hazlett, E. A., Buchsbaum, M. S., Goodman, M., Mitelman, S. A., Newmark, R., Trisdorfer, R., Haznedar, M. M., Koenigsberg, H. W., Flory, J., & Siever, L. J. (2007). Amygdala-prefrontal disconnection in borderline personality disorder. *Neuropsychopharmacology, 32*, 1629–1640.

New, A. S., Hazlett, E. A., Buchsbaum, M. S., Goodman, M., Reynolds, D., Mitropoulou, V., Sprung, L., Shaw R. B. Jr., Koenigsberg, H., Platholi, J., Silverman, J., & Siever, L. J. (2002). Blunted prefrontal cortical 18fluorodeoxyglucose positron emission tomography response to meta-chloropiperazine in impulsive aggression. *Arch Gen Psychiatry, 59*, 621–629.

Niedtfeld, I., Kirsch, P., Schulze, L., Herpertz, S. C., Bohus, M., & Schmahl, C. (2012). Functional connectivity of pain-mediated affect regulation in borderline personality disorder. *PLoS ONE, 7*(3), e33293.

Niedtfeld, I., Schulze, L., Kirsch, P., Herpertz, S. C., Bohus, M., & Schmahl, C. (2010). Affect regulation and pain in borderline personality disorder: a possible link to the understanding of self-injury. *Biol Psychiatry, 68*, 383–391.

Niedtfeld, I., Winter, D., Schmitt, R., Bohus, M., Schmahl, C., & Herpertz, S. C. (2017). Pain-mediated affect regulation is reduced after dialectical behavior therapy in borderline personality disorder: a longitudinal fMRI study. *SCAN, 12*(5), 739–747.

Nielen, M. M., Heslenfeld, D. J., Heinen, K., Van Strien, J. W., Witter, M. P., Jonker, C., & Veltman, D. J. (2009). Distinct brain systems underlie the processing of valence and arousal of affective pictures. *Brain Cognition, 71*, 387–396.

Ni, X. Q., Chan, D., Chan, K., McMain, S., & Kennedy, J. L. (2009). Serotonin genes and gene-gene interactions in borderline personality disorder in a matched case-control study. *Prog Neuropsychopharm Biol Psychiatry, 33*, 128–133.

Nunes, P. M., Wenzel, A., Borges, K. T., Porto, C. R., Caminha, R. M., & de Oliveira, I. R. (2009). Volumes of the hippocampus and amygdala in patients with borderline personality disorder: a meta-analysis. *J Pers Disord, 23*, 333–345.

Ochsner, K. N., Bunge, S. A., Gross, J. J., & Gabrieli, J. D. (2002). Rethinking feelings: an FMRI study of the cognitive regulation of emotion. *J Cogn Neurosci, 14*(8), 1215–1229.

Ochsner, K. N., & Gross, J. J. (2014). The neural bases of emotion and emotion regulation: a valuation perspective. In J. J. Gross (Ed.), *Handbook of emotion regulation* (2nd ed., pp. 23–42). New York: Guilford Press.

Ochsner, K. N., Gross, J. J. (2014). The neural bases of emotion and emotion regulation: a valuation perspective. In J. J. Gross, *Handbook of emotion regulation* (pp. 23–42). New York: Guilford Press.

Oldham, J. M., Skodol, A. E., & Bender, D. S. (2014). *Textbook of personality disorders*, 2nd ed. Washington, DC: American Psychiatric Publishing.

O'Neill, A., & Frodl, T. (2012). Brain structure and function in borderline personality disorder. *Brain Struct Funct, 217*, 767–782.

Panksepp, J., Herman, B. H., Vilberg, T., Bishop, P., & DeEskinazi, F. G. (1980). Endogenous opioids and social behavior. *Neurosci Biobehav Rev, 4*, 473–487.

Paret, C., Kluetsch, R., Zaehringer, J., Ruf, M., Demirakca, T., Bohus, M., Ende, G., & Schmahl, C. (2016). Alterations of amygdala-prefrontal connectivity with real-time fMRI neurofeedback in BPD patients. *Soc Cogn Affect Neurosci, 11*, 952–960.

Perez-Rodriguez, M. M., Hazlett, E. A., Rich, E. L., Ripoll, L. H., Weiner, D. M., Spence, N., Goodman, M., Koenigsberg, H. W., Siever, L. J., & New, A. (2012). Striatal activity in borderline personality disorder with comorbid intermittent explosive disorder: sex differences. *J Psychiatr Res, 46*, 797–804.

Perroud, N., Paoloni-Giacobino, A., Prada, P., Olie, E., Salzmann, A., Nicastro, R., Guillaume, S., Mouthon, D., Stouder, C., Dieben, K., Huguelet, P., Courtet, P., & Malfosse, A. (2011). Increased methylation of glucocorticoid receptor gene (NR3C1) in adults with a history of childhood maltreatment: a link with the severity and type of trauma. *Transl Psychiatry, 1*, e59. doi: 10.1038/tp.2011.60.

Perroud, N., Salzmann, A., Prada, P., Nicastro, R., Hoeppli, M., Furrer, S., Ardu, S., Krejci, I., Karege, F., & Malafosse, A. (2013). Response to psychotherapy in borderline personality disorder and methylation status of the BDNF gene. *Transl Psychiatry, 3*, e207.

Perroud, N., Zewdie, S., Stenz, L., Adouan, W., Bavamian, S., Prada, P., Nicastro, R., Hasler, R., Nallet, A., Piguet, C., Paoloni-Giacobino, A., Aubry, J. M., & Dayer A. (2016). Methylation of serotonin receptor 3A in ADHD, borderline personality, and bipolar disorders: link with severity of the disorders and childhood maltreatment. *Depress Anxiety, 33*, 45–55.

Pieper, S., Out, D., Bakermans-Kranenburg, M. J., & van IJzendoom, M. H. (2011). Behavioral molecular genetics of dissociation: the role of the serotonin transporter gene promoter polymorphism (5HTTLPR). *J Trauma Stress, 24*, 373–380.

Prados, J., Stenz, L., Courtet, P., Prada, P., Nicastro, R., Adouan, W., Guillaume, S., Olié, E., Aubry, J. M., Dayer, A., & Perroud, N. (2015). Borderline personality disorder and childhood maltreatment: a genome-wide methylation analysis. *Genes Brain Behav, 14*, 177–180.

Prossin, A. R., Love, T. M., Koeppe, R. A., Zubieta, J. K., & Silk, K. R. (2010). Dysregulation of regional endogenous opioid function in borderline personality disorder. *Am J Psychiatry, 167*, 925–933.

Reichborn-Kjennerud, T., Czajkowski, N., Roysamb, E., Ørstavik, R. E., Neale, M. C., Torgersen, S., & Kendler, K. S. (2010). Major depression and dimensional representations of DSM-IV personality disorders: a population-based twin study. *Psychol Medicine, 40*, 1475–1484.

Reichborn-Kjennerud, T., Ystrom, E., Neale, M. C., et al. (2013). Structure of genetic and environmental risk factors for symptoms of DSM-IV borderline personality disorder. *JAMA Psychiatry, 70*, 1206–1214.

Reitz, S., Kluetsch, R., Niedtfeld, I., Knorz, T., Lis, S., Paret, C., Kirsch, P., Meyer-Lindenberg, A., Treede, R.-D., Baumgaertner, U., Bohus, M., & Schmahl, C. (2015). Incision and stress regulation in borderline personality disorder: neurobiological mechanisms of self- injurious behavior. *Br J Psychiatry, 207*, 165–172.

Reitz, S., Krause-Utz, A., Pogatzki-Zahn, E. M., Ebner-Priemer, U., Bohus, M., & Schmahl, C. (2012). Stress regulation and incision in borderline personality disorder—a pilot study modeling cutting behavior. *J Pers Disord, 26*, 605–615.

Ruocco, A. C., Amirthavasagam, S., Choi-Kain, L. W., & McMain, S. F. (2013). Neural correlates of negative emotionality in borderline personality disorder: an activation-likelihood-estimation meta-analysis. *Biol Psychiatry, 73*, 153–160.

Ruocco, A. C., Amirthavasagam, S., & Zakzanis, K. K. (2012). Amygdala and hippocampal volume reductions as candidate endophenotypes for borderline personality disorder: a meta-analysis of magnetic resonance imaging studies. *Psychiatry Res, 201*, 245–252.

Ruocco, A. C., & Carcone, D. (2016). A neurobiological model of borderline personality disorder: systematic and integrative review. *Harv Rev Psychiatry, 24*, 31–329.

Rusch, N., Bracht, T., Kreher, B. W., Schnell. S., Glauche, V., Il'yasov, K. A., Ebert, D., Lieb, K., Hennig, J., Saur, D., & van Elst, L. T. (2010). Reduced interhemispheric structural connectivity between anterior cingulate cortices in borderline personality disorder. *Psychiatry Res, 181*, 151–184.

Rüsch, N., van Elst, L. T., Ludaescher, P., Wilke, M., Huppertz, J. J., Thiel, T., Schmahl, C., Bohus, M., Lieb, K., Hesslinger, B., Henning, J., & Ebert, D. (2003). A voxel-based morphometric MRI study in female patients with borderline personality disorder. *NeuroImage, 20*, 385–392.

Sadikaj, G., Moskowitz, D. S., Russell, J. J., Zuroff, D. C., & Paris, J. (2013). Quarrelsome behavior in borderline personality disorder: influence of behavioral and affective reactivity to perceptions of others. *J Abnorm Psychol, 122*, 195–207.

Sansone, R. A., & Sansone, L. A. (2011). Personality disorders: a nation-based perspective on prevalence. *Innov Clin Neurosci, 8*(4), 13–18.

Saunders, E. F., & Silk, K. R. (2009). Personality trait dimensions and the pharmacological treatment of borderline personality disorder. *J Clin Psychopharmacol, 29*(5), 461–467.

Scherpiet, S., Bruhl, A. B., Opialla, S., Roth, L., Jancke, L., & Herwig, U. (2013). Altered emotion processing circuits during the anticipation of emotional stimuli in women with borderline personality disorder. *Eur Arch Psychiatry Clin Neurosci, 264*, 45–60.

Schmahl, C., Arvastson, L., Tamm, J. A., Bohus, M., Abdourahman, A., & Antonijevic, I. (2013). Gene expression profiles in relation to tension and dissociation in borderline personality disorder. *PLoS ONE, 8*(8), e70787.

Schmahl, C., Berne, K. Krause, A., Kleindienst, N., Valerius, G., Vermetten, E., & Bohus, M. (2009). Hippocampus and amygdala volumes in patients with borderline personality disorder with or without posttraumatic stress disorder. *J Psychiatry Neurosci, 34*, 289–295.

Schmahl, C. G., Vermetten, E., Elzinga, B. M., & Douglas Bremner, J. (2003). Magnetic resonance imaging of hippocampal and amygdala volume in women with childhood abuse and borderline personality disorder. *Psychiatry Res, 122*, 193–198.

Schmitt, R., Winter, D., Niedtfeld, I., Herpertz, S., & Schmahl, C. (2016). Effects of psychotherapy on neuronal correlates of reappraisal in female patients with borderline personality disorder. *Biol Psychiatry Cogn Neurosci Neuroimag, 1*, 548–557.

Schnell, K., & Herpertz, S. C. (2007). Effects of dialectic-behavioral-therapy on the neural correlates of affective hyperarousal in borderline personality disorder. *J Psychiatr Res, 41*, 837–847.

Schulz, S. C., & Nelson, K. J. (2014). Somatic treatments. In J. M. Oldham, A. E. Skodol, D. S. Bender (Eds.), *Textbook of personality disorders* (2nd ed., p. 334). Washington, DC: American Psychiatric Publishing.

Schulze, L., Domes, G., Kruger, A., Berger, C., Fleischer, M., Prehn, K., Schmahl, C., Grossmann, A., Hauenstein, K., & Herpertz, S. C. (2011). Neuronal correlates of cognitive reappraisal in borderline patients with affective instability. *Biol Psychiatry, 69*, 564–573.

Schulze, L., Schmahl, C., & Niedtfeld, I. (2016). Neural correlates of disturbed emotion processing in borderline personality disorder: a multimodal meta-analysis. *Biol Psychiatry, 79*, 97–106

Seeman, P. (2002). Atypical antipsychotics: mechanism of action. *Can J Psychiatry, 47*, 27–38.

Seeman, P. (2013). Schizophrenia and dopamine receptors. *Eur Neuropsychopharmacol, 23*, 999–1009.

Silk, K. R., & Friedel, R. O. (2016). Psychopharmacological and neurobiological considerations in the integrated treatment of borderline personality disorder. In W. J. Livesley, G. Dimaggio, & J. F. Clarkin (Eds.), *The integrated treatment of personality disorders*. New York: Guilford Press.

Simeon, D., Bartz, J., Hamilton, H., Crystal, S., Braun, A., Ketay, S., & Hollander, E. (2011). Oxytocin administration attenuates stress reactivity in borderline personality disorder: a pilot study. *Psychoneuroendocrinology, 36*, 1418–1421.

Skodol, A. E., Grilo, C. M., Pagano, M. E., Bender, D. S., Gunderson, J. G., Shea, M. T, Yen, S., Zanarini, M. C., & McGlashan, T. H. (2005). Effects of personality disorders on functioning and well-being in major depressive disorder. *J Psychiatr Pract, 11*, 363–368.

Skodol, A. E., Gunderson, J. G., McGlashan, Dyck, I. R., Stout, R. L. Bender, D. S., Grilo, C. M., Shea, M. T., Zanarini, M. C., Morey, L. C., Sanislow, C. A., & Oldham, J. M. (2002). Functional impairment in patients with schizotypal, borderline, avoidant, or obsessive-compulsive personality disorder. *Am J Psychiatry, 159*(2), 278–283.

Soloff, P. H., George, A., Nathan, S., Schulz, P. M., Ulrich, R. F., & Perel, J. M. (1986). Progress in pharmacotherapy of borderline disorders: a double-blind study of amitriptyline, haloperidol, and placebo. *Arch Gen Psychiatry, 43*, 691–697.

Soloff, P., Nutche, J., Goradia, D., & Diwadkar, V. (2008). Structural brain abnormalities in borderline personality disorder: a voxel-based morphometry study. *Psychiatry Res, 164*, 223–236.

Soloff, P. H., Pruitt, P., Sharma, M., Radwan, J., White, R., & Diwadkar, V. A. (2012). Structural brain abnormalities and suicidal behavior in borderline personality disorder. *J Psychiatr Res, 46*, 516–525.

Spitzer, C., Barnow, S., Freyberger, H. J., & Grabe, H. J. (2007). Dissociation predicts symptom-related treatment outcome in short-term inpatient psychotherapy. *Aust N Z J Psychiatry, 41*, 682–687.

Stein, D. J., Hollander, E., DeCaria, C. M., Simeon, D., Cohen, L., & Aronowitz, B. (1996). m-Chlorophenylpiperazine challenge and borderline personality disorder: Relationship of neuroendocrine response, behavioral response, and clinical measures. *Biol Psychiatry, 15*, 508–513.

Stern, A. (1938) Psychoanalytic investigation of and therapy in the borderline group of neuroses. *Psychoanal Quarterly, 7*, 467–489.

Stiglmayr, C. E., Grathwol, T., Linehan, M. M., Ihorst, G., Fahrenberg, J., & Bohus, M. (2005). Aversive tension in patients with borderline personality disorder: a computer-based controlled field study. *Acta Psychiatr Scand, 111*, 372–379.

Stimpson, C. D., Tetreault, N. A., Allman, J. M., Jacobs, B., Butti, C., Hof, P. R., & Sherwood, C. C. (2011). Biochemical specificity of von Economo neurons in hominoids. *Am J Hum Biol, 23*, 22–28.

Stoffers, J. M., Völlm, B. A., Rücker, G., Timmer, A., Huband, N., & Lieb, K. (2012). Psychological therapies for people with borderline personality disorder. *Cochrane Database Syst Rev, 8.*

Stoffers, J., Völlm, B. A., Rücker, G., Timmer, A., & Lieb, K. (2010). Pharmacological interventions for borderline personality disorder. *Cochrane Database Syst Rev, 6.*

Svenningsson, P., Tzavara, E. T., Witkin, J. M., Fienberg, A. A., Nomikos, G. G., & Greengard, P. (2002b). Involvement of striatal and extrastriatal DARPP-32 in biochemical and behavioral effects of fluoxetine (Prozac). *Proc Natl Acad Sci U S A, 99,* 3182–3187.

Svenningsson, P., Tzavara, E. T., Witkin, J. M., Liu, F., Nomikos, G. G., & Greengard, P. (2002a). DARPP-32 mediates serotonergic neurotransmission in the forebrain. *Proc Natl Acad Sci U S A, 99,* 3188–3193.

Tadic, A., Victor, A., Baskaya, O., von Cube, R., Hoch, J., Kouti, I., Anicker, N. J., Hoppner, W., Lieb, K., & Dahmen, N. (2009). Interaction between gene variants of the serotonin transporter promoter region (5-HTTLPR) and catechol O-methyltransferase (COMT) in borderline personality disorder. *Am J Med Genet B Neuropsychiatr Genet, 150B,* 487–495.

Teschler, S., Bartkuhn, M., Kunzel, N., Schmidt, C., Kiehl, S., Dammann, G., & Dammann, R. (2013). Aberrant methylation of gene associated CpG sites occurs in borderline personality disorder. *PLoS ONE, 8*(12), e84180.

Thompson, R. R., & Walton, J. C. (2004). Peptide effects on social behavior: effects of vasotocin and isotocin on social approach behavior in male goldfish (Carassius auratus). *Behav Neurosci, 118,* 620–626.

Tomko, R. L., Trull, T. J., Wood, P. K., & Sher, K. J. (2013). Characteristics of borderline personality disorder in a community sample: comorbidity, treatment utilization, and general functioning. *J Pers Disord, 28,* 734–750.

Torgersen, S., Czajkowski, N., Jacobson, K., Reichborn-Kjennerud, T., Roysamb, E., Neale, M. C., & Kendler, K. S. (2008). Dimensional representations of DSM-IV cluster B personality disorders in a population-based sample of Norwegian twins: a multivariate study. *Psychol Med, 38,* 1617–1625.

Torgersen, S. M., Myers, J., Reichborn-Kjennerud, T., Roysamb, E., Kubarych, T. S., & Kendler, K. S. (2012). The heritability of cluster B personality disorders assessed both by personal interview and questionnaire. *J Personal Disord, 26*(6), 848–866.

Ungar, M., Ghazinour, M., & Richter, J. (2013). Annual research review: What is resilience within the social ecology of human development? *J Child Psychol Psychiatry, 54,* 348–366.

van Elst, T. L., Hesslinger, B., Thiel, T., Geiger, E., Haegele, K., Lemieux, L., Lieb, K., Bohus, M., Hennig, J., & Ebert, D. (2003). Frontolimbic brain abnormalities in patients with borderline personality disorder: a volumetric magnetic resonance imaging study. *Biol Psychiatry, 54,* 163–171.

van Elst, L. T., Thiel, T., Hesslinger, B., Lieb, K., Bohus, M., Hennig, J., & Ebert, D. (2001). Subtle prefrontal neuropathology in a pilot magnetic resonance spectroscopy study in patients with borderline personality disorder. *J Neuropsychiatry Clin Neurosci, 13,* 511–514.

van Erp, A. M., & Miczek, K. A. (2000). Aggressive behavior, increased accumbal dopamine, and decreased cortical serotonin in rats. *J Neurosci, 20,* 9320–9325.

Vermetten, E., & Spiegel, D. (2014). Trauma and dissociation: implications for borderline personality disorder. *Curr Psychiatry Rep, 16,* 434–438.

Visintin, E., De Panfilis, C., Amore, M., Balestrieri, M., Wolf, R. C., & Sambataro, F. (2016). Mapping the brain correlates of borderline personality disorder: a functional neuroimaging meta-analysis of resting state studies. *J Affect Disord, 204*, 262–269.

Vogel, F., Wagner, S., Başkaya, O., Leuenberger, B., Mobascher, A., Dahmen, N., Lieb, K, & Tadić, A. (2012). Variable number of tandem repeat polymorphisms of the arginine vasopressin receptor 1A gene and impulsive aggression in patients with borderline personality disorder. *Psychiatr Genet, 22*, 105–106.

Wang, G. Y., van Eljk, J., Demirakca, T., Sack, M., Krause-Utz, A., Cackowski, S., Schmahl, C., & Ende, G. (2016). ACC GABA levels are associated with functional activation and connectivity in the fronto-striatal network during interference inhibition in patients with borderline personality disorder. *NeuroImage, 147*, 164–174.

Whiteside, S. P., & Lynam, D. R. (2001). The five factor model and impulsivity: using a structural model of personality to understand impulsivity. *Personal Individual Diff, 30*, 669–689.

Wilson, S. T., Stanley, B., Brent, D. A., Oguendo, M. A., Huang, Y. Y., Haghighi, F., Hodgkinson, C. A., & Mann, J. J. (2012). Interaction between tryptophan hydroxylase I polymorphisms and childhood abuse is associated with increased risk for borderline personality disorder in adulthood. *Psychiatric Genetics, 22*(1), 15–24.

Wingenfeld, K., Spitzer, C., Rullkotter, N., & Lowe, B. (2010). Borderline personality disorder: hypothalamus pituitary adrenal axis and findings from neuroimaging studies. *Psychoneuroendocrinology, 35*(1), 154–170.

Winsper, C., Marwaha, S., Lereya, S. T., Thompson, A., Eyden, J., & Singh, S. P. (2016). A systematic review of the neurobiological underpinnings of borderline personality disorder (BPD) in childhood and adolescence. *Rev Neurosci, 27*, 827–847.

Zetzsche, T., Frodl, T., Preuss, U. W., Schmitt, G., Seifert, D., Leinsinger, G., Born, C., Reiser, M., Moller, H.J., & Meisenzahl, E. M. (2006). Amygdala volume and depressive symptoms in patients with borderline personality disorder. *Biol Psychiatry, 60*(3), 302–310.

Zubieta, J. K., Smith, Y. R., Bueller, J. A., Xu, Y., Kilbourn, M. R., Jewett, D. M., Meyer, C. R., Koeppe, R. A., & Stohler, C. S. (2001). Regional mu opioid receptor regulation of sensory and affective dimensions of pain. *Science, 293*, 311–315.

14 The Neurobiology of Antisocial Personality Disorders Focusing on Psychopathy

■ MICHAEL BALIOUSIS, NAJAT KHALIFA, AND BIRGIT VÖLLM

■ INTRODUCTION

Antisocial personality disorder (AsPD) is one of the 10 types of personality disorder described in the *Diagnostic and Statistical Manual of Mental Disorders* (*DSM-5*; American Psychiatric Association [APA], 2013). It is characterized by a pervasive pattern of disregard for, or violation of, the rights of others. Specific symptoms of APD include a failure to conform to social norms; deceitfulness, as indicated, for example, by repeated lying, use of aliases, or conning; impulsivity or failure to plan ahead; irritability and aggression; reckless disregard for the safely of self or others; consistent irresponsibility, as indicated by repeated failure to sustain consistent work or honor financial obligations; and a lack of remorse for the negative consequences of one's actions. Of these, three criteria have to be fulfilled in order to make the diagnosis; in addition, *DSM-5* requires the individual to have fulfilled criteria for conduct disorder as a child. The International Classification of Diseases, Tenth Edition (2010), describes a similar condition, dissocial personality disorder, the criteria for which overlap considerably with those for APD. Both diagnoses have been criticized for being circular and overinclusive and for focusing on deviant behaviors rather than underlying personality traits (Gunn, 2000).

APD is a relatively common condition with prevalence estimates of about 2% to 3% in the general population (Coid, 2006; Moran, 1999) but much higher rates in treatment, in particular forensic psychiatric and prison settings. For example, Singleton (1998) reported prevalences of 63% in male remand prisoners, 49% in male sentenced prisoners, and 31% in female prisoners. Not surprisingly, given the reliance on antisocial *behavior* in the diagnostic criteria, APD is associated with offending but also a range of other adverse outcomes such as homelessness, unemployment, relationship difficulties, substance use, and premature death (Robins, 1991).

Psychopathy is a related condition though not part of any of the current diagnostic manuals. The term has been used since the 19th century though its meaning has undergone considerable changes throughout history. Initially, it was rather vaguely defined to indicate a condition resulting in changes in conduct in the absence of obvious mental illness or retardation. The concept has been operationalized through the development of the Psychopathy Checklist (PCL) and its revised version, PCL-R (Hare, 1980, 2003), which is now the main tool employed to measure psychopathy. The 20 symptoms of the PCL-R have been modeled to describe two higher order factors: Factor 1, comprising interpersonal/affective traits, and Factor 2, capturing socially deviant behavior, though three- and four-factor models have also been advocated (e.g., Cooke & Michie, 2001).

Psychological interventions have been the main treatment approaches for APD and psychopathy though pharmacological interventions have also been tried. The evidence base for both is disappointing (for a summary of two Cochrane reviews on APD, see Gibbon et al., 2011), though there is some evidence for the effectiveness of cognitive-behaviorally based group therapies in APD. Psychopathy has been found to be even more difficult to treat, and some have argued that the condition is not treatable or that treatment even results in worse rather than better outcomes (however, for a review challenging this position, see d'Silva et al., 2004; Brown et al., 2014).

For advances to be made in the treatment of disorders associated with antisocial behavior, it is crucial to understand the etiology of these disorders. It is well known that a range of psychosocial factors are associated with antisocial behavior (for an overview, see, e.g., Glenn et al., 2013). The search for a biological basis for antisocial behavior first gained popularity with the 19th- century Italian criminologist Cesare Lombroso, who claimed to have found characteristics in the skulls of criminals indicating an evolutionary atavism rendering the individual more likely to act in an antisocial way, though this theory lacks a scientific basis.

Clues for a biological basis in the causation of APD come from a range of different observations, including heritability of antisocial traits and observations from individuals with brain injuries resulting in impulsivity, irritability, and violent behavior. This chapter reviews the evidence base for a range of biological factors in APD and psychopathy in adults (there is a substantial evidence base for children and adolescents with antisocial behavior as well, though the inclusion of these studies is outside our scope), including genetic factors, neurophysiological and neuropsychological findings, structural and functional brain changes, and transmitter and hormone aberrations. In order to summarize the evidence, we have systematically reviewed others' reviews and meta-analyses in the field but also refer to individual studies of particular relevance. We focus more on psychopathy than on APD because it provides a more narrow and less controversial concept, at least in relation to its use in research.

■ GENETIC FACTORS

Genetic studies posit to examine the etiological influences of genes on antisocial behavior constructs using behavioral and molecular genetic approaches. Additionally, genetic studies elucidate the gene–environment interplay in relation to these constructs, for instance by estimating the proportion of variance in phenotypic expressions that is related to genetic vulnerability and examining the moderating effects of environmental factors on genetic predisposition (Patrick, 2008; Ferguson, 2010).

Behavioral Genetic Approaches

Behavioral (quantitative) genetic approaches encompass family, twin, and adoption studies. Findings from these studies reveal that estimates of heritability of genetic influences on antisocial behavior is in the range of 40% to 50% (Viding et al., 2008). In a meta-analysis of 12 twin and adoption studies published between 1975 and 1994, Mason and Frick (1994) reported medium to large effect sizes for genetic influences, with approximately 50% of the variance in phenotypic expressions of antisocial behavior attributable to genetic influences. In another meta-analysis of 51 twin and adoption studies, Rhee and Waldman (2002) reported that 41% of the variance in the risk of antisocial behavior was attributed to genetic influences, 16% to shared environmental influences, and 43% to nonshared environmental influences. A more recent meta-analytical study (Ferguson, 2010) reported that 56% of the variance in the risk of antisocial behavior can be attributed to genetic influences, 11% to shared nongenetic influences, and 31% to individual specific influences. Further, in a study of 542 families participating in the Minnesota Twin Family Study, Hicks et al. (2004) reported that the transmission of a general vulnerability to all the externalizing disorders (conduct disorder, the adult criteria for APD, alcohol dependence, and drug dependence) accounted for most familial resemblance. This general vulnerability was highly heritable ($h^2 = 0.80$).

Genetics and Antisocial Personality Disorder

Studies conducted to date provide consistent evidence of a genetic contribution to APD (McGuffen & Thapar, 1992; Dahl, 1993). Family aggregation has been recorded for APD, with estimates of heritability in the range of 34% to 69% (Miles & Carey, 1997; Rhee & Waldman, 2002; Glatt et al., 2008; Mendoza & Casados, 2014). Higher prevalence rates for APD have been reported among adoptees with a family history of APD than for those without such history (Crowe, 1974; Cadoret, 1978). Cadoret and Stewart (1991) found that a combination of criminality in the biological parent and low socioeconomic status in the adoptive parent were strong predictors for antisocial personality and criminality. High prevalence rates of APD have also been reported among the biological and adoptive relatives of psychopathic probands (Schulsinger, 1982).

Twin studies reported higher concordance rates in monozygotic (MZ) than dizygotic (DZ) twins. For instance, McGuffin and Gottesman (1984) reported on the genetic influences on adult antisocial behavior in twins and found higher concordance rates in MZ (51%) than DZ (22%) twins. Further, a review of family, twin, and adoption studies of the third edition, revised edition of the *Diagnostic and Statistical Manual of Mental Disorders* (*DSM-III-R*)–defined APD reported that APD, alcoholism, and criminality run in families, with higher concordance in MZ than DZ twins (Dahl, 1993). Using cross-sectional and longitudinal data from 188 MZ and 101 DZ male twin pairs, Malone and colleagues (2006) found a moderate genetic influence on both symptoms of adult antisocial behavior and alcohol dependence at ages 17, 20, and 24, with a substantial proportion of this influence shared between the two disorders, suggesting that these disorders share susceptibility genes. In contrast, after controlling for alcoholism, Cadoret and colleagues (1985) found that antisocial behavior among biological parents predicted APD among adoptee probands, indicating that the estimate of heritability of APD does not necessarily reflect the heritability of alcoholism.

Genetics and Psychopathy

Twin studies of psychopathy and criminality indicate some influence for both genetic and nonshared environmental factors (Dolan, 1994; Waldman & Rhee, 2007; Taylor et al., 2003). In a study involving 353 male twins, Blonigen and colleagues (2003) found moderate heritability (h^2 = .29–.56) for the affect-based subscales of the Psychopathic Personality Inventory (Lilienfeld & Andrews, 1996). In another study involving 626 pairs of 17-year-old male and female twins, Blonigen and colleagues (2005) found significant heritability (h^2 = .46–.51) for two distinct psychopathic traits, namely fearless dominance and impulsive antisociality. Further, using data from over 1,000 MZ and DZ twins aged 16 to 17 years, Larsson et al. (2006) reported that large proportions of the variance (43%–56%) in the three psychopathic personality dimensions studied (grandiose/manipulative, callous/unemotional, and impulsive/irresponsible) were due to genetic factors. The remainder of the variance was due to nonshared environmental influences (e.g., different peer groups) among twin pairs, whereas shared environmental influences had a negligible influence.

The heritability of psychopathic traits in children and adolescents has been examined extensively in recent studies. For instance, in a study of 3,687 twin pairs from the Twins Early Development Study, Viding and colleagues (2005) used teachers' ratings of callous-unemotional traits, an analogue to psychopathy in children, and antisocial behavior to examine psychopathic tendencies in young children. They reported that (a) exhibiting high levels of callous-unemotional traits had strong genetic underpinnings; (b) antisocial behavior in children with high psychopathic tendencies was under extremely strong genetic influence, with no influence of shared environment; and (c) antisocial behavior in children with low psychopathic tendencies showed moderate genetic and shared environmental influences. Using a longitudinal twin study design involving 2,225 twins, Forsman and colleagues (2010) found that genetically influenced psychopathic personality was a robust predictor of adult antisocial behavior.

■ MOLECULAR GENETIC APPROACHES

Molecular genetic studies posit to examine the influences of genes on antisocial behavior through genotyping (identifying structural variation in the DNA), epigenetic (regulation of transcription), and gene expression (quantifying transcription) approaches. These approaches are either genome-wide or applied to specific (or candidate) genes (Gunter et al., 2010).

Genome-Wide Studies

While genome-wide linkage studies focus on alleles, genome-wide association studies focus on genes and haplotype blocks (Gunter et al., 2010). A review by Gunter et al. identified no genome-wide studies in which psychopathy and APD were the primary phenotypes under consideration. Nevertheless, the studies reviewed identified that areas worthy of consideration in future studies are within chromosomes 1, 2, 3, 9, 17, 19, and 20.

Candidate Gene Studies

Several candidate genes have shown a genetic contribution to antisocial behavior and the disorders of interest here, primarily those regulating the production of enzymes involving the production of amine neurotransmitters, such as monoamine oxidase A (MAOA) in maltreated children (Caspi et al., 2002), cataechole-O-methyltransferase (COMT) in children with attention deficit hyperactivity disorder (ADHD) who display aggressive behavior (Caspi et al., 2008), tryptophan hydroxylase (the rate-limiting enzyme in serotonin synthesis) in relation to aggression predisposition (Manuck et al., 1999), dopamine transporter in individuals with a history of adolescent-limited antisocial behavior (Burt & Mikolajewski, 2008), and the serotonin transporter (5HTT) in people with psychopathy (Glenn, 2011).

MAOA

Monoamine oxidase (MAO) isoenzymes A and B are neurotransmitter-metabolizing enzymes serving the catabolism of serotonin, norepinephrine, 2-phenylethylamine, other trace amines, and dopamine (Bortolato & Shih, 2011). The gene encoding their production is located on the X chromosome. A mutation of the MAOA gene was first implicated in antisocial behavior through observations by Brunner and colleagues (1993) following the identification of the defect in a large Dutch family whose male members were characterized by low IQ and impulsive aggression; the genetic disorder has since been named Brunner syndrome.

The MAOA gene also served as the focus of several genetic studies underscoring the role of interactions between genetic polymorphisms and negative childhood experiences in the development of antisocial behavior. In a landmark paper, using a large sample of males from the Dunedin Multidisciplinary Health and Development Study, Caspi and colleagues (2002) reported that a functional polymorphism in the gene encoding MAOA moderated the effect of childhood maltreatment on antisocial behavior, such that maltreated children with a genotype conferring high levels of MAOA expression were less likely to develop antisocial problems. This paper has since been cited over 4,400 times and prompted similar studies by other investigators, and the finding has been confirmed in an early meta-analysis of the original study and seven attempted replications (Taylor & Kim-Cohen, 2007).

More recent studies helped elucidate the role of MAOA activity further. For instance, using a sample of 538 participants from the Iowa Adoption Studies, Beach et al. (2010) found that high activity MAOA alleles predispose to symptoms of major depression in the context of child maltreatment, whereas low activity alleles predispose to symptoms of APD. Using data from 631 participants in a prospective cohort study involving court-substantiated cases of child abuse and neglect and a matched comparison group, Widom and Brzustowicz (2006) found that high levels of MAOA activity conferred protection to abused and neglected white participants from increased risk of becoming violent and/or antisocial in later life. This protective effect was not conferred to their non-white counterparts.

In a sample of 291 women (50% of whom experienced childhood sexual abuse), Ducci et al. (2008) found that the MAOA-linked polymorphic region (MAOA-LPR) low activity allele conferred increased vulnerability to APD and alcoholism in those with a history of childhood sexual abuse. Haplotype-based analysis revealed that MAOA haplotype containing the MAOA-LPR low activity allele was found in excess among individuals with alcoholism and those with alcoholism and antisocial behavior. Finally, a MAOB haplotype, termed haplotype C, was significantly associated with alcoholism and to a lesser extent with antisocial alcoholism.

In a study involving 841 individual twins from the Minnesota Twin Family Study assessed through to age 25, Derringer and colleagues (2010) studied the impact of MAOA genotype, childhood sexual assault, and harsh discipline on clinical externalizing symptoms (substance problems, adult antisocial behavior, and conduct disorder). These authors found evidence that childhood sexual assault interacted with MAOA genotype to predict antisocial behavior and conduct disorder symptoms, but not substance misuse problems, indicating that the interaction between MAOA and childhood maltreatment may be specific to specific subsets of externalizing disorders.

Though at least two studies (Huizinga et al., 2006; Haberstick et al., 2014) did not confirm an effect of MAOA activity on the relationship between childhood maltreatment and adolescent or adult antisocial behavior, findings from a recent meta-analysis of 27 studies involving nonclinical samples confirmed the interaction of childhood maltreatment, lesser MAOA activity, and development of antisocial behavior across 20 male cohorts. However, across 11 female cohorts, MAOA did not interact with combined early life adversities, but a weak association was found between maltreatment alone and antisocial behaviors in female subjects with high-activity MAOA genotype (Byrd & Manuck, 2014).

5HTT

The 5HTT gene (SLC6A4) is located on chromosome 17. It encodes a protein transporter responsible for moving the neurotransmitter serotonin from the synaptic space into the presynaptic neurons. The short allele of the gene is generally considered to increase the risk for a number of mental disorders, including depression and anxiety, as well as the development of externalizing psychopathology (Mendoza & Casados, 2014). The long allele has also been implicated in antisocial behavior. For instance, Sadeh et al. (2010) examined the relationship between SLC6A4 polymorphisms and psychopathic traits as a function of socioeconomic status in a community sample. The findings suggest that participants with the homozygous long allele variant of the 5-HT serotonin transporter protein and low socioeconomic status showed greater expression of psychopathic personality traits such as callous, unemotional, and narcissistic traits. Further, a review by Glenn (2011) examined findings from studies concerning the long allele variant of SLC6A4 which has received far less attention in the literature. The author argues that the presence of two long alleles may confer a risk for reduced emotional responding and psychopathic traits in the context of additional genetic and environmental factors.

COMT

Vevera et al. (2009) examined the relationship between COMT polymorphisms and violent behavior among 47 male violent offenders with APD and 43 healthy male controls matched on education. They found that the COMT Ala146Val polymorphism is more frequent among violent offenders with APD, lending further support to the role of COMT in determining interindividual variability in the proclivity for violent behavior. Using a case control study design involving 310 individuals with APD and 200 without APD, Cuartas Arias et al. (2011) examined gene–gene interactions and found that interactions between genetic variants in COMT, 5-HTR2A, and tryptophan hydroxylase gene were associated with APD. Regarding psychopathy, in a five-year follow-up study involving adolescents with ADHD, Fowler and colleagues reported on the link between psychopathy (measured using the PCL–Youth Version) and gene variants that affect COMT, MAOA, and 5HTT activity. They reported that all three gene variants were associated with the affective features of psychopathy while MAOA and 5HTT gene variants were associated with total psychopathy scores.

Other Genes

Several other genes have also been implicated in the etiology of APD and psychopathy though it would go beyond the scope of this chapter to describe these emerging findings (e.g., see Ponce et al., 2003, 2008, 2009; Mendoza & Casados, 2014; Cummings, 2015).

Conclusions and Limitations

Taken together, there is good evidence from quantitative genetic studies for heritability of antisocial behavior as well as the specific conditions of APD and psychopathy. Also, molecular genetic studies have focused on a number of candidate genes. Variability in estimates of heritability of genetic influences is partly due to variations in study design, assessment method, age, zygosity determination method, or gender (Rhee & Waldman, 2002) and partly to the use of different but overlapping phenotypic expressions of underlying genetic vulnerabilities (e.g., conduct disorder, APD, substance misuse disorders, impulsivity, psychopathy, or aggression) to index antisocial behavior (Mason & Frick, 1994; Slutske, 2001; Kreuger et al., 2002). Besides, the presence of comorbid conditions (such as ADHD, substance misuse, and impulse control disorders) and criminality bedevil the examination of heritability in APD (Dahl, 1993; Gunter et al., 2010). Further, definitions of psychopathy and antisocial spectrum disorder are not consistent across most studies (Gunter et al., 2010), and there is a dearth of published studies which clearly identify psychopathy in study participants, making it difficult to identify distinct genetic and environmental markers for psychopathy (Thompson & Ramos, 2014). Craig (2007) argued that the interaction between the neurotransmitter pathway genes leading to antisocial and/or violent behavior (particularly the MAOA and 5HTT encoding genes) and environmental stressors may provide protection against, or increase sensitivity to, adverse childhood maltreatment, an observation that may explain part of the variability in developmental outcomes associated with maltreatment. Nevertheless, our understanding of how the genes implicated in antisocial behavior interact with each other and the role of moderators of genetic risk factors remains limited (Slutske, 2001; Ferguson, 2010).

■ PSYCHOPHYSIOLOGICAL FINDINGS

Over the past few decades, the study of the psychophysiological underpinnings of antisocial behavior has attracted a fair deal of attention in the scientific literature, with electrodermal activity (EDA) and heart rate (HR) the most frequently used measures of autonomic functioning. Other indices of sympathetic (e.g., finger pulse volume, finger blood volume, pupillary dilation) and parasympathetic (e.g., pupillary constriction) nervous system activities have also been studied (Arnett, 1997). We focus here on the two most commonly used measures of autonomic activity, namely HR and EDA, which are thought to reflect emotional responses and motivational processes that underpin responses to internal and external stimuli (Gray, 1987; Fowles, 1988).

Findings in Antisocial Personality Disorder

There is a dearth of studies in which APD was the primary phenotype under consideration. Dinn and Harris (2000) compared subjects with APD presenting with prominent psychopathic personality features with matched control subjects on measures of frontal lobe dysfunction, personality questionnaires, clinical scales sensitive to APD, and electrodermal activity during the presentation of emotionally charged stimuli. Compared to controls, APD subjects showed greater deficits on measures of orbitofrontal dysfunction and lower EDA responses to aversive stimuli. Raine et al. (2000) found evidence of reduction in prefrontal grey matter volume in the absence of ostensible brain lesions and reduced autonomic activity during a social stressor in community volunteers with APD. These authors concluded that this prefrontal structural deficit may underlie the low arousal, poor fear conditioning, lack of conscience, and decision-making deficits that have been found to characterize antisocial, psychopathic behavior.

Findings in Psychopathy

Early studies of psychophysiological correlates of psychopathy used two main paradigms: paradigms assessing anticipatory responses to aversive (punishment) stimuli (e.g., an electric shock, unpleasant loud noise, white noise, negative social feedback) and paradigms assessing reactivity to aversive or orienting stimuli such as orienting tones or visual cues (Arnett, 1997). A consistent finding from these studies is that, compared to controls, people with psychopathy show evidence of electrodermal hyporeactivity in anticipation of punishment. Studies assessing their reactivity to punishment stimuli also reveal evidence of electrodermal hyporeactivity but only to very intense punishment stimuli (e.g., loud aversive tones). In contrast, they show no differences in autonomic reactivity to orienting stimuli (see reviews by Hare, 1978; Siddle & Trasler, 1981; Fowles & Missel, 1992; Arnett, 1997; Fowles, 2000). Additionally, there is evidence of greater heart rate acceleration in response to aversive stimuli (Arnett, 1997; Hare & Craigen, 1974; Hare et al., 1978; Ogloff & Wong, 1990).

Findings from recent studies show that people with psychopathy show evidence of (a) electrodermal hyporeactivity in a response-conflict paradigm, denoting reduced inhibitory processes in the face of conflict (Waid & Orne, 1982); (b) impaired differentiation in blink startle responses during presentations of affectively pleasant, unpleasant, and neutral slides, reflecting abnormal processing of emotional stimuli (Patrick et al., 1993); and (c) electrodermal hyporeactivity to fearful imagery (Patrick et al., 1994).

Taken together, these findings suggest that people with psychopathy may display abnormality in fear conditioning, inhibitory processes, and processing of emotional stimuli (Arnett, 1997; Fowles, 2000).

■ ELECTROENCEPHALOGRAPHY/EVENT-RELATED POTENTIALS

Electroencephalography (EEG) is regarded as a measure of arousal, attention, and cognitive activation. The units of analysis in EEG studies are EEG waveforms and event-related potentials (ERPs). EEG waveforms are influenced by mental and physiological states including deep sleep (delta), intake of sensory information and spatial memory (theta), wakeful relaxation and the synchronization of neuronal processes in the brain (alpha), working memory (beta), and alertness (gamma; Rudo-Hutt, 2015). In contrast, ERPs are small voltages on the EEG generated in response to time-locked events or stimuli (Dolan, 1994).

A review of early electrophysiological studies in psychopathy (Dolan, 1994) reported evidence of nonspecific EEG abnormalities (Ellingson, 1954), generalized excess theta activity (Howard, 1984), localized slow-wave activity in the temporal lobe in habitually aggressive psychopaths (Hill & Waterson, 1942), localized temporal lobe positive spiking in impulsive-aggressive psychopaths (Kurland et al., 1963), excess posterior temporal slow-wave activity (Blackburn, 1979; Howard, 1984), reduction in the amplitude of contingent negative variation (CNV; believed to reflect cortical preparatory activity; McCallum, 1973; Forth & Hare, 1989), correlations between CNV amplitude and sociability and CNV attenuation in secondary psychopathy (Howard et al., 1984), and small N100 responses (believed to reflect an orienting response which is elicited when an unexpected stimulus is presented) during task performance (Jutai & Hare, 1983). Studies examining the P300 ERP wave, which is sensitive to changes in allocation of attentional resources, show evidence of reduced P300 amplitude and prolonged P300 latency under conditions of distraction (Jutai et al., 1987).

More recently, in a meta-analysis of 38 studies, involving 2,616 subjects with antisocial behavior (i.e., aggression, APD, conduct disorder, oppositional-defiant disorder, psychopathy), Gao and Raine (2009) found evidence of reduced P300 amplitudes and prolonged P300 latencies. Compared to nonpsychopathic offenders, psychopathic offenders showed P300 amplitudes impairments only in standard oddball tasks (often used in ERP research to study the effects of stimulus novelty on information processing). The authors attributed the findings to impairment in deployment of neural resources in processing cognitive task-relevant information in individuals with antisocial behavior. Among a sample of personality-disordered patients detained at different levels of security who also met criteria for psychopathy ($N = 27$), Valmarov et al. (2010) reported that psychopathic patients showed a significantly reduced amplitude of an early frontal negative ERP component evoked by negative feedback and a high rate of errors of commission on a visual Go No-Go task. Findings are consistent with the idea that psychopathic patients' unsuccessful attempts to self-regulate reflect a cognitive deficit characterized by a failure to attend and respond to a mismatch between expected and obtained outcomes.

The finding of reduced P300 amplitude has been reported in a variety of other disorders (such as APD, alcoholism, and drug addiction), leading researchers to conclude that these disorders are underpinned by an overarching vulnerability (called externalizing) which is highly heritable (Kreuger et al., 2002). A significant inverse relationship between P300 and scores on externalizing has been documented (e.g., Patrick et al., 2006; Venables & Patrick, 2014).

Regarding EEG waves, a review by Rudo-Hutt (2015) found evidence of increased theta activity and decreased beta activity in people with APD. The results support the theory of cortical hypoarousal in externalizing disorders.

Conclusions and Limitations

The literature on the psychophysiological correlates of psychopathy is often complex and seemingly confusing. For instance, a meta-analysis of 95 studies of HR and EDA in people with aggression, psychopathy, and conduct problems (Lorber, 2004) revealed a complex constellation of interactive effects that varied with age, stimulus valence, and type of antisocial behavior construct (conduct disorder, psychopathy/sociopathy, aggression). Heterogeneities in behavior construct, experimental stimuli, age group, and outcome measures are major limitations of studies of psychophysiological functioning in antisocial spectrum disorders (Lorber, 2004). The issue is compounded further by the presence of criminality and comorbid conditions such as Axis I disorders and substance misuse.

■ NEUROPSYCHOLOGICAL FINDINGS

The neuropsychological literature on the presentations of APD has been largely theory-driven and has developed considerably over the years. It has focused heavily on psychopathy. Early accounts concentrated on general cognitive functioning such as IQ (Dolan, 1994; Flor-Henry, 1990), while more recent studies have increasingly focused on specific cognitive functions, such as emotion processing and response control, in explaining characteristics of psychopathy (e.g., emotional deficits and instrumental aggression; Blair, 2013; Kiehl, 2006; Marsh, 2016).

Generalized Neuropsychological Dysfunction

Earlier studies suggested that psychopathy and patterns of APD may be related to abnormal intelligence patterns, abnormal laterality of cognitive function, and frontal (executive) deficits (Dolan, 1994; Flor-Henry, 1990). Studies have reported that lower intelligence may predict violence and aggression and that individuals with psychopathy may demonstrate a pattern of higher performance (e.g., conceptual reasoning) compared to verbal IQ (e.g., verbal comprehension; Dolan, 1994; Gao, Glenn, Schug, Yang, & Raine, 2009; Golden, Jackson, Peterson-Rohne, & Gontkovsky, 1996; Kiehl, 2006). However, the link between lower IQ and psychopathy has not been supported over the years while a discrepancy between types of IQ is not unique to psychopathy and could reflect learning difficulties, as the effect has disappeared after controlling for reading ability (Dolan, 1994; Gao et al., 2009; Kiehl, 2006).

Left Hemisphere and Language Deficits

The suggestions that APD and psychopathy may be partly underpinned by impaired left hemisphere and language function comes from evidence suggesting relatively selective difficulties with semantic and verbal functions and lateral asymmetries. The literature on APD is limited, with some evidence of difference in story-telling (e.g., more verbosity) and in features of handwriting (e.g., shape of letter; Gawda, 2008a, 2008b). No impairments have been detected in fluency and concrete semantic processing, for example when participants were asked to generate words beginning with specific letters or to distinguish between concrete words and non-words (Deckel, Hesselbrock, & Bauer, 1996; Kosson, Lorenz, & Newman, 2006; Lorenz & Newman, 2002c; Stevens, Kaplan, & Hesselbrock, 2003).

Compared to individuals without psychopathy, individuals with psychopathy perform poorly on some lateralized divided attention tasks (particularly in connection with verbal stimuli) such as counting visual targets while responding to auditory targets (Jurado & Junque, 1996; Kosson, 1998; Kosson & Newman, 1986). They also perform poorly on a range of functions implicating conceptual use of language including aspects of verbal expression such as slower speech, less conceptual coherence, incongruent hand gestures and speech content, and difficulties with semantic comprehension of abstract words and metaphors (Blair, 2005b; Brites, 2016; Dolan, 1994; Gao et al., 2009; Kiehl, 2006).

The left hemisphere and language processing deficit hypotheses are not sufficiently specific to explain these findings, however, as left hemisphere processing and language functions do not seem impaired overall or for all aspects of function, and other neuropsychological functions also seem implicated where deficits have been noted. For example, individuals with psychopathy have shown superior performance or no impairment when verbal stimuli were presented to the right hemisphere, and language function deficits have been more pronounced for affective and abstract materials (Dolan, 1994; Gao et al., 2009; Hare & Jutai, 1988; Hare & McPherson, 1984). Studies have failed to detect language deficits in terms of semantic processing of concrete words, fluency, and functional linguistic skills such as spelling, phonology, simple syntax, fluency, and reading (Blair, 2005b; Brites, 2016; Gao et al., 2009; Jurado & Junque, 1996). Furthermore, processing abstract material is thought to draw on right rather than left hemisphere resources (Kiehl, 2006). Studies have also documented differences in verbal expression in psychopathy (e.g., more colorful language, expressing dominance, verbosity), but these have also been observed in other personality disorders and could be partly explained by differences in intelligence and instrumental use of language rather than a deficit (Brites, 2016; Sneiderman, 2006).

Frontal Lobe and Generalized Executive Function Deficit

The frontal lobe has been associated to executive functions such as self-regulation, planning, self-awareness, and so forth (Lezak, Howieson, Bigler, & Tranel, 2012). It is, therefore, no surprise that the erratic presentations of individuals with APD and psychopathy have generated hypotheses about frontal lobe dysfunction with considerable relevant research. Whilst major meta-analyses have supported a generalized executive function impairment in both APD and psychopathy (Morgan & Lilienfeld, 2000; Ogilvie, Stewart, Chan, & Shum, 2011), the relevance of generalized executive function deficit to either remains questionable.

The difficulty concluding that a generalized executive deficit underpins APD and psychopathy is due to the patterns in the reported effect sizes, limitations in the aggregate evidence, and heterogeneity in the target populations and among executive functions (and executive deficits). Effect sizes indicate that generalized deficits are prevalent in antisocial populations more generally (e.g., offenders, individuals with history of physical aggression, conduct disorder) but are at best modest in psychopathy and even less prevailing in APD (Morgan & Lilienfeld, 2000; Ogilvie et al., 2011). The robustness of a suggestion that frontal lobe impairment underpins APD and psychopathy seems even less convincing in light of limitations to pooling the evidence, such as publication bias, confounding of APD and psychopathy with other variables (e.g., incarceration as indicator of limited ability, substance abuse, and medication use), nonequivalent controls (e.g., students), and diversity in how psychopathy was operationalized (e.g., self-reported vs. structured clinical interviews with nonequivalent results; Dolan, 1994; Kiehl, 2006; Morgan & Lilienfeld, 2000; Navas Collado & Munoz Garcia, 2004; Ogilvie et al., 2011). Indeed, conceptualizing psychopathy and executive functions as homogeneous is problematic for several reasons, while better controlled studies with clinical samples reveal a more complex picture of deficits, at least for psychopathy.

Specific executive deficits in APD have been noted in planning, cognitive flexibility, working memory, and response inhibition, with most research examining dorsolateral prefrontal cortex (DLPFC) functions (e.g., Barkataki et al., 2005; De Brito, Viding, Kumari, Blackwood, & Hodgins, 2013; Dinn & Harris, 2000; Dolan, 2012; Dolan & Park, 2002; Stevens et al., 2003). However, these deficits have not been consistently reported and may reflect offending history more generally or presence of psychopathy rather than APD as the studies that found deficits compared offenders with APD versus nonoffending controls or had confounded APD with psychopathy. This conclusion is also in line with the findings from meta-analyses discussed.

Executive functions are diverse and heavily implicate other neuropsychological functions (Golden et al., 1996; Lezak et al., 2012). The relevant literature on psychopathy, which is more extensive than the literature in APD in terms of range of cognitive tests used and replication, presents more robust evidence of poor performance in specific executive functions. Studies have generally supported difficulties in complex tasks integrating cognitive and motor control such as planning in Porteus Mazes (Dolan & Park, 2002; Gao et al., 2009; Herpertz & Sass, 2000; Jurado & Junque, 1996; Kiehl, 2006). Deficits in response control in particular have been well documented (Blair, 2013). However, deficits in DLPFC or general frontal lobe functioning such as perseveration, cognitive flexibility, fluency, visuomotor control, and working memory (e.g., as assessed by the Wisconsin Card Sorting Test [WCST], Trail Making Test, set-shifting tests, the Digit Span) have not been supported consistently, particularly not in well-controlled studies with clinical samples (Blair, 2004, 2005b; Dolan, 1994; Fitzgerald & Demakis, 2007; Gao et al., 2009; Jurado & Junque, 1996; Maes & Brazil, 2013; Navas Collado & Munoz Garcia, 2004; Seguin, 2004; Smith, Arnett, & Newman, 1992; Sommer et al., 2006).

Psychopathy encompasses a heterogeneous group of individuals (Blackburn, 2009), and some of the discrepancies in the literature could reflect this diversity (Dolan,

1994; Fitzgerald & Demakis, 2007; Gao et al., 2009; Maes & Brazil, 2013). For example, deficits in visuomotor control and cognitive flexibility may be specific to low-anxious individuals with psychopathy or those scoring highly on the antisocial lifestyle factor (Maes & Brazil, 2013; Smith et al., 1992). Furthermore, individuals with psychopathy but without forensic history ("successful psychopaths"), or those with higher scores on the interpersonal/affective factors, have even shown superior executive performance (e.g., less perseveration on the WCST) relative to controls (Ishikawa, Raine, Lencz, Bihrle, & Lacasse, 2001; Maes & Brazil, 2013).

Overall, hypotheses relating to generalized cognitive impairment have generated considerable research. However, they have also increasingly appeared to be oversimplifications in light of the evidence, which reveals complex patterns of neuro-psychological functioning. Executive deficits in APD may reflect criminality more generally. In psychopathy, impairments appear more robust in relation to response control and integrating cognitive and motor control. Overall, the literature does not support a frontal or generalized executive dysfunction hypothesis in APD or psychopathy.

■ AFFECT-RELATED DEFICITS

There is a large body of research on the role of affective functions in psychopathy for which callousness and unemotionality are considered defining features (Hare, 2003). This research documents deficits in the processing of affective information, emotion recognition, and empathy.

Affective Processing

Several neuropsychological studies highlight a deficit in processing affective information in individuals with psychopathy, often tied in with the electrophysiological evidence discussed. The relevant literature in APD is limited compared to psychopathy, but studies have not highlighted affective processing deficits and have even indicated that the performance of women with APD may be influenced *more* by affective stimuli compared to controls when distinguishing between emotional words and non-words (heightened affective processing; Kosson et al., 2006; Lorenz & Newman, 2002c).

Unlike APD, the evidence relating to psychopathy stems from diverse paradigms indicating that individuals with psychopathy are influenced less in their performance by emotional context and content (particularly when it is negatively laden) compared to individuals without psychopathy. Relevant paradigms involve distinguishing between words and non-words, performing sustained attention tasks bracketed by or involving emotional stimuli, encoding affectively laden stimuli to memory, and attenuated affect when expressing emotional content (Blair, 2006, 2008b; Blair & Mitchell, 2009; Blair, Peschardt, Budhani, Mitchell, & Pine, 2006; Brites, 2016; Gao et al., 2009; Herpertz, 2003; Herpertz & Sass, 2000; Kiehl, 2006; Sobhani & Bechara, 2011; Sommer et al., 2006; Yildirim & Derksen, 2015). These deficits do not seem to be underpinned by lack of semantic awareness of the general affective content of stimuli (e.g., positive or negative; Lorenz & Newman, 2002a; Müller et al., 2008; Sommer et al., 2006) and have been contrasted with the heightened sensitivity to similar stimuli observed in populations with anxiety-related difficulties such as posttraumatic stress disorder (Blair & Mitchell, 2009).

Conclusions regarding the role of affective processing deficits in psychopathy remain tempered due to confounding with language and lateralized function. Much of the evidence uses verbal material, and there are reports of the strongest effects with such material or when tasks draw on left hemisphere resources (e.g., right-hand responses to stimuli; Herpertz & Sass, 2000; Kiehl, 2006; Lorenz & Newman, 2002a). Furthermore, visual stimuli and tasks are likely to be associated to some extent with verbal representations (Lezak et al., 2012; Törneke, 2010), which may have influenced findings on affective processing in psychopathy.

Emotion Recognition

Emotion recognition deficits in individuals with APD and psychopathy have emerged with some degree of reliability, though they may be partly underpinned by affective processing. The literature in APD is very limited compared to psychopathy but shows deficits in distinguishing facial emotional cues for distress and guilt and recognizing facial cues for sadness (potentially exacerbated as psychopathic traits increase; Dolan & Fullam, 2004, 2006).

The evidence on psychopathy indicates modest deficits across modalities (facial, vocal), which tend to be strongest for facial recognition of fear and sadness and potentially happiness (Blair, 2006, 2013; Dawel, O'Kearney, McKone, & Palermo, 2012; Marsh, 2016; Marsh & Blair, 2008; Wilson, Juodis, & Porter, 2011). These deficits generalize to broader emotion recognition deficits, for example identifying emotional content in verbal materials such as words, metaphors, and stories (Brites, 2016; Gao et al., 2009; Kiehl, 2006), and could reflect semantic rather than connotative processing of the stimuli (Day & Wong, 1996; Herpertz & Sass, 2000; Kosson, Suchy, Mayer, & Libby, 2002). The deficits seem mostly associated with the affective/interpersonal features of psychopathy (Dawel et al., 2012; Marsh, 2013).

Overall emotion recognition seems impaired in psychopathy according to a number of meta-analyses, but the deficits do not generalize across individual emotions and modalities consistently, especially in adult samples (Dawel et al., 2012; Marsh, 2016; Marsh & Blair, 2008; Wilson et al., 2011). Inconsistencies in the findings could be due to the focus of different studies and methodological limitations. Effect sizes on fear and sadness recognition are reported more frequently (Dawel et al., 2012; Wilson et al., 2011), hence meta-analyses have more power. However, aggregating studies from the same research group and with potentially overlapping samples may have overestimated effect sizes (e.g., Dawel et al., 2012). Discrepant results may also be due to sampling and methodological biases (e.g., college students, self-reported measures; Del Gaizo & Falkenbach, 2008; Gordon, Baird, & End, 2004; Wilson et al., 2011), ceiling effects in some emotion recognition tasks, and lack of power or limitations to the reliability of measurement in many studies (Dawel et al., 2012).

Conceptually, language deficits also seem implicated in performance on verbal emotion recognition tasks and the impairment may partly involve naming rather than recognizing relevant emotions (Marsh & Blair, 2008; Wilson et al., 2011). If individuals with psychopathy process emotion semantically, then difficulties processing abstract verbal material may partly underpin emotion recognition deficits. Notably, deficits do not seem unique to psychopathy as those in facial recognition appear comparable to findings from antisocial populations without psychopathy (e.g., offenders) in meta-analyses (Marsh & Blair, 2008). Consequently, emotion recognition deficits may partly explain some psychopathic traits but do not seem sufficiently robust as a core explanation of the syndrome.

Empathy

Emotion recognition deficits could partly account for deficits in empathy, the lack of which is a key feature in the antisocial personality. The literature is limited compared to that of emotion recognition, but authors conclude that APD and psychopathy are associated with difficulties empathizing with others' feelings (emotional empathy, extending beyond emotion recognition) but not with difficulties understanding others' perspectives and mental states (cognitive empathy; Anderson & Kiehl, 2014; Blair, 2005a, 2006, 2008a; Blair et al., 1996; Hansman-Wijnands & Hummelen, 2006; Krippl & Karim, 2011; Richell et al., 2003). For example, this deficit was reflected in difficulties with the more complex, second-order empathy (inference about someone else's understanding of another person's emotional state; Shamay-Tsoory, Harari, Aharon-Peretz, & Levkovitz, 2010) or with understanding how someone may have felt emotionally following a faux pas (but with no difficulties in understanding the faux pas; Dolan & Fullam, 2004). Intact cognitive empathy is consistent with the notion of relying on semantic rather than connotative content in affect recognition.

Conclusions regarding empathy impairments in psychopathy require further substantiation for several reasons. Of the studies cited in the literature, few are in adult populations (Anderson & Kiehl, 2014; Krippl & Karim, 2011; Marsh, 2013). Furthermore, APD and psychopathy are confounded with each other, and there may be ceiling effects in some tasks of cognitive empathy which could have made it difficult to detect further deficits or differences between APD and psychopathy (e.g., Dolan & Fullam, 2004). Also, studying empathy in psychopathy is circular and therefore potentially flawed altogether, since lack of emotional empathy but ability to deceive (intact cognitive empathy) are part of the syndrome's definition.

■ ATTENTION AND RESPONSE CONTROL

The literature on attention in APD is very limited compared to psychopathy and not driven by a coherent theoretical framework. Studies have associated APD with increased interference during Stroop paradigms (impaired selective attention) but with no other reliable deficits (e.g., continuous performance tasks assessing sustained attention; Barkataki et al., 2005; Dinn & Harris, 2000; Swann, Lijffijt, Lane, Steinberg, & Moeller, 2009). The literature on psychopathy has linked attentional processes to difficulties with response modulation (Newman, 2011), but in APD deficits in response reversal and response control have not been replicated sufficiently and remain confounded with offending (Barkataki et al., 2008; De Brito et al., 2013; Dinn & Harris, 2000; Dolan, 2012; Dolan & Park, 2002).

The literature on attention in psychopathy implicates primarily selective and divided attention processes. Some evidence indicates superior selective attention (unlike in APD), where the performance of individuals with psychopathy does not seem negatively affected by peripheral information in conflict-monitoring tasks (Blair & Mitchell, 2009; Gao et al., 2009). For example, individuals with psychopathy do not show increased interference during standard Stroop tasks and show less interference with picture-word, spatially separated, and numerical stimuli, compared to individuals without psychopathy (Blair & Mitchell, 2009; Gao et al., 2009; Maes & Brazil, 2013). Individuals with psychopathy have also shown impaired performance during tasks where they are required to divide or shift their attention (especially when more processing is required by the left hemisphere), which is consistent with reduced breadth of attention (Jurado & Junque, 1996; Kosson, 1998; Llanes & Kosson, 2006). Sustained attention does not seem reliably impaired in psychopathy (like APD) as evidenced by studies using single, continuous performance tasks (Kiehl, Bates, Laurens, Hare, & Liddle, 2006; Kiehl, Hare, Liddle, & McDonald, 1999; Kosson, 1996, 1998; Maes & Brazil, 2013).

The findings on selective and divided attention in psychopathy have led to the hypothesis that the syndrome may be underpinned by heightened deliberate focus of attention and difficulty processing secondary information (Baskin-Sommers, Curtin, & Newman, 2011; Blair, 2013; Blair & Mitchell, 2009; Gao et al., 2009; Newman, Curtin, Bertsch, & Baskin-Sommers, 2010). Newman and colleagues have led on this hypothesis to explain findings of impaired response control where individuals with psychopathy fail to adjust goal-directed behavior in light of changing peripheral information (Baskin-Sommers et al., 2011; Blair, 2005b, 2008b, 2013; Blair & Mitchell, 2009; Blair et al., 2006; Jurado & Junque, 1996; Kiehl, 2006; Newman et al., 2010). The literature primarily discusses difficulties with adjusting outcome expectancies and reversing or withholding responses to stimuli appropriately as contingencies of reinforcement change, potentially leading to frustration regarding lack of success obtaining rewards, aggression, and utilitarian behavior (Blair, 2005b, 2007b, 2008b, 2010b, 2013; Blair & Mitchell, 2009; Kuin, Masthoff, Kramer, & Scherder, 2015; Sobhani & Bechara, 2011; Sommer et al., 2006). Paradigms usually involve responses to stimuli that are no longer rewarded (extinction) or when the stimuli start being punished (passive avoidance, response inhibition; the subtler the change the larger the impairment). Difficulties seem specific to paradigms involving shifts in reinforcement or punishment rather than explicit shift in responses (i.e., based on being able to discriminate between different stimuli; Blair, 2006).

However, findings remain equivocal due to confounding of different factors involved. For example, deficits may relate to moderators such as low anxiety and immediacy of feedback while attentional processes and stimulus-reinforcement learning are confounded with each other (Alcazar-Corcoles, Verdejo-Garcia, & Bouso-Saiz, 2008; Gao et al., 2009; Sobhani & Bechara, 2011; Sommer et al., 2006). Crucially, a purely attentional account does not explain unequal deficits in processing different emotions, impairment in some but not all Stroop tasks, and unimpaired processing of distracters in some studies while a stimulus-reinforcement learning deficit cannot explain the generalized attentional focus, for example during Stroop tasks (Blair, 2005b, 2013). Both accounts seem necessary for an account of psychopathy, but the level and nature of contribution between attentional processes and stimulus-reinforcement learning remain unclear. Both accounts also need further development to account for language difficulties, such as those relating to abstract word processing.

■ OTHER FUNCTIONS

Other neuropsychological functions examined in APD but not falling within the major strands of literature discussed include simple motor control, such as moving fingers following a pattern, and memory, for example recall of story or numerical digits and recognition of patterns (Barkataki et al., 2005; Deckel et al., 1996; Dolan & Park, 2002;

Herpertz & Sass, 2000; Stevens et al., 2003). However, results do not suggest striking or reliable deficits, and, once again, there is cofounding with offending.

In psychopathy, additional functions include memory and learning, odor identification, mental rotation, simple motor control, and moral reasoning (Blair, 2005b; Herpertz & Sass, 2000; Jurado & Junque, 1996; Kiehl, 2006; Sommer et al., 2006). Deficits have been noted in odor identification (indicating orbitofrontal cortex [OFC] dysfunction), time estimation, and moral reasoning (Blair, 2013; Lapierre, Braun, & Hodgins, 1995; Moreira, Pinto, Almeida, & Barbosa, 2016; Tassy, 2011; Yildirim & Derksen, 2015). Regarding the latter, individuals with psychopathy (especially those low in anxiety) may be more likely to accept unintentional harm and transgressions involving harm (and endorse the latter in light of utilitarian gains) compared to individuals without psychopathy (Blair, 2013; Tassy, 2011; Yildirim & Derksen, 2015). This literature suggests that deficits in moral reasoning could be linked to reduced sensitivity to others' distress and personal cost. However, there are some conflicting findings which could be due to methodological factors (even methods of analysis; e.g., Cima, Tonnaer, & Hauser, 2010; Koenigs, Kruepke, Zeier, & Newman, 2012) and call for further replication. The deficits in time estimation are new in the literature and may contribute to impulsiveness in psychopathy (Moreira et al., 2016). They could reflect a mixture of neuropsychological deficits (including response control; Lezak et al., 2012; Perbal-Hatif, 2012), but replication in clinical samples is required.

Conclusions and Limitations

The literature on APD is limited compared to psychopathy, and the two presentations appear to be underpinned by different neuropsychological mechanisms. Executive deficits relating to DLPFC function (e.g., planning, inhibition, cognitive flexibility, and working memory) may partly underpin APD, but their influence appears small. There is no evidence of affective processing deficit in APD, but some impairments in emotion recognition and empathy have been noted. Studies indicate poor selective attention, but findings suggesting response control deficits do not appear to be robust as yet. Further research needs to address confounding of APD with offending history (due to nonequivalent control groups) and with psychopathy.

A large body of research has focused on the neuropsychological functions in psychopathy. Hypotheses of broad deficit, such as general cognitive impairment, left hemisphere dysfunction, and executive dysfunction, do not appear convincing. On the other hand, affect-related deficits, heightened selective attention, and difficulties with response control in line with changing consequences of responses have been more consistently (and extensively) documented. However, in light of inconsistencies, further research needs to take subtypes of psychopathy into account, aim to use well-validated measures of psychopathy, and extend recruitment beyond forensic and student settings. Attempts to dissociate (a) language and abstract information processing functions from affect processing and (b) attentional functions from response control appear necessary to aid further theoretical clarification.

▪ NEUROIMAGING STUDIES

Acquired brain injury studies and case studies of patients with diseases affecting the brain indicate associations between the development of antisocial behavior and brain damage particularly in prefrontal and temporal brain regions (e.g., Blair & Cipolotti, 2000; Tonkonogy, 1991). Neuropsychological findings in antisocial groups, as reviewed, also indicate potential functional deficits, particularly in the dorsolateral prefrontal cortex in APD (Dolan & Park, 2012), and in the orbitofrontal and ventromedial prefrontal cortex, and in the amygdala in psychopathy (Blair, 2013).

Brain imaging allows for the study of structural and functional brain changes in individuals with APD and psychopathy in the absence of neurological injury. A number of brain imaging techniques are available: Computer tomography (CT) uses X-ray techniques to produce cross-sectional images. Magnetic resonance imaging (MRI) studies are superior to CT scanning due to the improved spatial resolution and the use of magnetic fields rather than hazardous radiation. Both techniques provide data on structure but not function. Positron emission tomography (PET) and single-photon emission computer tomography (SPECT) studies allow for the study of brain function, both resting brain activity and task-related activations. Both techniques involve the injection of radioactive substances which are detected when distributed in the brain. Another disadvantage is their low spatial resolution (compared to functional MRI [fMRI]); they are therefore not the method of choice in research, although their neurotransmitter mapping ability might be useful in some studies. While there are some early PET and SPECT studies in antisocial populations, these are not reviewed here due to their poor methodological quality due to lack of control for confounding factors and as more recent research has mainly used MRI scanning to identify structural and fMRI scanning to describe functional abnormalities.

fMRI is the most widely used functional brain imaging technique. It is completely noninvasive and has high spatial (though poor temporal) resolution. fMRI relies on the different magnetic properties of oxygenated and deoxygenated hemoglobin in the blood. During the completion of a neurocognitive task, blood flow to brain regions involved in this task increases; this in turn increases the ratio of oxygenated versus deoxygenated blood. The strong magnetic field applied in the scanner results in alignment of nuclei of atoms (of relevance here are the hydrogen nuclei of tissue water) that generate a detectable signal which varies according to the magnetic properties of the blood.

■ STRUCTURAL IMAGING STUDIES

Early studies, using CT and MRI scanning, selected participants mainly by reference to behavior, rather than clinical diagnosis, such as serious offending or violent behavior (for a review of early studies, see Völlm, 2005). One of the earliest such studies was by Chesterman et al. (1994) who examined 10 patients in a high-security setting who had committed serious acts of violence and had been referred for neuropsychiatric assessment. The authors found abnormalities, including generalized and focal atrophy, in half of the subjects using CT scanning and all but one patient using MRI. Localized pathology was mainly located in the hippocampus, and the left brain was disproportionately more affected. Given the small sample size and highly selective sample, findings cannot be extrapolated to APD or psychopathy samples more generally. Similar early studies (e.g., Sakuta & Fukushima, 1998; Aigner et al., 2000; Soderstrom et al., 2000; Soderstrom et al., 2002) also showed high prevalences of brain abnormalities primarily in frontal and temporal regions (e.g., atrophies, cysts, infarctions) but are compromised by their selection of subjects with serious offenses and the potential of other confounding factors, such as brain injury and substance misuse. None of these studies included control groups in their design.

There have been few structural imaging studies focusing specifically on individuals identified by their diagnosis of APD. A number of studies have focused on individuals with alcoholism and comorbid APD and have produced inconsistent findings (Kuroglu et al., 1996; Laasko et al., 2000; Laasko et al., 2001; Laasko et al., 2002). Kuroglu et al., using CT scanning, did not find any correlation between antisocial personality traits and structural brain abnormalities. Laasko et al. (2000) studied only hippocampal volumes in two groups of violent offenders, one with type 1 alcoholism and one with type 2 alcoholism and APD, and a healthy control group using MRI scanning. Both patient groups showed reduced right hippocampal volumes compared to the control group. As a positive (rather than the expected negative) correlation between age and hippocampal volumes was found in the type 2 alcoholism/APD group, the authors suggested that findings cannot be attributed to cumulative toxic effects of alcohol but might instead be attributed to APD pathology. This interpretation is supported by the finding of a negative correlation between PCL-R (total and factor 1 [comprising interpersonal/affective traits]) scores and hippocampi volumes (Laasko et al., 2001). A later study by the same group (Laasko et al., 2002) expanded the line of inquiry to other brain areas and identified reduced volumes in the left OFC, DLPFC, and medial frontal cortex (MPFC) in individuals with type 2 alcoholism/APD compared to a healthy control group, though these findings were no longer significant after controlling for education and duration of alcoholism. Dolan et al. (2002) did also not find prefrontal cortex (PFC) volume deficits in a group of impulsive-aggressive personality-disordered patients though a temporal lobe volume reduction of 20% was found compared to the healthy control group. Barkataki et al. (2006) similarly reported reduced temporal but not frontal lobe volumes in a group of violent APD offenders compared to healthy controls.

The first methodologically robust MRI study on APD was conducted by Raine et al. (2000). The authors compared a group of 21 APD patients with 21 psychiatric patients with a mix of diagnoses, 27 patients with substance abuse disorders, and 34 healthy controls, all recruited from the community and matched for a range of sociodemographic and clinical factors. The study only looked at PFC volumes and found reduced volumes in the APD compared to all control groups. Later work by the same group identified abnormalities in the corpus callosum in a group of individuals with APD and high psychopathy scores (Raine et al., 2003) and increased hippocampal asymmetry in unsuccessful versus successful psychopaths (Raine et al., 2004), results suggestive of potential developmental abnormalities in these groups.

Studies specifically looking at psychopathic individuals have found structural abnormalities in frontal and temporal lobe regions, specifically the amygdala. For example, Müller et al. (2008) investigated forensic patients with high psychopathy scores, compared to healthy control subjects, and found significant gray matter reductions in both frontal and temporal brain regions, in particular the right superior temporal gyrus (STG). Oliveira-Souza et al. (2008) found that volume deficits in OFC, frontal polar cortex, and STG were negatively correlated with the affective features of psychopathy. Yang et al. (2009) reported a negative correlation between amygdala volumes and psychopathy scores, particularly the affective and interpersonal features, while Glenn at al. (2010) reported positive correlations with caudate body volumes while caudate head volumes were associated with the impulsive elements of the construct. These findings suggest that studies should differentiate between different groups within psychopathic individuals as certain symptoms might be related to specific brain pathology.

A number of reviews have been published on the imaging literature in antisocial groups. Yang and Raine (2009) reviewed and meta-analyzed imaging studies in violent, antisocial, and psychopathic individuals, though they only focused on prefrontal changes. Their review included 43 imaging studies, of which 31 were functional and 12 were structural imaging studies. The combined meta-analysis of structural and functional imaging studies found both reduced structure and functional deficits in the PFC. An analysis by region concluded these deficits were most profound in the right OFC, left DLPFC, and right anterior cingulate cortex (ACC) while no deficits were found in ventrolateral PFC and MPFC. Potentially moderating factors for sample characteristics were all nonsignificant, indicating effect sizes did not differ between violent and nonviolent, incarcerated and community, and psychopathic and nonpsychopathic samples. Effect sizes were, however, greater for functional than for structural imaging studies. A later meta-analysis (Nickerson, 2014) provided an update, including 58 studies using different imaging modalities. Fifteen of these studies had not been included in the earlier review described, of which all but two focused on individuals with psychopathy. This meta-analysis largely confirmed findings of the earlier review though found effect sizes to be larger for structural compared to functional imaging studies. Aoki et al. (2014) reviewed and meta-analyzed studies in antisocial groups using a particular technique of analyzing structural imaging data, voxel-based morphometry; 12 studies were included. Results suggest reduced volumes in parts of the basal ganglia, left insula, and left frontopolar cortex while volume increases were identified primarily in parts of the parietal lobe. The authors suggests that these deficits might be related to difficulties in allocating attention during emotional processing. Finally, Santana (2016) narratively reviewed 35 structural imaging studies in psychopathy and other groups with antisocial behavior. Volume deficits were found in a range of areas, though those reported by a larger number of individual studies included OFC, frontopolar cortex, VMPFC, MPFC, and ACC within the frontal and temporal pole, STG, amygdala, hippocampus, and insula with the temporal lobe. A study completed since the publication of this latest review identified increased volumes in striatal areas in individuals with psychopathy which were positively correlated with factor 2 scores (capturing socially deviant behavior; Korponay et al., 2017).

■ FUNCTIONAL IMAGING STUDIES

Functional imaging studies have focused on a range of different tasks, for example, those assessing instrumental learning, emotional and attentional processing, moral decision-making, and semantic and affective verbal processing. fMRI studies in antisocial groups have been published from the beginning of the 21st century onwards. The vast majority of fMRI studies have focused on psychopathy rather than APD, and emotional processing tasks have most commonly been used. In the following we describe some examples of such studies, before outlining the evidence from meta-analyses in this field.

One of the first fMRI studies in psychopathy was by Kiehl et al. (2001), comparing criminal and noncriminal psychopaths to normal control participants. The task used was an affective memory task in which subjects had to recognize neutral and negative verbal stimuli. Interestingly, task performance did not differ between groups in terms of accurately identifying stimuli as neutral or emotional, and recall was better for the emotional as opposed to the neutral stimuli in all groups. However, differences were found in brain activation patterns associated with the task; specifically, criminal psychopaths showed decreased activation in affect-related regions (amygdala, hippocampus, parahippocampus, striatum, cingulate) and increased activation in fronto-temporal regions. The authors interpreted this finding as evidence that the psychopathic group compensates the dysfunction in affect processing by employing more cognitive strategies to process affective material. However, the activation pattern was only found in psychopathic individuals with a criminal history and not in nonoffending psychopaths, calling into question the suggestion that it is related to the core pathology of the disorder.

Müller et al. (2003) described complex patterns of activations and deactivations during the processing of emotional stimuli in the absence of behavioral rating differences in individuals with high scores of psychopathy compared to healthy controls using pictures from the International Affective Picture System. They interpreted their findings as evidence for a disturbed interaction between "top-down" and "bottom-up" signals. Gordon et al. (2004), similarly, using an emotional recognition task in a group of college students divided into high and low scorers on a psychopathy instrument, found no behavioral differences though reduced brain activations were identified in right inferior frontal gyrus, MPFC, and amygdala while enhanced activations were shown in DLFPC and in the visual cortex and dorsolateral cortex, again supporting the notion of a potential cognitive compensation mechanism.

The finding of reduced activation in affect-related areas, particularly the amygdala, has been supported by a number of studies since, for example, in violent patients with schizophrenia and high psychopathy scores using fearful faces (Dolan & Fullam, 2009), and in psychopathy using tasks of social cooperation (Rilling et al., 2007) and moral decision-making (Glenn at al., 2009).

fMRI studies investigating aversive conditioning in individuals with psychopathy have yielded less consistent findings. Schneider et al. (2000), for example, found signal increases in DLPFC and amygdala while others (e.g., Birbaumer et al., 2005; Veit et al., 2002) reported reduced activations in OFC, insula, anterior cingulate, and right amygdala. Both reduced and enhanced activation patterns have been interpreted as evidence for dysfunction, the latter in the context of the proposed additional effort needed for tasks completed in psychopathic groups. Such findings have also been described in individuals with APD using an impulsivity task (Völlm et al., 2004).

A number of reviews have summarized findings from fMRI studies in antisocial groups. Yang and Raine (2009) identified 31 fMRI studies in their review, using different patient groups and tasks. Within the PFC, reduced activation was identified in right OFC, left DLPFC, and right ACC in their meta-analysis with no evidence that psychopathic and other antisocial, but not psychopathic, groups differed significantly in that respect. Comparable effect sizes were found for emotional and cognitive tasks. Blair (2010b) identified that almost all fMRI studies in psychopathy found reduced amygdala and OFC activations to a variety of tasks, including stimulus reinforcement based decision-making, reversal learning, aversive conditioning, emotional memory, and moral reasoning. His review also found evidence for dysfunctional responses in areas strongly connected to the amygdala and OFC, including insula, cingulate, parahippocampus, and anterior superior temporal gyrus. Blair (2010a) differentiated between types of aggression in their review. They found that studies looking at individuals with impulsive aggression showed increased, rather than decreased, subcortical and amygdala activity in response to emotional material, while frontal structures showed increased activations. The authors interpreted this finding in the context of emotional overreactivity and subsequent behavioral dyscontrol. On the contrary, in psychopathic individuals displaying instrumental aggression, reduced activity in emotion-processing structures were found, though not consistently. This could be related to the lack of empathy in the condition.

None of these reviews included more recent studies investigating not only structure and function of specific regions but also their connectivity. Contreras-Rodríguez et al. (2015) investigated connectivity in emotional and cognitive brain areas in offending individuals with psychopathy. Their results revealed reduced functional connectivity of prefrontal areas with limbic-paralimbic structures (e.g., insula, amygdala, hypothalamus, posterior cingulate cortex) but enhanced connectivity within the DLPFC, suggesting again weaker emotional but compensatory cognitive processing in psychopathy. Yoder et al. (2015) investigated amygdala connectivity and found decreased coupling with ACC, insula, striatum, and VMPFC, suggesting disrupted neural coupling within the salience network in psychopathy. Korponay et al. (2017) identified abnormal connectivity between striatal areas and DLPFC and midbrain (reduced) as well as parietal and occipital areas (increased). The authors interpreted their findings in the context of increased reward dependency in impulsive psychopathic individuals.

Conclusions and Limitations

There is strongest support from imaging studies in individuals with antisocial behavior for structural and functional abnormality in OFC, DLPFC, ACC, STG, hippocampus, insula, and amygdala. These findings support the notion of dysfunctional processing of emotion in antisocial groups. However, many of the imaging studies have suffered from insufficient attention to potentially confounding factors such as comorbidity, alcohol and substance abuse, medication, intellectual functioning, and effect of incarceration. In addition, APD and psychopathy have a range of clinical features, and future research needs to pay more attention to the relationship between structural and functional abnormalities and subtypes of the disorders, for example, the emotional and antisocial facets of psychopathy or different types of aggression. In addition, connectivity between brain areas warrant further attention.

■ NEUROTRANSMITTERS

Studies, both animal and human, suggest the involvement of multiple neurotransmitters in the modulation of antisocial, impulsive, and aggressive behavior. The most intensely studied neurotransmitter system in this regard is serotonin (5-HT), and the inverse relationship between 5-HT function and aggression and/or impulsivity is a constituent finding across different population samples and methodologies (for a review, see Dolan & Völlm, 2014).

5-HT

Serotonin is mainly implicated in mood regulation and impulse control. A number of measures have been used to index serotonin functioning. Central 5-HT function measures include the concentration of 5-HIAA, a serotonin metabolite in CSF and neuroendocrine drug challenges (e.g., with fenfluramine). Increased 5-HT activity at serotonin receptor sites in the hypothalamus increases the production of cortisol, which can be measured in the blood, thus providing a less invasive measure of central 5-HT function compared to CSF (Dolan, 1994; Glenn & Raine, 2008). Peripheral measures such blood levels of 5-HT, platelet MAO activity, and 5-HT binding sites provide a proxy of central 5-HT function.

Investigations of the role of neurotransmitter systems in the antisocial behavior spectrum have attracted a fair deal of attention in the scientific literature (Buchheim et al., 2013). However, there is a relative dearth of studies that have specifically investigated the role of neurotransmitter systems in the development and maintenance of APD or psychopathy (Glenn & Raine, 2008). A review of early studies investigating the association between 5-HT function and aggressive behavior demonstrated inverse relationships between the CSF concentration of 5-HIAA and measures of aggression, irritability, hostility, and criminality; between platelet MAO activity and sensation-seeking and impulsivity; and between prolactin response to fenfluramine and *DSM-III-R* impulsive-aggressive personality disorders (Dolan, 1994).

A study by Dolan et al. (2001) investigated relationships between impulsivity, aggression, 5-HT function, and testosterone in male offenders with personality disorders. The results showed reduced 5-HT function in offenders with borderline personality disorder, and 5-HT function was inversely correlated more strongly with impulsivity than with aggression. Recent studies demonstrated a positive association between increased impulsivity and impulsive aggression and 5-HT dysregulation in frontal brain areas (Buchheim et al., 2013). Taken together, this evidence suggests a role for 5-HT particularly in aggression driven by impulsivity or lack of inhibition. This suggestion is supported by observations in forensic populations showing that CSF 5-HIAA concentrations differentiated impulsive offenders from those with premeditated crimes and recidivists from nonrecidivists (Virkkunen et al., 1989, 1997). Impaired 5-HT functioning has also been implicated in both APD (Deakin, 2003) and psychopathy (Dolan, 1994; Glenn & Raine, 2008).

The role of the interaction between 5-HT dysregulation and other hormones has also been examined. A link between hypoglycemia and low 5-HT activity among habitually violent men has been suggested (Virkkunen, 1986). The low cortisol levels observed in psychopathy (Dolan, 1994) have been attributed to dysregulation of 5-HT function in the brain (Glenn & Raine, 2008). It has also been argued that the combination of low 5-HT and high testosterone levels may increase the tendency for violent aggression (Glenn & Raine, 2008). A genetic contribution to the relationship between 5-HT function and impulsive aggression has also been examined. This is supported by studies involving the 5-HT transporter gene, tryptophan hydroxylase gene, and the allelic variant of the MAOA polymorphism coding for high MAOA activity (for an overview, see Buchheim, 2013).

Dopamine

Specific psychopathic traits may also be linked to alterations in the mesolimbic dopamine reward and reinforcement system. For instance, in a neuroimaging study of community participants, Buckholtz et al. (2010) measured dopamine release in the mesolimbic system after treatment with amphetamine or participation in a monetary reward anticipation task. The authors found a correlation between the extent of dopamine release and scores on the Impulsive-Antisociality subscale of the Psychopathic Personality Inventory but not the Fearless-Dominance subscale. Given the significant role of the mesolimbic reward system in the development of substance abuse disorders, the authors suggest that mesolimbic dopamine hypersensitivity may act as a nexus between the impulsive and antisocial features of psychopathy and risk for substance abuse. Further, Soderstrom et al. (2001, 2003) found a positive association between psychopathy and increased homovanillic acid (a dopamine metabolite)/5-HIAA ratio. This increased ratio is thought to reflect impaired serotonergic regulation of dopamine, which leads to disinhibition of aggressive impulses (Glenn & Raine, 2008).

Other Neurotransmitters

Reduced catecholamine output in response to stress has been reported in psychopathic men awaiting trial (Lidberg et al., 1978), indicating less stress. Other studies have linked abnormalities in CSF and serum and urinary concentrations of catecholamines to indices of sensation-seeking, disinhibition, and aggression (e.g., Brown et al., 1979; Buchsbaum et al., 1981).

Conclusions and Limitations

Existing literature suggests that dysregulation of neurotransmitter systems may be implicated in the antisocial behavior spectrum. There is also evidence that neurotransmitter dysregulation can interact with certain genes and neuroendocrine systems and affect the functioning of certain brain regions. Therefore, understanding the interplay between these systems can help elucidate the mechanisms involved in the development of psychopathy and APD (Glenn & Raine, 2008).

■ HORMONES

The activities of the hypothalamic–pituitary–adrenal (HPA) and the hypothalamic–pituitary–gonadal axes have been studied in antisocial populations using cortisol (a marker of stress reactivity) and testosterone (a sex hormone) essays, respectively.

Hormones and Antisocial Personality Disorder

Raised testosterone levels have been associated with a range of antisocial behaviors, psychosocial problems, psychoactive substance misuse, and violence (Mazur & Booth, 1998). Few studies have examined the role of hormones in APD. Räsänen and colleagues (1999) examined associations between serum testosterone levels and criminal behavior in a sample of offenders with mental disorders and found higher serum testosterone levels among those with personality disorder than those with schizophrenia. In contrast, Aromäki et al. (1999) found no differences in testosterone levels between violent men (most with APD) and controls, but testosterone levels were significantly correlated with hostility. Lindberg and colleagues (2003) examined the relationship between serum testosterone level and sleep using polysomnography and spectral power analysis in 16 male subjects charged with highly violent offenses and ordered for a pretrial forensic psychiatric examination. They found that individuals with APD and comorbid borderline personality disorder had significantly more awakenings and lower sleep efficiency compared to those with APD alone. In a sample of 89 prisoners, Aluja and Garcia (2007) reported strong correlations between sex hormone-binding globulin (SHGB), total testosterone, and free bioavailable testosterone. Raised SHGB levels were only reported in those with a high probability of APD and those who scored highly on aggressiveness. These findings suggest that the relationship between testosterone and APD and aggressiveness may be mediated by SHBG.

A relatively new line of inquiry examines the role of autoantibodies in the regulation of the HPA axis. For example, a study by Fetissov and colleagues (2006) found high levels of adrenocorticotrophic hormone, oxytocin, and vasopressin-reactive autoantibodies in blood samples of prisoners and conduct-disordered subjects, indicating that these may be implicated in aggressive behavior through interference with the neuroendocrine mechanisms of stress and motivated behavior.

Hormones and Psychopathy

Only a few studies have examined the relation between testosterone levels and psychopathy (for an overview, see Glenn & Raine, 2008). Dolan et al. (2001) found a positive correlation between plasma testosterone concentration and aggressive acts and lower initial cortisol and higher testosterone concentrations in subjects with primary psychopathy compared to controls. In a sample of men undergoing forensic psychiatric examinations ($n = 61$), Stålenheim and colleagues (1998) found that elevated testosterone and SHGB levels were related to PCL-R–diagnosed psychopathy and *Diagnostic and Statistical Manual of Mental Disorders* (fourth edition [DSM-IV]; APA, 1994) diagnosed APD. A putative link between emotional deficits observed in psychopathy and a hormonal imbalance affecting testosterone and cortisol hormones has been proposed (Van Honk et al., 2005; van Honk & Schutter, 2006). Glenn and colleagues (2011) examined cortisol and testosterone levels in a community sample of 178 subjects with a wide range of psychopathy scores. The authors found no significant association between psychopathy and either of these measures independently but reported that psychopathy scores were associated with an increased ratio of testosterone (baseline) to cortisol responsivity to a stressor. These findings suggest that interconnected hormone systems may work in concert to predispose to psychopathy.

The role of thyroid hormones in the development of psychopathy has also been examined. For instance, Stålenheim and colleagues (1998) found that elevated levels of triiodothyronine (T3) were related to PCL-R–diagnosed psychopathy and DSM-IV (APA, 1994) diagnosed APD. However, findings from an earlier study did not support an association between increased T3 and psychopathic traits (Alm et al., 1996).

Conclusions and Limitations

Taken together, studies of testosterone levels have yielded mixed results in antisocial populations, and some have suggested that testosterone is a marker of social dominance rather than aggressive behavior in male subjects (Schug et al., 2010). However, Yildirim and colleagues (2012) proposed a model to explain the role of testosterone in the development of life-course persistent antisocial behavior. The model posits that raised foetal/circulating testosterone influences the development of the mesolimbic dopaminergic circuitry, right OFC, and cortico-subcortical connectivity, resulting in a strong reward motivation, low social sensitivity, and dampened regulation of strong motivational/emotional processes. These testosterone-induced endophenotypes can follow two distinct trajectories, antisocial or prosocial. The antisocial trajectory is likely to emerge when their effects are moderated by genetic factors and psychosocial adversities that increase the risk of antisocial behavior. The prosocial trajectory is more likely to emerge in the context of positive social experiences that promote prosocial behaviors.

■ OVERALL CONCLUSIONS

There is as yet no model of APD/psychopathy that accounts for all the different aspects of neurobiological findings reviewed in this chapter. Most models have focused on findings from imaging studies. One of the most prominent models in this respect is the Integrated Emotions Systems model proposed by Blair (e.g., Blair, 2007b). This model proposes that two brain regions are of particular relevance, the amygdala and the OFC. The model accounts for the deficits found in processing emotional information and stimulus-reinforcement learning, both functions relying on the amygdala. The amygdala has strong connections with the OFC, which is involved in decision-making based on the information received by the amygdala. Dysfunction in OFC accounts for deficits in reversal leaning and behavioral extinction, that is, failing to learn from previous experience and adapt behavioral choices accordingly. Evidence from recent studies also suggests that there is a lack of connectivity between these two regions in psychopathic individuals (e.g., Motzkin et al., 2011). Another model by Kiehl (e.g., Kiehl, 2006) additionally takes into account deficits found in limbic and paralimbic regions, including ACC, which plays a role in pain perception, emotional regulation, response conflict, error monitoring, as well as concern for others. The Kiehl model also includes the temporal lobes which have been shown to play a role in moral decision-making (e.g., Harenski et al., 2010). Other authors have emphasized attentional bias to account for the deficits in processing of emotional material in psychopathy (e.g., Baskin-Sommers et al., 2011). This theory proposes that psychopathic individuals have an abnormal attention bottleneck which reduces their capacity to process information peripheral to their goal-directed focus of attention. Interestingly, authors favoring this model of psychopathy have shown that affective processing in individuals with psychopathy can be improved if instructed to specifically focus on the affective stimulus; this could have implications for the development of therapeutic interventions in the condition. Clearly much more work is needed to synthesize the different neurobiological findings in psychopathy, including genetic findings. Citing the work of Thompson et al. (2001) and Meyer-Lindenberg et al. (2006), Raine (2008) underscored the importance of identifying the genes that have been associated with antisocial behavior and are thought to influence brain structure. Thompson et al. (2001) found that 90% of the variation in the volume of prefrontal gray matter in humans can be explained by genetic influences. Meyer-Lindenberg et al. (2006) reported that individuals with the MAOA polymorphism have an 8% reduction in the volume of the amygdala, anterior cingulate, and orbitofrontal (ventral prefrontal) cortex. Such work is promising in order to understand the pathway from genes over brain structure to function and outward behavior and to identify specific biomarkers which could form the focus of neurobiologically informed interventions in the future.

■ REFERENCES

Aigner, M., Eher, R., Fruehwald, S., Frottier, P., Gutierrez-Lobos, K., & Dwyer, S. M. (2000). Brain abnormalities and violent behaviour. *J Psychol Hum Sexual, 11*, 57–64.

Alcazar-Corcoles, M. A., Verdejo-Garcia, A., & Bouso-Saiz, J. C. (2008). [Forensic neuropsychology at the challenge of the relationship between cognition and emotion in psychopathy]. *Rev Neurol, 47*(11), 607–612.

Alm, P. O., af-Klinteberg, B., Humble, K., Leppert, J., Sorensen, S., Tegelman, R., Thorell, L. R., & Lidberg, L. (1996). Criminality and psychopathy as related to thyroid activity in former juvenile delinquents. *Acta Psychiatr Scand, 94*, 112–117.

Aluja, A., & Garcia, L.F. (2007). Role of sex hormone-binding globulin in the relationship between sex hormones and antisocial and aggressive personality in inmates. *Psychiatry Res, 152*(2–3), 189–196.

Anderson, N. E., & Kiehl, K. A. (2014). Psychopathy: developmental perspectives and their implications for treatment. *Restor Neurol Neurosci, 32*(1), 103–117.

Aoki, Y., Inokuchi, R., Nakao, T., & Yamasue, H. (2014). Neural bases of antisocial behavior, a voxel-based analysis. *Soc Cogn Affect Neurosci, 9*(8), 1223–1231.

American Psychiatric Association. (1994). *Diagnostic and statistical manual of mental disorders* (4th rev. ed.). Washington, DC: Author.

American Psychiatric Association. (2013). *Diagnostic and statistical manual of mental disorders* (5th ed.). Washington, DC: Author.

Arnett, P. A. (1997). Autonomic responsivity in psychopaths: a critical review and theoretical proposal. *Clin Psychol Rev, 17*, 903–936.

Aromäki, S. A., Lindman, E. R., & Eriksson, P. C. J. (1999).Testosterone, aggressiveness, and antisocial personality. *Aggress Behav, 25*(2), 113–123.

Barkataki, I., Kumari, V., Das, M., Hill, M., Morris, R., O'Connell, P., . . . Sharma, T. (2005). A neuropsychological investigation into violence and mental illness. *Schizophr Res, 74*(1), 1–13.

Barkataki, I., Kumari, V., Das, M., Sumich, A., Taylor, P., & Sharma, T. (2008). Neural correlates of deficient response inhibition in mentally disordered violent individuals. *Behav Sci Law, 26*(1), 51–64.

Barkataki, I., Kumari, V., Das, M., Taylor, P., & Sharma, T. (2006). Volumetric structural brain abnormalities in men with schizophrenia or antisocial personality disorder. *Behav Brain Res, 169*, 239 247.

Baskin-Sommers, A. R., Curtin, J. J., & Newman, J. P. (2011). Specifying the attentional selection that moderates the fearlessness of psychopathic offenders. *Psychol Sci, 22*(2), 226–234. doi:doi:10.1177/0956797610396227

Beach, S. R. H., Brody, G. H., Gunter, T. D., Packer, H., Wernett, P., & Philibert, R. A. (2010). Child maltreatment moderates the association of MAOA with symptoms of depression and antisocial personality disorder. *J Fam Psychol, 24*, 12–20.

Birbaumer, N., Veit, R., Lotze, M., Erb, M., Hermann, C., Grodd, W., & Flor, H. (2005). Deficient fear conditioning in psychopathy: a functional magnetic resonance imaging study. *Arch Gen Psychiatry, 62*, 799–805.

Blackburn, R. (2009). Subtypes of psychopath. In M. McMurran & R. Howard (Eds.), *Personality, personality disorder and violence* (pp. 113–132). Chichester, UK: Wiley Blackwell.

Blackburn, R. B. (1979). Cortical and autonomic arousal in primary and secondary psychopaths. *Psychophysiology, 16*, 143–150.

Blair, J., Sellars, C., Strickland, I., Clark, F., Williams, A., Smith, M., & Jones, L. (1996). Theory of mind in the psychopath. *J Forensic Psychiatry, 7*, 1525.

Blair, R. J. (2004). The roles of orbital frontal cortex in the modulation of antisocial behaviour. *Brain Cogn, 55*(1), 198–208.

Blair, R. J. (2005a). Applying a cognitive neuroscience perspective to the disorder of psychopathy. *Dev Psychopathol, 17*(3), 865–891.

Blair, R. J. (2005b). Responding to the emotions of others: dissociating forms of empathy through the study of typical and psychiatric populations. *Conscious Cogn, 14*(4), 698–718.

Blair, R. J. (2006). The emergence of psychopathy: implications for the neuropsychological approach to developmental disorders. *Cognition, 101*(2), 414–442.

Blair, J. (2007a). Aggression, psychopathy and free will from a cognitive neuroscience perspective. *Behav Sci Law, 25*(1), 321–331.

Blair, R. J. (2007b). The amygdala and ventromedial prefrontal cortex in morality and psychopathy. *Trend Cogn Sci, 11*(9), 387–392.

Blair, R. J. (2008a). Fine cuts of empathy and the amygdala: dissociable deficits in psychopathy and autism. *Q J Exp Psychol, 61*(1), 157–170.

Blair, R. J. (2008b). The amygdala and ventromedial prefrontal cortex: functional contributions and dysfunction in psychopathy. *Philos Trans R Soc Lond B Biol Sci, 363*(1503), 2557–2565.

Blair, R. J. (2010a). Neuroimaging of psychopathy and antisocial behavior: a targeted review. *Curr Psychiatry Rep, 12,* 76–82.

Blair, R. J. (2010b). Psychopathy, frustration, and reactive aggression: the role of ventromedial prefrontal cortex. *Br J Psychol, 101*(Pt 3), 383–399.

Blair, R. J. (2013). Psychopathy: cognitive and neural dysfunction. *Dialogues Clin Neurosci, 15*(2), 181–190.

Blair, R. J., & Mitchell, D. G. (2009). Psychopathy, attention and emotion. *Psychol Med, 39*(4), 543–555.

Blair, R. J., Peschardt, K. S., Budhani, S., Mitchell, D. G., & Pine, D. S. (2006). The development of psychopathy. *J Child Psychol Psychiatry, 47,* 262–276.

Blair, R. J. R. (2007). Aggression, psychopathy and free will from a cognitive neuroscience perspective. *Behav Sci Law, 25,* 321–331.

Blair, R. J. R., & Cipolotti, L. (2000). Impaired social response reversal. A case of "acquired sociopathy". *Brain, 123,* 1122–1141.

Blonigen, D. M., Carlson, S. R., Krueger, R. F., & Patrick, C. J. (2003). A twin study of self-reported psychopathic personality traits. *Pers Individ Dif, 35,* 179–197.

Blonigen, D. M., Hicks, B. M., Krueger, R. F., Patrick, C. J., & Iacono, W. G. (2005). Psychopathic personality traits: heritability and genetic overlap with internalizing and externalizing psychopathology. *Psychol Med, 35,* 637–648.

Bortolato, M., & Shih, J. C. (2011). Behavioural outcomes of monoamine oxidase deficiency: preclinical and clinical evidence. *Int Rev Neurobiol, 100,* 13–42. doi:10.1016/B978-0-12-386467-3.00002-9

Brites, J. A. (2016). The language of psychopaths: a systematic review. *Aggress Violent Behav, 27,* 50–54.

Brown, D., Larkin, F., Sengupta, S., Romero-Ureclay, J., Ross, C., . . . Das, M. (2014). Clozapine: an effective treatment for seriously violent and psychopathic men with antisocial personality disorder in a UK high-security hospital. *CNS Spectr, 19*(1), 391–402.

Brown, G. L., Goodwin, F. K., Ballenger, J. C., Goyer, P. F., & Major, L. F. (1979). Aggression in humans correlates with cerebrospinal fluid amine metabolites. *Psychiatry Res, 1,* 131–139.

Brunner, H. G., Nelen, M., Breakefield, X. O., Ropers, H. H., & van Oost, B.A. (1993). Abnormal behavior associated with a point mutation in the structural gene for monoamine oxidase A. *Science, 262*(5133), 578–580.

Buchheim, A., Rothb, G., Schiepek, G., Pogarelld, O., & Karchd, S. (2013). Neurobiology of borderline personality disorder (BPD) and antisocial personality disorder (AsPD). *Schweiz Arch Neurol Psychiatr, 164*(4), 115–122.

Buchsbaum, M. S., Goodwin, F. K., & Muscettola, G. (1981). Urinary MHPG, stress response, personality factors and somatosensory evoked potentials in normal subjects and patients with affective disorders. *Neuropsychobiology, 7*, 212–224.

Buckholtz, J. W., Treadway, M. T., Cowan, R. L, Woodward, N. D., Benning, S. D., Ansari, M. S., . . . Zald, D. H. (2010). Mesolimbic dopamine reward system hypersensitivity in individuals with psychopathic traits. *Nature Neurosci, 13*, 419–421.

Burt, S. A., & Mikolajewski, A. J. (2008). Preliminary evidence that specific candidate genes are associated with adolescent-onset antisocial behaviour. *Aggress Behav, 34*, 437–445.

Byrd, A. L., & Manuck, S. B. (2014). MAOA, childhood maltreatment, and antisocial behaviour: meta-analysis of a gene-environment interaction. *Biol Psychiatry, 75*(1), 9–17.

Cadoret, R. J. (1978). Psychopathology in adopted-away offspring of biologic parents with antisocial behaviour. *Arch Gen Psychiatry, 35*(2), 176–184. doi:10.1001/archpsyc.1978.01770260054005

Cadoret, R. J., O'Gorman, T. W., Troughton, E., & Heywood, E. (1985). Alcoholism and antisocial personality interrelationships, genetic and environmental factors. *Arch Gen Psychiatry, 42*(2), 161–167. doi:10.1001/archpsyc.1985.01790250055007

Cadoret, R. J., & Stewart, M. A. (1991). An adoption study of attention deficit/hyperactivity/aggression and their relationship to adult antisocial personality. *Compr Psychiatry, 32*, 73–82.

Caspi, A., Langley, K., Milne, B., Moffitt, T. E., O'Donovan, M., Owen, M. J., . . . Thapar, A. (2008). A replicated molecular genetic basis for subtyping antisocial Behaviour in children with attention-deficit/hyperactivity disorder. *Arch Gen Psychiatry, 65*(2), 203–210.

Caspi, A., McClay, J., Moffitt, T. E., Mill, J., Martin, J., Craig, I. W., . . . Poulton, R. (2002). Role of genotype in the cycle of violence in maltreated children. *Science, 297*, 851–854.

Chesterman, L. P., Taylor, P. J., Cox, T., Hill, M., & Lumsden, J. (1994). Multiple measures of cerebral state in dangerous mentally disordered inpatients. *Crim Behav Ment Health, 4*, 228–239.

Cima, M., Tonnaer, F., & Hauser, M. D. (2010). Psychopaths know right from wrong but don't care. *Soc Affect Cogn Neurosci, 5*, 59–67.

Coid, J. (1992). DSM-III diagnosis in criminal psychopaths: a way forward. *Crim Behav Ment Health, 2*, 78–94.

Cooke, D. J., & Michie, C. (2001). Refining the construct of psychopathy: towards a hierarchical model. *Psychol Assess, 13*, 171–188.

Craig, I. W. (2007). The importance of stress and genetic variation in human aggression. *Bio Essays, 29*, 227–236.

Crowe, R. R. (1974). An adoption study of antisocial personality. *Arch Gen Psychiatry, 31*(6), 785–791. doi:10.1001/archpsyc.1974.01760180027003

Cuartas Arias, J. M., Palacio Acosta, C. A., Valencia, J. G., Montoya, G. J., Arango Viana, J. C., Nieto, O. C., . . . Ruiz-Linares, A. (2011). Exploring epistasis in candidate genes for antisocial personality disorder. *Psychiatr Genet, 21*, 115–124. http://dx.doi.org/10.1097/YPG.0b013e3283437175

Cummings, M. A. (2015). The neurobiology of psychopathy: recent developments and new directions in research and treatment. *CNS Spectr, 20*, 200–206. doi:10.1017/S1092852914000741

Dahl, A. A. (1993). The personality disorders: a critical review of family and twin studies. *J Personal Disord, 7*(Suppl.), 86–99.

Dawel, A., O'Kearney, R., McKone, E., & Palermo, R. (2012). Not just fear and sadness: meta-analytic evidence of pervasive emotion recognition deficits for facial and vocal expressions in psychopathy. *Neurosci Biobehav Rev, 36*(10), 2288–2304.

Day, R., & Wong, S. (1996). Anomalous perceptual asymmetries for negative emotional stimuli in the psychopath. *J Abnorm Psychol, 105*(4), 648–652.

De Brito, S. A., Viding, E., Kumari, V., Blackwood, N., & Hodgins, S. (2013). Cool and hot executive function impairments in violent offenders with antisocial personality disorder with and without psychopathy. *PLoS ONE, 8*(6), e65566. doi:10.1371/journal.pone.0065566

Deakin, J. F. W. (2003). Depression and antisocial personality disorder: two contrasting disorders of 5HT function. *J Neural Transm, 64*(Suppl.), 79–93.

Deckel, A. W., Hesselbrock, V., & Bauer, L. (1996). Antisocial personality disorder, childhood delinquency, and frontal brain functioning: EEG and neuropsychological findings. *J Clin Psychol, 52*(6), 639–650. doi:10.1002/(SICI)1097-4679(199611)52:6<639::AID-JCLP6>3.0.CO;2-F

Deckel, A. W., Hesselbrock, V., & Bauer, L. (1996). Antisocial personality disorder, childhood delinquency, and frontal brain functioning: EEG and neuropsychological findings. *J Clin Psychol, 52*, 639–650.

Del Gaizo, A. L., & Falkenbach, D. M. (2008). Primary and secondary psychopathic-traits and their relationship to perception and experience of emotion. *Pers Individ Dif, 45*(3), 206–212. http://dx.doi.org/10.1016/j.paid.2008.03.019

Derringer, J., Krueger, R. F., Irons, D. E., & Iacono, W. G. (2010). Harsh discipline, childhood sexual assault, and MAOA genotype: an investigation of main and interactive effects on diverse clinical externalizing outcomes. *Behav Genet, 40*, 639–648. doi:10.1007/s10519-010-9358-9

Dinn, W. M., & Harris, C. L. (2000). Neurocognitive function in antisocial personality disorder. *Psychiatry Res, 97*(2–3), 173–190. http://dx.doi.org/10.1016/j.neubiorev.2007.08.003

Dolan, M. (1994). Psychopathy—a neurobiological perspective. *Br J Psychiatry, 165*(2), 151–159.

Dolan, M. (2012). The neuropsychology of prefrontal function in antisocial personality disordered offenders with varying degrees of psychopathy. *Psychol Med, 42*(8), 1715–1725. doi:10.1017/S0033291711002686

Dolan, M., & Fullam, R. (2004). Theory of mind and mentalizing ability in antisocial personality disorders with and without psychopathy. *Psychol Med, 34*(6), 1093–1102.

Dolan, M., & Fullam, R. (2006). Face affect recognition deficits in personality-disordered offenders: association with psychopathy. *Psychol Med, 36*(11), 1563–1569.

Dolan, M., & Fullam, R. (2009). Psychopathy and functional magnetic resonance imaging blood oxygenation level-dependent responses to emotional faces in violent patients with schizophrenia. *Biol Psychiatry, 66*(1), 570–577.

Dolan, M., & Park, I. (2002). The neuropsychology of antisocial personality disorder. *Psychol Med, 32*, 417–427.

Dolan, M., & Völlm, B. (2014). Disorder of brain structure and function and crime. In J. Gunn, C. Johnson, & P. Taylor (Eds.), *Forensic psychiatry, clinical, legal and ethical issues* (pp. 306–312). Abingdon, UK: Taylor and Francis.

Ducci, F., Enoch, M., Hodgkinson, C., Xu, K., Catena, M., Robin, R. W., & Goldman, D. (2008). Interaction between a functional MAOA locus and childhood sexual abuse predicts alcoholism and antisocial personality disorder in adult women. *Mol Psychiatry, 13*, 334–347.

Ellingson, R. J. (1954). The incidence of EEG abnormality among patients with mental disorders of apparently non organic origin: a critical review. *Am J Psychiatry, 3*, 263–275.

Ferguson, C. J. (2010). Genetic contributions to antisocial personality and behaviour: a meta-analytic review from an evolutionary perspective. *J Soc Psychol, 150*(2), 160–180.

Fetissov, S. O., Hallman, J., Nilsson, I., Lefvert, A. K., Oreland, L., & Hökfelt, T. (2006). Aggressive behaviour linked to corticotropin-reactive autoantibodies. *Biol Psychiatry, 60*, 799–802.

Fitzgerald, K. L., & Demakis, G. J. (2007). The neuropsychology of antisocial personality disorder. *Disease-a-Month, 53*(3), 177–183.

Flor-Henry, P. (1990). Neuropsychology and psychopathology: a progress report. *Neuropsychol Rev, 1*(2), 103–123.

Forsman, M., Lichtenstein, P., Andershed, H., & Larsson, H. (2010). A longitudinal twin study of the direction of effects between psychopathic personality and antisocial behaviour. *J Child Psychol Psychiatry, 51*(1), 39–47.

Forth, A., & Hare, R. D. (1989). The contingent negative variation in psychopaths. *Psychophysiology, 26*, 676–682.

Fowles, D. C. (1988). Psychophysiology and psychopathology: a motivational approach. *Psychophysiology, 25*, 373–391.

Fowles, D. C. (2000). Electrodermal hyporeactivity and antisocial behaviour: does anxiety mediate the relationship? *J Affect Disord, 61*, 177–189.

Fowles, D. C., & Missel, K. A. (1992). Electrodermal hyporeactivity, motivation, and psychopathy: theoretical issues. In E. F. Walker, R. H. Dworkin, & B. A. Cornblatt (Eds.). *Progress in experimental personality & psychopathology research.* New York: Springer Pub. Co.

Gao, Y., Glenn, A., Schug, R., Yang, Y., & Raine, A. (2009). The neurobiology of psychopathy: a neurodevelopmental perspective. *Can J Psychiatry, 54*, 813–823.

Gao, Y., & Raine, A. (2009). P3 event-related potential impairments in antisocial and psychopathic individuals: a meta-analysis. *Biol Psychol, 82*, 199–210.

Gawda, B. (2008a). A graphical analysis of handwriting of prisoners diagnosed with antisocial personality. *Percept Mot Skills, 107*(3), 862–872.

Gawda, B. (2008b). Love scripts of persons with antisocial personality. *Psychol Rep, 103*(2), 371–380.

Gibbon, S., Völlm, B. A., Khalifa, N., Duggan, C., Stoffers, J., Huband, N., Ferriter, M., & Lieb, K. (2011). Cochrane reviews of pharmacological and psychological interventions for antisocial personality disorder. *Eur Psychiatry, 4*(1), 48–54.

Glatt, S., Faraone, S., & Tsuang, M. (2008). Psychiatric genetics: a primer. In J. Smoller, B. Sheidley, & M. Tsuang (Eds.), *Psychiatric genetics. Applications in clinical practices* (pp. 3–26). Arlington, VA: American Psychiatric Publishing.

Glenn, A., Johnson, A., & Raine, A. (2013). Antisocial personality disorder: a current review. *Curr Psychiatry Rep, 15*(1), 427.

Glenn, A. L. (2011). The other allele: exploring the long allele of the serotonin transporter gene as a potential risk factor for psychopathy: a review of the parallels in findings. *Neurosci Biobehav Rev, 35,* 612–620.

Glenn, A. L., & Raine, A. (2008). The neurobiology of psychopathy. *Psychiatr Clin North Am, 31,* 463–475.

Glenn, A. L., Raine, A., Schug, R. A., Gao, Y., & Granger, D. A. (2011). Increased testosterone-to-cortisol ratio in psychopathy. *J Abnorm Psychol, 120*(2), 389–399.

Golden, C. J., Jackson, M. L., Peterson-Rohne, A., & Gontkovsky, S. T. (1996). Neuropsychological correlates of violence and aggression: a review of the clinical literature. *Aggress Violent Behav, 1*(1), 3–25. http://dx.doi.org/10.1016/1359-1789%2895%2900002-X

Gordon, H. L., Baird, A. A., & End, A. (2004). Functional differences among those high and low on a trait measure of psychopathy. *Biol Psychiatry, 56*(7), 516–521. http://dx.doi.org/10.1016/j.biopsych.2004.06.030

Gray, J. A. (1987). *The psychophysiology of fear and stress.* New York: Cambridge University Press.

Gunn, J. (2000). Politics and personality disorder: the demise of psychiatry. *Curr Opin Psychiatry, 13,* 545–547.

Gunter, T. D., Vaughn, M. G., & Philibert, R. A. (2010). Behavioural genetics in antisocial spectrum disorders and psychopathy: a review of the recent literature. *Behav Sci Law, 28,* 148–173. doi:10.1002/bsl.923

Haberstick, B. C., Lessem, J. M., Hewitt, J. K., Smolen, A., Hopfer, C. J., Halpern, C. T., . . . Harris, K. M. (2014). MAOA genotype, childhood maltreatment, and their interaction in the etiology of adult antisocial behaviours. *Biol Psychiatry, 75*(1), 25–30.

Hansman-Wijnands, M., & Hummelen, J. (2006). Differential diagnosis of psychopathy and autism spectrum disorders in adults: empathie deficit as a core symptom. *Tijdschrift voor Psychiatrie, 48*(8), 627–636.

Hare, R. D. (1978). Electrodermal and cardiovascular correlates of psychopathy. In R. D. Hare & D. Schalling (Eds.), *Psychopathic behaviour: approaches to research* (pp. 107–144). New York: John Wiley.

Hare, R. D. (1980). A research scale for the assessment of psychopathy in criminal populations. *Pers Individ Dif, 1,* 111–119.

Hare, R. D. (2003). *Hare Psychopathy Checklist–Revised (PCL-R)* (2nd ed.). Toronto: Multi-Health Systems.

Hare, R. D., & Craigen, D. (1974). Psychopathy and physiological activity in a mixed-motive game situation. *Psychophysiology, 11,* 197–206.

Hare, R. D., Frazelle, J., & Cox, D. N. (1978). Psychopathy and physiological responses to threat of an aversive stimulus. *Psychophysiology, 15,* 165–172.

Hare, R. D., & Jutai, J. W. (1988). Psychopathy and cerebral asymmetry in semantic processing. *Pers Individ Dif, 9*(2), 329–337.

Hare, R. D., & McPherson, L. M. (1984). Psychopathy and perceptual asymmetry during verbal dichotic listening. *J Abnorm Psychol, 93*(2), 141–149. doi:10.1037/0021-843X.93.2.141

Harenski, C., Harenski, K., Shane, M., & Kiehl, K. (2010). Aberrant neural processing of moral violations in criminal psychopaths. *J Abnorm Psychol, 119*(1), 863–874.

Herpertz, S. C. (2003). Emotional processing in personality disorder. *Curr Psychiatry Rep, 5*(1), 23–27.

Herpertz, S. C., & Sass, H. (2000). Emotional deficiency and psychopathy. *Behav Sci Law, 18*(5), 567–580.

Hicks, B. M., Krueger, R. F., Iacono, W. G., McGue, M., & Patrick, C. J. (2004). Family transmission and heritability of externalizing disorders: a twin-family study. *Arch Gen Psychiatry, 61*, 922–928.

Hill, J. D., & Waterson, D. (1942). EEG studies of psychopathic personalities. *J Neurol Neurosurg Psychiatry, 5*, 47–65.

Howard, R. C. (1984). The clinical EEG and personality in mentally abnormal offenders. *Psychol Med, 14*, 569–580.

Howard, R. C., Fenton, G. W., & Fenwick, B. (1984). The contingent negative variation, personality and antisocial behaviour. *Br J Psychiatry, 144*, 463–474.

Huizinga, D., Haberstick, B. C., Smolen, A., Menard, S., Young, S. E., Corley, R. P., . . . Hewitt, J. K. (2006). Childhood maltreatment, subsequent antisocial behaviour, and the role of monoamine oxidase A genotype. *Biol Psychiatry, 60*, 677–683.

Ishikawa, S. S., Raine, A., Lencz, T., Bihrle, S., & Lacasse, L. (2001). Autonomic stress reactivity and executive functions in successful and unsuccessful criminal psychopaths from the community. *J Abnorm Psychol, 110*(3), 423–432.

Jurado, M. A., & Junque, C. (1996). [Psychopathy and neuropsychology of the prefrontal cortex]. *Actas Luso-Esp Neurol Psiquiatr Cienc Afines, 24*(3), 148–155.

Jutai, J. W., & Hare, R. D. (1983). Psychopathy and selective attention during performance of a complex perceptual-motor task. *Psychophysiology, 20*, 146–151.

Jutai, J. W., Connolly, J. F., & Hare, R. D. (1987). Psychopathy and event related brain potentials (ERPs) associated with attention to speech stimuli. *Pers Individ Diff, 8*, 175–184.

Kiehl, K. A. (2006). A cognitive neuroscience perspective on psychopathy: evidence for paralimbic system dysfunction. *Psychiatry Res, 142*(2–3), 107–128.

Kiehl, K. A., Bates, A. T., Laurens, K. R., Hare, R. D., & Liddle, P. F. (2006). Brain potentials implicate temporal lobe abnormalities in criminal psychopaths. *J Abnorm Psychol, 115*(3), 443–453.

Kiehl, K. A., Hare, R. D., Liddle, P. F., & McDonald, J. J. (1999). Reduced P300 responses in criminal psychopaths during a visual oddball task. *Biol Psychiatry, 45*(11), 1498–1507.

Kiehl, K. A., Smith, A. M., Hare, R. D., Mendrek, A., Forster, B. B., Brink, J., & Liddle, P. F. (2001). Limbic abnormalities in affective processing by criminal psychopaths as revealed by functional magnetic resonance imaging. *Biol Psychiatry, 50*, 677–684.

Korponay, C., Pujara, M., Deming, P., Philippi, C., Decety, J., Kosson, D., Kiehl, K., & Koenigs, M. (2017). Impulsive-antisocial psychopathic traits linked to increase volume and functional connectivity within prefrontal cortex. *Soc Cogn Affect Neurosci, 12*(1), 1169–1178.

Kosson, D. S. (1996). Psychopathy and dual-task performance under focusing conditions. *J Abnorm Psychol, 105*(3), 391–400.

Kosson, D. S. (1998). Divided visual attention in psychopathic and non-psychopathic offenders. *Pers Individ Dif, 24*(3), 373–391.

Kosson, D. S., Lorenz, A. R., & Newman, J. P. (2006). Effects of comorbid psychopathy on criminal offending and emotion processing in male offenders with antisocial personality disorder. *J Abnorm Psychol, 115*(4), 798–806.

Kosson, D. S., & Newman, J. P. (1986). Psychopathy and the allocation of attentional capacity in a divided-attention situation. *J Abnorm Psychol, 95*(3), 257–263.

Kosson, D. S., Suchy, Y., Mayer, A. R., & Libby, J. (2002). Facial affect recognition in criminal psychopaths. *Emotion, 2*(4), 398–411.

Krippl, M., & Karim, A. (2011). "Theory of mind" and its neuronal correlates in forensically relevant disorders. *Der Nervenarzt, 82*(7), 843–852. doi:10.1007/s00115-010-3073-x

Krueger, R. F., Hicks, B. M., Patrick, C. J., Carlson, S. R., Iacono, W. G., & McGue, M. (2002). Etiologic connections among substance dependence, antisocial behavior, and personality: modeling the externalizing spectrum. *J Abnorm Psychol*, *111*(3), 411–424.

Kuin, N., Masthoff, E., Kramer, M., & Scherder, E. (2015). The role of risky decision-making in aggression: a systematic review. *Aggress Violent Behav A*, *25*, 159–172.

Kurland, H. D., Yaeger, C. T., & Arthur, R. J. (1963). Psychophysiological aspects of severe behaviour disorders. *Arch Gen Psychiatry*, *8*, 599–604.

Kuruoglu, A. C., Arikan, Z., Vural, G., Karatas, M., Arac, M., & Isik, E. (1996). Single photon emission computerised tomography in chronic alcoholism. Antisocial personality disorder may be associated with decreased frontal perfusion. *Br J Psychiatry*, *169*, 348–354.

Laakso, M. P., Gunning-Dixon, F., Vaurio, O., Repo-Tiihonen, E., Soininen, H., & Tiihonen, J. (2002). Prefrontal volumes in habitually violent subjects with antisocial personality disorder and type 2 alcoholism. *Psychiatry Res*, *114*, 95–102.

Laakso, M. P., Vaurio, O., Koivisto, E., Savolainen, L., Eronen, M., Aronen, H. J., . . . Tiihonen, J. (2001). Psychopathy and the posterior hippocampus. *Behav Brain Res*, *118*, 187–193.

Laakso, M. P., Vaurio, O., Savolainen, L., Repo, E., Soininen, H., Aronen, H. J., & Tiihonen, J. (2000). A volumetric MRI study of the hippocampus in type 1 and 2 alcoholism. *Behav Brain Res*, *109*, 177–186.

Lapierre, D., Braun, C. M., & Hodgins, S. (1995). Ventral frontal deficits in psychopathy: neuropsychological test findings. *Neuropsychologia*, *33*(2), 139–151.

Larsson, H., Andershed, H., & Lichtenstein, P. (2006). A genetic factor explains most of the variation in the psychopathic personality. *J Abnorm Psychol*, *115*, 221–230.

Lezak, M. D., Howieson, D. B., Bigler, E. D., & Tranel, D. (2012). *Neuropsychological assessment* (5th ed.). Oxford: Oxford University Press.

Lidberg, L., Levander, S., Schalling, D., & Lidberg, Y. (1978). Urinary catecholamines, stress, and psychopathy: a study of arrested men awaiting trial. *Psychosom Med*, *40*, 116–125.

Lilienfeld, S. O., & Andrews, B. P. (1996). Development and preliminary validation of a self-report measure of psychopathic personality traits in noncriminal populations. *J Personal Assess*, *66*, 488–524.

Lindberg, N., Tani, P., Appelberg, B., Naukkarinen, H., Rimón, R., Porkka-Heiskanen, T., & Virkkunen, M. (2003). Human impulsive aggression: a sleep research perspective. *J Psychiatr Res*, *37*, 313–324.

Llanes, S. J., & Kosson, D. S. (2006). Divided visual attention and left hemisphere activation among psychopathic and nonpsychopathic offenders. *J Psychopathol Behav Assess*, *28*(1), 9–18.

Lorber, M. F. (2004). Psychophysiology of aggression, psychopathy, and conduct problems: a meta-analysis. *Psychol Bull*, *130*(4), 531–552.

Lorenz, A. R., & Newman, J. P. (2002a). Deficient response modulation and emotion processing in low-anxious Caucasian psychopathic offenders: results from a lexical decision task. *Emotion*, *2*(2), 91–104.

Lorenz, A. R., & Newman, J. P. (2002b). Do emotion and information processing deficiencies found in Caucasian psychopaths generalize to African-American psychopaths? *Pers Individ Diff*, *32*, 1077–1086

Lorenz, A. R., & Newman, J. P. (2002c). Utilization of emotion cues in male and female offenders with antisocial personality disorder: results from a lexical decision task. *J Abnorm Psychol*, *111*(3), 513–516.

Maes, J. H., & Brazil, I. A. (2013). No clear evidence for a positive association between the interpersonal-affective aspects of psychopathy and executive functioning. *Psychiatry Res*, *210*(3), 1265–1274.

Malone, S., Taylor, J., Marmorstein, N., McGue, M., & Iacono, W. (2004). Genetic and environmental influences on antisocial behaviour and alcohol dependence from adolescence to early adulthood. *Dev Psychopathol*, *16*, 943–966.

Manuck, S. B., Flory, J. D., Ferrell, R. E., Dent, K. M., Mann, J., & Muldoo, M. F. (1999). Aggression and anger-related traits associated with a polymorphism of the tryptophan hydroxylase gene. *Biol Psychiatry*, *45*(5), 603–614.

Marsh, A. A. (2013). What can we learn about emotion by studying psychopathy? *Front Hum Neurosci*, *10*(7), 181.

Marsh, A. A. (2016). Understanding amygdala responsiveness to fearful expressions through the lens of psychopathy and altruism. *J Neurosci Res*, *94*(6), 513–525. http://dx.doi.org/10.1002/jnr.23668

Marsh, A. A., & Blair, R. (2008). Deficits in facial affect recognition among antisocial populations: a meta-analysis. *Neurosci Biobehav Rev*, *32*(3), 454–465.

Mason, D. A., & Frick, P. J. (2014). The heritability of antisocial behaviour: a meta-analysis of twin and adoption studies. *J Psychopathol Behav Assess*, *16* (4), 301–323.

McCallum, W. C. (1973). The CNV and conditionability in psychopaths. *Electroencephalogr Clin Neurophysiol*, *33*(Suppl.), 337–343.

McGuffin, P., & Gottesman, I. I. (1984). Genetic influences on normal and abnormal development. In M. Rutter & L. Hersov (Eds.), *Child psychiatry: modern approaches* (2nd ed., pp. 17–33). London: Blackwell.

McGuffin, P., & Thapar, A. (1992). The genetics of personality disorder. *Br J Psychiatry*, *160*, 12–23.

Mendoza, T. E. H., & Casados, J. J. P. (2014). Genetics of antisocial personality disorder: literature review. *Salud Mental*, *37*, 83–91.

Meyer-Lindenberg, A., Buckholtz, J. W., Kolachana, B. R., Hariri, A., Pezawas, L., Blasi, G., . . . Weinberger, D. R. (2006). Neural mechanisms of genetic risk for impulsivity and violence in humans. *Proc Natl Acad Sci U S A*, *103*, 6269–6274.

Miles, D., & Carey, G. (1997). Genetic and environmental architecture on human aggression. *J Person Soc Psychol*, *72*, 207–217.

Moran, P. (1999). *Antisocial personality disorder: an epidemiological perspective*. London: Gaskell.

Moreira, D., Pinto, M., Almeida, F., & Barbosa, F. (2016). Time perception deficits in impulsivity disorders: a systematic review. *Aggress Violent Behav*, *27*, 87–92.

Morgan, A. B., & Lilienfeld, S. O. (2000). A meta-analytic review of the relation between antisocial behaviour and neuropsychological measures of executive function. *Clin Psychol Rev*, *20*(1), 113–136.

Motzkin, J., Newman, J., Kiehl, K., & Koenigs, M. (2011). Reduced prefrontal connectivity in psychopathy. *J Neurosci*, *31*(48), 17348–17357. https://doi.org/10.1523/JNEUROSCI.4215-11.2011

Müller, J. L., Sommer, M., Dohnel, K., Weber, T., Schmidt-Wilcke, T., & Hajak, G. (2008). Disturbed prefrontal and temporal brain function during emotion and cognition interaction in criminal psychopathy. *Behav Sci Law*, *26*(1), 131–150.

Muller, J. L., Sommer, M., Wagner, V., Lange, K., Taschler, H., Roder, C. H., . . . Hajak, G. (2003). Abnormalities in emotion processing within cortical and subcortical regions in criminal psychopaths: evidence from a functional magnetic resonance imaging study using pictures with emotional content. *Biol Psychiatry*, *54*, 152–162.

Munafo, M. R., Clark, T. G., Moore, L. R., Payne, E., Walton, R., & Flint, J. (2003). Genetic polymorphisms and personality in healthy adults: a systematic review and meta-analysis. *Mol Psychiatry, 8*, 471–484.

Navas Collado, E., & Munoz Garcia, J. J. (2004). [Disexecutive syndrome in psychopathy]. *Rev Neurol, 38*(6), 582–590.

Newman, J. P., Curtin, J. J., Bertsch, J. D., & Baskin-Sommers, A. R. (2010). Attention moderates the fearlessness of psychopathic offenders. *Biol Psychiatry, 67*(1), 66–70. http://doi.org/10.1016/j.biopsych.2009.07.035

Nickerson, S. (2014). Brain abnormalities in psychopaths, A meta-analysis. *N Am J Psychol, 16*(1), 63–77.

Ogilvie, J. M., Stewart, A. L., Chan, R. C., & Shum, D. H. (2011). Neuropsychological measures of executive function and antisocial behaviour: a meta-analysis. *Criminology, 49*(4), 1063–1107. http://dx.doi.org/10.1111/j.1745-9125.2011.00252.x

Ogloff, J. R., & Wong, S. (1990). Electrodermal and cardiovascular evidence of a coping response in psychopaths. *Crim Just Behav, 17*, 231–245.

Oliveira-Souza, R., Hare, R., Bramati, I., Garrido, G., Ignácio, F., Tavor-Moll, F., & Moll, J. (2008). Psychopathy as a disorder of the moral brain: fronto-temporal grey matter reductions demonstrated by voxel-based morphometry. *NeuroImage, 40*(3), 1202–1213.

Patrick, C. J. (2008). Psychophysiological correlates of aggression and violence: an integrative review. *Philos Trans R Soc Lond B, 363*, 2543–2555. doi:10.1098/rstb.2008.0028

Patrick, C. J., Bradley, M. M., & Lang, P. J. (1993). Emotion in the criminal psychopath: startle reflex modulation. *J Abnorm Psychol, 102*, 82–92.

Patrick, C. J., Cuthbert, B. N., & Lang, P. J. (1994). Emotion-in the criminal psychopath: fear image processing. *J Abnorm Psychol, 103*, 523–534.

Perbal-Hatif, S. (2012). A neuropsychological approach to time estimation. *Dialogues Clin Neurosci, 14*(4), 425–432.

Ponce, G., Hoenicka, J., Jimenez-Arriero, M. A., Rodriguez-Jimenez, R., Aragues, M., Martin-Sune, N., . . . Palomo, T. (2008). DRD2 and ANKK1 genotype in alcohol-dependent patients with psychopathic traits: association and interaction study. *Br J Psychiatry, 193*(2), 121–125.

Ponce, G., Jimenez-Arriero, M. A., Rubio, G., Hoenicka, J., Ampuero, I., Ramos, J. A., & Palomo, T. (2003). The A1 allele of the DRD2 gene (TaqI A polymorphisms) is associated with antisocial personality in a sample of alcohol-dependent patients. *Eur Psychiatry, 18*(7), 356–360.

Ponce, G., Perez-Gonzalez, R., Aragues, M., Palomo, T., Rodriguez-Jimenez, R., Jimenez-Arriero, M. A., & Hoenicka, J. (2009). The ANKK1 kinase gene and psychiatric disorders. *Neurotox Res, 16*(1), 50–59.

Raine, A. (2008). From genes to brain to antisocial behaviour. *Curr Direct Psychol Sci, 17*(5), 323–328.

Raine, A., Bihrle, S., & LaCasse, L. (2000). Reduced prefrontal gray matter volume and reduced autonomic activity in antisocial personality disorder. *Arch Gen Psychiatry, 57*, 119–127.

Raine, A., Ishikawa, S. S., Arce, E., Lencz, T., Knuth, K. H., Bihrle, S., LaCasse, L., & Colletti, P. (2004). Hippocampal structural asymmetry in unsuccessful psychopaths. *Biol Psychiatry, 55*, 185–191.

Raine, A., Lencz, T., Bihrle, S., LaCasse, L., & Colletti, P. (2000). Reduced prefrontal gray matter volume and reduced autonomic activity in antisocial personality disorder. *Arch Gen Psychiatry, 57*, 119–127.

Raine, A., Lencz, T., Taylor, K., Hellige, J. B., Bihrle, S., LaCasse, L., . . . Colletti, P. (2003). Corpus callosum abnormalities in psychopathic antisocial individuals. *Arch Gen Psychiatry*, *60*, 1134–1142.

Räsänen, P., Hakko, H., Visuri, S., Paanila, J., Kapanen, P., Suomela, T., & Tiihonen, J. (1999). Serum testosterone levels, mental disorders and criminal behaviour. *Acta Psychiatr Scand*, *99*(5), 348–352.

Rhee, S. H., & Waldman, I. D. (2002). Genetic and environmental influences on antisocial behaviour: a meta-analysis of twin and adoption studies. *Psychol Bull*, *128*(3), 490–529.

Richell, R., Mitchell, D., Newman, C., Leonard, A., Baron-Cohen, S., & Blair, R. (2003). Theory of mind and psychopathy: can psychopathic individuals read the "language of the eyes"? *Neuropsychologia*, *41*(5), 523–526.

Rilling, J., Glenn, A., Jairam, M., Pagnoni, G., Goldsmith, D., Elfenbein, H., & Lilienfeld, S. (2007). Neural correlates of social cooperation and non-cooperation as a function of psychopathy. *Biol Psychiatry*, *11*(1), 1260–1271.

Robins, L., Locke, B., & Regier, D. (1991). An overview of psychiatric disorders in America. In L. Robins & D. Regier (Eds.), *Psychiatric disorders in America: the epidemiological catchment area study* (pp. 328–366). New York: Free Press.

Rudo-Hutt, A. S. (2015). Electroencephalography and externalizing behaviour: a meta-analysis. *Biol Psychol*, *105*, 1–19.

Sadeh, N., Javandi, S., Jackson, J., Reynolds, E. K., Potenza, M., Gelernter, J., . . . Verona, E. (2010). Serotonin transporter gene associations with psychopathic traits in youth vary as a function of socioeconomic resources. *J Abnorm Psychol*, *119*, 604–609.

Sakuta, A., & Fukushima A. (1998). A study on abnormal findings pertaining to the brain in criminals. *Internat Med J*, *5*, 283–292.

Santana, E. (2016). The brain of the psychopaths: a systematic review of structural neuroimaging studies. *Psychol Neurosci*, *9*(1), 420–443.

Schneider, F., Habel, U., Kessler, C., Posse, S., Grodd, W., & Muller-Gartner, H. W. (2000). Functional imaging of conditioned aversive emotional responses in antisocial personality disorder. *Neuropsychobiology*, *42*, 192–201.

Schug, R. A., Gao, Y., Glenn, A. L., Peskin, M., Yang, Y., & Raine, A. (2010). The developmental evidence base: neurobiological research and forensic applications. In G. J. Towl & D. A. Crighton (Eds.), *Forensic psychology*. Chichester, UK: Blackwell.

Schulsinger, F. (1982). Psychopathy, heredity and environment. *Internat J Ment Health*, *1*, 190–206.

Seguin, J. R. (2004). Neurocognitive elements of antisocial behaviour: relevance of an orbitofrontal cortex account. *Brain Cogn*, *55*(1), 185–197.

Shamay-Tsoory, S. G., Harari, H., Aharon-Peretz, J., & Levkovitz, Y. (2010). The role of the orbitofrontal cortex in affective theory of mind deficits in criminal offenders with psychopathic tendencies. *Cortex*, *46*(5), 668–677.

Siddle, D. A. T., & Trasler, G. B. (1981). The psychophysiology of psychopathic behaviour. In M. J. Christie & P. G. Mellett (Eds.), *Foundations of psychosomatics* (pp. 283–303). Chichester, UK: John Wiley.

Singleton, N., Meltzer, H., Gatward, R., Coid, J., & Deasy, D. (1998). *Psychiatric morbidity among prisoners in England and Wales*. London: HMSO.

Slutske, W. S. (2001). The genetics of antisocial behaviour. *Curr Psychiatry Rep*, *3*, 158–162.

Smith, S. S., Arnett, P. A., & Newman, J. P. (1992). Neuropsychological differentiation of psychopathic and nonpsychopathic criminal offenders. *Pers Individ Diff*, *13*(11), 1233–1243.

Sneiderman, A. (2006). *Word usage patterns in psychopathic jail inmates* (Unpublished doctoral dissertation). George Mason University, Washington, DC.

Sobhani, M., & Bechara, A. (2011). A somatic marker perspective of immoral and corrupt behaviour. *Soc Neurosci, 6*(5–6), 640–652.

Soderstrom, H., Blennow, K., Manhem, A., & Forsman, A. (2001). CSF studies in violent offenders. I. 5-HIAA as a negative and HVA as a positive predictor of psychopathy. *J Neur Transm, 108*, 869–878.

Soderstrom, H., Blennow, K., Sjodin, A., & Forsman, A. (2003). New evidence for an association between the CSF HVA: 5-HIAA ratio and psychopathic traits. *J Neurol Neurosurg Psychiatry, 74*, 918–921.

Soderstrom, H., Hultin, L., Tullberg, M., Wikkelso, C., Ekholm, S., & Forsman, A. (2002). Reduced frontotemporal perfusion in psychopathic personality. *Psychiatry Res, 114*, 81–94.

Soderstrom H., Tullberg M., Wikkelsö, C., Ekholm, S., & Forsman, A. (2000). Reduced regional cerebral blood flow in non-psychotic violent offenders. *Psychiatry Res Neuroimag Sec, 98*, 29–41.

Sommer, M., Hajak, G., Dohnel, K., Schwerdtner, J., Meinhardt, J., & Muller, J. L. (2006). Integration of emotion and cognition in patients with psychopathy. *Prog Brain Res, 156*, 457–466.

Stålenheim, E. G., Eriksson, E., Von Knorring, L., & Wide, L. (1998). Testosterone as a biological marker in psychopathy and alcoholism. *Psychiatry Res, 9*, 79–88.

Stevens, D., Charman, T., & Blair, R. J. (2001). Recognition of emotion in facial expressions and vocal tones in children with psychopathic tendencies. *J Genet Psychol, 162*, 201–211.

Stevens, M. C., Kaplan, R. F., & Hesselbrock, V. M. (2003). Executive-cognitive functioning in the development of antisocial personality disorder. *Addict Behav, 28*(2), 285–300.

Swann, A. C., Lijffijt, M., Lane, S. D., Steinberg, J. L., & Moeller, F. (2009). Trait impulsivity and response inhibition in antisocial personality disorder. *J Psychiatr Res, 43*(12), 1057–1063.

Tassy, S. (2011). La nécessité de distinguer le jugement et le choix subjectif dans les neurosciences cognitives de la morale. *Med Sci, 27*(10), 889–894.

Taylor, A., & Kim-Cohen, J. (2007). Meta-analysis of gene-environment interactions in developmental psychopathology. *Dev Psychopathol, 19*, 1029–1037.

Taylor, J., Loney, B. R., Bobadillo, L., Iacono, W. G., & McGue, M. (2003). Genetic and environmental influence on psychopathy trait dimensions in a community sample of male twins. *J Abnorm Child Psychol, 31*, 633–645.

Thompson, D. F., & Ramos, C. L. (2014). Psychopathy: clinical features, developmental basis and therapeutic challenges. *J Clin Pharm Ther, 39*, 485–495.

Thompson, P. M., Cannon, T. D., Narr, K. L., van Erp, T., Poutanen, V. P., & Huttunen, M. (2001). Genetic influences on brain structure. *Nature Neurosci, 4*, 1253–1258.

Tonkonogy, J. M. (1991). Violence and temporal lobe lesion: Head CT and MRI data. *J Neuropsychiatry, 3*, 189–196.

Törneke, N. (2010). *Learning RFT: an introduction to relational frame theory and its clinical application.* Oakland, CA: New Harbinger.

van Honk, J., Peper, J. S., & Schutter, D. J. L. G. (2005). Testosterone reduces unconscious fear but not consciously experienced anxiety: implications for the disorders of fear and anxiety. *Biol Psychiatry, 58*, 218–225.

van Honk, J., & Schutter, D. J. L. G. (2006). Unmasking feigned sanity: a neurobiological model of emotion processing in primary psychopathy. *Cogn Neuropsychiatry*, *11*(3), 285–306.

Varlamov, A., Khalifa, N., Liddle, P., Duggan, C., & Howard, R. (2011). Cortical correlates of impaired self-regulation in personality disordered patients with traits of psychopathy. *J Personal Disord*, *25*(1), 75–88. doi:10.1521/pedi.2011.25.1.75

Veit, R., Flor, H., Erb, M., Hermann, C., Lotze, M., Grodd, W., & Birbaumer, N. (2002). Brain circuits involved in emotional learning in antisocial behaviour and social phobia in humans. *Neurosci Lett*, *328*, 233–236.

Venables, N. C., & Patrick, C. J. (2014). Reconciling discrepant findings for P3 brain response in criminal psychopathy through reference to the concept of externalizing proneness. *Psychophysiology*, *51*(5), 427–436.

Vevera, J., Stopkova, R., Bes, M., Albrecht, T., Papezova, H., Zukov, I., Raboch, J., & Stopka, P. (2009). COMT polymorphisms in impulsively violent offenders with antisocial personality disorder. *Neuroendocrinol Lett*, *30*, 753–756.

Viding, E., Blair, R. J. R., Moffitt, T. E., & Plomin, R. (2005). Evidence for substantial genetic risk for psychopathy in 7-year-olds. *J Child Psychol Psychiatry*, *46*, 592–597.

Viding, E., Larsson, H., & Jones, A. J. (2008). Quantitative genetic studies of antisocial behaviour. *Philos Trans R Soc Lond B*, *363*, 2519–2527. doi:10.1098/rstb.2008.0037

Virkkunen, M. (1986). Reactive hypoglycaemic tendency among habitually violent offenders. *Nutr Rev* (Suppl.), May.

Virkkunen, M., De Jong, J., & Bartko, J. (1989). Relationship of psychosocial variables to recidivism in violent offenders and impulsive fire setters: a follow-up study. *Arch Gen Psychiatry*, *46*, 600–603.

Virkkunen, M., Eggert, M., Rawlings, R., & Linnoila, M. (1996). A prospective follow-up study of alcoholic violent offenders and fire setters. *Arch Gen Psychiatry*, *53*, 523–529.

Völlm, B. (2006). Neuroanatomical correlates of antisocial personality disorder and psychopathy. In F. J. Chen (Ed.), *Focus on brain mapping* (pp. 155–183). New York: Nova.

Völlm, B., Richardson, P., Stirling, J., Elliott, R., Dolan, M., Chaudry, I., . . . Deakin B. (2004). Neurobiological substrates of antisocial and borderline personality disorder—preliminary results of a functional fMRI study. *Crim Behav Ment Health*, *14*, 39–55.

Waid, W. M., & Orne, M. T. (1982). Reduced electrodermal response to conflict, failure to inhibit dominant behaviours, and delinquency proneness. *J Personal Soc Psychol*, *43*, 769–774.

Waldman, I. D., & Rhee, S. H. (2007). Genetic and environmental influences on psychopathy and antisocial behaviour. In C. Patrick (Ed.), *Handbook of psychopathy* (pp. 205–228). New York: Guilford Press.

Widom, C. S., & Brzustowicz, L. M. (2006). MAOA and the "cycle of violence": childhood abuse and neglect, MAOA genotype, and risk for violent and antisocial behaviour. *Biol Psychiatry*, *60*, 684–689.

Wilson, K., Juodis, M., & Porter, S. (2011). Fear and loathing in psychopaths: a meta-analytic investigation of the facial affect recognition deficit. *Crim Just Behav*, *38*(7), 659–668. http://dx.doi.org/10.1177/0093854811404120

Yang, Y., & Raine, A. (2009). Prefrontal structural and functional brain imaging findings in antisocial, violent, and psychopathic individuals, A meta-analysis. *Psychiatry Res Neuroimag*, *174*(2), 81–88.

Yang, Y., Raine, A., Narr, K., Colletti, P., & Toga, A. (2009). Localization of deformations within the amygdala in individuals with psychopathy. *Arch Gen Psychiatry*, *66*(1), 986–994.

Yildirim, B. O., & Derksen, J. J. (2015). Clarifying the heterogeneity in psychopathic samples: towards a new continuum of primary and secondary psychopathy. *Aggress Violent Behav*, *24*, 9–41. http://dx.doi.org/10.1016/j.avb.2015.05.001

Yoder, K., Porges, E., & Decety, J. (2015). Amygdala subnuclei connectivity in response to violence reveals unique influence of individual differences in psychopathic traits in a nonforensic sample. *Hum Brain Mapp*, *36*(1), 1417–1428.

15 The Neurobiological Basis of Avoidant Personality Disorder

■ THERESA WILBERG AND KENNETH SILK

Avoidant personality disorder (AvPD), a relatively recent diagnosis first introduced in the *Diagnostic and Statistical Manual of Mental Disorders* (third edition [*DSM-III*]; American Psychiatric Association [APA], 1980), was strongly influenced by Millon's (1981) description of a personality type characterized by social hypersensitivity and reactivity to others' affects and states of mind. This description originated in the early 20th century. Kretchmer (1925) described traits such as extreme shyness and efforts to avoid external stimuli as one of the polarities of a schizoid temperament. In *DSM-III* the anxious avoidance of AvPD was distinguished from the affective coldness and interpersonal indifference of schizoid personality disorder. AvPD also has some resemblance to the personality type described by Horney (1945) that was characterized by a tendency to move away from others, in contrast to moving toward or against people. Within the psychoanalytic tradition, a similar construct is found in the phobic character related to conflicts around longings for closeness combined with fear of intimacy.

In the fifth edition of the *DSM*, AvPD is described as a pervasive pattern of social inhibition, feelings of inadequacy, and hypersensitivity to negative evaluation (APA, 2013). The seven specific criteria of AvPD cover areas of social avoidance, novelty restriction, sensitivity to rejection and criticism, feelings of inferiority and inadequacy, and restraint within intimate relationships due to shame or fear of ridicule. Despite the high prevalence of AvPD in clinical settings as well as in the general population, AvPD is an underresearched diagnostic category. This holds not only for the phenomenological aspects of avoidant pathology, its prognosis, and its treatment but also with respect to the neurobiological underpinnings of the disorder.

As a diagnostic category AvPD has been subjected to the same general criticisms as those regarding the limitations of personality disorders as diagnostic categories. The validity of the diagnosis has been questioned further because of the overlap with social anxiety disorders (SAD), particularly the generalized type of social phobia. During past decades it has been disputed whether AvPD is just a more severe form of SAD (Bogels et al., 2010). This has probably contributed to the decreasing trend of research publications that directly address AvPD relative to publications on social phobia (Mendlowicz et al., 2006). When compared with social phobia, AvPD is associated with significantly more severe impairment in personality functioning and therefore deserves placement among the personality disorders (Hummelen et al., 2006; Marques et al., 2012; Eikenæs et al., 2013). The social fear associated with AvPD may be more related to problems with anxiety about intimacy and close relationships reinforced by insecure attachments, temperamentally based shyness, and an inclination toward behavioral avoidance than is the social anxiety found in social phobia. Nevertheless, research on social phobia, including its biological correlates, is highly relevant to the neurobiology of AvPD. As in SAD, attention bias toward potentially negative social cues, biased interpretation or deficits in social processing, and self-focused attention may apply also to many subjects with AvPD (Bowles & Meyer, 2008; Morrison & Heimberg, 2013).

Patients with AvPD constitute a heterogeneous group, a fact not immediately apparent in the formal definition of the disorder, which more or less seems to constitute a psychometrically one-dimensional construct (Hummelen et al., 2006). Co-occurring traits from other personality as well as symptom (old Axis I) disorders contribute to this heterogeneity. Co-occurring depression, substance misuse, and other anxiety disorders are frequent in clinical samples (Ralevski et al., 2005). However, some clinical characteristics of subjects with AvPD appear not well described in the current classification. While low self-esteem is a prominent feature of the disorder, in the clinical arena we find many subjects for whom the feelings of inferiority or inadequacy touch upon a more profound identity disturbance grounded in poor access to broader areas of mental life. Many patients present with constricted affective expression that suggests difficulty in appreciating the breadth of human emotional experience (one of the ways that avoidant and schizoid may have initially been confounded). The nature of this difficulty is not well understood currently but may lie in deficits in basic emotional systems or regulation processes involving both positive and negative affects (Taylor et al., 2004; Johansen et al., 2013). According to clinical observations AvPD is often associated with low affect consciousness or alexithymic features, that is, deficits in the cognitive processing of emotional experiences that suggest a limited capacity to symbolize emotions and to elaborate (mentally and experientially) upon emotional experiences (Nicolò et al., 2011). In combination with poor autobiographic memory, such features probably contribute to the poor sense of self, as well as to the low agency and self-directedness seen in many AvPD patients (Fivush et al., 2011).

Subjects at the moderate to severe end of the severity spectrum tend to have low metacognitive or mentalization capacities, not only of their own but also of others' minds, indicating that processes in the "social brain" are affected (DiMaggio et al., 2007). Social interaction may be confusing and anxiety provoking, ultimately stimulating behavioral and mental withdrawal as self-protective strategies. A salient feature of subjects with AvPD is their chronic feeling of alienation and loneliness.

In some patients, the social avoidance may be related to a lack of social skills due to milder forms of autistic traits (which in the past might have been labeled as mild Asperger's syndrome). Autism is a dimensional phenomenon and can be difficult to detect in subjects without striking peculiarities in appearance or habits. Adding to the heterogeneity of AvPD, and based on family studies and neurocognitive measures, is the suggestion that AvPD might be considered as part of the schizophrenia spectrum (Fogelson et al., 2010).

At the phenomenological level, then, AvPD comprises a wide array of traits and symptoms. Such features may correspond to different underlying neurobiological processes and dispositions. However, many of the dimensions underlying AvPD are not exclusive to AvPD but to a greater or lesser degree are shared with other disorders. This fits well with the Research Domain Criteria approach of the National Institute of Mental Health where the focus is on dimensions of observable behavior and neurobiological measures that cut across different diagnoses to increase our knowledge and appreciation of the possible neurobiological underpinnings of mental disorders.

■ OUTLINE OF CHAPTER

In the present chapter we report neurobiological findings with particular relevance to AvPD. Since the body of biologically oriented research that directly addresses AvPD is scarce, we also focus on some areas and dimensions assumed to be of special interest with respect to AvPD. But, as the introduction suggests, there are many different psychiatric disorders, cognitive styles, and interpersonal patterns that can impinge upon, overlap with, or influence the patient with AvPD. We then need to be selective in what areas we consider, knowing beforehand that we will be limited and less than thorough since we cannot review each possible biological underpinning for each overlapping or impinging influence on the ultimate clinical picture of AvPD.

We begin by reporting on biological findings that pertain to the diagnosis of AvPD, trying to summarize what has been done in the field of genetics, neurotransmitters, and neuroimaging. We then turn to areas of temperament, emotional dysfunction, attachment, and stress regulation. While these areas could apply across all personality disorders, we try to emphasize how they might apply more specifically to AvPD. There are phenomena such as attention, social processing, ruminations, autobiographical memory, self-esteem regulation, agency and self-direction, and social exclusion that may, at least in some people, either contribute to the development of AvPD and/or play a role in its maintenance, but neurobiological data in AvPD or social phobia are scarce. We bypass these not only because of space limitations but also because these issues are more general and cut across different diagnoses both within personality disorders as well as mental states (i.e., the old Axis I division). We leave discussion of biological issues in autism and schizophrenia to others.

■ NEUROBIOLOGICAL FINDINGS IN AvPD

Herpertz and coworkers (2000) investigated psychophysiological affect correlates in female patients with borderline personality disorder (BPD, $n = 24$), AvPD ($n = 23$), and normal controls ($n = 27$), while subjects viewed pictures with pleasant, unpleasant, and neutral emotional content. Psychophysiologic measures included skin conductance response (SCR), heart rate (HR), and startle response as assessed by electromyography (amplitude and latency), before and during the exposure. Despite no differences in self-ratings of emotional state before exposure to pictures, AvPD patients, compared with BPD patients and normal controls, had higher physiological base rate startle amplitude before beginning the experiment, but there were no between-group differences in baseline SCR or HR. During exposure there was a nonsignificant trend of higher mean startle amplitude among AvPD patients. The AvPD group had higher SCR than BPD subjects, though the response was not significantly different from normal controls. HR changes in AvPD subjects were not different from normal controls. The study actually focused on hyperresponsivity of BPD subjects (which was not confirmed). However, the authors speculate whether the higher baseline startle blinks in the AvPD group could reflect higher amounts of contextual fear, increased wariness of environmental events, and a general readiness to display defensive reactions to perceived aversive and threatening stimuli.

Joyce and coworkers (2003a) investigated eight genetic polymorphisms of the dopamine D4 receptor (DRD4) and three polymorphisms of the dopamine D3 receptor in a sample of 145 depressed patients. They found strong associations between both the two-repeat allele of the DRD4 exon III polymorphism and the T,T genotype of the DRD4–521 C>T polymorphism and AvPD, as well as obsessive personality disorder and traits, as assessed by Structured Diagnostic Interview for DSM-III-R. AvPD is usually associated with high levels of the temperament dimension harm avoidance and low levels of novelty seeking (Svrakic et al., 1993; Joyce et al., 2003a), but there were no associations between the DRD4 polymorphisms and any of Cloninger's temperament dimensions (i.e., harm avoidance, reward dependence, novelty seeking, or persistence; Cloninger et al., 1993). The authors suggest that the conflicting findings regarding genetic polymorphisms may arise from the problem of phenotype definition.

Bruce and coworkers (2004) compared serotonergic functioning in female patients with bulimia nervosa with ($n = 13$) or without ($n = 23$) co-occurring AvPD and normal eating controls without personality disorder ($n = 23$). Serotonin (5-HT) promotes prolactin secretion from the pituitary, and 5-HT-induced alterations in plasma prolactin is thought to reflect central serotonergic functioning. Plasma levels of prolactin were measured before and after administration of the partial 5-HT agonist meta-chlorophenylpiperazine (m-CPP). The patients also underwent a modified Go No-Go laboratory task to measure behavioral inhibition versus disinhibition in response to reward and punishment cues. Patients with bulimia and co-occurring AvPD had a blunted prolactin response following m-CPP challenge compared with the two other groups, indicating lower sensitivity to serotonergic activation. They also tended to be more behaviorally inhibited in response to cues for punishment. The authors suggest that co-occurring AvPD may contribute to the serotonergic dysregulation in patients with bulimia nervosa.

To test the hypothesis that the emotional reactivity characteristic of BPD may be related to anomalous habituation to emotional stimuli, Koenigsberg and coworkers (2014) investigated behavioral and neural correlates of habituation in patients with BPD ($n = 19$), AvPD ($n = 23$), and healthy controls ($n = 25$). The study focused on BPD, but it is also the first reported functional imaging study of AvPD. During functional magnetic resonance imaging (fMRI), the subjects viewed novel and repeated pictures with emotionally negative or neutral content. While the results indicated anomalous habituation in both diagnostic (personality-disordered) groups, there were some significant differences in neural activity. Unlike healthy subjects, neither BPD nor AvPD patients exhibited increased activity in the dorsal anterior cingulate cortex when viewing repeated versus novel pictures. Both diagnostic groups also exhibited smaller increases in insula-amygdala functional connectivity compared with healthy subjects, and both did not show habituation in self-report ratings of emotional intensity of the pictures. However, AvPD patients differed from the two other groups in some respects. Compared to the healthy controls, AvPD patients showed less increase in connectivity between insula and a broad region in middle frontal gyrus and posterior cingulate with more increase in connectivity to the cerebellum. Compared to BPD, the AvPD group showed less insula-ventral anterior cingulate functional connectivity and greater increases to the cerebellum. The authors emphasize that insula and anterior cingulate may be key nodes in a network dedicated to assessing salience of external and internal stimuli, allocation of attentional and control resources, and preparing for action. They state that the decreased connectivity to this region in AvPD patients suggests the possibility of a distinct mechanism accounting for the affective dysregulation in these patients.

While the reviewed studies include different levels of neurobiological data, they reveal that research on neurobiology of AvPD remains at a very early stage. AvPD has been included mainly as a comparison group in studies focusing on BPD. Hopefully, such studies may lay the groundwork for further research with AvPD as the primary focus to generate specific and more pertinent hypotheses rather than our current knowledge of neurobiological correlates of AvPD that is based on assumptions and indirect evidence.

Heredity

Results from heredity studies point toward a significant constitutional contribution to the development of AvPD. In two twin studies, the reported heritability estimates of AvPD were 28% in a clinical sample and 35% in a sample from the general population (Reichborn-Kjennerud, 2010). Results from this large population-based twin sample suggest that in females there may be a common genetic vulnerability to AvPD and social phobia and that individuals with high genetic liability may develop AvPD or social phobia as a result of environmental risk factors unique to each disorder (Reichborn-Kjennerud et al., 2007).

Personality Dimensions and Temperament

AvPD is related to neuroticism, introversion, harm avoidance, low novelty seeking, and behavioral inhibition (Samuel & Widiger, 2008; Svrakic et al., 1993; Joyce et al., 2003b; Meyer, 2002; Taylor et al., 2004; Claes et al., 2009; Pastor et al., 2007; Kimbrei et al., 2012). While these personality and temperament dimensions are derived from different sources of information and measurement (e.g., factor analyses of human vocabulary, animal research), they are significantly correlated when assessed by self-report in human subjects, probably due to some shared definitional characteristics.

Neuroticism as measured by the Revised NEO Personality Inventory (Costa & McCrae, 1992) is characterized by negative emotionality such as a tendency to experience anxiety, depression, vulnerability, and hostility. In Cloninger's psychobiological model, assessed by the Temperament and Character Inventory (Cloninger et al., 1993), harm avoidance (HA) reflects the tendency to respond strongly to aversive stimuli. HA is thought to play a role in inhibition or cessation of behaviors. In contrast, novelty seeking (NS) reflects the tendency to respond strongly to novelty and cues for reward, as well as relief from punishment. NS is thought to influence the activation and initiating of behaviors (Cloninger et al., 1993). The concept of NS overlaps to some extent with the behavioral activation system (BAS) in the revised Reinforcement Sensitivity Theory (RST; Corr, 2008). The BAS is defined as being sensitive to (activated by) reward and is thus associated with positive emotions and approach behavior. The behavioral inhibition system (BIS) of the RST, on the other hand, is activated by goal conflicts (e.g., approach-withdrawal conflicts) and is associated with risk assessment, avoidance, and negative emotions (Corr, 2008; Balconi et al., 2009). The most common measure of BIS and BAS is the BIS/BAS scales of Carver and White (1994). A higher BIS sensitivity has been suggested as a core vulnerability for Cluster C personality disorders, including AvPD (Caseras et al., 2001). A few studies have also found a relation between AvPD or Cluster C traits and lower scores on some BAS subscales (Meyer, 2002; Pastor et al., 2007).

Certainly a large number of biological processes undergird human temperament. Genetic studies have particularly focused on gene polymorphisms of neurotransmitter receptors and transporters, like serotonin, dopamine, and norepinephrine, glutamate, γ-aminobutyric acid, enzymes that degrade amines (e.g., monoamine oxidase), and catecholamine-O-methyltransferase (COMT), as well as opioids and hormones such as opiate peptides, oxytocin, and vasopressin (Kagan et al., 2007; Pelka-Wyisiecka et al., 2012).

Neuroticism and HA have in some studies been associated with a serotonin transporter promoter polymorphism, the 5-HTTLPR short allele, in line with Cloninger's original hypothesis that HA is associated with serotonergic function (Lesch et al., 1996; Schinka et al., 2004; Sen et al., 2004; Lahat et al., 2011), though there are studies that contradict these associations (Lang et al., 2004; Pelka-Wysiecka et al., 2012). The short allele is less efficient and leads to higher concentration of serotonin in the synaptic cleft. Interestingly Jacob and coworkers (2004) found an association between the 5-HTTLPR short allele and neuroticism/HA only in subjects with Cluster C disorders, in contrast to subjects with Cluster B disorders or healthy controls. Explorations of a relationship between anxious traits and polymorphisms in other 5-HT related genes, such as 5-HT1a and 5-HT2a, have yielded mixed or negative results (Serretti et al., 2007), but anxiety-related traits have in a few studies been associated with polymorphisms located on the tryptophan hydroxylase 2 gene (TPH2), the rate-limiting enzyme for serotonin synthesis that is thought to impact serotonin availability (Gutknecht et al., 2007; Reuter et al., 2007). A few studies point toward possible associations between anxious traits and introversion and various polymorphisms of the COMT gene, an enzyme responsible for degrading dopamine, epinephrine, and norepinephrine (Enoch et al., 2003; Stein et al., 2005).

It may be assumed that NS and BAS is influenced by dopaminergic activity, based on the hypothesis that the dopamine system mediates positive emotions and reward-related behaviors (Cloninger, 1993; Reuter, 2008). NS has been associated with DRD4 polymorphisms in some studies but not in others. Findings indicate that there may not be a simple association between dopamine-related polymorphisms and NS/BAS (Kluger et al., 2002). For example, in one study a DRD2 polymorphism interacted with a polymorphism of the COMT gene to predict BAS levels (Reuter et al., 2006). Genetic polymorphism may also interact with environmental influences like in the study of Das and coworkers (2001) where a certain DRD4 polymorphism moderated the effect of childhood adversities on resilience, possibly mediated by greater BAS sensitivity.

Thus some have found relationships between serotonin and dopamine functioning and personality and temperament dimensions found in AvPD, but results have been inconsistent and not easily replicable in genome-wide association studies (Shifman et al., 2008; Verweij et al., 2010; Terraciane et al., 2010; de Moore et al., 2012). Personality traits are complex phenotypes, and various traits are influenced by many genotypes with small effect sizes. Linking molecular genetics to personality traits and disorder is further complicated by age, race, and gender-specific effects and interactions of multiple genes and environmental factors (Stein et al., 2005; Caspi et al., 2010; Pelka-Wysiecka et al., 2012). More molecular genetic studies of thoroughly described subjects with AvPD are needed in our search for endophenotypes with clearer genetic connections. However, at this time there are methodological challenges and conceptual issues that present significant problems in performing molecular genetic studies of human behavior (Flint et al., 2010, pp. 206–214).

Temperament factors are thought to be related to distinct neuroanatomical pathways and processes involving regions such as the amygdala, the septohippocampal system, striatum and prefrontal cortex, as well as other structures such as the hypothalamus, cingulate, and periaqueductal grey (Cloninger et al., 1993; Reuter, 2008; Cherubin et al., 2008; De Pascalis et al., 2010). Still, the neuroanatomical correlates of temperament in humans remain incompletely understood, though we are slowly making some progress. Neuroticism has been related to structural brain variables such as smaller total brain volume, reduced thickness in specific prefrontal regions, smaller frontotemporal surface area, and widespread decrease in white matter microstructure (Wright et al., 2007; De Young et al., 2010; Bjørnebekk et al., 2013). Also, HA and NS have been associated with structural variance in specific brain areas and with reduced grey matter integrity in several regions such as in corticolimbic pathways, which has been interpreted as a possible mechanism to explain biased interpretation and sensitivity to social cues in individuals high on trait anxiety (Pujol et al., 2002; Gardini et al., 2009; Westlye et al., 2011). Only a limited number of studies have inconsistently demonstrated structural neuroanatomical relationships associated with the BIS/BAS system (Cherubin et al., 2008).

Expanding our knowledge of temperamental vulnerability through variations in basic brain-behavioral systems with measures of adult personality remains a challenge. Kagan and coworkers (1988) have approached the phenomenon of behavioral inhibition differently in their prospective observational studies of small infants. They use the term "behavioral inhibition" to describe the tendency of some infants to withdraw and show negative affect in response to new people, places, events, and objects (i.e., novelty). Such inhibited behavior may be rooted in the child's threshold for arousal evident as early as four month of age. Highly reactive babies, those showing more extreme levels of negative affect, motor activity, and irritability in response to novel stimuli, may reflect a distinct temperament type characterized by a lower threshold for limbic-hypothalamic arousal to novelty or unexpected changes in the environment, present in 20% of the population (Kagan & Snidman, 1999). Highly reactive babies tend to become inhibited children and have been modestly associated with peripheral biological measurements, that is, greater sympathetic tone in the cardiovascular system, increased salivary cortisol levels, and asymmetry of cortical activation in EEG, favoring a more active right frontal area, as well as greater general cortical activation, when compared to extremely low reactive or uninhibited children (Kagan & Snidman, 1999; Calkins et al., 1996).

Traits related to behavioral inhibition appear modestly stable over time from the second to the fifth year, but they are a risk for anxious symptoms, particularly SAD later in childhood and early adolescence (Swartz et al., 1999; Kagan & Snidman, 1999). But these children have not been examined for potential risk of AvPD in adulthood. However, Caspi and coworkers (1996) followed a group of children labeled "inhibited" in a large prospective general population study. At three years these children had been characterized as shy, fearful, and easily upset, based on behavioral observation and cognitive and motor tasks. At the age of 18 these "inhibited" children described themselves as overcontrolled, harm-avoidant, and nonassertive (Caspi et al., 1996). But no neurobiological data was reported.

Central to Kagan's model is reactivity in response to novelty in general, with the idea of "novelty" not restricted to people or negative emotional stimuli. Of note, therefore, is the study of Taylor and coworkers (2004) who examined samples of undergraduate students and found an association between AvPD and self-reported avoidance of novelty, as well as avoidance of non-social events. In order to study novelty Swartz and coworkers (2003a) developed a paradigm of novel versus familiar faces, all with emotionally neutral expressions. They investigated via fMRI 22 adults who in their second year of life had been categorized as inhibited or uninhibited. The inhibited in the past group showed a significantly greater response in both left and right amygdala to novel faces, while there were no group differences in response to familiar faces (Swartz et al., 2003b). The study of Koenigsberg and coworkers (2014) described previously found anomalous habituation to negative emotional pictures in subjects with AvPD, but so far no fMRI study has focused particularly on response to emotionally neutral novel stimuli in AvPD.

■ EMOTIONAL DYSFUNCTION

Many theories point to a dysfunction in the emotional domain in AvPD. Millon (1981) described individuals with AvPD as having low tolerance for painful feelings related to perceptions of inadequacy and negative self-worth, and interpersonal avoidance was proposed to serve as a protection against real and imagined psychic pain. Millon suggested that such protective strategies might pervade every facet of emotional life by producing a muddling of emotions or repression of all feelings, including positive feelings. Other clinical theories also hold the view that AvPD is associated with low affect tolerance or a general affect phobia (Beck & Freeman, 1990; McCullough et al., 2003). More recently, the metacognitive theory of DiMaggio and coworkers (2007) claims that patients with AvPD have more profound difficulty identifying their own mental states, both with respect to emotions and thoughts, with subsequent impaired ability to convey their experiences.

Although there are few empirical studies of emotions in individuals with AvPD, these notions have some support in a clinical study reporting a low level of affect consciousness in patients with AvPD compared to BPD, including conceptual expression of affects (Johansen et al., 2013), and in studies linking Cluster C personality disorders with higher levels of alexithymia and experiential avoidance, even though the specificity regarding the different Cluster C PDs is uncertain (Honkalampi et al., 2001; Nicolo et al., 2011). Investigating clinical and nonclinical samples Taylor and coworkers (2004) found associations between AvPD and self-reported avoidance of both positive and negative emotions. Further, a higher degree of negative affect and a lower degree of positive affect was reported in AvPD students compared to normal controls (Ye et al., 2011), supporting the relationships between AvPD and higher neuroticism/HA/negative emotionality and lower extroversion/NS/positive emotionality.

Thus emotional dysfunction appears significant in AvPD and could involve both positive and negative emotions, but so far research on specific affects is rare. Adaptive social functioning depends, in part, on the degree to which one is capable of recognizing and discriminating emotions expressed by others. The first study of facial recognition in AvPD applied morphing facial expressions of fear, anger, disgust, sadness, surprise, and happiness (Rosenthal et al., 2011). AvPD individuals made more errors in the classification of fear at full emotional expression compared to normal controls. There were no differences in the classification of the other emotions or regarding speed of emotions recognition. The findings point to an underlying deficit in processing of fear-related social cues, and the authors discuss whether individuals with AvPD may regulate fear-stimulated emotional arousal by directing attention away from the face and thereby impair perception accuracy. Less accuracy of fear recognition has also been reported in SAD, though studies of emotion recognition in SAD have mixed results (Garner et al., 2009).

Frontolimbic circuits are central for emotional processing and regulation, but several other networks are involved as well. The prefrontal frontal cortex, the orbitofrontal cortex, and the ventromedial prefrontal cortex, which are phylogenetically recent brain regions, regulate impulses, emotions, and behavior via inhibitory top-down control of emotional-processing structures (Martin et al., 2009). The phylogenetically older limbic system comprises structures such as the amygdala and hippocampus but also includes the cingulate and insular cortex that integrate sensory, affective, and cognitive components of pain and process information regarding internal bodily states. The amygdala has a key role in affective reactivity, and it is proposed that diminished communication between amygdala and prefrontal cortex may result in reduced capacity for integration of cognitive and behavioral emotional arousal (Aleman et al., 2008; Baur et al., 2011).

Consistent with this hypothesis, SAD has been associated with increased activation of the amygdala, decreased connectivity between amygdala and orbitofrontal cortex, and increased amygdala-medial prefrontal cortex connectivity. SAD has further been associated with increased insula reactivity, dorsal anterior cingulate hyporeactivity, and decreased insula-dorsal anterior cingulate cortex connectivity during exposure to fearful faces or anticipation of fear-provoking situations (Klump et al., 2012; Freitas-Ferrari et al., 2010). A comparison with the results of Koenigsberg and coworkers (2014) in AvPD is of course hampered by methodological differences but suggests a possibility for some functional similarities in emotional perception and cognitive regulation of fear and negative emotions between AvPD and SAD. More studies are needed. Greater amygdala hyperreactivity to emotional stimuli has been related to trait anxiety, but studies of AvPD are largely lacking (Hariri, 2009). However, in an ongoing study AvPD patients have shown greater right amygdala activity than healthy controls when viewing negative pictures relative to neutral pictures and greater bilateral amygdala activation during anticipation of carrying out a reappraisal task (Koenigsberg, unpublished data). The increases in amygdala activity were in proportion to subjects' self-reported state- and trait anxiety levels.

Recent findings suggest that patients with SAD may not only have altered processing of specific social fear related stimuli. Exposure to or anticipation of nonsocial emotional stimuli was related to increased activation in brain regions involved in both emotional arousal and in attention and perception processing, with decreased activation in orbitofrontal cortex in socially anxious patients compared to healthy controls (Brühl et al., 2011). One may assume that this could be the case for patients diagnosed with AvPD as well. Finally, knowledge of neural correlates of AvPD may be informed by research showing that self-criticism and self-reassurance seem to be associated with activation of distinct brain regions (Longe et al., 2010). Self-criticism and self-reassurance are assumed to involve a large range of processes including emotional states, self-monitoring, and self-reflection.

368 of Neurobiology of Personality Disorders

At the molecular genetic level, greater activity of the amygdala in response to fearful stimuli in 5-HTTLPR short allele carriers has been replicated in many studies of both healthy subjects and patients with anxiety disorders, including SAD (Hariri et al., 2002; Aleman et al., 2008). Moreover, while amygdala encodes both negative and positive emotions, there are indications that this genotype mainly modulates amygdala responsivity to negatively and not positively valenced cues (Dannlowski et al., 2010; Freitas-Ferrari et al., 2010; Homberg & Lesch, 2011). Thus overactivation of amygdala in short allele carriers could be indicative of oversensitivity to threat-related or other negative environmental stimuli. Modulation of amygdala activation has also been found in a polymorphism of the serotonin receptor type 3 gene, as well as in polymorphisms located on the TPH2 gene with greater amygdala activation for TPH2–703 T allele carriers (Aleman et al., 2008). Moreover a functional polymorphism on the COMT gene (COMPT Val108/158Met), with the low-activity Met allele leading to higher levels of prefrontal dopamine and the high-activity Val allele leading to lower levels of prefrontal dopamine, may be differentially involved in cognitive and emotional processes. Whereas the Met allele seems beneficial during the performance of cognitive tasks, the Val allele appears advantageous in processing aversive emotional stimuli. The Met allele has been associated with emotional dysregulation, increased corticolimbic reactivity, and higher negative bias (Aleman et al., 2008; Mier et al., 2010).

There has been less focus on positively valenced emotions in research relevant to AvPD. While an exaggerated amygdala response is fairly consistent with fearful faces in individuals with SAD, studies of amygdala alterations to positive/happy faces are limited or inconclusive (Freitas-Ferrari et al., 2010). Findings from psychophysiological and EEG studies support a relationship between BAS and greater sensitivity to positive emotions and greater left frontal activity, in contrast to a relationship between BIS and greater sensitivity to negative emotions and greater right frontal activity during exposure to emotional cues (De Pascalis et al., 2010; Balconi & Mazza, 2010). The hypothesis that the left hemisphere is generally dominant for positive emotions and the right for negative emotions may be too simple, however (Wager et al., 2003). Moreover, the concepts of positive versus negative emotions are criticized for being too vague, and it has been proposed that they be broken into a variety of specific emotions that will eventually map onto distinct brain systems (Burgdorf & Panksepp, 2006; Panksepp & Bliven, 2012). Also, the relative validity of the positive/negative emotion dichotomy compared with the approach/withdrawal dichotomy is still unresolved. In Wager and coworkers' (2003) meta-analysis of neuroimaging studies of emotions, the approach/withdrawal dichotomy yielded more significant results than the positive/negative emotions distinction. According to the RST, neurobiologically based behavioral approach/withdrawal processes might underlie all other affective experiences (Corr, 2008).

There is close overlap between the approach system/BAS/NS and the seek system proposed by Panksepp and Bliven (2012). All are assumed to depend in part on the ventral striatal dopaminergic system, as part of the basal ganglia and including the nucleus accumbens (Cloninger, 1993; Reuter, 2008; Burgdorf & Panksepp, 2006). The seek system is seen as one of seven distinct basic emotional systems that we share with other mammals. Of interest, therefore, is the finding that, compared to patients with BPD, patients with AvPD in particular had lower affect consciousness for the affect "interest/excitement" (Johansen et al., 2013). One may speculate if this reflects a disturbance of the seek system and a further indication of altered dopaminergic functioning in subjects with AvPD. Panksepp and Bliven argue that the seek system not only promotes exploration and investigation but also "energizes" all basic emotional systems with forms of appetitive and anticipatory arousal, including positively valenced emotions.

Neurobiological findings in subjects with AvPD may also vary as a function of alexithymic features in some individuals. Alexithymia is considered a trait-like disorder of affect regulation, usually measured by the Toronto Alexithymia Scale (Taylor et al., 1992), with heritability of 30% to 33% (Baughman et al., 2013). The defining features are difficulty in identifying and distinguishing between feelings and bodily sensations that are associated with emotional arousal, difficulty describing one's own emotions, poor imaginational processes, and externally oriented thinking.

Alexithymia is a multidimensional phenomenon covering both cognitive and emotional characteristics, and evidence from the literature suggests that alexithymic individuals could be characterized by a variety of coexisting functional brain anomalies (Reker et al., 2010). The question whether alexithymia is associated with hyporesponsiveness or hyperresponsiveness is still controversial and may depend on emotion type, valence, and brain region (Berthoz et al., 2002; Lee et al., 2011). However, despite some inconsistent findings, the data point to an automatic hyporesponsiveness of basic emotional processing, involving the limbic and ventral striatal systems, accompanied by reduced activation of prefrontal cortices and visual occipital-temporal structures during exposure to emotional pictures. Low activation has, for example, been reported in the amygdala, insula, anterior and posterior cingulate cortices, caudate, medial prefrontal cortex, orbitofrontal cortex, cuneus, and fusiform gyrus (Reker et al., 2010; Lee et al., 2011; Larsen et al., 2003; Mantani et al., 2005). These structures are differentially involved in the elicitation, awareness, and regulation of emotional experiences. While neurobiological aspects of alexithymia remain not fully understood, hypotheses include limbic hyporesponsiveness, inadequate neural connections in frontolimbic structures, right hemisphere weakness in processing of emotions, or a deficit in interhemispheric communication (resulting in emotional material becoming cut off from the verbally expressive left hemisphere and instead expressed via right hemisphere controlled physiological channels; Reker et al., 2010). More research is needed to clarify whether certain neurobiological aspect of alexithymia are relevant for patients with AvPD.

Attachment

Even if research is limited, there is incipient evidence that AvPD is associated with high levels of attachment avoidance and/or attachment anxiety in adult attachment relationships, as assessed by self-report (Tiliopoulos & Jiang, 2012). Attachment avoidance involves avoidance of intimacy, reluctance to self-disclosure, and preference for self-sufficiency. Attachment anxiety on the other hand, involves worry about rejection and abandonment, excessive need for approval from others, and distress when partner is unavailable. A substantial portion of AvPD patients might have a combination of attachment avoidance and anxiety, classified as fearful attachment (Wilberg, unpublished data). The degree of overlap between fearful attachment and the disorganized/unresolved attachment pattern within the classification based on the Adult Attachment Interview is still unclear, but these patterns may have shared characteristics. Fearful attachment could, however, reflect a conflict between approach and avoidance urges when the attachment system is activated, and this conflict may be resolved behaviorally by an avoidant reaction (Sheldon & West, 1990).

Attachment security versus insecurity is thought to have its roots in early years depending on the child's experiences with caregivers as sensitive and responsive to his or her needs and distress. Based on such experiences the child develops mental representations of self and others and relationships in general, so-called internal working models, which later influence the capacity to establish mutually nurturing relationships as an adult (Shaver & Hazan, 1993). Attachment style is believed to color how we perceive and interpret socially relevant information and attachment-related cues and to have a major influence on how we regulate our emotions and respond to the emotions of others. Avoidant attachment is associated with a downregulation of emotions and attachment anxiety with an upescalation of emotions in attachment contexts (Shaver & Mulincer, 2002). Therefore, neurobiological findings in attachment research may to a large degree overlap with the findings regarding social cognitive biases and emotional processing described earlier. Indeed, such processes may partly be mediated by individual differences in attachment styles. Fearfully attached individuals tend to view others more negatively (Niedenthal et al., 2002; Meyer et al., 2004). Highly anxious and avoidant attachment in individuals with AvPD may predispose them to appraise and interpret other people as rejecting, and such biases in social interpretation processes are thought to be critical for the maintenance of the pattern of active social withdrawal. As with SAD, there is emerging empirical evidence of negative biases in social cognition in individuals with AvPD features, and such biased information processing may be inflexible and context-unresponsive (Meyer et al., 2004; Bowles & Meyer, 2008). In some studies the attachment styles or avoidant cognitive schemas were better predictors of information-processing biases than the AvPD traits themselves (Meyer et al., 2004; Dressen et al., 1999).

Behavioral genetic studies in infants suggest that genetic factors play a minor role in attachment security and that both shared and nonshared environmental factors play a significant role (Bakermans-Kranenburg & van IJzendoorn, 2007). However, genetic factors may play a somewhat larger role in disorganized attachment. Some molecular genetic studies have found associations between polymorphisms of the 7-repeat DRD4 allele and attachment disorganization, particularly in interaction with DRD4–521 C/T promoter polymorphism (i.e., the T allele; Lakatos et al., 2002). However, such associations have not been replicated in many studies (Bakermans-Kranenburg & van IJzendoorn, 2007). The most important genetic effects on attachment may reside in interactions with environmental factors. There are some indications that the development of disorganized attachment in infants might be related to an interaction between 7-repeat DRD4 allele with environmental influences (e.g., parental unresolved loss and trauma or quality of care; van IJzendoorn & Bakermans-Kranenburg, 2006; Gervai et al., 2007). Some studies have also presented evidence for interactions between the 5-HTTLPR short allele and parental sensitivity on attachment security and disorganization (Barry et al., 2008; Spangler et al., 2009). On the other hand, Luijk and coworkers (2011) tested main and interaction effects of polymorphisms in DRD4, DRD2, COMT, 5-HT, and the oxytocin receptor gene (OXTR) in a two large birth cohorts. These are all candidate genes putatively involved in attachment. The only consistent evidence for additive genetic effects was that carriers of the COMT Val/Met genotype had higher disorganized scores compared with both Val/Val and Met/Met carriers. No gene–environment interaction was detected. Thus results from molecular genetic studies are somewhat inconsistent.

Interacting with different kinds of attachment figures normally activates reward and motivation-related brain structures, and insecure attachment could modulate such responses (Bora et al., 2009; Strathern, 2011). A few studies suggest that attachment avoidance may be related to lower activation in brain regions linked to dopaminergic function and reward in a socially rewarding interaction, including the ventral striatum and ventral tegmental area (Vrička et al., 2008; Laakso et al., 2000). Other fMRI findings are that individuals high on attachment avoidance were shown to exhibit weaker somatosensory activations in response to masked sad faces, interpreted in support of the hypothesized downregulation of emotions in avoidant people (Suslow et al., 2009). Attachment-related anxiety has, on the other hand, been connected with stronger neural responses to happy facial expressions in areas that are involved in the perception of facial emotion and the assessment of affective valence and social distance (Donges et al., 2012). Individuals high on anxious and avoidant attachment also seem to respond differently to social rejection. Anxious attachment may relate to heightened neural responses to cues of rejection in regions usually associated with social rejection, like the dorsal anterior cingulate cortex and anterior insula, whereas avoidant attachment may relate to less activation in these regions (DeWall et al., 2012). Although not consistent, insecure attachment has been related to increased activation of amygdala during experimentally induced socially relevant negative emotional stimuli (Lemche et al., 2006; Vrička et al., 2008; Riem et al., 2012). However, many studies have documented a relationship between insecure attachment and altered autonomic function, stress regulation, and immune responses (Gunnar et al., 1996; Gouin et al., 2009; Oosterman et al., 2010).

The hypothalamic neuropeptide oxytocin has emerged as an important biologic substrate modulating social cognition and affiliative behavior and is critical for development of attachment behavior. Oxytocin enhances interpersonal trust and processing of positive emotions and influences the evaluation of socially relevant cues and the ability to infer mental states from others' faces (Bora et al., 2009; Heinrich et al., 2009). Oxytocin has anxiolytic effects, modulates the autonomic nervous system, and may diminish hypothalamic–pituitary–adrenal (HPA) reactivity to psychosocial stress (Heinrich et al., 2009; Norman et al., 2012a). However, endogenous oxytocin levels influences HPA axis reactivity in a bidirectional manner and may also be released in response to stress (Tops et al., 2007). Oxytocin seems differently related to attachment anxiety and trait anxiety in males and females (Weisman et al., 2013). Oxytocin administration has shown several effects on brain activation, like decreased amygdala activation and attenuated amygdala-brainstem coupling, in response to threatening social stimuli (Norman et al., 2012a). Altogether oxytocin seems to increase the salience and processing of social approach related cues while simultaneously decreasing threat-related cues associated with social avoidance behavior. Some of the these effects may be genetically driven, as OXTR polymorphism has been shown to affect amygdala activation to emotionally salient social cues, brain structure alterations, and neurocardiac reactivity to social stress (Tost et al., 2010; Inoue et al., 2010; Norman et al., 2012a). Yet, the sensitivity of the oxytocinergic system is strongly influenced by early environmental factors (Strathern, 2011; Norman et al., 2012a).

Thus oxytocin, and possibly the less studied neuropeptide vasopressin, is of potential interest regarding neurobiological processes in AvPD (Shalev et al., 2011). Recent studies of generalized SAD have found modulated amygdala reactivity in response to fearful faces and altered activity in other areas in response to sad faces after intranasal administration of oxytocin (Labuschagne et al., 2010). No studies have so far focused on AvPD.

Finally, knowledge of neurobiological processes in AvPD may also be informed by research on loneliness and social isolation, including its correlations with somatic health problems. Individuals with AvPD tend to experience a lack of social support and social connectedness but also increased somatic problems (Olssøn & Dahl, 2012; Marques et al., 2012). Perceived loneliness is associated with increased cardiovascular risk factors, morbidity, and mortality. Such risks are related to health behavior but also to changes in physiological mechanisms involving autonomic, immune, and neuroendocrine functions, including the HPA axis (Hawkley & Cacioppo, 2010; Norman et al., 2012b).

HPA Axis, Childhood Abuse, Heart Rate Variability

The HPA axis in mammals plays a major role in the regulation of as well as the response to stress. It is well known that various stressors that are perceived or experienced as exceedingly stressful, including interpersonal events, can impact the HPA system, and some of these events are believed to cause permanent alterations in that system. Genetics or constitutional predisposition with respect to the reactivity of this system also plays a role. In applying these concepts to AvPD, we might consider that, if there are stressors, strains, or conflicts in the realm of attachment or attachment style directly or indirectly related to interpersonal experiences, these can have profound and perhaps lasting impacts on the HPA axis.

While much of what is written here could be considered speculative because it is based more on inference than hard data, it may be useful to elaborate upon how the HPA axis might function in AvPD. We may be able to connect altered reactivity of the HPA to issues of perceived harm or neglect during childhood. While we have little supporting data with respect to AvPD because of the paucity of research on this particular diagnosis, there is some information with regard to social phobia that could point us in an interesting direction.

Roelofs and colleagues (2009) explored HPA responsivity and its relationship to social avoidance behavior in people with social phobia. Earlier work by Sapolsky (1990) with primates revealed that dominant males had lower basal levels of cortisol than subordinates though both exhibited marked and similar increases in cortisol when stressed. The description of what types of stress subordinate male baboons underwent from dominant males would suggest that the subordinates were victims of bullying. The source of the increased basal cortisol concentrations in the subordinates appeared to be central (i.e., under control from the hypothalamus), and it was thought to be related to greater resistance to feedback because of diminished response to dexamethasone. It is known that repeated stress can downregulate glucocorticoid receptors culminating in resistance to feedback. Perhaps even more interesting for the study of personality and personality disorder is that dominant males with the lowest basal cortisol concentrations had a number of other characteristic traits; they could more readily distinguish between a threatening and a nonthreatening situation, and they had a greater likelihood of initiating as well as winning the fight(s) they initiated (Sapolsky & Ray, 1989). Thus social situation and stressors as well as personality characteristics come into play here.

Condren and coworkers (2002) found that in patients with generalized social phobia there was a greater cortisol response to a stressor (serial subtraction and digit span) without differences between patients and controls in baseline cortisol concentrations, suggesting a hyperresponsive adrenocortical response to stress. This hyperresponsivity of cortisol was found in socially phobic adults but only when the stressor was a social stressor and not a physical one (Furlan et al., 2001). Roelofs and coworkers (2009) in a somewhat ingenious experiment found that this elevated cortisol correlated with social avoidance to angry faces (the tendency to want to move away from those faces). Further, though there appeared to be no difference in baseline cortisol levels in subjects with SAD, the presence of a history of childhood abuse led to higher cortisol levels when exposed to a stressor (a mathematical challenge; Elzinga et al., 2010).

Before proceeding further, we might pause to examine the issue of abuse and/or neglect in subjects who have the diagnosis of AvPD or generalized social phobia. The Collaborative Longitudinal Personality Disorders Study (Skodol et al., 2005) compared subjects with AvPD to those with depression. They found no difference in a history of sexual abuse or physical neglect, but physical and emotional abuse occurred at a significantly higher rate in the childhoods of those with AvPD (Rettew et al., 2003). Yet the rate in the AvPD group was not significantly different from rates in the other personality disorder (OPD) group, and the results appeared to be confounded by comorbidity with BPD as well as PTSD. But the AvPD group did differ from the OPD group by having fewer adult relationships and poorer parental social ability. The social relationships of the AvPD individuals appeared to be dysfunctional as early as grade school. Nonetheless, Johnson and colleagues (1999) found that emotional neglect in children increased the risk for developing AvPD, and Joyce et al. (2003b) found that parental neglect as well as a high avoidant style in childhood combined with an early onset anxiety disorder appeared to increase the risk for future AvPD. Additional support comes from an ongoing study comparing patients with AvPD with patients with social phobia. Those with AvPD had experienced more childhood neglect, while the groups did not differ regarding sexual abuse (Eikenæs, unpublished data).

Children with high levels of internalizing symptoms (i.e., inhibitions) who were raised by mothers with depression revealed elevated cortisol levels after a startle response (Ashman et al., 2002). Further, the children of mothers with AvPD had higher adrenocorticotropic hormone (ACTH) response to corticotropic hormone,, though the increased ACTH response did not produce higher cortisol responses. These mothers were thought to be less supportive and less positively involved with their children than mothers without AvPD. This pattern of exaggerated ACTH without corresponding increase in cortisol has been shown in women with an early history of sexual abuse but no depression (Heim et al., 2001).

Meyer and Carver (2000) suggested "that negative childhood memories and a sensitive temperamental disposition each relate particularly strongly to AvPD features when combined with pessimistic expectations. Phrased differently, people who expect negative outcomes are generally more likely to withdraw and avoid, and this appears all the more true if they are highly sensitive, or if they recall rejection, isolation, and other negative experiences during their childhood" (p. 244).

One of the interesting findings here is that while baseline cortisol does not differentiate between healthy controls and avoidant and/or socially phobic individuals, if one looks at heart rate variability (HRV) in socially phobic subjects, a different pattern emerges. Socially phobic people appear to lack HRV in the resting state, and they are not very good at estimating their HR (Gabler et al., 2013). These patients appear to have less cardiovagal control. There was a reduced or inverse association between HRV and increased subjective anxiety over social interactions, as there was between HRV and greater psychological distress and alcohol use (Alvares et al., 2013). This inverse relationship between HRV and social anxiety has been shown by others as well (Boone et al., 1999). Yet there is often no difference in basal (resting) HR between people with social anxiety and controls, and there appears to be a disconnect between subjective anxiety and HR response (Hofman et al.,1995).

Concluding Comments and Future Directions

We place concluding comments and future directions together because each informs the other. Part of the difficulty we have in coming to any specific conclusions about the biology of AvPD rests not only in the scarcity of studies but also in the uncertainty of the AvPD diagnosis itself. Is AvPD a personality disorder, separate and distinct from what we call anxiety disorders (in the old Axis I *DSM* division), or does it overlap substantially with generalized social phobia or severe SAD? If we could more systematically tease apart these diagnoses, we then might be better able to know how much we can assume to apply from studies of the biology of SAD to AvPD.

This suggests that more work first needs to be done on the diagnostic issues. Or perhaps we need to explore biologic and genetic similarities across three different diagnostic groups, those with "simple" social phobia, those with generalized social phobia (or severe SAD), and those with AvPD. The challenge will come perhaps in finding an AvPD group that is free from other comorbidities, particularly but not limited to comorbidities in the personality disorder diagnostic realm. Comorbidity with the mood and anxiety disorders must be considered as well. In order to be able to form large enough cohorts in each of these groupings, these studies will probably demand coordination between various centers, because no single center can possibly make available sufficient numbers of subjects necessary to provide the power to distinguish between groups that probably on a number of neurobiological levels have substantial overlap. Also, as neurobiological processes seem to develop in interaction with environmental influences, there is a need for descriptions of study samples that go beyond diagnostic features.

We certainly have the tools to explore psychiatric patients across and within many aspects of neurobiology. But what we lack is the diagnostic precision to establish the cohorts more cleanly. Or perhaps we need to examine the individuals through studies of dimensions of biology and psychopathology that are most certainly more closely tied to the underlying biology, rather than exploring them through our current flawed diagnostic categories. The existing categories are clearly manmade, and while they often reflect how patients present to us as clinical phenotypes, they fail in too many instances to consistently represent common biological underpinnings.

■ REFERENCES

Aleman, A., Swart, M., & van Rijn, S. (2008). Brain imaging, genetics and emotion. *Biol Psychol, 79,* 58–69.

Alvares, G. A., Quintana, D. S., Kemp, A. H., Zwieten, A. V., Balleine, B. W., Hickie, I. B. et al. (2013). Reduced heart rate variability in social anxiety disorder: associations with gender and symptom severity. *PLoS ONE, 8,* e0468.

American Psychiatric Association. (1980). *Diagnostic and statistical manual of mental disorders* (3rd ed.). Washington, DC: American Psychiatric Association.

American Psychiatric Association. (2013). *Diagnostic and statistical manual of mental disorders* (5th ed.). Arlington, VA: American Psychiatric Association.

Ashman, S. B., Dawson, G., Panagiotides, H., Yamada, E., & Wilkerson, C. W. (2002). Stress hormone levels of children of depressed mothers. *Dev Psychopathol, 14*, 333–349.

Balconi, M., Falbo, L., & Brambilla, E. (2009). BIS/BAS responses to emotional cues: self-report, autonomic measure and alpha band modulation. *Pers Individ Diff, 47*, 858–863.

Balconi, M., & Mazza, G. (2010). Lateralization effect in comprehension of emotional facial expression: a comparison between EEG alpha band power and behavioral inhibition (BIS) and activation (BAS) systems. *Laterality, 15*, 361–384.

Bakermans-Kranenburg, M. J., & van IJzendoorn, M. H. (2007). Research review: Genetic vulnerability or differential susceptibility in child development: the case of attachment. *J Child Psychol Psychiatry, 48*, 1160–1173.

Barry, R. A., Kochanska, G., & Philibert, R. A. (2008). G x E interaction in the organization of attachment: Mothers' responsiveness as a moderator of children's genotypes. *J Child Psychol Psychiatry, 49*, 1313–1320.

Baughman, H. M., Schermer, J. A., Veselka, L., Harris, J., & Vernon, P. A. (2013). A behavior genetic analysis of trait emotional intelligence and alexithymia: A replication. *Twin Research and Human Genetics, 16*, 554–559.

Baur, V., Hänggi, J., Rufer, M., Delsignore, A., Jäncke, L., Hervig, U. et al. (2011). White matter alterations in social anxiety disorder. *J Psychiatr Res, 45*, 1366–1372.

Beck, A. T., & Freeman, A. (1990). *Cognitive therapy of personality disorders.* New York: Guilford Press.

Berthoz, S., Artiges, E., Van de Moortele, P. F., Poline, J. B., Rouquette, S., Consoli, S. M. et al. (2002). Effect of impaired recognition and expression of emotions on frontocingulate cortices: an fMRI study of men with alexithymia. *Am J Psychiatry, 159*, 961–967.

Bjørnebekk, A., Fjell, A. M., Walhovd, K. B., Grydeland, H., Torgersen, S., & Westlye, L. T. (2013). Neuronal correlates of the five factor model (FFM) of human personality: Multimodal imaging in a large healthy sample. *NeuroImage, 65*, 194–208.

Bogels, S. M., Alden, L., Beidel, D. C., Clark, L. A., Pine, D. S., Stein, M. B. et al. (2010). Social anxiety disorder: questions and answers for the DSM-V. *Depress Anx, 27*, 168–189.

Boone, M. L., McNeil, D. W., Turk, C. L., Carter, L. E., Ries, B. J., & Lewin, M. R. (1999). Multimodal comparisons of social phobia subtypes and avoidant personality disorder. *J Anx Disord, 13*, 271–292.

Bora, E., Yucel, M., & Allen, N. B. (2009). Neurobiology of human affiliative behavior: implications for psychiatric disorders. *Curr Opin Psychiatry, 22*, 320–325.

Bowles, D. P., & Meyer, B. (2008). Attachment priming and avoidant personality features as predictors of social-evaluation biases. *J Pers Disord, 22*, 72–88.

Bruce, K. R., Steiger, H., Koerner, N. M., Israel, M., & Young, S. N. (2004). Bulimia nervosa with co-morbid avoidant personality disorder: behavioural characteristics and serotonergic function. *Psychol Med, 34*, 113–124.

Brühl, A. B., Rufer, M., Delsignore, A., Kaffenberger, T., Jäncke, L., & Herwig, U. (2011). Neural correlates of altered general emotion processing in social anxiety disorder. *Brain Res, 1378*, 72–83.

Burgdorf, J., & Panksepp, J. (2006). The neurobiology of positive emotions. *Neurosci Biobehav Rev, 30*, 173–187.

Caceras, X., Torrubia, R., & Farré, J. M. (2001). Is the behavioural inhibition system the core vulnerability for Cluster C personality disorders? *Pers Individ Diff, 31*, 349–359.

Calkins, S. D., Fox, N. A., & Marshall, T. R. (1996). Physiological antecedents of inhibited and uninhibited behavior. *Child Dev, 67*, 523–540.

Carver, C. S., & White, T. L. (1994). Behavioral inhibition, behavioral activation, and affective responses to impending reward and punishment: the BIS/BAS scales. *J Person Soc Psychol, 67*, 319–333.

Caspi, A., Hariri, A. R., Holmes, A., Uher, R., & Moffitt, T. E. (2010). Genetic sensitivity to the environment: The case of the serotonin transporter gene and its implications for studying complex diseases and traits. *Am J Psychiatry, 167*, 509–527.

Caspi, A., Moffitt, T. E., Newman, D. L., & Silva, P. A. (1996). Behavioral observations at age 3 years predict adult psychiatric disorders. *Arch Gen Psychiatry, 53*, 1033–1039.

Cherbuin, N., Windsor, T. D., Anstey, K. J., Maller, J. J., Meslin, C., & Sachdev, P. S. (2008). Hippocampal volume is positively associated with behavioural inhibition (BIS) in a large community-based sample of mid-life adults: the PATH through life study. *SCAN, 3*, 262–269.

Claes, L., Vertommen, S., Smits, D., & Bijttebier, P. (2009). Emotional reactivity and self-regulation in relation to personality disorders. *Pers Individ Diff, 47*, 948–953.

Cloninger, C. R., Svrakic, D. M., & Przybeck, T. R. (1993). A psychobiological model of temperament and character. *Arch Gen Psychiatry, 50*, 975–990.

Condren, R. M., O'Neill, A., Ryan, M. C. M., Barrett, P., & Thakore, J. H. (2002). HPA axis response to a generalized stressor in generalized social phobia. *Psychoneuroendocrinology, 27*, 693–703.

Corr, P. J. (2008). Reinforcement sensitivity theory (RST): introduction. In P. J. Corr (Ed.), *The reinforcement sensitivity theory of personality* (pp. 1–43). Cambridge: Cambridge University Press.

Costa, P. T., & McCrae, R. R. (1992). *Revised NEO Personality Inventory (NEO-PI-R) and NEO Five Factor Inventory (NEO-FFI), professional manual.* Odessa, FL: Psychological Assessment Resources.

Dannlowski, U., Konrad, C., Kugel, H., Zwitserlood, P., Domschke, K., Schöning, S. et al. (2010). Emotion specific modulation of automatic amygdala responses by 5-HTTLPR genotype. *NeuroImage, 53*, 893–898.

Das, D., Cherbuin, N., Tan, X., Anstey, K. J., & Easteal, S. (2011). DRD4-exon III-VNTR moderates the effect of childhood adversities on emotional resilience in young-adults. *PLoS ONE, 6*, e20177.

De Moor, M. H. M., Costa, P. T., Terracciano, A., Krueger, R. F., de Geus, E. J. C., Toshiko, T. et al. (2012). Meta-analysis of genome-wide association studies for personality. *Mol Psychiatry, 17*, 337–349.

De Pascalis, V., Varriale, V., & D'Antuono, L. (2010). Event-related components of the punishment and reward sensitivity. *Clin Neurophysiol, 121*, 60–76.

DeWall, C. N., Masten, C. L., Powell, C., Combs, D., Schurtz, D. R. et al. (2012). Do neural responses to rejection depend on attachment style? An fMRI study. *SCAN, 7*, 184–192.

DeYoung, C. G., Hirsh, J. B., Shane, M. S., & Papademetris, X. (2010). Testing predictions from personality neuroscience: brain structure and the big five. *Psychol Sci, 21*, 820–828.

DiMaggio, G., Semerari, A., Carcione, A., Nicolò, G., & Procacci, M. (2007). *Psychotherapy of personality disorders. Metacognition, states of mind and interpersonal cycles.* London: Routledge.

Donges, U. S., Kugel, H., Stuhrmann, A., Grotegerd, D., Redlich, R., Lichev, V. et al. (2012) Adult attachment anxiety is associated with enhanced automatic neural response to positive facial expression. *Neuroscience, 220*, 149–157.

Dreessen, L., Arntz, A., Hendriks, T., Keune, N., & van den Heout, M. (1999). Avoidant personality disorder and implicit schema-congruent information processing bias: a pilot study with a pragmatic inference task. *Behav Res Ther, 37*, 619–632.

Eikenæs, I., Hummelen, B., Abrahamsen, G., Andrea, H., & Wilberg, T. (2013). Personality functioning in patients with avoidant personality disorder and social phobia. *J Pers Disord*, 27, 746–763.

Elzinga, B. M., Spinhoven, P., Berretty, E., de Jong, P., & Roelofs, K. (2010). The role of childhood abuse in HPA-reactivity in social anxiety disorder: a pilot study. *Biol Psychiatry*, 83, 1–6.

Enoch, M. A., Xu, K., Ferro, E., Harris, C. R., & Goldman, D. (2003). Genetic origins of anxiety in women: a role for a functional catechol-O-methyltransferase polymorphism. *Psychiatr Genet*, 13, 33–41.

Fivush, R., Habermas, T., Waters, T. E. A., & Zaman, W. (2011). The making of autobiographical memory: intersections of culture, narratives and identity. *Internat J Psychol*, 46, 321–345.

Flint, J., Greenspan, R. J., & Kendler, K. S. (2010). *How genes influence behavior.* New York: Oxford University Press.

Fogelson, D. L., Asarnow, R. A., Sugar, C. A., Subotnik, K. L., Jacobson, K. C., Neale, M. C. et al. (2010). Avoidant personality disorder symptoms in first-degree relatives of schizophrenia patients predict performance on neurocognitive measures: The UCLA family study. *Schizophr Res*, 120, 113–120.

Freitas-Ferrari, M. C., Hallak, J. E. C., Trzesniak, C., Filho, A. S., Machado-de-Sousa, J. P., Chagas, M. H. N. et al. (2010). Neuroimaging in social anxiety disorder: a systematic review of the literature. *Prog Neuropsychopharmacol Biol Psychiatry*, 34, 565–580.

Furlan, P. M., DeMartinis, N., Schweizer, E., Rickels, K., & Lucki, I. (2001). Abnormal salivary cortisol levels in social phobic patients in response to acute psychological but not physical stress. *Biol Psychiatry*, 50, 254–259.

Gabler, M., Daniels, J. K., Lamke, J. P., Fydrich, T., & Walter, H. (2013). Heart rate variability and its neuro correlates during emotional face processing in social anxiety disorder. *Biol Psychiatry*, 94, 319–330.

Gardini, S., Cloninger, C. R., & Venneri, A. (2009). Individual differences in personality traits reflect structural variance in specific brain regions. *Brain Res Bull*, 79, 265–279.

Garner, M., Baldwin, D. S., Bradley, B. P., & Mogg, K. (2009). Impaired identification of fearful faces in generalized social phobia. *J Affect Disord*, 115, 460–465.

Gervai, J., Novak, A., Lakatos, K., Toth, I., Danis, I., Ronai, Z. et al. (2007). Infant genotype may moderate sensitivity to maternal affective communications: attachment disorganization, quality of care, and the DRD4 polymorphism. *Soc Neurosci*, 2, 307–19.

Gouin, J. P., Glaser, R., Loving, T. J., Malarkey, W. B., Stowell, J., Houts, C. et al. (2009). Attachment avoidance predicts inflammatory responses to marital conflict. *Brain Behav Immun*, 23, 898–904.

Gunnar, M. R., Brodersen, L., Nachmias, M., Buss, K., & Rigatuso, J. (1996). Stress reactivity and attachment security. *Dev Psychobiol*, 29, 191–204.

Gutknecht, L., Jacob, C., Strobel, A., Kriegebaum, C., Müller, J., Zeng, Y. et al. (2007). Tryptophan hydroxylase-2 gene variation influences personality traits and disorders related to emotional dysregulation. *Internat J Neuropsychopharmacol*, 10, 309–320.

Hariri, A. R. (2009). The neurobiology of individual differences in complex behavioral traits. *Annu Rev Neurosci*, 32, 225–247.

Hariri, A. R., Mattay, V. S., Tessitore, A., Kolachana, B., Fera, F., Goldman, D. et al. (2002). Serotonin transporter genetic variation and the response of the human amygdala. *Science*, 297, 400–403.

Hawkley, L. C., & Cacioppo, J. T. (2010). Loneliness matters: a theoretical and empirical review of consequences and mechanisms. *Ann Behav Med*, 40, 218–27.

Heim, C., Newport, D. J., Bonsall, R., Miller, A. H., & Nemeroff, C. B. (2001). Altered pituitary-adrenal axis responses to provocative challenge tests in adult survivors of childhood sexual abuse. *Am J Psychiatry, 158,* 575–581.

Heinrichs, M., von Dawans, B., & Domes, G. (2009). Oxytocin, vasopressin, and human social behavior. *Front Neuroendocrinol, 30,* 548–557.

Herpertz, S. C., Schwenger, U. B., Kunert, H. J., Lukas, G., Gretzer, U., Nutzmann, J. et al. (2000). Emotional responses in patients with borderline personality as compared with avoidant personality disorder. *J Pers Disord, 14,* 339–351.

Hofmann, S. G., Newman, M. G., Ehler, A., & Roth, W. T. (1995). Psychophysiological differences between subgroups of social phobia. *J Abnorm Psychol, 104,* 224–231.

Homberg, J. R., & Lesch, K. L. (2011). Looking on the bright side of serotonin transporter gene variation. *Biol Psychiatry, 69,* 513–519.

Honkalampi, K., Hintikka, J., Antikainen, R., Lehtonen, J. & Viinamäki, H. (2001). Alexithymia in patients with major depressive disorder and comorbid Cluster C personality disorders: A 6-month follow-up study. *J Pers Disord, 3,* 245–254.

Horney, K. (1945). *Our inner conflicts.* Oxford: Norton.

Hummelen, B., Wilberg, T., Pedersen, G., & Karterud, S. (2006). An investigation of the validity of the Diagnostic and Statistical Manual of Mental Disorders, fourth edition avoidant personality disorder construct as a prototype category and the psychometric properties of the diagnostic criteria. *Compr Psychiatry, 47,* 376–383.

Inoue, H., Yamasue, H., Tochigi, M., Abe, O., Liu, X., Kawamura, Y. et al. (2010). Association between the oxytocin receptor gene and amygdalar volume in healthy adults. *Biol Psychiatry, 68,* 1066–1072.

Jacob, C. P., Strobel, A., Hohenberger, K., Ringel, T., Gutknecht, L., Reif, A. et al. (2004). Association between allelic variation of serotonin transporter function and neuroticism in anxious Cluster C personality disorders. *Am J Psychiatry, 161,* 569–572.

Johansen, M. S., Normann-Eide, E., Normann-Eide, T., & Wilberg, T. (2013). Emotional dysfunction in avoidant compared to borderline personality disorder: A study of affect consciousness. *Scand J Psychol, 54,* 515–521.

Johnson, J. G., Smailes, E. M., Cohen, P., Brown, J., & Bernstein, D. P. (1999). Associations between four types of childhood neglect and personality disorder symptoms during adolescence and early adulthood: findings of a community-based longitudinal study. *J Pers Disord, 14,* 171–187.

Joyce, P. R., McKenzie, J. M., Luty, S. E., Mulder, R. T., Carter, J. D., Sullivan, P. F. et al. (2003b). Temperament, childhood environment and psychopathology as risk factors for avoidant and borderline personality disorders. *Aust N Z J Psychiatry, 37,* 756–764.

Joyce, P. R., Rogers, G. R., Miller, A. L., Mulder, R. T., Luty, S. E., & Kennedy, M. A. (2003a). Polymorphisms of DRD4 and DRD3 and risk of avoidant and obsessive personality traits and disorders. *Psychiatr Res, 119,* 1–10.

Kagan, J., Reznick, J. S., & Snidman, N. (1988). Biological bases of childhood shyness. *Science, 240,* 167–171.

Kagan, J., & Snidman, N. (1999). Early childhood predictors of adult anxiety disorders. *Biol Psychiatry, 46,* 1536–1541.

Kagan, J., Snidman, N., Kahn, V., & Towsely, S. (2007). The preservation of two infant temperaments into adolescence. Introduction. *Monogr Soc Res Child Dev, 72,* 1–9.

Kimbrei, N. A., Mitchell, J. T., Hundt, N. E., Robertson, C. D., & Nelson-Gray, R. O. (2012). BIS and BAS interact with perceived parental affectionless control to predict personality disorder symptomatology. *J Pers Disord, 26,* 203–2012.

Kluger, A. N., Siegfried, Z., & Ebstein, R. P. (2002). A meta-analysis of the association between DRD4 polymorphism and novelty seeking. *Mol Psychiatry, 7,* 712–717.

Klump, H., Angstadt, M., & Phan, K. L. (2012). Insula reactivity and connectivity to anterior cingulate cortex when processing threat in generalized social anxiety disorder. *Biol Psychol*, *89*, 273–276.

Koenigsberg, H. W., Denny, B. T., Fan, J., Liu, X., Guerreri, S., Mayson, S. J. et al. (2014). The neural correlates of anomalous habituation to negative emotional pictures in borderline and avoidant personality disorder patients. *Am J Psychiatry*, *171*, 82–90.

Kretschmer, E. (1925). *Physique and character*. Oxford: Harcourt, Brace.

Laakso, A., Vilkman, H., Kajander, J., Bergman, J., Haaparanta, M., Solin, O. et al. (2000). Prediction of detached personality in healthy subjects by low dopamine transporter binding. *Am J Psychiatry*, *157*, 290–292.

Labuschagne, I., Phan, K. P., Wood, A., Angstadt, M., Chua, P., Heinrichs, M. et al. (2010). Oxytocin attenuates amygdala reactivity to fear in generalized social anxiety disorder. *Neuropsychopharmacology*, *35*, 2403–2413.

Lahat, A., Hong, M., & Fox, N. A. (2011). Behavioral inhibition: is it a risk factor for anxiety? *Internat Rev Psychiatry*, *23*, 248–257.

Lakatos, K., Nemoda, Z., Toth, I., Ronai, Z., Ney, K., Sasvari-Szekely, M. et al. (2002). Further evidence for the role of the dopamine D4 receptor (DRD4) gene in attachment disorganization: Interaction of the exon III 48-bp repeat and the 521 C/T promoter polymorphisms. *Mol Psychiatry*, *7*, 27–31.

Lang, U. E., Bajbouj, M., Wernicke, C., Rommelspacher, H., Danker-Hopfe, H., & Gallinat, J. (2004). No association of a functional polymorphism in the serotonin transporter gene promoter and anxiety-related personality traits. *Neuropsychobiology*, *49*, 182–184.

Larsen, J. K., Branda, N., Bermond, B., & Hijmanc, R. (2003). Cognitive and emotional characteristics of alexithymia. A review of neurobiological studies. *J Psychosomat Res*, *54*, 533–541.

Lee, B. T., Lee, H. Y., Sae-Ah Park, S. A., Lim, J. Y., Tae, W. S., Lee, M. S. et al. (2011). Neural substrates of affective face recognition in alexithymia: A functional magnetic resonance imaging study. *Neuropsychobiology*, *63*, 119–124.

Lemche, E., Giampietro, V. P., Surguladze, S. A., Amaro, E. J., Andrew, C. M., Williams, S. C. R. et al. (2006). Human attachment security is mediated by the amygdala: Evidence from combined fMRI and psychophysiological measures. *Hum Brain Mapp*, *27*, 623–635.

Lesch, K. P., Bengel, D., Heils, A., Sabol, S. Z., Greenberg, B. D., Petri, S. et al. (1996). Association of anxiety-related traits with a polymorphism in the serotonin transporter gene regulatory region. *Science*, *274*, 1527–1531.

Longe, O., Maratos, F. A., Gilbert, P., Evans, G., Volker, F., Rockliff, H. et al. (2010). Having a word with your self: neural correlates of self-criticism and self-reassurance. *NeuroImage*, *49*, 1849–1856.

Luijk, M. P., Roisman, G. I., Haltigan, J. D., Tiemeier, H., Booth-Laforce, C., van IJzendoorn, M. H. et al. (2011). Dopaminergic, serotonergic, and oxytonergic candidate genes associated with infant attachment security and disorganization? In search of main and interaction effects. *J Child Psychol Psychiatry*, *52*, 1295–307.

Mantani, T., Okamoto, Y., Shirao, N., Okada, G., & Yamawaki, S. (2005). Reduced activation of posterior cingulate cortex during imagery in subjects with high degrees of alexithymia: a functional magnetic resonance imaging study. *Biol Psychiatry*, *57*, 982–990.

Marques, L., Porter, E., Keshaviah, A., Pollack, M. H., Van Ameringen, M., Stein, M. B. et al. (2012). Avoidant personality disorder in individuals with generalized social anxiety disorder: what does it add? *J Anx Disord*, *26*, 665–672.

Martin, E. I., Ressler, K. J., Binder, E., & Nemeroff, C. B. (2009). The neurobiology of anxiety disorders: brain imaging, genetics, and psychoneuroendocrinology. *Psychiatr Clin North Am, 32,* 549–575.

McCullough, L., Kuhn, N., Andrews, S., Kaplan, A., Wolf, J., & Hurley, C. L. (2003). *Treating affect phobia. A manual for short-term dynamic psychotherapy.* New York: Guilford Press.

Mendlowicz, M. V., Braga, R. J., Cabizuca, M., Land, M. G., & Figueira, I. L. (2006). A comparison of publication trends on avoidant personality disorders and social phobia. *Psychiatry Res, 144,* 205–209.

Meyer, B. J. (2002). Personality and mood correlates of avoidant personality disorder. *J Pers Disord, 16,* 174–188.

Meyer, B. J., & Carver, C. S. (2000). Negative childhood accounts, sensitivity, and pessimism: a study of avoidant personality features in college students. *J Pers Disord, 14,* 233–248.

Meyer, B., Pilkonis, P. A., & Beevers, C. G. (2004). What's in a (neutral) face? Personality disorders, attachment styles, and the appraisal of ambiguous social cues. *J Pers Disord, 18,* 320–336.

Mier, D., Kirsch, P., & Meyer-Lindenberg, A. (2010). Neural substrates of pleiotropic action of genetic variation in COMT: a meta-analysis. *Mol Psychiatry, 15,* 918–927.

Millon, T. (1981). *Disorders of personality: DSM-III: axis II.* New York: Wiley.

Morrison, A. S., & Heimberg, R. G. (2013). Social anxiety and social anxiety disorder. *Annu Rev Clin Psychol, 9,* 249–274.

Nicolò, G., Semerari, A., Lysaker, P. H., DiMaggio, G., Conti, L., D'Angerio, S. et al. (2011). Alexithymia in personality disorders: correlations with symptoms and interpersonal functioning. *Psychiatry Res, 190,* 37–42.

Niedenthal, P. M., Brauer, M, Robin, L., & Innes-Ker, Å. H. (2002). Adult attachment and the perception of facial expression of emotion. *J Person Soc Psychol, 82,* 419–433.

Norman, G. J., Hawkley, L., Cole, S. W., Berntson, G. G., & Cacioppo, J. T. (2012b). Social neuroscience: the social brain, oxytocin, and health. *Soc Neurosci, 7,* 18–29.

Norman, G. J., Hawkley, L., Luhmann, M., Ball, A. B., Cole, S. W., Berntson, G. G. et al. (2012a). Variation in the oxytocin receptor gene influences neurocardiac reactivity to social stress and HPA function: A population based study. *Horm Behav, 61,* 134–139.

Olssøn, I., & Dahl, A. A. (2012). Avoidant personality problems—their association with somatic and mental health, lifestyle, and social network. A community-based study. *Compr Psychiatry, 53,* 813–821.

Oosterman, M., De Schipper, J. C., Fisher, P., Dozier, M., & Schuengel, C. (2010). Autonomic reactivity in relation to attachment and early adversity among foster children. *Dev Psychopathol, 22,* 109–18.

Panksepp, J., & Bliven, L. (2012). The evolution of affective consciousness: studying emotional feelings in other animals. In J. Panksepp & L. Bliven (Eds.), *The archeology of mind. Neuroevolutionary origins of human emotions* (pp.47–94). New York: Norton.

Pastor, M. C., Ross, S. R., Segarra, P., Montanés, S., Poy, R., & Moltó, J. (2007). Behavioral inhibition and activation dimensions: relationship to MMPI-2 indices of personality disorder. *Pers Individ Diff, 42,* 235–245.

Pelka-Wysiecka, J., Zietek, J., Grzywacz, A., Kucharska-Mazur, J., Bienkowski, P., & Samochowiec, J. (2012). Association of genetic polymorphisms with personality profile in individuals without psychiatric disorders. *Prog Neuropsychopharmacol Biol Psychiatry, 39,* 40–46.

Pujol, J., López, A., Deus, J., Cardoner, N., Vallejo, J., Capdevila, A. et al. (2002). Anatomical variability of the anterior cingulate gyrus and basic dimensions of human personality. *NeuroImage, 15,* 847–855.

Ralevski, E., Sanislow, C. A., Grilo, C. M., Skodol, A. E., Gunderson, J. G., Shea, M. T. et al. (2005). Avoidant personality disorder and social phobia: Distinct enough to be separate disorders? *Acta Psychiatr Scand, 112,* 208–214.

Reichborn-Kjennerud, T. (2010). Genetics of personality disorders. *Clin Lab Med, 30,* 893–910.

Reichborn-Kjennerud, T., Czajkowski, N., Torgersen, S., Neale, M. C., Orstavik, R. E., Tambs, K. et al. (2007). The relationship between avoidant personality disorder and social phobia: A population-based twin study. *Am J Psychiatry, 164,* 1722–1728.

Reker, M., Ohrmann, P., Rauch, A. V., Kugel, H., Bauer, J., Dannlowski, U. et al. (2010). Individual differences in alexithymia and brain response to masked emotional faces. *Cortex, 46,* 658–667.

Rettew, D. C., Zanarini, M. C., Yen, S., Grilo, C. M., Skodol, A. E., Shea, M. T. et al. (2003). *J Am Acad Child Psychiatry, 42,* 1122–1130.

Reuter, M. (2008). Neuro-imaging and genetics. In P. J. Corr (Ed.), *The reinforcement sensitivity theory of personality* (pp. 317–344). Cambridge: Cambridge University Press.

Reuter, M., Kuepper, Y., & Hennig, J. (2007). Association between a polymorphism in the promoter region of the TPH2 gene and the personality trait of harm avoidance. *Internat J Neuropsychopharmacol, 10,* 401–404.

Reuter, M., Schmitz, A., Corr, P., & Hennig, J. (2006). Molecular genetics support Gray's personality theory: the interaction of COMT and DRD2 polymorphisms predicts the behavioural approach system. *Internat J Neuropsychopharmacol, 9,* 155–166.

Riem, M. M. E., Bakermans-Kranenburg, M. J., IJzendoorn, M. H., Out, D., & Rombouts, S. A. (2012). Attachment in the brain: adult attachment representations predict amygdala and behavioral responses to infant crying. *Attach Hum Dev, 14,* 533–551.

Roelofs, K., van Peer, J., Berretty, E., de Jong, P., Spinhoven, P., & Elzinga, B. M. (2009). Hypothalamus-pituitary-adrenal axis hyper-responsiveness is associated with increased social avoidance behavior in social phobia. *Biol Psychiatry, 65,* 336–343.

Rosenthal, M. Z., Kim, K., Herr, N. R., Smoski, M. J., Cheavens, J. S., Lynch, T. R. et al. (2011). Speed and accuracy of facial expression classification in avoidant personality disorder: A preliminary study. *Personal Disord, 2,* 327–334.

Samuel, D. B., & Widiger, T. A. (2008). A meta-analytic review of the relationships between the five-factor model and DSM-IV-TR personality disorders: a facet level analysis. *Clin Psychol Rev, 28,* 1326–1342.

Sapolsky, R. (1990). Adrenocortical function, social rank, and personality among wild baboons. *Biol Psychiatry, 28,* 862–878.

Sapolsky, R., & Ray, J. (1989). Style of dominance and their physiological correlates among wild baboons. *Am J Primatol, 18,* 1–9.

Schinka, J. A., Busch, R. M., & Robichaux-Keene, N. (2004). A meta-analysis of the association between the serotonin transporter gene polymorphism (5-HTTLPR) and trait anxiety. *Mol Psychiatry, 9,* 197–202.

Sen, S., Burmeister, M., & Ghosh, D. Meta-analysis of the association between a serotonin transporter promoter polymorphism (5-HTTLPR) and anxiety-related personality traits. (2004). *Am J Med Genet, 127B,* 85–89.

Serretti, A., Calati, R., Giegling, I., Hartmann, A. M., Möller, H. J., Colombo, C. et al. (2007). 5-HT2A SNPs and the Temperament and Character Inventory. *Prog Neuropsychopharmacol Biol Psychiatry, 31,* 1275–1281.

Shalev, I., Israel, S., Uzefovsky, F., Inga Gritsenko, I., Kaitz, M., & Ebstein, R. P. (2011). Vasopressin needs an audience: Neuropeptide elicited stress responses are contingent upon perceived social evaluative threats. *Horm Behav, 60*, 121–127.

Shaver, P. R., & Hazan, C. (1993). Adult romantic attachment: Theory and evidence. In D. Perlman & W. Jones (Eds.), *Advances in personal relationships* (vol. 4, pp. 29–70). London: Jessica Kingsley.

Shaver, P. R., & Mukilincer, M. (2002). Attachment-related psychodynamics. *Attach Hum Dev, 4*, 133–161.

Sheldon, A. E. R., & West, M. (1990). Attachment pathology and low social skills in avoidant personality disorder: an exploratory study. *Can J Psychiatry, 35*, 596–599.

Shifman, S., Bhomra, A., Smiley, S., Wray, N. R., James, M. R., Martin, N. G. et al. (2008). A whole genome association study of neuroticism using DNA pooling. *Mol Psychiatry, 13*, 302–312.

Skodol, A. E., Gunderson, J. G., Shea, M. T., McGlashan, T. H., Morey, L. C., Sanislow, C. A. et al. (2005). The Collaborative Longitudinal Personality Disorders Study (CLPS): overview and implications. *J Pers Disord, 19*, 487–504.

Spangler, G., Johann, M., Ronai, Z., & Simmermann, P. (2009). Genetic and environmental influences on attachment disorganization. *J Child Psychol Psychiatry, 50*, 952–961.

Strathearn, L. (2011). Maternal neglect: Oxytocin, dopamine and the neurobiology of attachment. *J Neuroendocrinol, 23*, 1054–1065.

Stein, M. B., Fallin, M. D., Schork, N. J., & Gelernter, J. (2005). COMT polymorphisms and anxiety-related personality traits. *Neuropsychopharmacology, 30*, 2092–2102.

Suslow, T., Kugel, H., Rauch, A. V., Dannlowski, U., Bauer, J., Konrad, C. et al. (2009). Attachment avoidance modulates neural response to masked facial emotion. *Hum Brain Mapp, 30*, 3553–3562.

Svrakic, D. M., Whitehead, C., Przybeck, T. R., & Cloninger, R. (1993). Differential diagnosis of personality disorders by the seven-factor model of temperament and character. *Arch Gen Psychiatry, 50*, 991–999.

Swartz, C. E., Wright, C. I., Shin, L. M., Kagan, J., & Rauch, S. L. (2003b). Inhibited and uninhibited infants "grown up": adult amygdalar response to novelty. *Science, 300*, 1952–1953.

Swartz, C. E., Snidman, N., & Kagan, J. (1999). Adolescent social anxiety as an outcome of inhibited temperament in childhood. *J Am Acad Child Adol Psychiatry, 38*, 1008–1015.

Swartz, C. E., Wright, C. I., Shin, L. M., Kagan, J., Whalen, P. J., McMullin, K. G. et al. (2003a). Differential amygdalar response to novel versus newly familiar neutral faces: A functional MRI probe developed for studying inhibited temperament. *Biol Psychiatry, 53*, 854–862.

Taylor, C. T., Laposa, M. T., & Alden, L. E. (2004). Is avoidant personality disorder more than just social avoidance? *J Pers Disord, 18*, 571–594.

Taylor, G. J., Parker, J. D. A., Bagby, R. M., & Acklin, M. W. (1992). Alexithymia and somatic complaints in psychiatric out-patients. *J Psychosom Res, 36*, 417–424.

Terracciano, A., Sanna, S., Uda, M., Deiana, B., Usala, G., Busonero, F. et al. (2010). Genome-wide association scan for five major dimensions of personality. *Mol Psychiatry, 15*, 647–656.

Tiliopoulos, N., & Jiang, Y. (2012). The empirical (ir)relevance of attachment theory. *ACPARIAN, 4*, 14–23.

Tops, M., van Peer, J. M., Korf, J., Wijers, A. A., & Tucker, D. M. (2007). Anxiety, cortisol, and attachment predict plasma oxytocin. *Psychophysiology, 44*, 444–449.

Tost, H., Kolachana, B., Hakimi, S., Lemaitre, H., Verchinski, B. A., Mattay, V. S. et al. (2010). A common allele in the oxytocin receptor gene (OXTR) impacts prosocial temperament and human hypothalamic-limbic structure and function. *PNAS, 107,* 13936–13941.

van IJsendoorn, M. H., & Bakermans-Kranenburg, M. J. (2006). DRD4 7-repeat polymorphism moderates the associataion between maternal unresolved loss and trauma and infant disorganization. *Attach Hum Dev, 8,* 291–307.

Verweij, K. J. H., Zietsch, B. P., Medland, S. E., Gordon, S. D., Benyamin, B., Nyholt, D. R. et al. (2010). A genome-wide association study of Cloninger's temperament scales: Implications for the evolutionary genetics of personality. *Biol Psychol, 85,* 306–317.

Vrtička, P., Andersson, F., Grandjean, D., Sander, D., & Vuilleumier, P. (2008). Individual attachment style modulates human amygdala and striatum activation during social appraisal. *PLoS ONE, 3,* e2868.

Wager, T. D., Phan, K. L., Liberzon, I., & Taylor, S. F. (2003). Valence, gender, and lateralization of functional brain anatomy in emotion: a meta-analysis of findings from neuroimaging. *NeuroImage, 19,* 513–531.

Weisman, O., Zagoory-Sharon, O., Schneiderman, I., Gordon, I., & Ruth Feldman, R. (2013). Plasma oxytocin distributions in a large cohort of women and men and their gender-specific associations with anxiety. *Psychoneuroendocrinology, 38,* 694–701.

Westlye, L. T., Bjørnebekk, A., Grydeland, H., Fjell, A. M., & Walhovd, K. B. (2011). Linking anxiety-related personality trait to brain white matter microstructure. Diffusion tensor imaging and harm avoidance. *Arch Gen Psychiatry, 68,* 369–377.

Wright, C. I., Feczko, E., Dickerson, B., & Williams, D. (2007). Neuroanatomical correlates of personality in the elderly. *NeuroImage, 35,* 263–272.

Ye, G., Yao, F. M., Fu, W. Q., & Kong, M. (2011). The relationships of self-esteem and affect of university students with avoidant personality disorder. *Chin Ment Health J, 25,* 141–145.

Implications for Diagnostic Systems and Treatment

16 Established and Novel Pharmacological Approaches to the Treatment of Personality Disorders

■ S. CHARLES SCHULZ AND
ROBERT O. FRIEDEL

■ INTRODUCTION

Until the late 1970s, the prevailing belief among psychiatrists was that personality disorders (PDs) were only minimally responsive to psychotherapy and were unresponsive to medications. The latter position was challenged in 1979 by Brinkley et al. in a review of the literature on the pharmacological treatment of borderline personality disorder (BPD) and a presentation of five case studies from their clinical work. These data suggested that some patients with the disorder responded well, initially and long term, to low doses of a first-generation antipsychotic agent (FGA; D2 receptor antagonist). The evidence for the use of medications in the treatment of BPD became more credible when patients with BPD showed improvement in two randomized controlled trials (RCTs) utilizing the D2 receptor antagonists thiothixene (Goldberg et al., 1986) and haloperidol (Soloff et al., 1986), encouraging further studies of this and other classes of medications in this population of subjects. A review of these studies is presented in this chapter.

The purposes of this chapter are first, to review the current status of pharmacological treatments of PDs and second, to consider a number of novel pharmacological approaches that may yield additional beneficial results in the treatment of these disorders.

To help achieve these objectives and to enhance the coherency of this book, when appropriate we utilize the neuroscience-based nomenclature (NbN) for psychotropic agents that has been introduced recently (Zohar et al., 2014, 2015; also see Chapter 2 in this volume). In this system, the presumptive modes and mechanisms of action of each drug form the basis of the nomenclature rather than the name of the disorder or one or more symptoms. For example, in the NbN most FGAs are referred to as D2 receptor antagonists, the second-generation antipsychotics (SGAs) are referred to as D2 and 5-HT2A receptor antagonists, and aripiprazole is referred to as a D2, 5-HT1A receptor partial agonist. It is proposed by its authors that this nomenclature will begin to bring psychopharmacology in line in this respect with the rest of medicine.

■ ESTABLISHED PHARMACOLOGICAL APPROACHES TO THE TREATMENT OF PD

The current medication management of PDs has been reviewed recently by Silk and Friedel (2016) in the context of the recent integration of the psychotherapeutic treatment of PDs, especially BPD. This chapter approaches the issue from a neurobiological perspective, which is consistent with the intent of this book. As noted, an update in the nomenclature of psychotherapeutic agents has been proposed because "an earlier period of scientific understanding, failing to reflect contemporary developments and knowledge, does not aid clinicians in selecting the best medication for a given patient, and tends to confuse patients by prescribing a drug that does not reflect their identified diagnosis (e.g. prescribe 'antipsychotics' to depression)" (Zohar et al., 2014). We include some of the new terminology in this chapter because it serves to clarify the neurobiological basis of psychopharmacotherapy.

■ FGAs IN BPD

Seven years after the initial report of Brinkley et al. (1979), Goldberg et al. (1986) published one of the two initial RCTs testing the efficacy of FGAs in BPD. Thiothixene (FGA; D2 receptor antagonist) was administered at a mean daily dose of 8.7 mg for 12 weeks to subjects with symptoms that met the Gunderson and Singer (1975) criteria for BPD. The results of this study suggested that thiothixene was significantly effective in reducing illusions, ideas of reference, psychoticism, obsessive-compulsive symptoms, and phobic anxiety in BPD alone or when combined with symptoms of schizotypal personality disorder (SPD), which also falls within the Gunderson and Singer criteria, compared to the placebo-control group. The superiority of the medication over the placebo was most pronounced in those subjects with moderate to severe symptoms.

An article in the same issue of the journal reported the results of an RCT conducted by Paul Soloff and his colleagues on the use of several classes of medications in subjects with BPD meeting *Diagnostic and Statistical Manual of Mental Disorders* (*DSM*; third edition) criteria (Soloff et al., 1986). In this study, haloperidol (D2 receptor antagonist), at a mean daily dose of 7.24 mg., was found to be significantly more effective than placebo, initially supporting the findings with thiothixene that D2 receptor antagonists as a class may have efficacy in some symptoms of BPDs. However, the results with haloperidol at a mean daily dose of 4 mg did not replicate the prior study of haloperidol, possibly because a significantly lower dose was used in the second study (Soloff et al., 1993).

Following the 1986 reports, Cowdry and Gardner (1988) evaluated medications in four different pharmacological classes in volunteers with BPD. Cross-medication comparisons demonstrated significant improvement in those who completed the whole period on trifluoperazine (D2 receptor antagonist), consistent with the finding in thiothixene noted. An open-label, 12-week trial on thioridazine, another D2 receptor antagonist, demonstrated reductions on Symptom Checklist–90 (SCL-90) scales in the areas of hostility and depressive features (Teicher et al., 1989). These data suggested that the class of D2 receptor antagonists may have a therapeutic effect on some symptoms of BPD, not all of which fall into the antipsychotic-defined cognitive/perceptual symptom domain of the disorder (e.g., anxiety and depression). These clinical treatment results are consistent with the neurobiological aberrations observed in subjects with BPD (see Chapter 15) and underscore the relevance of the NbN of Zohar et al. (2015).

The encouraging results of these studies were followed by other RCTs that examined a broad number of classes of psychotropic medications in the treatment of subjects with certain PDs, especially BPD (Stoffers et al., 2010). The positive results of some of these studies contributed to the growing body of literature on the pharmacological treatment of PDs and to the biological basis of these disorders reported in Chapters 14 through 17.

▪ SGAs IN BPD

SGAs (D2/5-HT2A receptor antagonists) emerged in the 1990s as a result of reports indicating fewer movement disorders than experienced with D2 receptor antagonists. Consequently, studies in the treatment of BPD with antipsychotic agents turned to the D2/5-HT2A receptor antagonists.

The first published study of a medication in this class in BPD reported the effects of olanzapine in a case series of 11 BPD subjects (Schulz et al., 1999). Systematic evaluation of effects reveled a significant reduction in measures including symptoms of anger, psychoticism, and interpersonal sensitivity. No movement disorder symptoms were noted. Since then, multiple RCTs of this class of medications have been conducted and support the contention that some SGAs, especially aripiprazole, effectively reduce some core symptoms of BPD (Lieb et al., 2010).

Aripiprazole, though not a true SGA by pharmacological definition, has demonstrated the broadest effects on BPD symptom profiles of all SGAs studied in an RCT (Nickel et al., 2006, 2007; Lieb et al., 2010). It has significant effects on at least one core symptom in each of the four dimensions of the disorder, including anger, impulsivity, specific cognitive symptoms, and interpersonal problems, and in co-occurring symptoms of depression, anxiety, and the general level of psychiatric pathology. Nickel et al. (2007) then examined the long-term use of aripiprazole versus placebo over 18 months and found that it continued to demonstrate efficacy and safety on all rating scales used. It should be noted that aripiprazole is not a normal atypical antipsychotic agent because it is simultaneously a dopaminergic agonist and antagonist and a 5-HT2A receptor antagonist, otherwise termed a "partial agonist" (Stahl, 2008, pp. 375–376).

Six RCTs have compared olanzapine to placebo in subjects with BPD. In three of these studies, involving 631 subjects, the pooled data revealed significant inferiority of placebo compared to olanzapine for affective instability, anger, anxiety, and psychotic symptoms (Lieb et al., 2010). Inconsistent differences were found for suicidal ideation. In the remaining three trials, two found olanzapine inferior to placebo for self-injurious behavior. Food and Drug Administration (FDA) approval of BPD as an indication for olanzapine was sought in two pivotal trials that included 765 subjects (Schulz et al., 2008; Zanarini et al., 2011). Of the two trials, placebo was not inferior to olanzapine in one (Schulz et al., 2008), but it was in the other, in which olanzapine demonstrated sustained effectiveness for at least 12 weeks (Zanarini et al., 2012). Of note, in the initial trial, there was a statistically significant advantage of olanzapine compared to placebo until the last rating ($p = 0.062$). This prevented the FDA from approving the categorical diagnosis of BPD as an indication for the use of olanzapine.

The efficacy of quetiapine, another D2/5-HT2A receptor antagonist, approved by the FDA for schizophrenia and both manic and depressive episodes of bipolar disorder, was found to be effective in the treatment of paranoia and other psychotic symptoms of BPD in five open-label trials with daily doses ranging from 250 mg to 500 mg. These studies led to the first placebo-controlled RCT of long-acting quetiapine at two fixed daily doses in 95 subjects (Black et al., 2014). The results showed that the placebo was significantly inferior to quetiapine at the 150 mg dose in the reduction of symptoms of the disorder. Side effects included sedation, change in appetite, and dry mouth. Because of suggestions to examine symptom domains of BPD in medication trials, Lee et al. (2016) analyzed SCL-90 measures in 95 subjects from this study and reported the reduction of interpersonal sensitivity, depression, and hostility.

Peculiarly, ziprasidone appeared effective when administered intramuscularly for acute agitation associated with BPD in an emergency room setting (Pascual et al., 2006), but the medication used orally did not demonstrate a significant therapeutic effect on symptoms of the disorder in an RCT (Pascual et al., 2008). This may be the result of inadequate oral dosing and administration in the absence of food, common problems in the treatment of patients with ziprasidone (Stahl, 2008, pp. 416–417).

In the most recent and comprehensive meta-analyses of the responses of BPD to medications, Stoffers et al. (2010) concluded that the D2, 5-HT1A receptor partial agonist aripiprazole, olanzapine, a D2/5-HT2A receptor antagonist, and the D2 receptor antagonist haloperidol appear to reduce certain symptoms of cognitive-perceptual impairment, particularly excessive suspiciousness and paranoid ideation, and also appear to reduce affective dysregulation and impulse dyscontrol.

■ MOOD STABILIZERS

Meta-analyses of the mood stabilizers studied in RCTs in subjects with BPD demonstrated efficacy for valproate, lamotrigine, and topiramate (see Stoffers et al., 2010; Lieb et al., 2010). Valproate blocks the hydrolysis of phosphatidylinositol 4,5-bisphosphate to its secondary messengers, interferes with voltage-sensitive sodium channels (VSSCs), and may increase gamma-aminobutyric acid (GABA) activity (see Stahl, 2008, pp. 672–689, and Chapter 2). The analyses suggested varying levels of efficacy of valproate for anger, depression, and interpersonal problems. Lamotrigine, which may work by blocking the alpha-subunit of the VSSCs and thereby the release of glutamate, was superior to placebo for reduction of anger and impulsivity. Topiramate, which appears to reduce glutamate function and enhance GABA function by interfering with sodium and/or calcium channels, was superior to placebo for impulsivity and interpersonal problems and had a greater effect on females than males in the reduction of anger. This is an unusual finding because topiramate typically does not demonstrate mood stabilization of other disorders in studies or in clinical practice (Stahl, 2008, pp. 686–687).

■ ANTIDEPRESSANTS

Low mood and thoughts and self-injurious behaviors (SIBs) are common in individuals with BPD and have led to examining antidepressant treatment in these patients. Consequently, after the first selective serotonin reuptake inhibitor (SSRI; fluoxetine) was released in the late 1980s, its effect on subjects with BPD was examined promptly. In the first RCT of an SSRI in BPD (Salzman et al., 1995), placebo was inferior to fluoxetine in the reduction of anger in subjects with mild to moderate but not with severe

BPD. A second RCT of an SSRI (fluvoxamine) in 38 female patients with BPD resulted in improvement only in rapid mood shifts (Rinne et al., 2002). Subsequent surveys of BPD patients indicate that SSRIs, in keeping with the now-outdated American Psychiatric Association (APA, 2001) guideline are used frequently. However, meta-analyses of the data (Stoffers et al., 2010; Lieb et al., 2010) do not support the efficacy of SSRIs for symptoms of this disorder. The tricyclic antidepressant amitriptyline was *inferior* to placebo in BPD subjects (Soloff et al., 1986).

■ LITHIUM

The second edition of the *DSM* did not include the diagnosis of BPD (APA, 1968). Inpatients labeled as "emotionally unstable character disorder," some of whom may have met current criteria for BPD, studied in a controlled trial appeared to benefit from lithium (Rifkin et al., 1972). Latter studies did not confirm the initial finding (Goldberg, 1989).

■ BENZODIAZEPINES

Cowdry and Gardner (1988) reported that alprazolam did not lead to improvement of symptoms of BPD; subjects actually became more disinhibited and engaged in more SIBs. Nonetheless, a survey of psychiatrists found that some still prescribe this class of medications for patients with BPD (Knappich et al., 2014). However, there may be some advantage to using benzodiazepines to "lead in" or "top up" antipsychotics (Stahl, 2008, p. 434).

■ INTEGRATED USE OF MEDICATION AND PSYCHOTHERAPY

The first report of a BPD study that tested the interaction of medications with psychotherapy evaluated the effects of dialectical behavior therapy (DBT) and fluoxetine (Simpson et al., 2004). There were no benefits found by the addition of fluoxetine to DBT, which is consistent with the findings noted that SSRIs have shown no benefit in BPD. However, Soler and colleagues (2005) in a placebo-controlled trial of DBT with or without olanzapine, found that subjects receiving DBT and olanzapine (mean = 8.83 mg/day) demonstrated an improvement that was superior compared to either treatment alone and that this group had fewer drop-outs. A second olanzapine/DBT study (Linehan et al., 2008) reported that the integration of both therapies resulted in a greater reduction in anger symptoms. Both studies confirmed and extended the benefits of olanzapine in BPD, suggesting that an effective medication enhances psychotherapy in BPD (Silk & Friedel, 2016).

■ PREDICTION OF RESPONSE TO MEDIATION WITH BRAIN IMAGING

Brain imaging of subjects with significant illnesses—schizophrenia and bipolar disorder—began in the 1970s and early 1980s with measures on computed tomography scans. After comparing patients to controls, Weinberger et al. (1980) examined the measure of ventricular brain ratio in patients with the diagnosis of schizophrenia and compared those who were responders to antipsychotic medication versus those who were not. The patients with enlarged ventricles responded more poorly to treatment. To determine if this was present at the outset of the illness, Schulz et al. (1983) performed the study in adolescents with recent-onset schizophrenia and confirmed that the patients with enlarged ventricles had an inferior response to those with normal size ventricles. Now this area of research has moved to very sophisticated studies, including the use of connectivity magnetic resonance imaging in first-episode patients, and also demonstrates a significant difference in functional measures (Sarpal et al., 2016).

Such studies in schizophrenia suggest a potential benefit in examining biological endophenotypes of BPD to explore variations in treatment response. Currently, a pilot, positron emission tomography scan study is underway to determine response to olanzapine in BPD subjects. Preliminary results suggest that a number of regions of interest are associated with statistically significant response to olanzapine treatment in BPD subjects (Schlesinger et al., 2012).

■ CONCLUSIONS ON THE CURRENT USE OF MEDICATIONS FOR BPD

We conclude that certain medications are therapeutic for some symptoms of BPD and that aripiprazole and D2/5-HT receptor antagonists may enhance the benefits of psychotherapy. The known mechanisms of actions of the medications effective in BPD are consistent with the data related to the pathophysiology of the disorder as it is currently understood (see Chapter 15). The APA (2001) guideline for the pharmacological treatment of BPD is now considered out of date, and a switch from the use of SSRIs and SGAs to mood stabilizers and antipsychotic agents is indicated (Abraham & Calabrese, 2008; Lieb et al., 2010; Feurino & Silk, 2011).

The APA (2001) guideline was developed before many of the current studies were reported. However, this is not the case for the guideline of the National Institute for Health Care and Excellence (NICE 2009) in the United Kingdom. This guideline stated that "treatment should not be used specifically for borderline personality disorder or for the individual symptoms or behavior associated with the disorder (for example, repeated self harm, marked emotional instability, risk taking behavior and transient psychotic symptoms)." In a review of the Cochrane meta-analyses, Lieb et al. (2010) state, "We suggest considering a reassessment of these [the NICE] recommendations, as there actually is encouraging evidence of the effectiveness of treatment for individual symptoms of borderline personality disorder."

■ NOVEL PHARMACOLOGICAL APPROACHES TO THE TREATMENT OF PDS

With the exception of BPD, there is minimal or no information on the efficacy of the pharmacological treatment of most PDs. To a significant degree, this is the result of a relative lack of academic and scientific enthusiasm for the area of PDs compared with other mental disorders. To confirm this suggestion, one need only review a number of clinical psychiatric evaluations to realize how seldom the diagnosis of a PD is made, even in most academic departments of psychiatry. During the use of the various *DSM* (fourth edition) series, the most common Axis II diagnoses were "deferred" and "none." Therefore, identification of suitable subjects for scientific investigation of PDs is difficult. Also, as was recognized in former DSM terminology, PDs were often "ego-syntonic" (denied by the symptomatic individual). Finally, there has been a lack of consensus regarding the specification of the essential research methodologies in this population of subjects (Zanarini et al., 2010).

One major methodological problem focuses on the existing diagnostic categorical method vs. the proposed alternative, multidimensional personality trait diagnostic model (*DSM-5*, pp. 761–781). A main problem with the categorical diagnostic method is evident when one considers the heterogeneity of symptoms in the categorical method among patients with the same PD diagnosis. For example, there are nine discrete criteria of BPD that are listed in *DSM-5*. Only five of these criteria are required to make the diagnosis of the disorder when using the categorical approach. Applying the standard equation for the calculation of combinations, $C = n!/r! \, (n - r)!$, in which n = the number of total criteria and r = the number required to make the diagnosis, there are 126 different ways that five of the nine criteria for BPD can be combined that will result in a diagnosis of the disorder. This is a minimal number because many criteria contain more than one symptom. To our knowledge, no study of the pharmacological or psychotherapeutic treatment of BPD has controlled for this obviously important, confounding variable.

Another less evident and discussed, and presently incalculable, variable is exemplified again by the heterogeneity of individuals with BPD. The source of this variable is the multiple neurobiological factors that underlie the phenotypic expressions (e.g., symptoms) of PDs. Even a cursory reading of the material presented indicates clearly that this is so. For example, if each of the nine *DSM* criteria of BPD is the result of only two of numerous biological variables potentially involved in each symptom, either of which may result in the symptom, then n in this equation increases to at least 18 while the required criteria remain at five. Doubling the number of possible criteria-related variables results in a mathematical increase in the heterogeneity of the disorder to 8,568 different combinations of biological variables that may result in the diagnosis of BPD. While this is a considerable oversimplification of the situation, it does underscore present, valid conceptual and practical difficulties in study design. A recent genetic finding in BPD, however, may prove helpful in simplifying this particular methodological dilemma. As noted in Chapter 15, multivariate genetic analyses of the 9 *DSM-IV* BPD criteria have found that one highly heritable BPD factor influences all nine BPD criteria, regardless of the degree to which each was influenced themselves by genetic and environmental factors (e.g., Reichborn-Kjennerud et al., 2013). This could reduce considerably the number of critical, symptom-related factors and medication-sensitive targets of treatment of BPD.

It is beyond the scope of this chapter to address the large number of research strategies and current leads that could be pursued to identify and increase the number of pharmacological agents effective in the treatment of PDs. There are so many possibilities that it is difficult to select from those described, stimulated by or inferred from the material presented in the preceding chapters or other sources. Also, researchers experienced in the fields of neural science and clinical psychopharmacology do not require any guidance from the authors of this chapter on how best to apply the information contained in this book.

However, we discuss four approaches that demonstrate some evidence-based merit worthy of consideration: (a) further investigations of the efficacy of clozapine, especially in BPD, SPD, and antisocial personality disorder (AsPD); (b) investigative strategies based on advances in pharmacogenetics and epigenetics; (c) exploration of the neuroanatomical and neurochemical advances in synaptic function; and (d) scientifically-controlled studies of psychedelic substances such as psilocybin (magic mushrooms), methylenedioxy-methamphetamine (Ecstasy or Molly), and N-methyltyramine.

Before discussing these issues in more detail, we underscore the central role of technological advances that are now being used in such studies. The material in this book strongly suggest that the next, most successful advances in the pharmacological treatment of PDs, whatever they may be, will be based on the use of advanced technologies. Currently used variations of neuroimaging especially have enabled many of the recent advances in our knowledge of brain structure and function, including those in the areas of the chemistry and physiology of synaptic function and network connectivity and integration. Recently introduced techniques, such as optogenetics (Deisseroth et al., 2015), will expand our knowledge more rapidly. These and other technological advances have provided researchers for the first time with access to the structural integrity and the functional activity of specific brain pathways in the living, human brain in healthy and diseased states. Such information is refocusing pharmacotherapy research and clinical care from heterogeneous, categorically diagnosed individuals to those with objectively verifiable, biologically based symptoms.

Clozapine

Clozapine was developed by Sandoz in 1961 and first released in Switzerland in 1972 for the treatment of schizophrenia. Although a number of other SGAs have been developed since then, it remains the "gold standard" of medications in this class (see Zink & Correll, 2015; Stahl, 2008, pp. 409–410). Clozapine has one of the most complex sets of pharmacological properties of any of the SGAs. In addition to its D2 and 5-HT2A antagonisms, it has at least 13 other pharmacological actions (Stahl, 2008, pp. 409–410), but the precise reason for its superiority is unknown. It is especially effective in reducing aggression and violence, is the only antipsychotic agent shown to reduce the risk of suicide, causes few extrapyramidal symptoms, and does not seem to produce tardive dyskinesia. However, it continues to be considerably underutilized for schizophrenia, its primary indication. After reports of agranulocytosis caused by the use of clozapine appeared in 1975, resulting in death in some cases, it was withdrawn voluntarily by the manufacturer. After 10 years, due to its clear superiority over other atypical antipsychotics, it was reapproved for use only in treatment-resistant schizophrenia and with strict hematological monitoring. Its indications were expanded and blood monitoring requirements were refined by the FDA in 2002 and again in 2005. In late 2015, because of the evidence that clozapine was still significantly underutilized in the United States compared to other countries, in an effort to enhance its appropriate clinical use, the FDA again clarified and simplified the proper use of clozapine in the Clozapine Risk Evaluation and Mitigation Strategy Program (www.clozapinerems.com).

We believe that clozapine is the "low-hanging pharmacological fruit" available to advance rapidly the pharmacological treatment of individuals with PDs who present a clear risk of harm to themselves or others. First, as will be documented, it may be used now with some confidence, but great caution, in those cases of BPD that are otherwise medication-resistant, present a significant risk of harm, and require frequent hospitalizations. Second, it may be administered in certain cases and in preliminary trials by psychiatrists experienced in its use in patients with SPD and AsPD who are at risk as noted and where there is modest evidence that SGAs may possess efficacy as discussed later. Third, It provides additional opportunities to determine the features of clozapine that result in its superior efficacy compared to other SGAs in specific symptoms of BPD and other disorders, such as anger, aggression, and cognitive disturbances (Stoffers et al., 2010). Finally, such studies should provide further insights into the neuropathology of BPD and other PDs and the development of new medications in their treatment. Therefore, clozapine will receive more detailed attention in this chapter than other, more novel approaches that may have considerable heuristic value but less data to support their clinical use.

Clozapine Treatment of PDs

The initial data on D2 receptor antagonists discussed suggested they may be of value in the treatment of some symptoms of BPD. Subsequently, a number of RCTs have since supported the proposal that D2/5-HT2A receptor antagonists, and similar compounds like aripiprazole, have verifiable but mild to moderate beneficial effects for some symptoms of the disorder (Stoffers et al., 2010; Lieb et al., 2010; Stoffers & Lieb, 2015). Therefore, it appears reasonable to attempt to enhance the efficacy of these medications in PDs by investigating further the use of clozapine.

The Use of Clozapine in BPD

A review of the literature revealed 16 studies of the efficacy of clozapine in BPD. (As will be noted, we could identify only one other report of clozapine in subjects with any other PD.) The first reported clinical trial of clozapine on patients with BPD was conducted by Frankenburg and Zanarini in 1993. It is discussed here with the other three largest studies of this topic.

Of the remaining 12 reported studies of the effects of clozapine in BPD, eight are single case reports, all demonstrating moderate to large improvement (see Beri et al., 2014). However, as noted by Beri et al., publication bias can be a significant confounding factor in the interpretation of case studies, especially individual reports. Of interest though is one of a 17-year-old girl, to our knowledge the only adolescent with BPD treated with clozapine reported in the literature (Argent & Hill, 2014).

Four case studies with fewer than 10 subjects each have been reported, involving four (Zarzar & McEvoy, 2013), five (Swinton, 2001), seven (Chengapappa et al., 1999) and eight (Parker, 2002) subjects. All reported moderate to large therapeutic effects in subjects previously treatment-resistant to one or more antipsychotic agents. In these studies, mean daily doses of clozapine ranged from 150 to 421 mg. In studies of other disorders, clozapine plasma levels of 350 to 420 ng/ml are reported to be associated with the likelihood of good clinical response (Mauri et al., 2014). Unfortunately, none of these four studies reported clozapine blood levels. Therapeutic effects of clozapine were determined by the authors using structured and nonstructured methods of evaluation of varied features of the disorder. Most prominent of these were self- and other-directed physical aggression, number of days on enhanced observation, and frequency and length of hospitalization. Taken together, these four studies, which involve a total of 24 previously SGA-resistant subjects with BPD, may be considered to provide at least modest evidence that clozapine has therapeutic benefits in aggressive symptoms, severity of illness, and number of relapses of BPD in these SGA-resistant subjects.

The remaining four studies of clozapine in BPD are more informative, having utilized different methodological approaches and larger and more varied samples of subjects than the other 12 reports. As noted, Frankenburg and Zanarini (1993) performed a trial of the effects of clozapine in 15 inpatients with BPD, all of whom had prolonged and/or pronounced atypical psychotic symptoms. Clozapine was titrated as needed, achieving a mean daily dose of 253.3 mg. Efficacy was rated blind to baseline symptoms on the Brief Psychiatric Rating Scale (BPRS) and the Global Assessment Scale (GAS) after two to nine months of treatment. The BPRS decreased significantly from a mean of 57.0 to 37.8 ($P = .001$), and the GAS improved significantly from a mean of 30.8 to 43.1 ($P = .001$). Positive, negative, and general symptoms also decreased significantly.

Benedetti et al. (1998) performed an open-label trial of low-dose clozapine in 12 BPD patients with severe, psychotic-like symptoms. All had previously failed to improve on a four-month therapeutic program, including antipsychotics in 9 of the 12 subjects. Those with comorbid Axis I and medical pathologies were excluded. Clinician-rated scales included the BPRS, the Hamilton Rating Scale for Depression, and the Global Assessment of Functioning Scale at baseline and after 4 and 16 weeks. Each subject, treated as an inpatient, was administered clozapine from 25 to 100 mg/ day (mean = 43.8 mg) for 16 weeks. A significant decrease in psychotic symptoms was observed in the first two weeks associated with a significant reduction in affective instability, physical aggression, suicidality, impulsivity, depression, and frequency of rehospitalization and an increase in global functioning. The main side effects of sedation, hypersalivation, and decreased white blood count were transient and did not interrupt clozapine therapy.

To date, Haw and Stubbs (2011) have reported the largest study of clozapine in BPD in a cross-sectional survey of the use of antipsychotics for BPD in a secure, UK hospital setting. The results were determined from interviews with the treating psychiatrists. Seventy-nine of 231 (34%) hospitalized patients were diagnosed with *DSM-IV-TR* BPD, severe enough that almost all patients were detained. Only two of the BPD patients exhibited psychotic symptoms. Eighty percent of the patients were receiving one or more antipsychotic agents at baseline and 48% were receiving two or more. Antipsychotic medications were the most frequently prescribed medications for these patients (55 of 79; 70%), and clozapine was the most commonly prescribed antipsychotic (30 of 55; 55%). It was reported by the treating psychiatrists as the most likely medication to result in major improvements in target symptoms. Other medications resulted in minor improvement or no change. The final daily dose of clozapine was that estimated by the psychiatrists to result in the most improvement (median = 275 mg; range = 100–600 mg). All but one of the 15 psychiatrists involved knew they were not following the United Kingdom's National Institute for Health and Clinical Excellence (NICE, 2009) Guideline for BPD to *not* use antipsychotic agents for any symptoms of BPD, but they did so because they perceived the need to treat effectively severe and complex cases.

The second largest and the longest study to date of clozapine treatment in BPD was an examination of a case series of 22 women with high-risk, severe BPD who were inpatients at St. Andrew's Healthcare in Northampton, UK, a secure psychiatric hospital (Frogley et al., 2013). All were or had been previously detained for care by court or civil order. Exclusion criteria included a learning disability (IQ <70) and a diagnosis of any Axis I psychotic disorder. An extensive list of demographic and clinical information was collected at baseline. All participants had received previously at least one antipsychotic agent; the mode was three, and some had received six. The mean daily dose of clozapine during the study was <300 mg, and mean clozapine plasma levels were 430 ng/ml at 6 months, 410 ng/ml at 12 months, and 360 ng/ml at 18 months, reflecting decreased dosing over this interval. This is the only study of clozapine in BPD to date which reports plasma levels, all of which were essentially within the therapeutic range of 350 to 420 ng/ml noted. Outcome measures were the Brief Psychotic Rating Scale, GAF, days on one-to-one observation, the number of therapeutic sessions attended, risk incidents over a four-week baseline period, self- and other-directed injurious behaviors, and a modified Overt Aggression Scale. The study hypotheses were that clozapine would reduce the frequency and severity of risk behaviors, severity of symptoms, and concomitant pharmacological treatment and improve functioning and nonpharmacological therapeutic engagement. The results of the study indicated a highly significant improvement in all outcome measures, with only one not achieving a $P < .001$. There was also reported an improvement in both internal and external symptoms, though these are not defined specifically. Over the 18-month duration of the study, weight increased by an average of 7.8 kg and glucose by 12.2 mg/dL to a final level of 88.9. Continuation rates of subjects on clozapine in the study were 95.5%.

Taken together, the results of the studies reported to date on the use of clozapine in BPD provide a modest to moderate degree of preliminary evidence that clozapine produces consistently a broad range of significant improvement in some of the core symptoms of the disorder in SGA-resistant subjects with a moderate to marked range of severity. In addition, in those studies reported to date, there appears to be no greater risk of neutropenia, increased weight, and glucose intolerance than that reported in schizophrenia or schizoaffective disorder. Because of the amount of the evidence and the time over which these data were reported, clozapine cannot accurately be considered a *novel* pharmacological approach to the treatment of BPD. However, the significant underutilization of this medication, especially in the United States, even for its indicated uses, strongly suggests that the use of clozapine in the treatment of BPD may well offer the most promising opportunity to bring significant relief of suffering immediately to many individuals with BPD and their families. To our knowledge, no other antipsychotic agent with this amount of evidence supporting its efficacy in BPD has not undergone one or more RCTs to rigorously test its efficacy, safety, and tolerability. Such studies with clozapine are long overdue.

Clozapine in Antisocial PD

Only one study conducted in the past 40 years could be identified that has examined the effects of clozapine on AsPD. Brown et al. (2014) conducted a retrospective review of case notes and evaluated the effects of clozapine in a series of seven patients with primary AsPD and high psychopathic traits of serious violence who were detained in a high-security hospital in the United Kingdom. Outcome measures focused on impairment in the cognitive-perceptual, impulsive-behavioral control, and affective regulation symptom domains of AsPD. Clinical Global Impression scores and metabolic parameters were also evaluated. Over the term of the study, all seven patients showed significant improvement in each symptom domain, especially in impulse-dyscontrol and in anger, with a significant decreased risk of violence in six of seven patients. The effects occurred especially at low doses of clozapine producing serum levels < 350 ng/mL. Clozapine serum levels in six of the seven patients were 150 to 350 ng/mL.

Considering the enormous personal and social dysfunction experienced and caused by individuals with AsPD, especially those with moderate to severe psychopathic tendencies, it would seem worth pursuing this lead. The obstacles to doing so are surely formidable, but the potential benefits to the individuals involved and to society certainly seem to justify the effort.

Clozapine in SPD

As noted in this chapter, there is evidence that FGAs and SGAs have efficacy in relieving some of the symptoms of SPD. Given the positive results of SGAs in SPD, of clozapine in preliminary studies of BPD, and in one study of AsPD, one would expect that more preliminary and follow-up trials would have already been performed with clozapine in subjects with medication-resistant SPD, but this has not been the case. One may speculate about the reasons for this, but it remains a research opportunity in PDs that is searching for a place to happen.

Concluding Thoughts on Clozapine

The superiority of clozapine over other SGAs in the treatment of patients at high risk with schizophrenia, schizoaffective disorders, and other disorders suggests it may prove beneficial to individuals with PDs. As noted, the mechanism of action of FGAs is mainly considered to be related mainly to D2 receptor antagonism, while SGAs demonstrate both D2 antagonism and much greater 5-HT2A receptor antagonistic properties than the FGAs (Mauri et al., 2014). Clozapine, the prototypic SGA, has significantly greater antagonism at 5-HT2A receptors than at D2 receptors and additional effects at GABA and glycine receptors. These, and the numerous other pharmacological characteristics of clozapine noted earlier, appear to make it unique among SGAs (Stahl, 2008, pp. 409–410; Zink & Correll, 2015).

It has been thought that the main action that differentiates the efficacy, tolerability, and adverse reactions of SGAs from FGAs is the additional 5-HT2A receptor inhibition (Meltzer, 1994). There is emerging evidence that this initial hypothesis needs to be broadened to include other modulator systems, and especially those involving the glutamatergic, mood stabilizer systems (Zink & Corell, 2015). The lower rate and degree of extrapyramidal symptoms (EPS) among the SGAs compared to FGAs has been proposed to be a function of the degree of 5-HT2A receptor antagonism and the rate of binding and release of SGAs to D2 receptors, with clozapine having the fastest binding and release ("skipping") rate and the lowest occurrence of EPSs (Seeman, 2013). Continued research in these areas suggests a promising proliferation of the next generations of antipsychotic agents.

▪ PHARMACOGENETICS AND EPIGENETICS

At this time, there is no clear evidence that polymorphisms of one or more specific genetic sites are involved in enhancing the risk of developing symptoms of any PD. However, there is preliminary evidence that suggest polymorphisms of certain candidate genes such as those producing the D2, 5-HT2A or other neurotransmitter receptors, and the promotor genes that up- or downregulate their production (Delvecchio et al., 2016; Brennan, 2014). Another candidate gene is that of the brain-derived neurotropic factor (BDNF). BDNF is a key synaptogenic molecule that enhances synaptic repair and may serve as a sensitive functional marker and pharmacotherapeutic target. Its activity is detectable in early clinical development by electroencephalography markers that permits examination of target engagement or drug-related efficacy of synaptic repair (Soltesz et al., 2014).

▪ EPIGENETICS AND PROMOTOR GENE TARGETS

The importance of psychosocial risk factors in the development and treatment of PDs is well established (see Chapter 20). These risk factors appear to play a central role in the environmental influences that modify inherent psychological traits and behaviors. These effects seem to be mediated by up- or downregulation of specific promotor genes as a result of DNA methylation and associated processes. For example, Guidotti and Grayson (2014) have recently summarized evidence suggesting that altered DNA methylation is involved in the pathogenesis of schizophrenia and bipolar disorder. Methylation/demethylation processes are influenced by antipsychotic agents that are dibenzepine derivatives (clozapine, quetiapine, and olanzapine) but not by the butyrophenone derivative haloperidol and the piperidal-benzisoxazole derivative risperidone. The dibenzepine derivatives and valproate activate DNA-demethylation of GABAnergic and glutamatergic promotors and induce chromatin remodeling that helps to correct dysregulation of transmission in these pathways in schizophrenia and bipolar disorder. Interestingly, clozapine and valproate correct the *RELN and GAD67* promotor hypermethylation in methionine-treated mice and the offspring of prenatally stressed mice. Valproate combined with clozapine, but not haloperidol, also corrects the hyperactivity and impaired social interactions in these animal models.

Given the importance of psychosocial factors in the psychopathology and psychotherapy of PDs, further exploration of the specific mechanisms of epigenetic influences on brain functioning offers a promising approach to the pharmacological enhancement of psychosocial interventions in these disorders.

▪ PSYCHEDELIC AGENTS

Anthropological evidence suggest that psychedelic agents derived from plants have been used by humans for thousands of years, presumably as a means to expand external and internal sensory perceptions and cognitive experiences (Halberstadt, 2015). Drugs in this class (e.g., LSD, DMT, mescaline, psilocybin, and ibogaine) have been defined by the FDA as Schedule I Controlled Substances: they have no accepted medical use in the United States; they are considered unsafe for use under medical supervision; and they have a high potential for abuse (Title 21 Code of Federal Regulations (C.F.R.) §§ 1308.11 through 1308.15). However, there is increasing evidence that these and similar, chemically synthesized substances have the capacity to be useful in the management of a number of serious physical and mental symptoms. For example, a review of the efficacy of endocannabinoids suggests that targeting this system presents a novel approach to the treatment of anxiety disorders, especially posttraumatic stress disorder (Korem et al., 2015) and cancer care (Abrams & Guzman, 2015).

A cursory review of the large number of scientific articles on this topic suggests that this field may yield significant advances in the development of new pharmacotherapeutic agents that are useful in the treatment of PDs. For example, there are data that suggest some psychedelic substances increase awareness of one's environment and enhance empathy of other individuals. These brain functions are central features of psychosis and AsPD. Nonetheless, not until the neurobiological mechanisms of these disturbances and the effects on them of psychedelic agents are better understood will the psychedelics be able to provide guidance in the development of effective treatments for borderline, schizotypal, antisocial, and other PDs. For this to occur, the pervasive, negative attitude toward the rigorous and cautious scientific evaluation of such substances must continue to diminish.

■ REFERENCES

Abraham, P. F., & Calabrese, J. R. (2008). Evidenced-based pharmacologic treatment of borderline personality disorder: a shift from SSRIs to anticonvulsants and atypical antipsychotics? *J Affect Dis, 111*, 21–30.

Abrams D. I., & Guzman, M. (2015). Cannabis in cancer care. *Clin Pharmacol Ther, 97*, 575–586.

American Psychiatric Association. (1968). *Diagnostic and statistical manual of mental disorders* (2nd ed.). Washington, DC: American Psychiatric Association.

American Psychiatric Association. (2001). Practice guideline for the treatment of patients with borderline personality disorder. *Am J Psychiatry, 158*(suppl):1–52.

Argent S. E., & Hill, S. A. (2014). The novel use of clozapine in an adolescent with borderline personality disorder. *Ther Advan Psychopharmacol, 4*, 149–155.

Benedetti, F., Sforzini, L., Colombo, C., Maffei, C., & Smeraldi, E. (1998). Low-dose clozapine in acute and continuation treatment of severe borderline personality disorder. *J Clin Psychiatry, 59*(3), 103–107.

Beri, A., & Boydell, J. (2014). Clozapine in borderline personality disorder: a review of the evidence. *Ann Clin Psychiatry, 26*, 139–144.

Black, D. W., Zanarini, M. C., Romine, A., Shaw, M., Allen, J., & Schulz, S. C. (2014). Comparison of low and moderate dosages of extended-release quetiapine in borderline personality disorder: a randomized, double-blind, placebo-controlled trial. *Am J Psychiatry, 171*, 1174–1182.

Brennan, M. D. (2014). Pharmacogenetics of second-generation antipsychotics. *Pharmacogenomics, 15* 869–884.

Brinkley, J. R., Beitman, B. D., & Friedel, R. O. (1979). Low-dose neuroleptic regimens in the treatment of borderline patients. *Arch Gen Psychiatry, 65*, 319–326.

Brown, D., Larkin, F., Sengupta, S., Romero-Ureclay, J. L., Ross, C. C., Gupta, N., Vinestock, M., & Das, M. (2014). Clozapine: an effective treatment for seriously violent and psychopathic men with antisocial personality disorder in a UK high-security hospital. *CNS Spectr, 19*, 391–402.

Chengapappa, K. N., Ebeling, T., Kang, J. S., Levine, J., & Parepally, H. (1999). Clozapine reduces severe self-mutilation and aggression in psychotic patients with borderline personality disorder. *J Clin Psychiatry, 60*, 477–484.

Cowdry, R. W., & Gardner, D. L. (1988). Pharmacotherapy of borderline personality disorder: alprazolam, carbamazepine, trifluoperazine, and tranylcypromine. *Arch Gen Psychiatry, 45*, 111–119.

Deisseroth, K., Etkin, A., & Malenka, R. C. (2015). Optogenetics and the circuit dynamics of psychiatric disease. *JAMA, 313*, 2019–2020.

Delvecchio, G., Bellani, M., Altamura, A. C., & Brambilla, P. (2016). The association between the serotonin and dopamine neurotransmitters and personality traits. *Epidemiol Psychiatr Sci, 25*, 109–112.

Feurino, L., & Silk, K. R. (2011). State of the art in the pharmacologic treatment of borderline personality disorder. *Curr Psychiatry Rep, 13*, 69–75.

Frankenburg, F. R., & Zanarini, M. C. (1993). Clozapine treatment of borderline patients: a preliminary study. *Comp Psychiatry, 34*, 402–405.

Frogley, C., Anagnostakis, K., Mitchell, S., Mason, F., Taylor, D., Dickens, G., & Picchioni, M.M. (2013). A case series of clozapine for borderline personality disorder. *Ann Clin Psychiatry, 25*, 125–134.

Goldberg, S. C. (1989). Prediction of change in borderline personality disorder. *Psychopharmacol Bull, 25*, 550–555.

Goldberg, S. C., Schulz, S. C., Schulz, P. M., Resnick, R. J., Hamer, R. M., & Friedel, R. O. (1986). Borderline and schizotypal personality disorders treated with low-dose thiothixene vs. placebo. *Arch Gen Psychiatry, 43*, 680–686.

Guidotti, A., & Grayson, D. R. (2014). DNA methylation and demethylation as targets for antipsychotic therapy. *Dialogues Clin Neurosci, 16*, 419–429.

Gunderson, J., & Singer, M. (1975). Defining borderline patients: an overview. *Am J Psychiatry, 132*, 1–10.

Halberstadt, A. L. (2015). Recent advances in the neuropsychopharmacology of serotonergic hallucinogens. *Behav Brain Res, 277*, 99–120.

Haw, C., & Stubbs, J. (2011). Medication for borderline personality disorder: a survey at a secure hospital. Int *J Psychiatry Clin Pract, 15*, 280–285.

Knappich, M., Horz-Sagstetter, S., Schwerthoffer, D., Leucht, S., & Rentrop, M. (2014). Pharmacotherapy in the treatment of patients with borderline personality disorder: results of a survey among psychiatrists in private practices. *Int Clin Psychopharmacol, 29*, 224–228.

Korem, N., Zer-Aviv, T. M., Ganon-Elazar, E., Abush, H., & Akirav, I. (2015). Targeting the endocannabinoid system to treat anxiety-related disorders. *J Basic Clin Physiol Pharmacol, 27*, 193–202.

Lee, S. S,. Allen, J., Black, D. W., Zanarini, M. C., & Schulz, S. C. (2016). Quetiapine's effect on the SCL-90-R domains in patients with borderline personality disorder. *Ann Clin Psychiatry, 28*, 4–10.

Lieb, K., Völlm, B., Rücker, G., Timmer, A., & Stoffers, J. M. (2010). Pharmacotherapy for borderline personality disorder: Cochrane systematic review of randomised trials. *Brit J Psychiatry, 196*, 4–12.

Linehan, M. M., McDavid, J. P., Brown, M. Z., Sayrs, J. H. R., & Gallop, R. J. (2008). Olanzapine plus dialectical behavior therapy for women with high irritability who met criteria for borderline personality disorder. A double-blind, placebo-controlled pilot study. *J Clin Psychiatry, 69*, 999–1005.

Mauri, M. C., Paletta, S., Maffini, M., Colasanti, A., Dgogna, F., Di Pace, C., Altamura, A. C. (2014). Clinical pharmacology of atypical antipsychotics: an update. *EXCLI J, 13*, 1163–1191.

Meltzer, H. Y. (1994). An overview of the mechanism of action of clozapine. *J Clin Psychiatry, 55* Suppl B, 47–52.

National Institute for Health and Clinical Excellence. (2009). Borderline personality disorder: treatment and management. National Collaborating Centre for Mental Health. Leicester, UK: British Psychological Society, p. 297.

Nickel, M. K., Loew, T. H., & Pedrosa, G. F. (2007). Aripiprazole in treatment of borderline patients, part II: an 18-month follow-up. *Psychopharmacol, 191*, 1023–1026.

Nickel, M. K., Muehlbacher, M., Nickel, C., KIettler, C., Pedrosa, G.F., Bachler, E., Buschmann, W., Rother, N., Fartacek, R., Egger, C., Anvar, J., Rother, W. K., Loew, T. H., Kaplan, P. (2006). Aripiprazole in the treatment of patients with borderline personality disorder: a double-blind, placebo-controlled study. *Am J Psychiatry, 163*, 833–838.

Parker, G. F. (2002). Clozapine and borderline personality disorder. *Psychiat Serv, 53*, 348–349.

Pascual, J. C., Soler, J., Puigdemont, D., Perez-Egea, R., Tiana, T., Alvarez, E., & Perez, V. (2008). Ziprasidone in the treatment of borderline personality disorder: a double-blind, placebo-controlled, randomized study. *J Clin Psychiatry, 69*(4), 603–608.

Pascual, J.C., Soler, M.J., Barrachina, J., Campins, M.J., Alvarez, E., & Perez, V. (2006). Injectable typical antipsychotics for agitation in borderline personality disorder. *Pharmacopsychiatry, 39*(3), 117–118.

Reichborn-Kjennerud, T., Ystrom, E., Neale, M. C., Aggen, S.H., Mazzeo, Knudsen, G.P., Tambs, K., Czajkowski, N., & Kendler, K. S. (2013). Structure of genetic and environmental risk factors for symptoms of DSM-IV borderline personality disorder. *JAMA Psychiatry, 70*,1206–1214.

Rifkin, A., Quitkin, F., Carrillo, C., Blumberg, A.G., & Klein, D.F. (1972). Lithium carbonate in emotionally unstable character disorder. *Arch Gen Psychiatry, 163*, 519–523.

Rinne, T., van den Brink, W., Wouters, L., & van Dyck, R. (2002). SSRI treatment of borderline personality disorder: a randomized, placebo-controlled clinical trial for female patients with borderline personality disorder. *Am J Psychiatry, 159*, 2048–2054.

Salzman, C., Wolfson, A.N., Schatzberg, A., Looper, J., Henke, R., Albanese, M., Schwartz, J., & Miyawaki, E. (1995). Effect of fluoxetine on anger in symptomatic volunteers with borderline personality disorder. *J Clin Psychopharmacol, 15*(1), 23–29.

Sarpal, D. K., Argyelan, M., Robinson, D. G., Szeszko, P. R., Karlsgodt, K. H., John, M., Weissman, N., Gallego, J. A., Kane, J. M., Lencz, T., & Malhotra, A.K. (2016). Baseline striatal function connectivity as a predictor of response to antipsychotic drug treatment. *Am J Psychiatry, 173*, 69–77.

Schulz, S. C., Camlin, K. L., Berry, S. A., & Jesberger, J. A. (1999). Olanzapine safety and efficacy in patients with borderline personality disorder and comorbid dysthymia. *Biol Psychiatry, 46*, 1429–1435.

Schulz, S. C., Sinicrope, P., Kishore, P., & Friedel, R. O. (1983). Treatment response and ventricular brain enlargement in young schizophrenic patients. *Psychopharmacol Bull, 19*, 510–512.

Schulz, S. C., Zanarini, M. C., Bateman, A., Bohus, M., Detke, H. C., Trzaskoma, Q., Tanaka, Y., Lin, D., Deberdt, W., & Corya, S. (2008). Olanzapine for the treatment of borderline personality disorder: variable dose 12-week randomized double-blind placebo-controlled study. *Br J Psychiatry, 193*, 584–592.

Seeman, P. (2013). Schizophrenia and dopamine receptors. *Eur Neuropsychopharmacol*, *23*, 999–1009.

Silk, K. S., & Friedel, R. O. (2016). Psychopharmacological considerations in integrated modular treatment. In W. J. Livesley, G. Dimaggio & J.F. Clarkin (Eds.), *Integrated treatment for personality disorders: a modular approach* (pp. 211–231). New York: Guilford Press.

Simpson, E. B., Yen, S., Costello, E., et al. (2004). Combined dialectical behavior therapy and fluoxetine in the treatment of borderline personality disorder. *J Clin Psychiatry*, *65*, 379–385.

Soler, J., Pascual, J. C., Campins, J., et al. (2005). Double-blind, placebo-controlled study of dialectical behavior therapy plus olanzapine for borderline personality disorder. *Am J Psychiatry*, *162*, 1221–1224.

Soloff, P. H., Cornelius, J. R., George, A., Nathan, S., Perel, J.M., & Ulrich, R. F. (1993). Efficacy of phenelzine and haloperidol in borderline personality disorder. *Arch Gen Psychiatry*, *50*, 377–385.

Soloff, P.H., George, A., Nathan, S., Schulz, P.M., Ulrich, R.F., & Perel, J.M. (1986). Progress in pharmacotherapy of borderline disorders: a double-blind study of amitriptyline, haloperidol, and placebo. *Arch Gen Psychiatry*, *43*, 691–697.

Soltesz, F., Suckling, J., Lawrence, P., et al. (2014). Identification of BDNF sensitive electrophysiological markers of synaptic activity and their structural correlates in healthy subjects using a genetic approach utilizing the functional BDNF Val66Met polymorphism. *PLoS ONE*, *9*(4), e95558. doi:10.1371/ journal.pone.0095558

Stahl, S. M. (2008). *Stahl's essential psychopharmacology*. New York: Cambridge University Press.

Stoffers, J. M., & Lieb, K. (2015). Pharmacotherapy for borderline personality disorder—current evidence and recent trends. *Curr Psychiatry Rep*, *17*, 534.

Stoffers, J. M., Völlm, B. A., Rücker, G., Timmer, A., Huband, N., & Lieb, K. (2012). Psychological therapies for people with borderline personality disorder. *Cochrane Database Syst Rev*, *15*, 8, CD005652. doi: 10.1002/14651858.CD005652.pub2

Stoffers, J., Völlm, B. A., Rücker, G., Timmer, A., & Lieb, K. (2010). Pharmacological interventions for borderline personality disorder. *Cochrane Database Syst Rev* 2010 *16*, 6:CD005653. doi: 10.1002/14651858.CD005653.pub2

Swinton, M. (2001). Clozapine in severe borderline personality disorder. *J Forens Psychiatry*, *12*, 580–591.

Teicher, M. H., Glod, C. A., Aaronson, S. T., Gunter, P. A., Schatzberg, A. F., & Cole, J. O. (1989). Open assessment of the safety and efficacy of thioridazine in the treatment of patients with borderline personality disorder. *Psychopharmacol Bull*, *25*, 535–549.

Weinberger, D. R., Bigelow, L. B., Kleinman, J. E., Klein, S. T., Rosenblatt, J. E., & Wyatt, R. J. (1980). Cerebral ventricular enlargement in chronic schizophrenia: an association with poor response to treatment. *Arch Gen Psychiatry*, *37*, 11–13.

Zanarini, M. C., Schulz, S. C., Detke, H. C., Tanaka, Y., Zhao, F., Lin, D., Deberdt, W., Kryzhanovskaya, L., & Corya, S. (2011). A dose comparison of olanzapine for the treatment of borderline personality disorder: a 12-week randomized, double-blind, placebo-controlled study. *J Clin Psychiatry*, *10*, 1353–1365.

Zanarini, M. C., Schulz, S. C., Detke, H., Zhao, F., Lin, D., Pritchard, M., Deberdt, W., Fitzmaurice, G., & Corya, S. (2012). Open-label treatment with olanzapine for patients with borderline personality disorder. *J Clin Psychopharmacol*, *32*, 398–402.

Zanarini, M. C., Stanley, B., Black, D. W., Markowitz, J. C., Goodman, M., Lynch, T. R., Levy, K., Fonagy, P., Bohus, M., Farrell, J., & Sanislow, C. (2010). Methodological considerations for treatment trials for persons with borderline personality disorder. *Ann Clin Psychiatry*, *22*, 75–83.

Zarzar, T., & McEvoy, J. (2013). Clozapine for self-injurious behavior in individuals with borderline personality disorder. *Ther Adv Psychopharmacol, 3*, 272–274.

Zink, M., & Correll, C. U. (2015). Glutamatergic agents for schizophrenia: current evidence and perspectives. *Expert Rev Clin Pharmacol, 8*, 335–352.

Zohar, J., Nutt, D., Kupfer, D., Moller, H. J., Yamawaki, S., Spedding, M., & Stahl, S. M. (2014). A proposal for an updated neuropsychopharmacological nomenclature. *Eur Neuropsychopharmacol, 24*, 1005–1014.

Zohar, J., Stahl, S., Moller, H. J., Blier, P., Kupfer, D., Yamawaki, S., Uchida, H., Spedding, M., Goodwin, G. M., & Nutt, D. (2015). A review of the current nomenclature for psychotropic agents and an introduction to the neuroscience-based nomenclature. *Eur Neuropsychopharmacol, 25*, 2318–23.

17 Neurobiological Underpinnings of Psychosocial Treatment in Personality Disorders

■ MARIANNE GOODMAN, JENNIFER CHEN, AND ERIN A. HAZLETT

■ INTRODUCTION: GENERAL PSYCHOTHERAPY CONCEPTS

Psychotherapy derives from the Greek words "psyche" defined as spirit or soul and "therapeia," denoting healing and medical treatment. Over the past 100 years, there has been a robust interest in the practice of psychotherapy and clarifying its mechanism of change. While all psychotherapies aim to ameliorate psychic pain, through the exploration of feelings, behaviors, and thoughts, over 250 approaches have proliferated, targeting and emphasizing differing cognitive, emotional, and relational processes. This chapter focuses on the psychotherapies with the largest empirical basis and that are most relevant to personality dysfunction; these include behavioral therapy, cognitive-behavioral therapy (CBT), interpersonal psychotherapy (IPT), psychodynamic psychotherapy, and psychoanalytic psychotherapy.

Behavioral therapy focuses on behavioral actions and aims to modify the reinforcers and conditioning of behavioral patterns. CBT centers on modifying maladaptive thoughts, cognitions, and thinking patterns and includes formats such as dialectical behavioral therapy (DBT). IPT emphasizes the interpersonal context in relationship to psychological distress and stresses the building of interpersonal skills to improve relationships and mood. Psychodynamic psychotherapy examines views of the self and other, and psychoanalytic approaches address unconscious beliefs and interaction patterns with the goal of developing insight. In trying to best understand mechanisms of psychotherapeutic change, initial efforts conducted across psychotherapy orientations focused on process evaluation from therapist and patient interactions (Johansson & Høglend, 2007) and highlight the importance of safety within a psychotherapeutic relationship. From this relationship, the ability to develop new psychological awareness is thought to be a core requirement for change (Levitt & Williams, 2010).

Other theorists hypothesize alternative critical elements underlying psychotherapeutic change including mindfulness of emotion (Corrigan, 2004). Mindful processing of emotion is a component of CBT, IPT, DBT, and psychodynamic approaches. While there are distinctions between how this mechanism of change functions in each different therapy modality, mindfulness of emotions allows patients to acknowledge and observe emotional processes as they occur, moment to moment, rather than avoid or immediately escape painful affect. In CBT, patients are taught how to distinguish between feelings and thoughts and to identify any distorted thinking and misinterpretation that may lead to negative emotions as they become consciously aware of unhelpful thought patterns. Similarly, IPT teaches patients to identify and correctly express emotions in the context of relationships for symptom alleviation. DBT takes into account core mindfulness skills of describing emotions as they are being experienced, rather than impulsively acting on them, to bring about distress tolerance and emotion regulation. In psychodynamic therapy, mindfulness of emotion may manifest as exploration of the transference and countertransference elements in the therapy room as it is occurring. In each of these modalities, the ability to withhold self-judgment of the emotional state (i.e., not feeling guilty, ashamed, angry about the primary emotion) is a core component of the process of observing, reflecting, and describing emotional states and reconciling opposing states, which contribute to effective change in psychotherapy.

The therapeutic alliance has received a great deal of attention in the literature across all treatment modalities (Horvath & Symonds, 1991) as a mechanism of change. Indeed, research has shown that a stronger therapeutic alliance leads to more positive treatment outcome (Horvath & Symonds, 1991; Kaufman, 2000; Summers & Barber, 2003). Not surprisingly, a successful therapeutic alliance offers a dynamic and collaborative relationship to the patient to experience empathic understanding, emotional expression, and corrective interpersonal connection within a therapeutic frame. This framework provides a mutual understanding of goals and tasks that are shared by both therapist and patient, and this bond between therapist and patient continues to evolve and strengthen from session to session. Although treatment modalities may differ in the approach and process, each modality presented also relies on a strong therapeutic alliance that shares more commonalities than differences. Additionally, Cozolino (2002) found that the therapeutic alliance may be the key to developing new neural networks through learning and integrating thoughts, feelings, and actions throughout the therapy process. A study by Stratford et al. (2012) examined neurophysiological correlates of high therapeutic alliance by examining electroencephalography (EEG) activity and skin conductance in clients during sessions with their therapist. Findings indicated prefrontal, parietal, and occipital EEG was associated with therapeutic alliance and anxiety and heart rate decreased after therapy.

More recently, another mechanism of change that has emerged is that of skills acquisition and practice. Gibbons et al. (2009) found that compensatory skills acquisition (i.e., development of new coping skills) and changes in actual versus ideal self-discrepancy were also instrumental components of psychotherapeutic change across both cognitive and psychodynamic modalities. The underlying biological substrates of these mechanisms are just beginning to emerge. However, there remains a deficit in our understanding of the neurobiological correlates and how these translate to therapeutic change.

■ NEUROBIOLOGY OF PSYCHOTHERAPY

In a highly influential paper delineating the neurobiological basis of psychotherapy, Gabbard (2000) builds on Kandel's (1998) idea that psychotherapy is a "form of learning" that leverages the brain's plasticity and capacity for change. Just as Kandel demonstrated in Aplysia snails, learning from the environment resulted in alterations of synaptic connections and involved changes in gene expression. These processes facilitate the organism's ability to adapt to environmental change. Psychotherapy is posited as another environmental influence with the potential to affect neurotransmission patterns and genetic expression. Following this line of thinking, psychotherapy, as conceptualized by Etkin and colleagues (2005), is *new learning in the context of a therapeutic relationship*. By framing psychotherapy as a "learned process," we may develop a better understanding of how psychotherapy acts on brain functioning.

Research over the last few decades has shown that learning occurs on multiple levels and in various memory systems in the brain. As the brain learns new information, the neurological process of memory consolidation takes what is learned in short-term memory and encodes and stores it into long-term memory to be retrieved at a later time. As patients in a psychotherapeutic context begin treatment, there is often novel information (i.e., new schemas, new skills, new self-beliefs) to be learned and consolidated. As these new data are acquired and practiced, they become synthesized into memory systems to be retrieved at a later time.

Memory consolidation consists of two specific processes of synaptic consolidation and system consolidation. Synaptic consolidation occurs directly after the initial acquisition of information, usually within the first few hours after learning. System consolidation is the process by which memories dependent on the hippocampus become independent of the hippocampus over the time span of weeks to years.

Consolidation requires a neurochemical process called *long-term potentiation*, in which synapses increase in strength as more signals are transmitted between two neurons each time learning occurs. As these two neurons begin firing together over time, they become more synchronized and sensitized to one another through the mechanism of potentiation, making it more likely that they will continue to fire together in the future. Hippocampal long-term potentiation has been linked to memory formation.

With each new experience or data, the brain creates more connections between neurons at the synaptic level, reorganizing and rerouting previous connections and pruning connections that are not used as frequently, known as *associability* (Jeffery & Reid, 1997). The strengthened connections create lasting neural networks that become stronger and more familiar through the use of frequent rehearsal, repetition, and recall over a span of time. As a result, the brain is able to reconsolidate memories each time new information is gathered. This ability to change the strength and efficiency between neurons is known as *neural plasticity*. The phrase, "cells that fire together wire together" is often used to summarize the Hebbian theory of brain plasticity. In the context of psychotherapy, what is learned and discovered in a therapeutic context oftentimes requires practice, repetition, and rehearsal in order for new habits or thought patterns to be formed. As patients become more insightful, memories may be reorganized and reconsolidated. Consequently, effective memory consolidation of psychotherapeutic skills and insight can bring about lasting change, as rehearsal of learned skills creates mastery and increases agency.

In psychotherapy, these alterations increase the strength of synaptic connections and point to the brain's plasticity even into adulthood. Psychotherapy acts to reorganize neural networks within the brain, allowing the brain to be altered intentionally (Flores, 2010). There is also research that shows that emotionally enriching environments, such as psychotherapy, play a part in developing positive brain change (Flores, 2010) as positive emotions and memory circuits become linked together. Post and Weiss (1997) suggest that emotional memory requires neuroplasticity that utilizes a larger number of synapses and requires more complexity and self-organization. Synapses in the hippocampus and neocortex show neuroplasticity in that they are bidirectionally malleable, and these changes persist until they are part of long-term memory storage.

The neuroscience of memory has made significant strides in the last decade, building from the hypothesis of long-term potentiation, or the reinforcement of synaptic connections, to now encompass epigenetic mechanisms (Guan et al., 2015). Epigenetics involves cellular processes that alter gene expression though the addition or subtraction of methyl groups to DNA, modify histone groups, or interfere with amino acid production by binding to mRNA. These epigenetic processes can either increase or decrease the expression of genes that code for proteins important in memory formation, consolidation, and even extinction. While this field is still in its infancy, a deeper understanding of these processes may lead to improved psychotherapeutic outcomes involving memory and learning (e.g., extinguishing traumatic memories in posttraumatic stress disorder [PTSD], facilitating the recovery of lost memories, and slowing the loss of age-related decline in memory; Zovkic et al., 2013).

Memory can be thought of as both explicit and implicit, two distinct systems implicating different brain function and relying on different neural structures. The explicit memory system utilizes the temporal lobe, particularly the hippocampus, in recording and later recalling experiences (Liggan & Kay, 1999). The implicit memory system relies on the basal ganglia and is thought to exist based on the influence of early attachment experiences on emotional behavior (Liggan & Kay, 1999). These two systems are significant in the course of neurodevelopment and memory development through the life span. At birth, infants have a functional memory system and exhibit more implicit learning rather than explicit memory (Amini et al., 1996). This system creates and stores prototypes and rules that are following and not conscious. These learned behaviors may not be available for conscious processing but guide behavior. In psychotherapy, the learned implicit rules stored in memory become revealed through awareness and insight, and change occurs through learning new patterns via the explicit memory system until they become habitual and part of the implicit memory system (Liggan & Kay, 1999).

As discussed previously, the therapeutic alliance is a new attachment relationship between therapist and patient, which is capable of regulating neurophysiology through restructuring of the attachment-related implicit memory system (Liggan & Kay, 1999). Participation in psychotherapy is thought to activate the implicit memory system and allow for implicitly stored material to be accessed, modified, and reconsolidated.

These findings point to the importance of viewing psychotherapy through a biopsychosocial lens, as psychological interventions can alter the brain on a biological level just as much as offer "psychological benefits" of feeling better and developing sense of agency and control. Psychotherapy affects glucose metabolism rates in the brain, as demonstrated by Baxter et al. (1992) and Schwartz et al. (1996), who showed psychotherapy and fluoxetine successfully decreased metabolic rates in the right caudate nucleus in obsessive–compulsive disorder (OCD) treatment responders. Similarly, van der Kolk (1997) found increased prefrontal metabolism in patients with PTSD after a trial of eye movement desensitization and reprocessing. A study from Finland found that psychodynamic therapy may have a significant impact on increasing serotonin metabolism (Viinamaki et al., 1998). CBT has been shown to change the lactate levels in people suffering from panic disorder (Shear et al., 1991) and has also impacted thyroid hormone levels in people diagnosed with major depressive disorder (MDD; Joffe et al., 1996).

Early life stress and traumatic experiences have been implicated as risk factors in the etiology and persistence of psychological disorders. Studies have examined the hypothalamic–pituitary–adrenal (HPA) axis, which acts to regulate stress responses in the brain. After being exposed to stress, the hypothalamus releases corticotropin-releasing factor, which is then transported to the anterior pituitary. This stimulates the release of adrenocorticotropin, which then stimulates glucocorticoids to be synthesized and secreted from the adrenal cortex. This stress response is counterregulated by a negative feedback mechanism that targets the pituitary gland, hypothalamus, and hippocampus. Dysregulation of the HPA axis is associated with many disorders. Hyperactivity of the HPA axis has been found in melancholic depression, eating disorders, and alcoholism. Hypoactivity of the HPA axis has been implicated in PTSD, chronic fatigue syndrome, and idiopathic pain disorders.

Stress has been found to have long-lasting damaging consequences on the brain, particularly on the hippocampus, which contains many glucocorticoid receptors. While psychopharmacological interventions such as antidepressants have been found to normalize HPA axis activity, the impact of psychotherapy treatments on HPA activity such as CBT are just beginning to be recognized (Kim et al., 2009). The neurobiological study of psychotherapy, however, significantly lags behind research on pharmacotherapy.

■ NEUROIMAGING AND PSYCHOSOCIAL TREATMENT

Psychotherapy provides learning through exploration of affect-laden memories and experience, which gives increased synaptic field potentials, suggesting the formation of new synapses and brain plasticity (Liggan & Kay, 1999). Psychotherapy allows for changes in long-term memory storage. Liggan and Kay conceptualize parallels between brain structures and schools of psychotherapy. The brain's plasticity is able to show changes in various brain regions, depending on the modality of treatment. Behavioral therapy, for instance, focuses on disturbances of learning and memory related to motor behavior. Thus the brain structures implicated are the amygdala, basal ganglia, and hippocampus. In cognitive therapy, the focus is on identifying and modifying negative cognitions and schemas, and brain areas predicted to be affected include the neocortex and frontal cortex. In psychodynamic therapy, the focus is on interpersonal representations that were engrained in childhood. It is surmised that the brain regions implicated include the lateralized cerebral hemisphere and subcortical areas.

As described, there is growing appreciation that the mental processes involved in psychotherapy affect brain activity, and, with the advent of more sophisticated neuroimaging methodology, the viewing of brain changes with psychotherapy is now feasible. Longitudinal neuroimaging permits not only the visualization of specific brain region involvement and change but also identifies modifications in connectivity between regions and alterations in network circuitry. Such data are invaluable in the development of improved treatments and outcome, elucidating underlying disease processes, and may offer neurobiological markers for both prodromal features and therapeutic response. Additionally, using biological measures of brain changes with treatment augments self-report clinical symptomatology data by providing an objective metric of change. Neuroimaging studies of psychotherapy exist for multiple disorders including MDD, OCD, and anxiety disorders, including PTSD, and phobias, and there are preliminary findings for DBT and CBT in personality disorders.

The role of unconscious processes is a critically important element of psychoanalytic treatment approaches. Thoughts and actions occurring outside of the patient's awareness are targets for the treatment with insight as the end goal. The underlying brain processes involved in conscious and unconscious thought has been investigated in functional magnetic resonance imaging (fMRI) paradigms by Etkin (2004) with a backward masking paradigm of fearful faces, essentially emotion threats seen so briefly and then followed by a neutral face, which they do not register as conscious thought. The fearful faces are believed to be unconsciously processed. Interestingly, heightened activity in the amygdala was seen only with the fearful faces, suggesting a separate network of brain activity for unconscious versus conscious processing. The authors speculate that emotional disorders may be caused by unconscious biases and that the rostral anterior cingulate cortex (ACC) hypoactivity and amygdala hyperactivity are influenced by unconscious processing (Etkin et al., 2004). Furthermore, certain psychotherapies that effectively target these unconscious biases may be successfully altering ACC circuitry.

■ **NEUROIMAGING PREDICTORS OF PSYCHOSOCIAL INTERVENTIONS ACROSS DISORDERS**

Etkin and colleagues (2005) propose that predictions of who responds to a particular therapeutic approach may rely on factors other than psychiatric diagnosis and instead rely on individual differences in brain processing which are quantified through brain activation patterns to various stimuli. These stimuli may be related to the particular psychosocial approach. This reflection of brain activity is believed to underlie the mechanism of disease more than clinical symptomatology. They propose the need to develop a "cognitive behavioral stress test" that will provide information on prognosis, inform treatment selection, and monitor treatment outcome based on neuroimaging parameters. The development of such a paradigm is in its beginning stages.

Visualization of pretreatment brain activity has been found to be a potent predictor of treatment outcome for medication trials in MDD and OCD, as well as CBT in MDD (Siegle et al., 2012). Elevated pretreatment rostral ACC activity distinguished responders from nonresponders in several studies (Mayberg et al., 1997; Saxena et al., 2003; Davidson et al., 2003). Rostral ACC, responsible for detection of emotional conflict and exercising cognitive control, is thereby executing important integrative functions necessary for emotion regulation, and higher levels of pretreatment suggest a capacity to engage these processes. In contrast, patients with OCD who have lower activation of the orbitalfrontal cortex (OFC) responded better to medication interventions, but individuals with higher OFC pretreatment activation responded better to psychotherapy (Brody et al., 1998). For CBT treatments, Siegle and colleagues (2012) found that lower pretreatment subgenual cingulate activity in response to negative words predicted more favorable outcome across two different scanners and differing patient characteristics. While these findings require replication with larger, better controlled studies, the notion that functionality of key components of the circuitry provide predictive value will be an area of growing emphasis.

■ NEUROBIOLOGICAL UNDERPINNINGS OF PSYCHOSOCIAL TREATMENT SPECIFIC TO PERSONALITY DISORDERS

Cloninger et al. (1993) created a psychobiological model of personality with four dimensions encompassing "temperament" and three dimensions of "character." Their findings indicate that temperament is 50% to 60% heritable, manifest in childhood, and have biases in perceptual memory. These dimensions include novelty seeking, harm avoidance, reward dependence, and persistence. The other 40% to 50% of personality is considered "character," which includes self-directedness, cooperativeness, and self-transcendence. These dimensions are shaped more by environmental factors, such as family, social relationships, and insight into the self as one matures as an adult. They found that personality disorders scored low in two character variables across the board: self-directedness and cooperativeness. Temperament appeared to be highly stable over time and is generally nonresponsive to psychotherapy. Alternatively, character variables appeared more flexible and respond more favorably to psychotherapy. Thus, being neurobiologically informed has become crucial to effective treatment of personality disorders (Gabbard, 2000).

There is a growing appreciation of the efficacy of psychosocial interventions for treatment of personality disorder, as evidenced by the burgeoning evidence base for treatments for BPD including DBT, CBT, mentalization-based psychotherapy, transference-based psychotherapy, schema-based psychotherapy, and CBT for antisocial personality disorder (Lieb et al., 2010). Despite this recognition of effective outcomes, there is limited data pertaining to clarifying the underlying biological mechanisms of psychosocial treatment effect in personality disorders For instance, within the transference-focused psychotherapy literature, success treatment in borderline personality disorder (BPD) was associated with personality change through changes in attachment and reflective functioning (Levy et al., 2005) with DBT treatment effect believed to rely on increased skill acquisition (Neacsiu et al., 2010). This information is essential for deepening an understanding of therapeutic response and disease processes and the development of future, more effective treatment and personalized medicine approaches.

■ NEUROIMAGING STUDIES OF PSYCHOSOCIAL INTERVENTIONS IN PERSONALITY DISORDERS

To date, there is a paucity of published brain imaging research on psychotherapeutic trials in BPD, which includes only a clinical report (van Elst, 2001), one study with a small sample (Schnell & Herpertz, 2007), and an open DBT trial from our lab (Goodman et al., 2014). Schnell and Herpertz (2010) examined fMRI in six BPD and six healthy controls participants during five time points, with a "passive viewing" of photographic images from the International Affective Picture Show (IAPS; Lang et al., 1997). BPD subjects received a 12-week inpatient DBT program. DBT treatment decreased the BOLD response to unpleasant pictures in the ACC, posterior cingulate, and insula. DBT responders (four of six) also showed less activation in the amygdala and both hippocampi. These findings are limited by the small sample size, lack of standardized treatment protocol, and absence of a standardized definition of treatment responder.

Our lab examined the effects of 12 months of DBT treatment on amygdala fMRI activity and habituation to unpleasant, neutral, and pleasant IAPS pictures in BPD patients. Event-related fMRI was obtained pre- and post-12-months of standard DBT in unmedicated BPD patients. Healthy controls were studied as a benchmark for normal amygdala activity and change over time ($n = 11$ per diagnostic group). Change in emotion regulation was measured with the Difficulty in Emotion Regulation (DERS) scale (Gratz & Roemer, 2004). During each scan, participants viewed an intermixed series of unpleasant, neutral, and pleasant pictures presented twice (termed "novel" and "repeat"). Emotion regulation measured with the DERS significantly improved in the BPD group. fMRI results showed the predicted Group × Time interaction: compared with yoked controls scanned at baseline and 12 months, the BPD group exhibited a pattern of amygdala activation that decreased with treatment. This reduction in amygdala activation posttreatment in BPD was present for all three pictures types but was particularly notable in the left hemisphere and during the repeated emotional picture conditions (i.e., unpleasant and pleasant). Examination of individual differences among the BPD patients showed that improved amygdala habituation to repeated unpleasant pictures was associated with improvement on the DERS in terms of (a) overall emotional regulation and (b) emotion regulation strategy (DERS subscale on emotion regulation). These findings have promising treatment implications and support the notion that DBT targets amygdala hyperactivity which is part of the disturbed neural circuitry underlying emotional dysregulation.

■ CONCLUSION

Etkin and colleagues (2005) theorize the importance of new learning within a context of a therapeutic relationship as fundamental to the basis of psychotherapy effect. A growing body of neurobiological data in the fields of memory and learning, psychotherapy treatment effect, attachment, and neuroimaging supports this notion. While still in its infancy, and far behind research in psychopharmacological interventions, understanding how psychotherapy acts on brain function is critical in order to continue to develop more effective strategies and chose which psychosocial interventions will benefit which patients.

Future work examining biological underpinnings is sorely needed in order to better understand dysfunction specific to particular personality disorders and also across psychotherapy interventions to elucidate mechanisms specific to a particular modality. It will be necessary to delineate therapeutic effect derived from factors general to all treatment approaches (e.g., therapeutic alliance), as well as features unique to a particular psychosocial treatment approach.

■ REFERENCES

Amini, F., Lewis, T., Lannon, R., et al. (1996). Affect, attachment, memory: contributions towards psychobiologic integration. *Psychiatry, 59,* 213–223.
Baxter, L. R., Schwartz, J. M., Bergman, K. S., et al. (1992). Caudate glucose metabolism rate changes with both drug and behavior therapy for obsessive-compulsive disorder. *Arch Gen Psychiatry, 49,* 681–689.

Brody, A. L., Saxena, S., Schwartz, J. M., et al. (1998). FDG-PET predictors of response to behavioral therapy and pharmacotherapy in obsessive compulsive disorder. *Psychiatry Res*, *84*(1), 1–6.

Cloninger, C. R., Svrakic, D. M., & Pryzbeck, T. R. (1993). A psychobiological model of temperament and character. *Arch Gen Psychiatry*, *50*, 975–990.

Corrigan, F. M. (2004). Psychotherapy as assisted homeostasis: Activation of emotional processing mediated by the anterior cingulate cortex. *Med Hypoth*, *63*, 968–973.

Cozolino, L. (2002). *The neuroscience of psychotherapy: building and rebuilding the human brain*. New York: W.W. Norton.

Davidson, R. J., Irwin, W., Anderle, M. J., et al. (2003). The neural substrates of affective processing in depressed patients treated with venlafaxine. *Am J Psychiatry*, *160*(1), 64–75.

Etkin, A., Klemenhagen, K. C., Dudman, J. T., et al. (2004). Individual differences in trait anxiety predict the response of the basolateral amygdala to unconsciously processed fearful faces. *Neuron*, *44*(6), 1043–1055.

Etkin, A., Pittenger, C., Polan, H. J., & Kandel, E. R. (2005) Toward a neurobiology of psychotherapy: basic science and clinical applications. *J Neuropsychiatry Clin Neurosci*, *17*(2), 145–158.

Flores, P. J. (2010). Group psychotherapy and neuro-plasticity: an attachment theory perspective. *Int J Group Psychother*, *60*(4), 546–570.

Gabbard, G. O. (2000). A neurobiologically informed perspective on psychotherapy. *Br J Psychiatry*, *177*, 117–122.

Gibbons, M., Crits-Christoph, P., Ring-Kurtz, S., et al. (2009). Unique and common mechanisms of change across cognitive and dynamic psychotherapies. *J Consult Clin Psychol*, *77*(5), 801–813.

Goodman, M., Carpenter, D., Tang, C. Y., Goldstein, K. E., Avedon, J., Fernandez, N., Mascitelli, K. A., Blair, N. J., New, A. S., Triebwasser, J., Siever, L. J., & Hazlett, E. A. (2014). Dialectical behavior therapy alters emotion regulation and amygdala activity in patients with borderline personality disorder. *J Psychiatr Res*, *57*, 108–116.

Gratz, K. L., & Roemer, L. (2004). Multidimensional assessment of emotion regulation and dysregulation: development, factor structure, and initial validation of the difficulties in emotion regulation scale. *J Psychopathol Behav Assess*, *26*(1), 41–54.

Guan, J., Xie, H., & Ding, X. (2015). The role of epigenetic regulation in learning and memory. *Exp Neurol*, *268*, 30–36.

Horvath, A. O., & Symonds, B. D. (1991). Relation between working alliance and outcome in psychotherapy: A meta-analysis. *J Couns Psychol*, *38*(2), 139–149.

Jeffery, K. J., & Reid, I. C. (1997). Modifiable neuronal connections: an overview for psychiatrists. *Am J Psychiatry*, *154*, 156–164.

Joffe, R., Segal, Z., & Singer, W. (1996). Change in thyroid hormone levels following response to cognitive therapy for major depression. *Am J Psychiatry*, *153*, 411–413.

Johansson, P., & Høglend, P. (2007). Identifying mechanisms of change in psychotherapy: mediators of treatment outcome. *Clin. Psychol Psychother*, *14*, 1–9.

Kandel, E. R. (1998). A new intellectual framework for psychiatry. *Am J Psychiatry*, *155*, 457–469.

Kaufman, M. (2000). Effects of therapist self-monitoring on therapeutic alliance and subsequent therapeutic outcome. *Clin Supervisor*, *19*, 41.

Kim, W., Lim, S. K., Chung, E. J., & Woo, J. M. (2009). The effect of cognitive behavior therapy-based psychotherapy applied in a forest environment on physiological changes and remission of major depressive disorder. *Psychiatry Investig*, *6*, 245–254.

Lang, P. J., Bradley, M. M., & Cuthbert, B. N. (1997). International Affective Picture System (IAPS): Technical Manual and Affective Ratings. NIMH Center for the Study of Emotion and Attention.

Lieb, K., Völlm, B., Rücker, G., Timmer, A., & Stoffers, J. M. (2010). Pharmacotherapy for borderline personality disorder: Cochrane systematic review of randomized trials. *Br J Psychiatry*, *196*(1), 4–12.

Levitt, H. M., & Williams, D. C. (2010). Facilitating client change: principles based upon the experience of eminent psychotherapists. *Psychother Res*, *20*(3), 337–352.

Levy, K. (2006). The mechanisms of change in the treatment of borderline personality disorder with transference focused psychotherapy. *J Clin Psychol*, *62*(4), 481–501.

Liggan, D. Y., & Kay, J. (1999). Some neurobiological aspects of psychotherapy: a review. *J Psychother Pract Res*, *8*(2), 103–114.

Mayberg, H. S., Brannan, S. K., Mahurin, R. K., et al. (1997). Cingulate function in depression: a potential predictor of treatment response. *Neuroreport*, *8*(4), 1057–1061.

Neacsiu, A. D., Rizvi, S. L., & Linehan, M. M. (2010). Dialectical behavior therapy skills use as a mediator and outcome of treatment for borderline personality disorder. *Behav Res Ther*, *48*(9), 832–839.

Post, R. M., & Weiss, S. R. (1997). Emergent properties of neural systems: how focal molecular neurobiological alterations can affect behavior. *Dev Psychopathol*, *9*, 907–929.

Saxena, S., Brody, A. L., Ho, M. L., et al. (2003). Differential brain metabolic predictors of response to paroxetine in obsessive-compulsive disorder versus major depression. *Am J Psychiatry*, *160*(3), 522–532.

Schnell, K., & Herpertz, S. (2007). Effects of dialectic-behavioral-therapy on the neural correlates of affective hyperarousal in borderline personality disorder. *J Psychiatr Res*, *41*, 837–847.

Schwartz, J., Stoessel, P., Baxter, L., et al. (1996). Systematic changes in cerebral glucose metabolic rate after successful behavior modification treatment of obsessive compulsive behavior. *Arch Gen Psychiatry*, *53*, 109–113.

Shear, M. K., Fyer, A. J., Ball, G., et al. (1991). Vulnerability to sodium lactate in panic disorder patients given cognitive-behavioral therapy. *Am J Psychiatry*, *148*, 795–797.

Siegle, G. J., Thompson, W. K., Collier, A., Berman, S. R., Feldmiller, J., Thase, M. E., & Friedman, E. S. (2012). Toward clinically useful neuroimaging in depression treatment: prognostic utility of subgenual cingulate activity for determining depression outcome in cognitive therapy across studies, scanners, and patient characteristics. *Arch Gen Psychiatry*, *69*(9), 913–924.

Stratford, T. (2012). Neuroanalysis of therapeutic alliance in the symptomatically anxious: the physiological connection revealed between therapist and client. *Am J Psychother*, *66*(1), 1–21.

Summers, M. D., & Barber, J. P. (2003). Therapeutic alliance as a measurable psychotherapy skill. *Acad Psychiatry*, *27*, 160–165.

van der Kolk, B. A. (1997). The psychobiology of posttraumatic stress disorder. *J Clin Psychiatry*, *58*(suppl 9), 16–24.

van Elst, L. T. (2001). Subtle prefrontal neuropathology in a pilot magnetic resonance spectroscopy study in patients with borderline personality disorder. *J Neuropsychiatry Clin Neurosci*, *13*(4), 511–514.

Viinamaki, H., Kuikka, J., Tiihonnen, J., et al. (1998). Changes in monoamine transport density related to clinical treatment: a case controlled study. *Nord J Psychiatry*, *55*, 39–44.

Zovkic, I. B., Guzman-Karlsson, M. C., & Sweatt, J. D. (2013). Epigenetic regulation of memory formation and maintenance. *Learn Mem*, *20*, 61–74.

18 Conclusions and Future Directions

■ CHRISTIAN SCHMAHL, K. LUAN PHAN,
AND ROBERT O. FRIEDEL

Personality disorders (PDs) are characterized along multiple interacting domains of aberrant behavior: cognition, affect, impulsivity, and interpersonal relations. Cognitive impairment cuts across multiple PDs and include problems with memory, attention and other higher order executive functions. Affective dysfunction manifests as difficulty processing emotionally salient information or difficulty with recognition of social cues. Problems with impulse control also relate to poor decision-making and cognitive control/inhibition. Together, these deficits lead to problems in social interactions, which rely on the integrated function of cognition, emotion, and impulse regulation. At the neural level, these domains are thought to be instantiated by discreet brain structures and neurochemistry. Both genetic, neuroimaging (functional, structural, neurochemical), and pharmacologic studies have elucidated the key elements that govern personality, emotional and cognitive function.

However, many gaps remain that should be addressed by future research. First, more studies are needed to better understand how cognition, emotion, and social interactions relate to one another at the behavioral and neural levels. For example, much of the existing literature probe socioemotional brain function using static stimuli, rather than paradigms that utilize dynamic social interactions, which may better reflect the difficulty patients with PDs have in real-world relationships. Second, little is known about how brain structure and function are related to the underlying neurochemical or molecular processes that give rise to behavior in vivo in humans, in the laboratory or in the real world. Relatedly, because PDs are thought to arise early in life, more research is needed to better understand how developmental pathways, both normal and disrupted, such as following environmental adversity, affect brain structure, function, and chemistry over time, from birth through adolescence. Third, although behavioral and molecular genetics are clearly linked to personality traits, less is known about how they interact to lead to the development of PDs, in general or particularly to certain kinds of PDs. Fourth, although PDs have been characterized categorically (schizotypal vs. borderline vs. antisocial), there may be shared underlying genetic, neurochemical, and anatomical abnormalities that are shared across these "distinct" categories. Moreover, these aberrant social, cognitive, and emotional processes and the associated limbic-prefrontal brain and underlying neurochemistry (serotonin, dopamine, opioids) are also implicated in other forms of psychopathology (depression, bipolar disorder, anxiety disorder, addiction). Understanding how these systems—for example, dopamine and cognitive control—may lead to impulsive actions and poor decision-making across multiple PDs and comorbid conditions is critical.

As noted below, the debate whether a categorical or a dimensional model best suits PDs is robust and ongoing. A dimensional model that incorporates genetic/ molecular-neural-behavioral domains to explain and integrate cognition-emotion-social interactions could lead to the development of common, shared biologically based endophenotypes that refines the current nosology of PDs and to new prevention and therapeutic strategies that may "target" a common underlying construct (e.g., cognitive training, emotion regulation training, social skills training). Finally, the emergence of translational, data-driven, computational approaches to molecular/ genetic and cognitive-affective neuroscience promises to delineate a more accurate model of cognition, motivation, and emotion which will better inform our understanding of the basis of personality and PDs.

The overarching aim of PD research over the next ten years should be to elucidate central pathological mechanisms, e.g. of emotion processing and social interaction, on the subjective, behavioral, and neurobiological levels, and to link these mechanisms to existing and novel interventions. Ultimately, the clarification of these central mechanisms should improve strategies for primary and secondary prevention and help to optimize assessment and treatments on both a psychotherapeutic and a pharmacotherapeutic level. The first step should be for researchers to investigate central mechanisms such as disturbed emotion processing and its implications on social interaction, impulsivity and aggression, or non-suicidal self-injury. The second step should be to seek validation of identified key mechanisms as potential endophenotypes and to use these to tailor specific therapeutic interventions.

Some of these mechanisms could potentially be used to define endophenotypes, which should be closer to the site of the primary causes (whether genetic or environmental) than to the diagnostic category of personality disorder. Endophenotypes for mental disorders are, among other criteria, primarily state-independent; that is, they manifest themselves whether or not the illness is active. This view also suggests that endophenotypes are related to the development of the disorder and do not mimic long-term consequences or secondary manifestations of co-occurring Axis I disorders. Including remitted patients and adolescent patients in research projects could address these issues.

■ THE DIMENSIONAL DIAGNOSTIC MODEL OF PDs

In the years preceding and since the publication of the current edition of the *Diagnostic and Statistical Manual of Mental Disorders* (fifth edition [*DSM-5*]), published by the American Psychiatric Association (APA) in 2013, there has been considerable controversy over the diagnostic approach that should be utilized for defining PDs. It is beyond the intent and scope of this book to describe in detail the reasons for proposals to change the existing categorical format to a format employing evaluation of dimensional features of these disorders. For those readers interested in pursuing this issue in more depth, there are multiple publications and one book (Oldham et al., 2014) in the literature that will provide the arguments and the evidence on both sides of this issue. In addition, the issue is well described in a condensed form in Chapter 3.

It may be that, in part, that rationale for the proposed dimensional model of PDs could be enhanced if the supporting evidence of phenomenological data were balanced by addressing more thoroughly than has yet occurred data on the neurobiological factors that contribute to these disorders. It is a well-accepted truism in modern medicine that knowledge of the biological basis of human disease forms the foundation for accurate diagnoses and provides the rationale for effective treatment. In those diseases that affect the human brain, Ledoux (1996) has framed this position clearly and succinctly as follows: "the proper level of analysis of a psychological function is the level at which that function is represented in the brain."

In response to the *DSM-5* Task Force's and the Personality and Personality Disorders Work Group's proposal that a dimensional approach to PDs be adopted, the APA Board of Trustees decided to continue with the existing categorical model of diagnosis of these disorders until further research supporting a dimensional approach is available. Data from the neurobiological literature on PDs is continuing to be increasingly available. For example, since the publication of *DSM-5*, the data from quantitative genetic studies of PDs has provided additional evidence that there are significant, but different, degrees of inherent risk factors that contribute to the developments of PDs (see Chapter 3).

This can be appreciated readily by examination of the results of recent quantitative genetic studies of these disorders (see Chapter 3). For example, such studies now provide quantitative estimates of the heritability of individual dimensions (endophenotypes) of BPD and the descriptions of the complex interplay between genetic and environmental factors of the disorder. Also, some of the strongest evidence to support the hypothesis that PDs are a maladaptive variant of normal personality may be derived from *quantitative* genetic studies, especially of endophenotypes (Flint et al., 2010). This may be true for some time because valid and replicable data from *molecular* genetic approaches require very large sample sizes to produce valid and replicable results (Flint et al., 2010, pp. 91–93). This is just one important example of how some of the information on the neurobiological basis of PDs may be of practical importance sooner than one might expect.

■ NEW TREATMENT APPROACHES

One example of a mechanism-based psychotherapy approach is real-time functional magnetic resonance imaging neurofeedback (rtfMRI). rtfMRI has recently come to be a focus of clinical psychiatry and psychotherapy research (deCharms et al., 2005; Linden, 2014; Linden et al., 2012; Ruiz, Birbaumer, & Sitaram, 2013; Ruiz, Lee, et al., 2013; Young et al., 2014; Zilverstand, Sorger, Sarkheil, & Goebel, 2014), with pioneering studies providing initial evidence that it might play a promising role in future therapies for chronic pain and mental disorders such as depression, schizophrenia, and phobias. Several studies conducted in healthy participants have demonstrated improvement in control over key areas of emotional responding (Brühl et al., 2014; Caria, Sitaram, Veit, Begliomini, & Birbaumer, 2010; Hamilton, Glover, Hsu, Johnson, & Gotlib, 2011; Johnston, Boehm, Healy, Goebel, & Linden, 2010; Lawrence et al., 2013; Paret et al., 2014; Scheinost et al., 2013; Sulzer et al., 2013; Veit et al., 2012; Zotev et al., 2011). This literature supports the feasibility of using neurofeedback to target brain regions of the affective system, such as the amygdala, as an alternative or at least an add-on to psychotherapy for mental disorders that are associated with emotion dysregulation.

We investigated whether participants would be able to downregulate their amygdala response to aversive pictures when they were provided with continuous feedback from this region. The first study was conducted in healthy controls (Paret et al., 2014). Healthy female participants ($N = 32$) completed one session of training that comprised four runs, with each run presenting aversive pictures under three different conditions. In the REGULATE condition, participants were provided with continuous visual feedback on brain activation via a thermometer display and were instructed to use this feedback to try to consciously downregulate the thermometer. Half the participants received feedback on activation in the amygdala, while the other half received it from a control region located in the basal ganglia. In the VIEW condition, they were instructed to respond naturally to the aversive pictures, that is, to not make any attempt to regulate the thermometer. In the fourth run, they were given the same instructions about downregulation that they had been given in the REGULATE condition, but this time they did not receive feedback on brain activation, in order to assess the transfer of the regulation training. fMRI neurofeedback was associated with successful downregulation of the amygdala response in both groups. During transfer, we found evidence for a differential influence of group on brain self-regulation and of downregulation of the right amygdala response in the experimental group.

In a second study (Paret et al., 2016a), we applied the same protocol to borderline patients (N = 10) to see if down-regulation of amygdala activation could be achieved in this population as well. Participants underwent 4 training sessions over 2 weeks. We found a reduced amygdala response in the REGULATE condition as contrasted with the VIEW condition, with reduction already seen in the first session and a further decrease in the group mean seen over the course of the four sessions. Borderline patients also showed an increase of amygdala-prefrontal connectivity over the course of the four sessions, a pattern which was also observed in healthy subjects after one session of rtfMRI (Paret et al., 2016b).

Another area which could be an interesting target of a mechanism-based approach is social interaction. Taken together, data from the currently established treatment programs in BPD converge to some beneficial impact on social integration but leaving up to 50% of the treated clients with a Global Assessment of Functioning score lower than 60, indicating persistent serious social problems (see Lis & Bohus, 2013). Possible explanations for the unsatisfactory treatment effects in the domain of social functioning may be that (a) the implemented interventions do not target with sufficient specificity those social cognitive processes that are actually impaired in PDs and/ or that (b) the available interventions do not allow for a sufficiently intense training. It may be assumed that a change of disadvantageous processing styles and the linked behaviors requires an intensive training of the affected social cognitive processes to allow for an automation of these processes and a use of behaviors acquired during therapy in everyday life. As a consequence, interventions are required which address impairments in social cognition and which allow for an intensive training of the impaired domains of social functioning as it is possible in a cost-efficient manner by computer-assisted trainings.

Although during the past years an increasing effort has been invested in the development of social cognitive interventions, the available approaches have primarily been designed for individuals suffering from schizophrenia. A recent meta-analysis suggests beneficial effects on emotion recognition abilities and theory of mind; however, no effects on attribution style (aggression, hostility, and blame biases) or on social perception measures were found (see Kurtz & Richardson, 2012; Statucka & Walder, 2013; Wolwer, Combs, Frommann, & Penn, 2010). Most of the available interventions such as social cognition and interaction training (Penn, Roberts, Combs, & Sterne, 2007; Roberts & Penn, 2009) are group-based trainings which are time- and effort-intensive in nature. In contrast to trainings of cognitive functions such as COGPACK or "My Brain Training," only a few computer-assisted trainings for social cognition exist to date. A limitation of these existing social cognition trainings is that they rather train cognitive processes with social emotional stimuli (see, e.g., brainhq.com, which provides modules to train perception for and memory of facial stimuli via matching tasks) or focus on single, very circumscribed functions such as affect control during emotional working memory tasks (Schweizer & Dalgleish, 2011; Schweizer, Grahn, Hampshire, Mobbs, & Dalgleish, 2013; Schweizer, Hampshire, & Dalgleish, 2011).

As an example of such an intervention in the field of PDs, in the German Clinical Research Unit on BPD, a computerized social interaction training program has been developed. It targets six symptom domains: (I) Perception of Positive Emotions, (II) Memorizing Positive Emotions, (III) Social Coaxing, (IV) Cooperation and Competition (V) Social Domains, (VI) Social Cooperation under Stress. In order to maximize motivation and compliance, all modules are designed according to gamification principles (e.g., Werbach & Hunter, 2012; Hamari et al., 2014); that is, elements and designs of computer games are used such as challenges, points, badges, and leader boards. Different game levels can be achieved; credits within each level and positive feedback of performance in the manner of accuracy and speed of performance is given. This allows the participant to monitor his or her trainings successes and to compare it to other "players." Each module is designed in an adaptive manner; that is, the difficulty is increased or decreased depending on the participant's performance to sustain motivation.

These examples of neurobiology-inspired therapeutic approaches may help to elucidate new avensues in the often difficult treatment of severly ill patients with personality disorders in the future.

▪ **REFERENCES**

Brühl, A. B., Scherpiet, S., Sulzer, J., Stampfli, P., Seifritz, E., & Herwig, U. (2014). Real-time neurofeedback using functional MRI could improve down-regulation of amygdala activity during emotional stimulation: a proof-of-concept study. *Brain Topogr, 27*(1), 138–148. doi: 10.1007/s10548-013-0331-9

Caria, A., Sitaram, R., Veit, R., Begliomini, C., & Birbaumer, N. (2010). Volitional control of anterior insula activity modulates the response to aversive stimuli. A real-time functional magnetic resonance imaging study. *Biol Psychiatry, 68*(5), 425–432. doi: 10.1016/j.biopsych.2010.04.020

deCharms, R. C., Maeda, F., Glover, G. H., Ludlow, D., Pauly, J. M., Soneji, D., . . . Mackey, S. C. (2005). Control over brain activation and pain learned by using real-time functional MRI. *Proc Natl Acad Sci U S A, 102*(51), 18626–18631. doi: 10.1073/pnas.0505210102

Flint, J., Greenspan, R. J., & Kendler, K. S. (2010). *How genes influence behavior.* New York: Oxford University Press, pp. 89–92.

Hamari, J., Koivisto, J., & Sarsa, H. (2014). Does gamification work? A literature review of empirical studies on gamification. Proceedings of the 47th Hawaii International Conference on System Sciences, January 6–9.

Hamilton, J. P., Glover, G. H., Hsu, J. J., Johnson, R. F., & Gotlib, I. H. (2011). Modulation of subgenual anterior cingulate cortex activity with real-time neurofeedback. *Hum Brain Mapp, 32*(1), 22–31. doi: 10.1002/hbm.20997

40 ■ Neurobiology of Personality Disorders

Johnston, S. J., Boehm, S. G., Healy, D., Goebel, R., & Linden, D. E. (2010). Neurofeedback: a promising tool for the self-regulation of emotion networks. *Neuroimage, 49*(1), 1066–1072. doi: 10.1016/j.neuroimage.2009.07.056

Kurtz, M. M., & Richardson, C. L. (2012). Social cognitive training for schizophrenia: a meta-analytic investigation of controlled research. *Schizophr Bull, 38*, 1092–1104.

Lawrence, E. J., Su, L., Barker, G. J., Medford, N., Dalton, J., Williams, S. C., . . . David, A. S. (2013). Self-regulation of the anterior insula: reinforcement learning using real-time fMRI neurofeedback. *Neuroimage, 88C*, 113–124. doi: 10.1016/j.neuroimage.2013.10.069

LeDoux, J. (1996). *The emotional brain*. New York: Touchstone, p. 16.

Linden, D. E. (2014). Neurofeedback and networks of depression. *Dialogues Clin Neurosci, 16*(1), 103–112.

Linden, D. E., Habes, I., Johnston, S. J., Linden, S., Tatineni, R., Subramanian, L., . . . Goebel, R. (2012). Real-time self-regulation of emotion networks in patients with depression. *PLoS One, 7*(6), e38115. doi: 10.1371/journal.pone.0038115

Lis, S., & Bohus, M. (2013). Social interaction in borderline personality disorder. *Curr Psychiatry Rep, 15*, 338.

Oldham, J. M., Skodol, A. E., & Bender, D. S. (2014). *Textbook of personality disorders*. (2nd ed.). Washington, DC: American Psychiatric Publishing.

Paret, C., Kluetsch, R. C., Ruf, M., Demirakca, T., Hösterey, S., Ende, G., & Schmahl, C. (2014). Down-regulation of amygdala activation in response to aversive pictures with real-time fMRI neurofeedback *Front Behav Neurosci, 8*, 299.

Paret, C., Kluetsch, R., Zaehringer, J., Ruf, M., Demirakca, T., Bohus, M., . . . Schmahl, C. (2016a). Alterations of amygdala-prefrontal connectivity with real-time fMRI neurofeedback in BPD patients. *SCAN, 11*, 952–960.

Paret, C., Ruf, M., Gerchen, M. F., Kluetsch, R., Demirakca, T., Jungkunz, M., . . . Ende, G. (2016b). fMRI neurofeedback of amygdala response to aversive stimuli enhances prefrontal-limbic brain connectivity. *Neuroimage, 125*, 182–188.

Penn, D. L., Roberts, D. L., Combs, D., & Sterne, A. (2007). Best practices: the development of the Social Cognition and Interaction Training program for schizophrenia spectrum disorders. *Psychiatric Serv, 58*, 449–451. doi: 10.1176/appi.ps.58.4.449

Roberts, D. L., & Penn, D. L. (2009). Social cognition and interaction training (SCIT) for outpatients with schizophrenia: a preliminary study. *Psychiatry Res, 166*, 141–147.

Ruiz, S., Birbaumer, N., & Sitaram, R. (2013). Abnormal neural connectivity in schizophrenia and fMRI-brain-computer interface as a potential therapeutic approach. *Front Psychiatry, 4*, 17. doi: 10.3389/fpsyt.2013.00017

Ruiz, S., Lee, S., Soekadar, S. R., Caria, A., Veit, R., Kircher, T., . . . Sitaram, R. (2013). Acquired self-control of insula cortex modulates emotion recognition and brain network connectivity in schizophrenia. *Hum Brain Mapp, 34*(1), 200–212. doi: 10.1002/hbm.21427

Scheinost, D., Stoica, T., Saksa, J., Papademetris, X., Constable, R. T., Pittenger, C., & Hampson, M. (2013). Orbitofrontal cortex neurofeedback produces lasting changes in contamination anxiety and resting-state connectivity. *Transl Psychiatry, 3*(4), e250. doi: 10.1038/tp.2013.24

Schweizer, S., & Dalgleish, T. (2011). Emotional working memory capacity in posttraumatic stress disorder (PTSD). *Behav Res Ther, 49*, 498–504.

Schweizer, S., Grahn, J., Hampshire, A., Mobbs, D., & Dalgleish, T. (2013). Training the emotional brain: improving affective control through emotional working memory training. *J Neurosci, 33*, 5301–5311.

Schweizer, S., Hampshire, A., & Dalgleish, T. (2011). Extending brain-training to the affective domain: increasing cognitive and affective executive control through emotional working memory training. *PLoS One, 6*, e24372.

Statucka, M., & Walder, D. J. (2013). Efficacy of social cognition remediation programs targeting facial affect recognition deficits in schizophrenia: a review and consideration of high-risk samples and sex differences. *Psychiatry Res, 206,* 125–139.

Sulzer, J., Sitaram, R., Blefari, M. L., Kollias, S., Birbaumer, N., Stephan, K. E., . . . Gassert, R. (2013). Neurofeedback-mediated self-regulation of the dopaminergic midbrain. *Neuroimage, 83,* 817–825. doi: 10.1016/j.neuroimage.2013.05.115

Veit, R., Singh, V., Sitaram, R., Caria, A., Rauss, K., & Birbaumer, N. (2012). Using real-time fMRI to learn voluntary regulation of the anterior insula in the presence of threat-related stimuli. *Soc Cogn Affect Neurosci, 7*(6), 623–634. doi: 10.1093/scan/nsr061

Werbach, K., & Hunter, D. (2012). *For the win: how game thinking can revolutionize your business.* Philadelphia: Wharton Digital Press.

Wolwer, W., Combs, D. R., Frommann, N., & Penn, D. L. (2010). Treatment approaches with a special focus on social cognition: overview and empirical results. In V. Roder & A. Medalia (Eds.), *Neurocognition and social cognition in schizophrenia patients* (pp. 61–78). Basel: Karger.

Young, K. D., Zotev, V., Phillips, R., Misaki, M., Yuan, H., Drevets, W. C., & Bodurka, J. (2014). Real-time FMRI neurofeedback training of amygdala activity in patients with major depressive disorder. *PLoS One, 9*(2), e88785. doi: 10.1371/journal.pone.0088785

Zilverstand, A., Sorger, B., Sarkheil, P., & Goebel, R. (2014). Towards therapy in the scanner: enhancing fear regulation in spider phobia through fMRI neurofeedback. Paper presented at the Human Brain Mapping meeting, Hamburg.

Zotev, V., Krueger, F., Phillips, R., Alvarez, R. P., Simmons, W. K., Bellgowan, P., . . . Bodurka, J. (2011). Self-regulation of amygdala activation using real-time FMRI neurofeedback. *PLoS One, 6*(9), e24522. doi: 10.1371/journal.pone.0024522

■ INDEX